T0245096

This compact yet comprehensive handbook provides an essential source of expert practical advice for trainees and residents in pediatrics. It covers the full range of pediatric problems likely to be encountered in the hospital setting. It has been written by a highly experienced team of subspecialists, based at the internationally renowned BC Children's Hospital in Vancouver. Their vast wealth of teaching experience has been distilled in this volume to provide the most up-to-date and authoritative advice available on the care of the sick child. The style of presentation is designed to facilitate quick and easy reference, which can be so essential in emergency cases.

This clear and concise handbook will be an essential source of information and reference for all who are involved in pediatric health care, from resident and trainee pediatricians, through to medical students and nursing staff.

The pocket pediatrician

The pocket pediatrician

Edited by M. Seear

*British Columbia's Children's
Hospital, Vancouver*

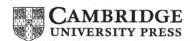
CAMBRIDGE
UNIVERSITY PRESS

CAMBRIDGE UNIVERSITY PRESS
Cambridge, New York, Melbourne, Madrid, Cape Town, Singapore, São Paulo

Cambridge University Press
The Edinburgh Building, Cambridge CB2 8RU, UK

Published in the United States of America by Cambridge University Press, New York

www.cambridge.org
Information on this title: www.cambridge.org/9780521568814

First published 1996

A catalogue record for this publication is available from the British Library

Library of Congress Cataloguing in Publication data

The pocket pediatrician / edited by M. Seear.
  p. cm.
  Includes index
  ISBN 0 521 56881 1 (pb)
  1. Pediatrics – handbooks, manuals, etc. I. Seear, M.
RJ48.P63 1996
618.92–dc20   95–52606 CIP

ISBN 978-0-521-56881-4 paperback

Transferred to digital printing 2008

Every effort has been made in preparing this book to provide accurate and
up-to-date information which is in accord with accepted standards and
practice at the time of publication. Although case histories are drawn
from actual cases, every effort has been made to disguise the identities of
the individuals involved. Nevertheless, the authors, editors and publishers
can make no warranties that the information contained herein is totally
free from error, not least because clinical standards are constantly
changing through research and regulation. The authors, editors and
publishers therefore disclaim all liability for direct or consequential
damages resulting from the use of material contained in this book. Readers
are strongly advised to pay careful attention to information provided by
the manufacturer of any drugs or equipment that they plan to use.

This book is for
the memory of
MICHAEL SWALLOW

CONTENTS

ANALYTICAL CONTENTS LIST

PREFACE

Although this is the first published edition of the British Columbia's Children's Hospital manual, it is based on an in-house resident's handbook that has been continuously updated for the past 10 years. Each chapter has been written by a pediatric subspecialist with extensive experience in that area of medicine. These sections represent the lessons learned from years of pediatric practice in a referral Children's Hospital. The manual is not aimed solely at pediatric housestaff. It will hopefully be of value to all health workers concerned with the care of sick children, whether practicing in hospital or out in the community.

We have tried to balance space limitations with the need to cover a subject in sufficient detail, by using point form for many topics. English grammar takes a beating but a lot of information can be presented quickly. Wherever possible, some background notes are given, especially for common medical problems.

Apart from individual authors, I am grateful to all the staff of British Columbia's Children's Hospital who made suggestions and helped with the preparation of this manual. I am particularly grateful to Ms. Julia Mark who typed and organized the entire manuscript single-handedly. The project would certainly not have been possible without her efforts.

We wish all your patients the best of health and hope you enjoy the manual.

Mike Seear

CARDIOLOGY   CHAPTER 1
Derek Human

HEART DISEASE IN INFANCY

Congenital heart disease represents the commonest major structural malformation. It occurs in roughly 12:1,000 live born infants. Under normal circumstances, 8:1,000 will be recognized during the first year of life; two of these will present with critical heart disease requiring some form of intervention in the first few months of life. The presentation of heart disease usually comes in one of three forms: congestive heart failure, cyanosis and/or cardiac murmur.

Although expensive studies such as angiography and gated MRI's have a part to play in the investigation of children with heart disease, it is possible to make a diagnosis using little more than clinical skills, an electrocardiogram (ECG) and a chest radiograph.

Heart failure

The classical signs of heart failure are cardiomegaly, tachypnea and hepatomegaly. Left–sided failure causes pulmonary vascular congestion, interstitial edema and decreased compliance. The child's response is to develop rapid shallow breathing. Early heart failure can easily be confused with respiratory disease. Lymphatic obstruction can cause small airway obstruction with hyperinflation and wheeze (so called "cardiac asthma"). Pulmonary crackles are a late sign and are rarely heard. Right–sided failure causes systemic venous congestion, which is generally accommodated by a distended liver. Peripheral edema is a very late sign of right–sided failure. In practice, either pure right or left–sided failure is uncommon since the distended failing ventricle rapidly impedes the function of the other ventricle.

1. Presentation
The presenting features may develop slowly and mimic other diseases, especially respiratory disease. Some of the major presenting signs and symptoms are:
• Respiratory: wheeze, tachypnea, cough, retractions.
• Cardiac: hypotension, poor pulses, tachycardia, gallop, cardiomegaly.
• Peripheral perfusion: pale, mottled, cyanosed, cool peripheries.
• Others: hepatomegaly, failure to thrive, easy sweating, poor feeding.

2. Causes
There are many causes of pump failure, but they can be classified under four headings:
• Myocardial failure: cardiomyopathy, viral infection, ischemia, storage diseases, prolonged arrhythmias.
• Volume overload: excessive fluid administration, renal failure, recirculating load (bidirectional shunts), regurgitant load (valvular incompetence).
• Increased afterload: pulmonary or systemic hypertension, valvular obstruction (AS, PS), coarctation.
• Impaired cardiac filling: valvular obstruction (TS, MS), pericardial tamponade or constriction, restrictive cardiomyopathy, obstructed pulmonary veins.

3. Diagnosis
Once the diagnosis of congestive heart failure has been made on clinical grounds, it is possible
to get a good idea of the underlying cause using two noninvasive investigations (chest X–ray and
ECG). Using the chest X–ray to estimate pulmonary blood flow (decreased, normal or increased)
and the ECG to indicate ventricular dominance (right, left or biventricular hypertrophy), it is
possible to gain a good idea of the cause of the heart failure using Table I:

Table I: Causes of cardiac failure with normal saturation

Chest X–ray, pulmonary flow	Normal		Increased	
ECG	Right	Left	Right	Left or both
Cardiac defect	PS, MS	MR, AS, coarctation, cardiomyopathy	ASD, large L → R shunt, early pulmonary hypertension	VSD, PDA, AV canal

4. Management
Management remains the same for all ages:
• Reduce congestion with diuretics.
• Improve cardiac output with inotropes.
• Reduce afterload with vasodilators.
• Surgical correction of structural anomalies.
A detailed outline of the treatment of heart failure is given in chapter 11 (Intensive Care and
Continuous Infusion Drugs).

Heart failure in older children

The clinical presentation of heart failure in older children is similar to the neonatal presentation
except that pulmonary crackles and peripheral edema become more common with increasing size.

The age at presentation of heart failure gives some clue to the etiology:
• First 2 weeks:
    Volume overload: shunts (PDA, rarely VSD or cushion defects), valvular regurgitation, AV
    fistulae (cardiac, cranial).
    Left heart obstruction: coarctation, AS, hypoplastic left heart.
    Right heart obstruction: TAPVD, double outlet right ventricle.
    Others: myocarditis (coxsackievirus, rubella, toxoplasmosis), arrhythmias (congenital heart
    block, SVT, WPW).
• Two weeks to end of first year:
    Volume overload: PDA, large VSD, single ventricle, truncus, TAPVD, AV canal, TGA with
    VSD.
    Pressure overload: pulmonary hypertension, PS (rare in tetralogy).
    Myocarditis: EF, Pompe's disease, viral infection, anomalous coronary arteries.
    Arrhythmias.
• One year and above:
    Bacterial endocarditis ± underlying heart disease.

Hypertension: systemic or pulmonary.
Cor pulmonale: cystic fibrosis, bronchopulmonary dysplasia.
Myocarditis: viral, rarely rheumatic fever, very rarely diphtheria.
Cardiomyopathies.
Late structural: PDA, coarctation, ASD.
Nonstructural: when looking after children who have had open heart surgery, it should be remembered that there are many nonstructural causes of heart failure. Hypoglycemia, acidosis, hypocalcemia, anemia, asphyxia and septicemia should all be considered when searching for a cause of poor pump function.

Cyanosis

Oxygen desaturation is reasonably well tolerated. Many children with cyanotic heart disease are able to grow and develop normally in their first year with saturations as low as 70%. In older children, the cause of cyanosis is almost always due to respiratory problems (pneumonia, pneumothorax, thoracic trauma). In the neonate, the differential diagnosis of cyanosis is large and it can be surprisingly difficult to distinguish between respiratory and cardiac disease.
Mild cyanosis is difficult to detect clinically and, if there is any doubt, it is sensible to use a pulse oximeter. Cyanosis is clinically underestimated in anemic children because there is a smaller quantity of desaturated blue hemoglobin circulating in the body. It is overestimated in polycythemic children because sluggish capillary flow gives the child a bluish coloration. In the absence of an oximeter, central oxygen saturation is best indicated by the color of the tongue.

1. Differential diagnosis
It is important not to concentrate totally on congenital heart disease when confronted with a cyanosed newborn. The differential diagnosis includes many acute noncardiac emergencies which must not be overlooked:
• Respiratory: hyaline membrane disease, pneumonia, pneumothorax, diaphragmatic hernia, tracheoesophageal fistula, lobar emphysema.
• CNS: respiratory depression due to seizures, ventricular hemorrhage, drugs, trauma, asphyxia.
• Cardiac: transposition, pulmonary stenosis, truncus arteriosus, tricuspid atresia, tetralogy, Ebstein's anomaly, TAPVD.
• Persistent fetal circulation: pulmonary hypertension due to sepsis, acidosis, hypoglycemia, polycythemia.
• Miscellaneous: transient tachypnea of the newborn, meconium aspiration syndrome, severe hyaline membrane disease, diaphragmatic hernia, methemoglobinemia.

2. Management
The main steps in managing a cyanosed neonate are as follows:
• Acute resuscitation: neonates have very little cardiorespiratory reserve so cyanosis should be considered as an emergency. Unless the child is particularly stable, consideration should be given to intubating the child and supporting the circulation with colloids and inotropes.
• Hyperoxic test: place the child in 100% oxygen for at least 10 minutes. Monitor oxygen saturation and, if possible, arterial oxygen tension.
  Normal child: PaO_2 > 500 mm Hg.
  Pure pulmonary disease: PaO_2 usually > 100 mm Hg.

Right to left shunt: usually well below 100 mm Hg.
- Unfortunately, once a child with congenital heart disease is intubated because of persistent pulmonary hypertension, the hyperoxic test will rarely be of value.
- Other investigations: the most urgent investigation following stabilization is a chest X–ray, followed by an ECG and echocardiogram to rule out cardiac malformations.
- Prostaglandin test: if working in a peripheral hospital, prior to transporting a cyanosed child to a referral center, it is usually safe to give a trial of prostaglandin E_1 (0.05–0.1 µg/kg per min). The main side effect in roughly 20% of cases is apnea. Children usually respond to stimulation but intubation equipment should be readily available.

3. Diagnostic algorithm
The following algorithm for cyanotic children (Table II) is based on an estimate of pulmonary flow from a chest X–ray and an estimate of ventricular dominance from an ECG. It can be used to determine the most likely structural defects before the echocardiography technician arrives.

Table II: Causes of neonatal cyanosis

Chest X–ray, pulmonary flow	Decreased			Increased	
ECG, ventricular dominance	Right	Left	Both	Right	Left or both
Cardiac defect	Tetralogy, Eisenmenger's complex, Ebstein's anomaly, PFC	Tricuspid atresia, pulmonary atresia	TGA plus PS	TAPVD, hypoplastic, left TGA	TGA or VSD, single ventricle, truncus

4. Treatment
Specific treatment will obviously depend on the underlying abnormality but, in all cases, it is sensible to treat the child for septicemia. Persistent fetal circulation is a common complication of neonatal septicemia and most physicians would cover the child with ampicillin and gentamicin until a blood culture has been negative for 2 days.

Persistent fetal circulation

Many of the problems that cause cyanosis will also be complicated by persistent fetal circulation. Consequently, there is a good deal of overlap in presentation. As the child adapts to air breathing following birth, the oxygen saturation increases and pulmonary artery pressure falls. Once the systemic pressure is greater than pulmonary pressure, then right to left shunting across the ductus arteriosus is reduced. The ductus does not close immediately so some bidirectional shunting can occur over the next few days if the child cries. If the pulmonary pressure remains higher than systemic pressure for a variety of reasons, then right to left shunting continues and the child remains cyanosed. This situation is usually referred to as persistent fetal circulation (PFC) or persistent pulmonary hypertension (PPH).

There are many reasons for pulmonary hypertension in the newborn but the major ones are:
- Respiratory disease: meconium aspiration, severe hyaline membrane disease, pulmonary

hypoplasia (usually with diaphragmatic hernia).
* Miscellaneous: septicemia (particularly group B *Streptococcus*), asphyxia, polycythemia.

Management consists of removing the underlying cause and reversing the shunt, both by increasing the systemic pressure and decreasing the pulmonary artery pressure.
Apart from normal standards for resuscitation, there is little that can be done to remove most of the causes. However, all children with PFC should be treated for septicemia with ampicillin and gentamicin until blood cultures have returned.
Blood pressure should be maintained vigorously with infusions of colloids and inotropes. Isuprel is a good choice as long as the side effect of tachycardia can be tolerated. Its beta action has some degree of pulmonary vasodilation. Inotropes with alpha–agonist activity, such as adrenalin, may make matters worse by aggravating the pulmonary hypertension.
The pulmonary vasculature of these children is sensitive to irritation. Children should be intubated, sedated and nursed by the most experienced person available. Pulmonary pressure will also be reduced by improved oxygenation, alkalosis (mild hyperventilation plus bicarbonate infusion) and inhaled nitric oxide. The dose range is not yet established but many physicians start at 80 ppm and rapidly reduce it to 20 ppm once an effect has been obtained. Powerful vasodilators, such as tolazoline and phenoxybenzamine, have been used in the past. They reduce pulmonary pressure but usually also reduce systemic pressure in the same ratio. Systemic hypotension is a serious risk and their use is largely abandoned in favor of nitric oxide.

HEART DISEASE OF OLDER CHILDREN

Cardiac murmurs

Even meeting the oxygen demand at rest requires the movement of large amounts of blood through small vessels and trabeculated cardiac chambers. It is hardly surprising that this produces benign flow murmurs.

Only clinical experience can give the ability to distinguish between benign and significant murmurs but a few pointers might help:
* Heart murmurs heard from the time of birth are most likely to be organic.
* The initial murmur of infancy is usually caused by peripheral pulmonary stenosis. The noise radiates widely and gets softer as the child grows.
* The innocent murmurs of childhood are usually heard after the first year. They are often characterized by the following features: systolic, sternal, soft sounds are normal, softens on sitting.

Rheumatic fever

The incidence of measles and tuberculosis was dropping rapidly, well before respective vaccinations for these illnesses were introduced. In the same way, rheumatic fever was becoming less common well before anyone thought of treating it with penicillin. The eradication of group A *Streptococcus* by penicillin is certainly not the reason for the rarity of rheumatic fever, since about 20% of children still carry pharyngeal *Streptococcus* without developing any problems whatsoever. There are many other examples of improved health, ranging from pertussis to dental caries, that probably have less to do with advances in medicine than many doctors would admit.

Why does life expectancy improve or perinatal mortality fall? Why does birth weight increase and why do university students get taller? The common denominator is probably improved social conditions. The exact causes are impossible to determine but the fact remains that if a population is clean, well fed and housed, many of the traditional scourges of humanity simply disappear (to be replaced, it must be admitted by diseases of affluence).

Rheumatic fever may be down but it certainly is not out. The diagnosis is based on criteria put forward by Jones and subsequently revised. A firm diagnosis of rheumatic fever can be made if there are two major manifestations or one major and two minor manifestations in addition to evidence of recent streptococcal infection.

The modified Jones criteria are as follows:
- Major criteria: flitting polyarthritis, carditis, erythema marginatum, subcutaneous nodules, Sydenham's chorea.
- Minor criteria: previous history of rheumatic fever, arthralgia, elevated acute phase reactants (ESR; C–reactive protein, WBC), prolonged PR or QT interval, fever, evidence of streptococcal infection, positive culture, scarlatiniform rash, elevated streptococcal antibodies.

Cyanotic spells, tetralogy of Fallot

Depending on the severity of the lesion, most children with tetralogy of Fallot are cyanosed in room air because of right to left shunting at ventricular level secondary to partial outflow obstruction.

Acute hypercyanosis (Tet spells) can occur at any age, beginning in the neonatal period. These are characterized by:
- Rapid onset of severe cyanosis.
- Accompanying dyspnea.
- Subsequent effects of hypoxia such as lethargy, unconsciousness and seizures.

The characteristic rough systolic murmur of tetralogy usually lessens or disappears, suggesting that these spells are probably due to an increase in outflow obstruction. Treatments are aimed at reducing infundibular spasm or increasing systemic resistance in an attempt to reverse the right to left shunt.

There is usually no time for detailed investigations and the management consists of the following:
- Place the child in the knee–chest or squatting position. (Older children who do not have access to surgical correction often learn to adopt a squatting position in response to an attack.)
- Administer oxygen by face mask.
- Give morphine (0.1 mg/kg i.v.).
- If there is no recovery at this stage, try sodium bicarbonate (1 mEq/kg i.v.).
- Propranolol is of value in relieving infundibular spasm (0.05 mg/kg by slow i.v. push); the side effect is hypotension.
- Phenylephrine (0.1 mg i.m.) can be tried in an attempt to increase systemic resistance.

Hypertension

The investigation and management of hypertension is covered in chapter 19 (Renal).

Kawasaki's disease

Mucocutaneous lymph node syndrome (Kawasaki's disease) is an acute febrile disease of children. The disease is discussed in chapter 22 (Rheumatology).

The major features are as follows:
• Prolonged fever, unresponsive to antibiotics or antipyretics.
• Conjunctivitis.
• Cracked lips with inflamed mucous membranes.
• Cervical lymphadenopathy.
• Truncal rash including hands and feet.
• Peripheral edema.

The most important complication is coronary vasculitis. This can lead to coronary dilatation, subsequent aneurysm formation, thrombosis, rupture or myocardial ischemia. It affects roughly 20% of children and may occur within 1 or 2 weeks of the fever. All children suspected of having the disease should be examined with two–dimensional echocardiography.

Apart from coronary vasculitis, cardiovascular complications can include: endocarditis, heart failure, pericarditis, myocarditis and arrhythmias. Cardiovascular complications affect roughly 20% of all patients with Kawasaki's disease; 1–2% of these children die from their complications. Many aneurysms settle with time but some children require coronary artery bypass surgery. Others may develop early coronary artery disease.

Therapy consists of the following:
• Intravenous gamma globulin (2 g/kg over 12 h). Early therapy has been shown to limit coronary vascular complications.
• High dose aspirin (100 mg/kg per 24 h) is recommended for the first 2 weeks of the illness, followed by a low dose (5 mg/kg per d) for another 2 months, even if the echocardiogram is normal.

CARDIAC INVESTIGATIONS

Although expensive MRI's and echocardiography have a place in the investigation of complex congenital heart disease, it must be stressed that the basic workup of a child with cardiac complaints relies on a physical examination, a chest X–ray and an ECG. Careful use of these three techniques will limit the use of expensive investigations in children who do not need them.

Electrocardiography

The ECG has been around for nearly 100 years so there is an enormous literature surrounding its interpretation. However, with an orderly approach, it is possible to get a lot of information from a standard 12 lead tracing with minimal experience.

A suggested approach is as follows:

1. Rate (at the standard ECG paper speed of 25 mm/s)
- 1 mm (1 small square) = 0.04 second.
- 5 mm (1 large square) = 0.2 second.
- Heart rate = 60/R–R interval in seconds.
- If there is complete AV block, it is helpful to calculate an atrial and a ventricular rate.

2. P–wave
The P–wave represents atrial depolarization and, in normal sinus rhythm, precedes the QRS complex. First check whether P–waves exist at all (junctional rhythm). If P–waves exist, examine their morphology (flutter, fibrillation or hypertrophy) and whether they consistently precede a QRS complex.
- P–wave criteria for atrial hypertrophy:
  Left atrial hypertrophy:
  Broad or notched P–wave.
  P–wave duration > 0.08 second.
  Inverted P–wave in V_1.
  Right atrial hypertrophy:
  Peaked P–wave > 3 mm in any lead.

3. PR interval
This interval is the time taken for the atrial impulse to be conducted to the ventricle. It is measured from the beginning of the P–wave to the beginning of QRS complex. The average value is 0.11 second from birth to school age, after which it rises to 0.14 second by adolescence. It should not be > 0.18 second at any age.

4. QRS complex
This complex represents the depolarization of the ventricles. It gives information on ventricular hypertrophy, infarction or abnormal conduction. Based on QRS morphology, several criteria exist for the definition of ventricular hypertrophy. They may not be applicable to premature infants or to children with complex malformations or heart block. Criteria for ventricular hypertrophy are:
- Left ventricular hypertrophy, one or more of the following:
  R–wave in V_6:
  > 16 mm at 0–6 months.
  > 19 mm at 6–12 months.
  > 21 mm at > 12 months.
  S–wave in V_1: > 20 mm at all ages.
  Q–wave in V_5 to V_7: > 4 mm.
- Right ventricular hypertrophy, one or more of the following:
  R–wave in V_1:
  > 14 mm at first week.
  > 10 mm at first month.
  > 7 mm at first year.
  > 5 mm at > 1 year.

S–wave in V₆:
> 14 mm at first week.
> 10 mm at first month.
> 5 mm at > 1 month.
qR pattern in lead V_1 (normal variant in 10%).
• Cardiac axis is best calculated for the QRS complexes in lead I and aVF using Figure I. The same figure can be used to calculate an axis for the T and P waves.

5. QT interval
This interval is measured from the beginning of the QRS complex to the end of the T–wave. It is affected by heart rate and is corrected by dividing the QT interval by the square root of the R–R interval (both measured in seconds). QTc should be < 0.45 in infants, 0.44 in children and 0.43 in adolescence.

Figure I: Calculation of cardiac axis

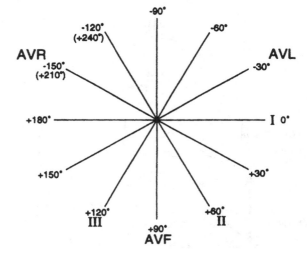

Echocardiography

Modern echocardiography began with the development of the m–mode ultrasound, which was based on the image produced by bouncing a single narrow beam of ultrasound off the cardiac structures. The next development was two–dimensional echocardiography. In this technique, the original beam is rotated through an arc, which enables a wedge–shaped slice of the heart to be viewed. The most recent advance has been Doppler echocardiography, which uses the Doppler principle to interrogate a small area of the heart and give information on flow velocities.

1. M–mode echocardiography
The thin pencil of sound is reflected from the structures of the heart to give a characteristic pattern when printed out over time. Various indices of ventricular function and valvular function can be derived from the m–mode tracing (Figure II).

Figure II: M–mode echocardiography

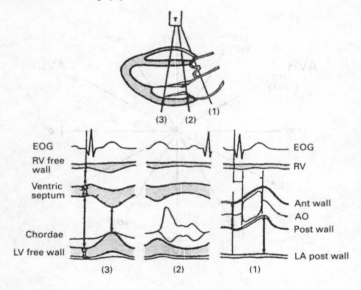

2. Two–dimensional echocardiography
The transducer head is rotated rapidly, backwards and forwards, so that a wedge–shaped, cross–sectional view of the heart is obtained. The image is confusing to the uninitiated since it is necessary to have a good knowledge of cardiac anatomy before the flickering images on the screen can be interpreted. Figure III represents what is shown in a parasternal long axis view.

Figure III: Two–dimensional echocardiogram (long axis view)

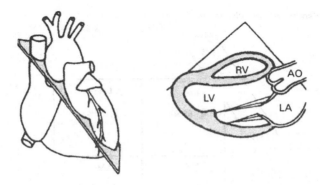

3. Doppler ultrasound
A small (2 × 4 mm) segment of the two–dimensional image can be sampled to provide information on direction and velocity of blood flow using the Doppler principle. Under some circumstances, an estimate of intravascular pressure can also be obtained. Typical areas of interest are the pulmonary outflow tract and the ductus arteriosus. Some machines display different velocities or different directions of flow as varying colors. This makes it easier to detect small areas of turbulence caused by a VSD or area of stenosis.

Cardiac catheterization

Echocardiography has not entirely removed the need for cardiac catheterization. In fact, the relatively recent development of balloon dilatation for suitable forms of valvular stenosis and coarctation has made therapeutic catheterization quite a common procedure in many centers. Earlier enthusiasm for the closure of ASD's and PDA's using various expandable devices has not been maintained. Figure IV gives chamber pressures and saturations for a structurally normal heart.

Figure IV: Cardiac catheterization values

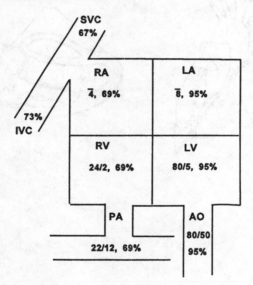

Pressures and oxygen saturations are displayed for a structurally normal heart.
SVC: superior vena cava
IVC: inferior vena cava
RA: right arium
LA: left atrium
RV: right ventricle
LV: left ventricle
PA: pulmonary artery
AO: aorta

DEATH AND DYING
Andrew Macnab

CHAPTER 2

TERMINAL ILLNESS/DEATH

In most sections of this book, death is not mentioned, although terminal illness can and does occur in many of the conditions described. In the Intensive Care Unit (ICU), 6% of the patients die, and this is likely the highest proportion within the hospital. However, transfer to ICU is not obligatory prior to death nor for that matter is being in hospital. If everything appropriate has been done in an attempt to diagnose and treat the child, it may well be that (s)he and the family will be more than happy for death to occur at home, provided all appropriate support measures are in place.

Hopefully, when a child dies, the possibility has been anticipated and there has been time for those close to the child to discuss the prospect of death with the patient and with members of the immediate family. As with the grieving process, an individual's concept of death and the approach and reactions to it will vary with age, culture and upbringing. However, it is safe to say that in the majority of cases, the opportunity to talk about the likelihood of death is welcomed, providing the moment is appropriate and the words are well chosen. It is often a good technique to encourage the child to ask you questions. Your perception of his or her fears may be considerably off mark, and it may well be that some reassurance that the child will not be alone and will not be allowed to be in pain is what they most want to hear.

As a junior doctor, it is easy to shy away from death and stand on the sidelines while it is dealt with by somebody more senior. Death, however, is a situation that requires a comparable degree of good care, skillful management, appropriate communication and empathy, as in many other acute medical situations. For this reason, it is good for you to be involved, at first passively with a physician experienced in dealing with death and then more actively as your confidence develops. Hopefully, when a child dies, physicians are present or readily available who know the child and family well and can communicate appropriately prior to, during and after death. However, as with other acute medical problems, death has a knack of happening out of hours and at weekends or when the relevant people are not available. While the tendency, these days, is for numerous support individuals to be present at certain times, in the acute event, the resident often finds himself or herself essentially alone. This is a testing time and it is important for all residents to be involved with death under more optimal circumstance early in their training. This is particularly true when death is sudden or unexpected (e.g. sudden infant death syndrome presenting in the Emergency Room).

Death is always a dramatic event for all concerned but is all the more so when it occurs unexpectedly. Under these circumstances, the physicians caring for the patient rarely know the patient or his/her family well, and this can compound the difficulties of diagnosis, care and communication.

It is important to remember that there are five stages in the grieving process, as described by Elizabeth Khubler–Ross. They are: prolonged denial and isolation, anger, guilt and bargaining, depression, and acceptance and reinvestment.

When death is an acute event, the first stages of anger, denial and guilt are commonly encountered together. Consequently, communication should be done with care and forethought, and the most senior and empathetic staff available should do it. This is not a job to delegate to junior residents or nurses. Research shows that the effectiveness of the initial intervention determines, in significant part, how well individuals progress through the grieving process and whether it is completed adequately. Clumsy management may delay acceptance as well as reinvestment.

The emotional effect on you personally and your colleagues of dealing with a child who dies should not be underestimated. The stress produced needs to be addressed consciously by you. Talking about it helps but, in some instances, the circumstances will be such that you may need more assistance.

Critical incident stress is now a recognized entity and individuals trained in helping to alleviate its effects exist in most hospitals. See chapter 20 (Resident/Fellow Training). Have a low threshold for seeking their advice.

Contact with parents

When possible, parents should be notified of death or impending death in person but sometimes telephone calls are necessary. When this is the case, begin by identifying yourself and the hospital. Tell the parents that there has been an acute problem, deterioration or accident (depending on the actual events that have occurred) and ask them if they can come to the hospital. If they can come, it is important to know how long it will take them. Give them the name of the physician to ask for on arrival, repeat again where their child is and to which ward or department they should come. Consider suggesting to parents that they be accompanied by a friend or relative.

Ideally, a call should always be made while resuscitation is still in progress so that parents can be warned of a potentially fatal outcome. If sudden death occurs without an opportunity for a warning call, whenever possible, try to avoid giving the news of actual death over the telephone, but if this cannot be avoided or if you are specifically asked, it is of course important to tell the truth and explain simply what has happened. At the end of the call, repeat who you are and from where you are calling. For Emergency Room patients, give parents the hospital telephone number as well.

If death is not sudden but is expected, communication by telephone is much simpler and can be more direct.

Arrival of parents

Ward staff or Emergency Room staff should be told to expect parents and should also be informed if the child has already died. Parents need a place of privacy available when they arrive. Make early contact with them. If possible, meet them prior to the child's actual death so that you can forewarn them again of the seriousness of their child's condition and the probability of death. If you are unable to leave the resuscitation, this responsibility should be delegated. Also ensure that someone continues to see the parents at least every 5–10 minutes with an update. Parents are often comforted if they know that their child has been told they are near by. In some centers now, parents are allowed to be present during cardiopulmonary resuscitation. Generally speaking, they are reported to find this experience helpful in their long–term grieving and acceptance. Certainly when death is imminent, parents should be allowed to visit and be with their child.

News of death

This is never easy or pleasant. It is important to recognize your own feelings at this time and to organize your thoughts before speaking to parents. However, news of death should never be unduly delayed.

Parents find it helpful if the events are repeated in chronological order, using simple, compassionate language. Eye contact and touch are appropriate and helpful. It is usually a good idea to ask extraneous family members to wait outside the room. If it is honest to do so, provide parents with the reassurance that everything possible was done and that their child was not in pain. Tell them what actions were taken in an attempt to help their child. Be prepared to repeat this information several times if necessary but do not labor points unnecessarily. Give parents time alone but return shortly. Offer them the opportunity to visit their child. Once the immediate family is notified, information can be shared with other family members. This is an important aspect of care for the grieving family as a whole.

The grief response

The stages of grief are outlined above but each individual will express their grief in a variety of ways. There is no right or wrong way. This is a time when you need to be a good listener. Demonstrations of emotion are normal and acceptable, both your own and those of the grieving family. Both parties likely need reassurance of this. Tears for example hurt no one. Do not take emotional outbursts or expressions of anger personally. Concentrate on trying to answer parents' questions like "if only..." or "why...." These questions are particularly common after sudden death. Where possible, reassure parents that things would not have been different had they acted in some other way.

Your own feelings and those of the other medical and nursing staff members involved with the family also need to be addressed. It is important to have time to discuss these feelings so that the staff can grieve appropriately as well. It requires a great deal for a nurse to be at the bedside of a dying child throughout a shift. Any sense of failure or error among the staff should be aired. No matter how often one deals with the death of a child, it never becomes easy and some degree of grief is always involved. See how other residents, nurses and physicians are as soon as you have dealt appropriately with the needs of the family.

Viewing the body

Most parents want to see their child and should be encouraged to do so to say good–bye. It is important at these times to refer to the child by name and not as "it" or "the body." It is kind to prepare the parents for what they will see, particularly if they have not been in the ward or Emergency Room before. You can do this by explaining the child's condition and the presence of equipment and other staff. The team caring for the child should make every effort to have the child looking as tidy and as free from resuscitation equipment as possible. Although parents generally manage the sight of equipment well, connecting it with everything possible being done for their child, they do not cope well with blood, vomit and tape on the child's body. Give the parents as long as they require with their child. Allow other relatives in to visit. Where possible, have the child in a side room where the parents can have some degree of privacy and other patients and their families are not disturbed. This is usually the time when additional support staff such as clergy, other physicians, etc., can be notified.

Arrangements

Parents should be told about plans for autopsy. Sometimes this will have been discussed prior to the child's death and consent forms may even have been signed. Autopsy reveals a great deal of information relevant to diagnosis and future care of other patients. Where parents decline autopsy consent, the attending physician should be notified as well as the Department of Pathology so that additional discussions can be undertaken with the parents. It is the responsibility of the physician in charge of the patient's care to notify the coroner of any death which should be reported. These include deaths within 48 hours of surgery, deaths following accidents and deaths where the cause of death is unclear. If the coroner is to be involved, it is kind to notify the parents at the time of death as funeral arrangements may be delayed. Document in the chart that the coroner has been notified, which coroner was spoken to, and what the decison was regarding this becoming a coroner's case or not.

Most parents will need to be advised to contact a funeral home. They should be given the telephone number of the Terminal Case Registry for help with any questions regarding arrangements, documents, etc. Notification of the other physicians involved with the child's care is very important. It is a good idea to list in the chart who has been notified and when. The family practitioner should be included on this list. There is nothing more unfortunate than a physician meeting parents and asking them, in ignorance, how their child is hours, days or weeks after death has occurred. The attending physician will usually complete the medical certificate of death at the Terminal Case Registry. This may also be done by the physician pronouncing death. This document lists the cause(s) of death and indicates if more information will be available later following autopsy. The funeral home takes this to Vital Statistics, who register the death and issue a burial permit.

It is generally not a good idea to prescribe sedative agents for parents because the ongoing care of the grieving adult is best managed by the family physician. However, families can find it helpful to be warned of the symptoms of grief such as mood change, depression, sleep disturbance, tearfulness, loss of concentration and poor appetite; sometimes medication is required for a relative who is particularly distressed. Ativan in a dose of 0.05–0.1 mg sublingually is probably the best medication as it is effective promptly and has a relatively short duration of action.

If a parent has to cope with the death of a child alone, it is helpful to arrange with someone to drive him or her home. All parents should be given a telephone number and a physician's name to contact in case of further questions. If there are other children in the family, help the parents to make plans to discuss the death of their child in an appropriate way with these children. Any inappropriate delay can complicate the grieving process for the dead child's siblings. Parents should be warned that younger children have a very different concept of death and may say things in response to the news which seem uncaring but are not intended to be hurtful.

Managing death effectively is one of the ongoing challenges of medicine. The needs of the child, the family, you and other staff must all be considered in order for the grieving process to be completed as effectively as possible.

Nowadays, the issue of organ donation comes up in connection with many deaths. Where brain death occurs or sudden death follows an accident, the heart, lungs, liver, kidneys and cornea are all organs which can be potentially donated. With increasing awareness of the benefits of organ transplant, some parents will raise the question themselves. In other cases, gentle inquiry should be made as to the family's feelings. One approach is to mention that under these circumstances some families derive comfort from the knowledge that their child has helped another by donation, but the exact approach has to depend on the individuals involved. When parents do express interest or give consent directly, the attending physician will likely notify the local agency which deals with organ transplant. These individuals can answer transplant related questions, have access to details of the current tests required and are in contact with the agencies capable of harvesting and transplanting specific organs. Once involved, they will coordinate the necessary tests and arrangements with the medical staff involved. Harvesting organs is expensive and it will not be undertaken without a reasonable chance of success. Prolonged hypoxia–ischemia, systemic sepsis and doubt about the cause of death will prevent the child from being an organ donor. However, if any possibility exists, this should be discussed with the attending staff and the transplant program representative at the earliest opportunity. Life support is continued in the interim with particular attention paid to maintaining oxygenation, blood pressure and urine output.

DEFINITION OF BRAIN DEATH

Rules concerning the definition of brain death vary considerably around the world. In British Columbia, the following information is valid.

A child may be diagnosed as clinically brain dead by two independent consultants, one of whom is a neurosurgeon or neurologist. This diagnosis is made on the basis of absent brain stem reflexes and a demonstrated absence of any spontaneous respiratory effort in the presence of a rising PCO_2 while the patient is adequately oxygenated (apnea test). The brain stem reflexes checked are: corneal reflexes, pupillary responses to light, doll's eye reflex, gag reflex, cold caloric responses and response to pain. The patient must be normothermic and free from sedative drugs, particularly phenobarbital.

The examination must take place when the patient is not medicated with a paralyzing agent and has levels of sedative or anticonvulsant agents (such as phenobarbital) which are, at most, at the lower end of the therapeutic range. An alternative means of establishing brain death is to have consecutive EEG studies which are isoelectric. Once again, these studies must be done when metabolic and drug parameters are within realistic limits.

When brain dead patients are involved as organ donors, ventilatory and circulatory support continues, pending harvesting of the donated organs. The time of clinical brain death is reported to the Health Records Department and the status of the child is then changed from "patient" to "donor." Under these circumstances, when the medical registration of death is completed, it is the date and time of clinical brain death that is entered and not the date and time when the heart finally stopped.

CARDIOPULMONARY ARREST

Most pediatric cardiac arrests are secondary to hypoxia, resulting from respiratory arrest. Because children have a healthy myocardium, prompt attention to airway, breathing and O_2 is usually all the resuscitation that is required.

Sequence of events

1. Establish diagnosis
- Shake and shout.
- Check respirations and pulse (brachial/carotid).
- Activate the resuscitation team.

2. Start ABC's
- Airway:
    Extend head and lift jaw.
    Suction airway if necessary.
    Place oral airway if necessary.
    Administer O_2.
- Breathing:
    Begin artificial ventilation (mouth to mouth or bag and mask to mouth).
    Respiratory rate: neonate, 40/min, infant/child, 20/min, teenager, 15/min.
    Tidal volume: about 10–15 mL/kg (assessed clinically by adequate chest movements).
    Indications for intubation:
    Inability to adequately ventilate by bag and mask.
    Full cardiac arrest.
- Circulation:
    Establish if there is a heart rate and blood pressure.
    With patient on a firm surface, begin external cardiac massage (ECM) at a ratio of 1:5 (ventilations to compressions) if: in neonate, heart rate < 60/min or heart rate of 60–80/min and not increasing with ventilation; in older child, there is asystole or any other nonperfusing rhythm.
    Assess adequacy of compressions by palpation of femoral pulse.
    Attach ECG monitor and oximeter.
- Intravenous access:
    Establish i.v. access if not already available.
    Peripheral venous access may be difficult in severe shock or full cardiac arrest. Consider external jugular vein or femoral vein access. Intraosseous access can usually be established much faster than venous cut down, therefore, should be considered the method of choice in children < 6 years of age who are in full cardiac arrest.
    Insert a #16 to #20 gauge bone marrow biopsy needle or spinal needle with stylet into the anteromedial surface of tibia 1–3 cm below the tibial tubercle.

Immediately give 20 mL/kg normal saline or Ringer's lactate over 20 min. Deliver colloid (5% albumin or plasma) and whole blood if there is blood loss.
- Drugs: epinephrine, atropine, lidocaine and naloxone may be given with 2 mL normal saline via endotracheal tube.
- Specific indications (there is only one drug to remember):
  Asystole: epinephrine.
  Bradycardia: epinephrine/atropine.
  EMD: epinephrine and treat the cause (hypoxemia, tension pneumothorax, hypovolemia, tamponade).
  Ventricular fibrillation: epinephrine + defibrillate 2 J/kg (asynch); then 4 J/kg and lidocaine 1 mg/kg + infusion 20–50 µg/kg per min.
  Ventricular tachycardia: if stable, lidocaine 1 mg/kg and infusion; if unstable, cardioversion 0.5–1 J/kg, then 2 J/kg.

SHOCK

Shock occurs when there is inadequate blood flow to meet the metabolic needs of the vital organs. The key to diagnosis is clinical anticipation and suspicion. More than one factor may be present.

Etiology

- Hypovolemic: trauma, surgery, diabetic ketoacidosis, burns, adrenal insufficiency.
- Cardiogenic: congenital heart disease, congenital heart failure, arrhythmias, tamponade, tension pneumothorax.
- Distributive: septic, anaphylactic, drug intoxication, neurogenic.

Diagnosis

- Cardiovascular: tachycardia with small volume pulse. Hypotension is often a late sign in children. Lower limit blood pressure is 70 + (2 × age in years).
- Neurological: agitation, confusion, decreased level of consciousness.
- Renal: decreased urine output (< 1 mL/kg per h).
- Skin: pale, cool, clammy skin with decreased capillary refill. Patients with septic shock may be flushed and warm.

Management

- All patients at risk should have vital signs and urine output monitored closely.
- Early aggressive attention to ABC's: O_2 and i.v. access 10–20 mL/kg normal saline or Ringer's lactate.
- Early use of colloid such as 5% albumin or plasma. Whole blood should be considered if there is significant blood loss.
- Children with septic shock may require large volumes of fluid (60–80 mL/kg) before rise in blood pressure is seen.
- Consider central venous pressure (CVP) monitoring in ICU setting.

- Lumbar puncture should be deferred until initial shock is controlled especially if there is evidence of disseminated intravascular coagulation (DIC).
- Foley catheter to monitor urine output.
- If sepsis is suspected, then empiric antibiotic coverage should be commenced.

1. Inotropic support
- Dopamine: epinephrine precursor with both direct and indirect alpha– and beta–adrenergic activity.
  Indications: hypotension or poor perfusion with stable cardiac rhythm.
  Dose: low dose 1–5 µg/kg per min for increased renal and splanchic blood flow; 3–10 µg/kg per min beta effect predominates with increased CO; 10–20 µg/kg per min alpha effect predominates with peripheral vasoconstriction. Start at 2–5 µg/kg per min and titrate up according to effect.
- Dobutamine: direct–acting, relatively selective beta–adrenergic activity.
  Indications: hypotension or poor perfusion in the postarrest patient.
  Dose: 5–20 µg/kg per min.
- Epinephrine: direct–acting adrenergic activity, more beta at low dose (< 0.3 µg/kg per min) and more alpha at higher doses (> 0.3 µg/kg per min).
  Indications: hypotension or poor perfusion with stable rhythm or hemodynamically significant bradycardia in the young infant where lower diastolic pressure may not be tolerated.
  Dose: 0.1–1 µg/kg per min.
- Isoproterenol: pure beta–adrenergic activity (increased heart rate, contractility and pulse pressure).
  Indications: hemodynamically significant bradycardia.
  Dose: 0.1–1 µg/kg per min.

2. Workup is specific to suspected underlying diagnosis
- CBC, platelets, PT, PTT, cross–match blood, blood culture.
- Arterial blood gases, electrolytes, BUN, creatinine, glucose, calcium.
- Septic workup including urine culture, CSF culture, stool culture.
- Chest X–ray, ECG and cardiac monitor.

MULTIPLE TRAUMA

An organized step–by–step approach is essential in delivering proper medical care to the multiply injured child. Organize the "trauma team" as much in advance of the patient's arrival in the Emergency Room as possible. The trauma team leader should be clearly identified and will coordinate both patient management and subspecialty referrals.

Management

1. Primary survey (first 2 minutes)
- Airway and C–spine:
  Assume C–spine injury in any multiple trauma, especially with blunt injury above the chest.
  Immobilize with hard collar or sand bags.
  100% O_2 by mask.

Jaw thrust or chin lift.
Ensure airway is clear of debris.
Oral airway if patient is obtunded.
- Breathing:
  Ensure adequate ventilation; bag or mask as necessary.
  Endotracheal intubation should be performed during the primary survey only if an airway cannot be obtained or the patient cannot be adequately ventilated. Rapid sequence technique is preferred as all children should be assumed to have a full stomach.
  Seal open pneumothorax.
  Alleviate tension pneumothorax.
- Circulation:
  Assess continuously for signs of shock.
  Control external hemorrhage by compression.
  Obtain vascular access with two large bore peripheral i.v.'s; intraosseous infusions may be lifesaving until alternate vascular access is obtained.
  Simultaneously obtain blood for cross–match, CBC, electrolytes, BUN, creatinine, glucose, liver function tests, amylase and clotting studies.
  Initiate fluid resuscitation with 20 mL/kg normal saline or Ringer's lactate; may repeat up to three boluses, then give 10 mL/kg packed red blood cells if there has been blood loss.
- Disability:
  Rapid neurological assessing LOC → GCS.
  Alert.
  Voice response.
  Pain response.
  Unresponsive.
  Pupillary size and reaction.
- Exposure: completely undress the patient as occult injuries are easily missed.

2. Secondary survey and ongoing resuscitation
- Reassess vital signs including temperature as heat loss is a significant stressor in children due to the high body surface:volume ratio.
- Continuous monitoring throughout the resuscitation is essential (cardiac, oximetry, blood pressure, urinary output).
- Rapid sequence intubation:
  Assume all multiply injured children have a full stomach prior to intubation.
  Preoxygenate with 100% O_2 by mask. Allow the patient to breathe spontaneously or assist ventilation by gentle bagging if necessary. Ensure suction is available.
  Atropine 0.01–0.02 mg/kg i.v. (minimum 0.1 mg) 2 min prior to intubation.
  If significant head injury with suspected increased ICP: lidocaine 1 mg/kg i.v.
  Sedation: thiopental 3–5 mg/kg i.v. (much less if patient is in shock).
  Relaxation: succinylcholine 1–2 mg/kg i.v.
  Apply continuous cricoid pressure until intubation is complete and tube placement confirmed.
  Endotracheal intubation: oral intubation is the method of choice; tube size = age/4 + 4; uncuffed if < 8 years of age.

- Examination:
  Head and maxillofacial trauma: relatively large head makes injury frequent.
  C–spine: maintain immobilization until all C–spine films are reviewed by an experienced physician.
  Chest: children have a highly elastic chest wall, therefore, pulmonary contusion and hemorrhage are relatively more frequent.
  Abdomen: children have a greater propensity to develop gastric ileus following even minor trauma. Insert nasogastric tube if ileus or significant abdominal trauma suspected. Insert orogastric tube if head injury is a concern. Include rectal examination and insert Foley catheter if normal.
  Extremities: note obvious deformities and assess neurovascular function to all limbs.
  Neurological: reassess Glasgow Coma Scale and pupils.
- Radiology: obtain CT scan of the head, C–spine, abdomen or pelvis as appropriate. Obtain plain films of C–spine, chest, abdomen, pelvis and extremities as appropriate.
- Pain management: fentanyl 1 µg/kg per dose i.v.; morphine 0.1 mg/kg per dose i.v.

3. Definitive care
This will be determined by clinical evaluation and response to resuscitation. Appropriate subspecialty services will direct further investigation and management.

HEAD INJURY

Whatever the mechanism of head injury, the primary brain damage is irreversible. The aims of management are to preserve life and to prevent secondary brain injury. Secondary damage due to cerebral edema can be reduced by avoiding hypoxia, hypercarbia, hypotension, hypoglycemia and hyperglycemia. Careful neurological observations are vital so that intracranial hemorrhage and other complications can be detected and treated early.

Severe head injuries (unconscious)

- Follow ABCDE's as for multiple trauma.
- Obtain a rapid history while attending to the above to determine mechanism and severity of insult, other potential sites of injury and whether the clinical picture is consistent with the story.
- Consider all head injured patients as multiple trauma. In cases of major trauma, it is easy to focus on the head injury and miss associated problems such as a ruptured spleen or fractured femur. Assume C–spine injury and maintain immobilization until proven otherwise.
- Perform a rapid and focused neurological examination to determine need for immediate resuscitation and to establish a baseline for measuring subsequent neurological change.

Raised intracranial pressure

- If the initial assessment suggests raised intracranial pressure (ICP), then the best management is rapid sequence endotracheal intubation. Premedicate with lidocaine, given 1 minute before intubation.
- Mannitol 0.5–1 g/kg i.v. Patient must be catheterized.
- Urgent CT scan and neurosurgical consult.

Prevention of secondary brain injury

- Elevate head of bed 30° and keep head in midline.
- Monitor arterial blood gases to keep PaO_2 > 100 mm Hg and $PaCO_2$ 35–40 mm Hg. Do not hyperventilate unless patient is clinically deteriorating.
- Insert orogastric tube to low suction.
- Replace acute blood loss, then restrict maintenance fluids to two–thirds maintenance.
- Maintain normal temperature.
- Sedation may be necessary to reduce raised ICP associated with agitation. Diazepam 0.1 mg/kg and morphine 0.1 mg/kg q2–4h followed by infusions of both. Do not paralyze unless absolutely necessary since major monitoring signs are lost.
- Post–traumatic seizures should be treated with diazepam and dilantin as described for status epilepticus.
- Neurosurgical consult should be sought early, especially if there is any sign of depressed or basilar skull fracture, lateralizing neurological signs or intracranial hemorrhage with raised ICP.

ANAPHYLAXIS

Anaphylaxis is due to an immediate (type 1) hypersensitivity reaction that occurs soon after antigen exposure. The most common antigens are drugs, especially penicillins, insect stings, foods, contrast media and blood products.

Diagnosis (involves a spectrum from mild to severe)

- Cardiovascular: tachycardia, arrhythmias, hypotension.
- Respiratory: upper airway obstruction, bronchospasm.
- Skin: urticaria, angioedema.
- Gastrointestinal: hyperperistalsis, vomiting.

Treatment

- Discontinue or remove offending antigen.
- Airway/breathing: O_2 by mask. Laryngeal edema and bronchospasm are initially treated with subcutaneous epinephrine 1:1000 solution—0.01 mL/kg (0.05 mL/yr of life), minimum 0.1 mL, maximum 1 mL.
- Circulation: hypotension may be severe and require vigorous fluid resuscitation. Start with 10 mL/kg normal saline or Ringer's lactate. May require inotropic support.
- Other medications: diphenhydramine (benadryl) 1 mg/kg p.o., i.m. or i.v.; hydrocortisone (solucortef) 5–10 mg/kg i.v.; prednisone 1–2 mg p.o.
- Long–term: education (e.g. avoidance of antigen, treatment with epipen syringe, Medic Alert tag).

ADRENAL INSUFFICIENCY

The adrenal cortex produces two major hormones necessary for maintaining life: cortisol (glucocorticoid) and aldosterone (mineralocorticoid), although there is overlap between the two categories. Adrenal insufficiency can be primary in origin and caused by adrenal dysfunction, secondary related to lack of ACTH production by the pituitary or tertiary related to abnormal hypothalamic regulation. Primary adrenal insufficiency can be caused by autoimmune destruction, adrenal hemorrhage or infection. Patients will have manifestations of both glucocorticoid and mineralocorticoid deficiency. Patients with the salt losing form of congenital adrenal hyperplasia will have similar findings.

Secondary and tertiary adrenal insufficiency will manifest as cortisol deficiency. Aldosterone production is primarily regulated by the renin–angiotensin system. Causes of secondary and tertiary adrenal insufficiency include congenital hypopituitarism and damage to either the hypothalamus or pituitary by infection, neoplasm, hemorrhage or external radiation. Patients who have been on suppressive doses of steroids may have cortisol deficiency upon steroid withdrawal. This may occur even on therapy and under physical stress if steroid doses are not in the stress range.

Diagnosis

- Common presentation: nausea and vomiting which progresses to dehydration, decreased peripheral perfusion and hypotension → SHOCK.
- Consider the diagnosis:
  In infants with ambiguous genitalia.
  In children with hyperpigmentation, unexplained vomiting and dehydration, unexplained hyperkalemia or hyponatremia.
  In children with shock whose symptoms seem out of line with the precipitating event.
  All patients who have received or are receiving steroids.

Investigations

- Electrolytes, BUN, creatinine, glucose.
- Consider: ACTH, cortisol, renin, aldosterone, 17–hydroxyprogesterone.
- Characteristic findings: hyponatremia (< 130 mmol/L), hypochloremic acidosis, hyperkalemia (> 5), raised glucose, raised BUN.

Treatment

- ABC's: shock should be treated with supplemental O_2 and i.v. fluid resuscitation 10–20 mL/kg normal saline with 5% dextrose.
- Hypoglycemia 1 g/kg (2 mL/kg) 50% dextrose: dilute 1:1 with water to give 25% solution.
- Hyperkalemia will usually correct with fluid management and hydrocortisone therapy.

Steroid replacement

- Hydrocortisone 100–150 mg/m^2 i.v. immediately with 25 mg/m^2 q4h over next 24 h period.
- Mineralocorticoid: during the first day of treatment, high dose hydrocortisone therapy usually provides sufficient mineralocorticoid.
- Fluorocortisone (florinef) can be given orally once recovery from the acute illness has occurred.

Maintenance therapy

- Hydrocortisone 12–20 mg/m² per d p.o. div. t.i.d.
- Fluorocortisone (florinef) 50–100 µg p.o. once to twice daily.
- Monitor patient for suppression of adrenal androgens, growth and blood pressure.
- Salt intake must be maintained in patients with salt loss: 1–2 g/d.

UNDIAGNOSED COMA

- Priorities in management should begin with ABC's and monitoring.
- Rapid evaluation to focus on clinical category and potential underlying cause. Primary goal is to recognize and treat raised ICP, differentiate between nonstructural and structural disorder which may require rapid neurosurgical intervention, exclude reversible problems such as hypoglycemia and drug overdose.

Etiology

- Nonstructural (95%):
  Infection: meningitis, encephalitis, sepsis. CNS infection is the most common cause of unrecognized coma in children.
  Hypoxic–ischemic encephalopathy: suffocation, drowning, CO_2 poisoning, cardiorespiratory arrest, strangulation.
  Seizure or postictal state: epilepsy.
  Intoxication or poisoning: antihistamine and decongestant preparations, alcohol, opiates, sedatives, antipsychotics, ASA, anticonvulsants, heavy metals.
  Metabolic disorders: diabetic ketoacidosis, hypoglycemia, hepatic or renal encephalopathy, Reye's syndrome, inborn errors of metabolism.
- Structural (5%):
  Trauma: subdural or epidural hemorrhage.
  Tumor: posterior fossa tumors most common in children.
  Infection: abscess.
  Vascular: arteriovenous malformation, aneurysm.

History

- Recent: health, trauma, toxic exposures, available drugs at home, infectious contacts, foreign travel.
- Past: seizures, diabetes, drugs, heart disease, social conditions.

Examination

- Vitals: temperature, pulse, blood pressure, respiration.
- Neurosurgical: level of consciousness (Glasgow Coma Scale), pupillary reflexes, brain stem reflexes (gag, corneal, doll's eye), neck stiffness, lateralizing signs. Chart findings carefully for comparison over time.
- General: fontanelle, neck stiffness, signs of trauma, odor of breath, hydration.

Treatment

- ABC's:
    If raised ICP is suspected, the child should be treated as a head injury.
    Intubation should be performed in a controlled manner under protection of atropine, thiopentone and paralysis.
    Lidocaine 1 mg/kg i.v. should be given 1–2 min prior to intubation.
    Give mannitol 0.25 g/kg if not stabilized following intubation.
    Consult Neurosurgery immediately if structural lesion is suspected.
- Check dextrostix and draw blood for laboratory investigations:
    CBC, blood cultures.
    Glucose, electrolytes, BUN, creatinine, Ca, Mg, liver function tests.
    Arterial blood gases, serum lactate, ammonia.
    Toxicology screen: serum, urine or gastric aspirate.
    Serum amino acids, urine organic acids.
- Drugs:
    Glucose: neonate, 0.25 g/kg = 1 mL/kg 25% dextrose; child, 0.5–1 g/kg = 2 mL/kg 25% dextrose.
    Naloxone: 0.1 mg/kg i.v.
    Consider the administration of flumazenil 0.1–0.2 mg i.v. over 15 s; repeat 0.1 mg q1 min; up to 3 mg infusion may be required.
    Antibiotic and antiviral coverage if indicated.
- Carefully review history, physical examination and results of laboratory investigations. Watch closely for evolution of clinical state.

STATUS EPILEPTICUS

Although seizures must always be viewed as a symptom of underlying pathology, significant morbidity or death may result from the seizure itself.

The most common medical errors are: failure to give adequate dose of drug, failure to give a long–acting convulsant with short–acting benzodiazepine and failure to anesthetize the patient early if the seizure continues.

Treatment

- Stabilize with attention to ABC's.
- Oral airway or intubation as necessary; administer O_2; i.v. access.
- Draw blood for CBC, arterial blood gases, electrolytes, BUN, creatinine, Ca, Mg, glucose (with dextrostix), blood cultures.
- Drugs:
    Lorazepam 0.05–0.1 mg/kg i.v. over 2 min (maximum 4 mg), diazepam 0.3 mg/kg i.v. over 2 min (maximum 10 mg); may repeat dose in 5–10 min if seizures persist.
    If i.v. not established rapidly, diazepam may be given per rectum with a small feeding tube or a tuberculin syringe at a dose of 0.5 mg/kg.
    Phenytoin 20 mg/kg i.v. in normal saline i.v. over 20 min (rate not > 50 mg/min). Give even if seizures controlled with benzodiazepine.

If hypoglycemic (dextrostix < 3 mmol/L), give 1 mL/kg 50% dextrose.
- Other drug options include:
  Phenobarbital 10–150 mg/kg i.v. (rate not > 30 mg/min); may repeat dose in 10 min.
  Paraldehyde 0.3 mL/kg in an equal volume of mineral oil given rectally; may repeat dose in 20 min.
  (Caution: risk for respiratory depression increases with each new drug given.)
- If seizures are still not controlled, both Neurology and ICU should be consulted. Morbidity and mortality increase rapidly if seizures last longer than 30 minutes. Consideration should be given to induction, intubation and general anesthesia.
- Phenobarbital and phenytoin levels should be checked 1 hour postloading.
  Phenytoin: therapeutic range, 40–80 µmol/L; maintenance dose, 5–10 mg/kg per d div. q8–12h.
  Phenobarbital: therapeutic range, 65–170 µmol/L; maintenance dose, 3–5 mg/kg per d div. q12h.
- If CNS infection is suspected, then age appropriate antibiotics should be started once blood cultures have been drawn. A lumbar puncture should be deferred until the patient is stable. Pleocytosis of the CSF is unlikely to be affected by prior antibiotic administration. Urine should be sent for antigen analysis. The organism is usually obtained by blood culture in > 85% of cases.

ACUTE UPPER AIRWAY OBSTRUCTION

The first consideration with acute respiratory obstruction is to distinguish between upper and lower airway disease. Upper airway disease typically has inspiratory distress with stridor; lower airway obstruction has predominantly expiratory distress with wheeze.

Etiology

- Infection: acute epiglottitis, laryngotracheobronchitis (viral croup), retropharyngeal abscess, tonsillitis, peritonsillar abscess, bacterial tracheitis.
- Trauma: foreign body, upper airway burns, external trauma to the neck.
- Tumors: hemangioma, neoplasms.
- Other: angioedema, spasmodic croup, congenital malformations.

Acute epiglottitis

Consider this diagnosis in all cases of upper airway distress. This may be suggested by a child of any age who presents with rapid onset of inspiratory stridor with high fever and rapidly progressive respiratory distress with retractions. A fearful expression, pallor, lethargy, drooling and the inability to swallow may all be apparent. Clinical suspicion is sufficient.

1. Treatment
- Allow patient to adopt position of comfort.
- Avoid agitation with procedures such as intravenous starts.
- Be prepared for acute respiratory obstruction and have available a bag and mask and equipment for intubation. Remember, you can usually hand ventilate a child with epiglottitis.

- Notify ICU, ENT and Anesthesia with a view to a controlled, elective intubation in the Operating Room.

2. Early epiglottitis
- Beware of the patient with early epiglottitis who has not yet become severely ill and may be difficult to distinguish from other croup syndromes. The most distinguishing aspect of epiglottitis is the rapidity of onset with fever, lethargy and stridor, developing within 2–6 hours. Breathing is usually quiet with a reluctance to cough. A lateral X–ray of the neck may help in diagnosis (have Radiology come to you).
- Remember the mnemonic:
    Hypopharyngeal air space dilation.
    Epiglottic swelling (thumb sign).
    Aryepiglottic swelling.
    Tracheal air column disruption.
- Increased prevertebral soft tissues or air fluid levels may be seen with a retropharyngeal abscess, and subglottic narrowing (steeple sign) may be seen with croup.

3. Definitive treatment
- Secure airway.
- Establish i.v. and obtain blood cultures.
- Antibiotic therapy: aimed towards treatment of Haemophilus influenzae.
    Cefotaxime 200 mg/kg per d div. q6h.
    Or, ampicillin 100–200 mg/kg per d div. q6h and chloramphenicol 75 mg/kg per d div. q6h.
- Examine carefully for other manifestations of H. influenzae infection, including meningitis, pneumonia, otitis media, septic arthritis, pericarditis, DIC and septicemia.
- Prophylaxis: for patients and families where there is a sibling < 4 years of age. The family and patient should all receive rifampin to eradicate carrier state.

Laryngotracheobronchitis (Croup)

The usual etiological agents are parainfluenza, influenza, RSV and adenovirus.

1. Diagnosis
Although respiratory distress is the prominent feature, in contrast to the child with epiglottitis, these children are generally restless and a barky cough is prominent. High fever may be present initially, however, more commonly the fever is low grade. There is usually a coryzal phase followed by 1 or 2 days of stridor and barky cough.

2. Treatment
- Consider hospital management for the child with:
    Persistent stridor at rest, especially if associated with retractions.
    Decreased ability to drink or clinical manifestations of dehydration.
- Specific drug therapy may include:
    Racemic epinephrine delivered via nebulizer diluted with normal saline p.r.n.
    Dexamethasone 0.25 mg/kg i.v. or 0.8 mg p.o.; should be repeated q8h × 3 doses.
    In mild to moderate cases, inhaled budesonide 1 mg q12h × 2 doses.

ACUTE LOWER AIRWAY OBSTRUCTION

The common differential diagnoses of acute onset of wheezing are asthma, bronchiolitis, foreign body aspiration, acute anaphylaxis and exacerbation of chronic bronchopulmonary dysplasia. Less commonly, pneumonia or congestive heart failure may be confused with asthma.

ACUTE ASTHMA AND STATUS ASTHMATICUS

Asthma is characterized by recurrent episodes of reversible lower airway constriction. Status asthmaticus is the failure to respond to drugs that usually relieve bronchoconstriction.

Diagnosis

Although asthmatics usually present with respiratory distress and predominantly expiratory wheeze, the diagnosis should be considered in any child presenting with recurrent cough, shortness of breath or chest congestion. Previous response to bronchodilator therapy is characteristic. A trial of bronchodilator therapy may be both diagnostic and therapeutic.

History

- Determine the onset, duration and clinical course of the present illness.
- Determine severity of past attacks, including frequency, usual course, steroid usage and intensive care management, and number of hospitalizations. If a child had needed an ICU admission before, beware. Admit if at all worried.
- List present drug treatment regime and any recent changes.
- Determine usual triggers, including previous anaphylaxis.

Examination

- Severity is determined by close attention to the vital signs as well as to both the neurological and cardiorespiratory systems.
- Respiratory distress is manifested by tachypnea, using of accessory muscles, hyperinflation and prolongation of the expiratory phase of respiration.
- Ominous signs include an abrupt decline in respiratory rate, absent or markedly decreased breath sounds, inability to speak, cyanosis, fatigue and altered mental status (either agitation or depression).

Treatment

- Management should focus on immediate treatment with laboratory investigations minimized.
- Chest X–ray should be considered when pneumothorax, pneumomediastinum or pneumonia is suspected.
- Arterial blood gases are of minimal value, especially when the practical difficulties of arterial puncture are considered.
- Spirometry, especially the peak expiratory flow rate, may be useful in assessing severity and response to treatment.

General measures

- Avoid agitation as this will contribute to the child's respiratory distress.
- Position the child with the head of the bed up or sitting in the parent's lap.
- Deliver humidified O_2 30–40% by face mask or nasal prongs.
- Monitor the child with continuous oximetry if in moderate to severe distress.

Specific measures

1. Nebulized salbutamol (ventolin)
1 mL (5 mg/mL respirator solution) in 3 mL of normal saline with 100% O_2 at 6–8 L/min over 10 min. This dose is the same regardless of age or weight. Frequency of administration will vary depending on the severity of the attack and may be given continuously (changing the chamber every 10–15 minutes) until the bronchospasm has resolved.

2. Ipratropium bromide (atrovent) (0.5 mg/mL)
If patients are < 2 years of age, 0.25–0.5 mL may be added to the respirator solution as an adjunct to salbutamol on a q6–8h basis; if > 2 years of age, 0.5–1.0 mL may be added.

3. Epinephrine (1:1000 solution)
0.01 mg/kg may be given subcutaneously to those patients with a marked degree of bronchospasm or if an anaphylactic component is suspected. This dose may be repeated every 10 min if necessary. Cardiac monitoring is essential.

4. Intravenous fluids
Intravenous fluids should be started early in the severe asthmatic as these children are usually significantly dehydrated and will require intravenous access for drug therapy. Fluid requirements will be increased.

5. Steroids
Steroids should be given to all asthmatics whose acute attack is severe enough to prompt treatment in an Emergency Room. Methylprednisolone 2 mg/kg i.v. bolus and then 1 mg/kg q6h or hydrocortisone 5 mg/kg i.v. q6h. Avoid steroids in children who have recently been exposed to chickenpox. The patient may be changed to oral steroids once the clinical condition is more stable. A short course of steroids (< 7 days) may be discontinued abruptly; however, if longer courses are necessary or if the patient was recently on steroids, they should be tapered more slowly. Oral betamethasone 0.1–0.2 mg/kg per d is usually preferred to prednisone (1.0–2.0 mg/kg per d) because of its taste.

Additional drug therapy

Although the use of aminophylline is controversial, this drug may be of some use in the severe asthmatic who does not respond well to initial therapy. It is usually reserved for patients requiring ventolin more frequently than every hour. Loading dose of 6 mg/kg over 20–30 min followed by an infusion of 0.9 mg/kg per h for adolescents and 1.1 mg/kg per h for younger children. Reduce the load to 3 mg/kg if the patient has used theophylline products in the previous 12 hours.

Therapeutic range 55–110 µmol/L. Levels should be checked within 1 hour of the loading dose.

Complications

1. Pneumothorax
Pneumothorax, if under tension, should be immediately drained by inserting a large bore (#14G) intracath in the second intercostal space in the midclavicular line or in the fourth intercostal space in the anterior axillary line. Follow by chest tube insertion and connection to underwater seal.

2. Respiratory failure
Respiratory failure may necessitate intubation and assisted ventilation. This is best performed by an anesthetist or pediatric intensivist by either intravenous induction with ketamine or inhalation induction with halothane.

BACTERIAL MENINGITIS

Bacterial meningitis has a 5–10% mortality and 25% chance of neurological sequelae. The peak age group is 6 months to 2 years when classical symptoms of meningeal irritation are not easily elicited. Although irritability or lethargy are often present, no specific clinical picture has been shown to reliably identify all these children. Fever > 39 °C and white blood cell counts over 15,000/mm^3 are associated with a significantly greater risk of bacteremia and meningitis.

Diagnosis

Examination of the CSF is essential for diagnosis. However, in patients with signs of ICP, focal neurological signs, or progressive neurological impairment or shock, the lumbar puncture should be deferred. Life threatening problems should be dealt with immediately by instituting the ABC's and parenteral antibiotics should be administered urgently. The organism is recovered from the blood in over 85% of cases.

Investigations

• CBC, differential, blood culture, electrolytes, BUN, creatinine, glucose and coagulation studies.
• Urinalysis and urine culture.
• CSF cell count, differential, glucose, protein, culture and Gram stain. Antigen analysis may be done if available, especially if the lumbar puncture is delayed.

Management

• Strict attention to ABC's as approximately 10% of children may present with shock. Fluid resuscitation should continue until adequate circulation has been established. Inotropes and CVP monitoring may be necessary.
• Coma, progressive neurological deterioration or focal signs warrant urgent intubation and hyperventilation.
• Seizures should be treated immediately and hypoglycemia should be considered as a possible precipitating factor.

• Fluids should be restricted to two–thirds maintenance for the first 48 hours following initial stabilization and serum sodium should be followed closely. SIADH is common.

1. Medications
• Antibiotics: empiric coverage is started according to the most likely age specific organisms:
  0–2 months:
  Ampicillin: 200 mg/kg per d q4h.
  Gentamicin: 7.5 mg/kg per d q8h.
  Cefotaxime: 200 mg/kg per d q6h.
  2–4 months:
  Ampicillin: 200 mg/kg per d q4h.
  Cefotaxime: 200 mg/kg per d q6h.
  4 months–7 years:
  Cefotaxime: 200 mg/kg per d q8h.
  > 7 years:
  Ampicillin: 200–400 mg/kg per d q6h.
  Penicillin: 200,000 unit/kg per d q4h.
• Steroids: this remains a controversial issue in the management of bacterial meningitis. There is some evidence to suggest that in cases of *H. influenzae* meningitis, if given prior to antibiotics, there may be a beneficial effect on reducing the chance of neurological sequelae, especially sensorineural hearing loss. The recommended dose is dexamethasone 0.15 mg/kg i.v. every 6 h for 4 d.

2. Prophylaxis of contacts
This should be instituted as early as possible for meningococcal and *H. influenzae* type B cases.
• Meningococcal: treat all family members, irrespective of age, with rifampin 10 mg/kg (maximum 600 mg) p.o. twice daily for 2 d.
• *Haemophilus*: treat all family members if there is a child in the family < 4 years of age or if the index case is < 1 year. Give rifampin 20 mg/kg (maximum 600 mg) p.o. twice daily for 4 d.
All cases should be reported to the public health authorities, especially if the index case attends a daycare facility.

DIABETIC KETOACIDOSIS (DKA)

DKA remains the most common cause of death in the diabetic < 20 years of age. It may also be the first presentation of insulin dependent diabetes mellitus (IDDM). It should be remembered that the treatment of DKA is potentially dangerous. Overhydration or too rapid correction of hyperglycemia can lead to cerebral edema and death. Electrolyte disturbances, especially hypokalemia and hypoglycemia, can also be lethal.

History

• Common complaints may include polyuria, polydipsia, polyphagia, weight loss and abdominal pain.
• If the child is a known diabetic, ask about daily dose of insulin and recent changes, diet, previous episodes of DKA and precipitating causes (drugs, alcohol, concurrent illness,

noncompliance with drug regime or poor social setting).

Examination

- General examination.
- Assess level of consciousness, perfusion, blood pressure, pulse and hydration. These patients are generally significantly dehydrated.

Investigation

- Serum glucose (include dextrostix), electrolytes, BUN, creatinine, Ca, PO_4.
- CBC, arterial blood gases and urine for ketones, glucose and culture.

Management

1. Order of priority
- Rapid correction of shock with normal saline.
- Replacement of electrolyte deficits, especially potassium.
- Smooth control of hyperglycemia.
- Correction of any precipitating factors, if possible.

2. Fluid management
- Give 10 mL/kg normal saline rapidly. Repeat until perfusion and blood pressure are adequate. Calculate the total fluid deficit based on a clinical estimate (usually 100 mL/kg).
- Plan to give the total deficit plus maintenance over 24 hours.
- The initial fluid should be normal saline; when the serum glucose falls to 12–15 mmol/L, change to D5W one–half normal saline to prevent hypogycemia.

3. Electrolyte replacement
- Begin potassium replacement after the initial fluid bolus, provided urine output is confirmed. Add 15 mEq KCl and 15 mEq KPO_4 to 1 liter of i.v. solution.
- Sodium bicarbonate is generally not recommended as it may precipitate paradoxical CNS acidosis and cerebral edema. Acidosis generally improves with rehydration alone.

4. Insulin therapy
- Low dose short–acting intravenous insulin is the treatment of choice. It requires an accurate infusion pump and a separate infusion site from the fluid replacement site.
- Add 50 units regular insulin to 500 mL normal saline (solution 0.1 unit/mL).
- Run the solution through the i.v. tubing to saturate insulin binding sites.
- Give insulin 0.1 unit/kg bolus followed by 0.1 unit/kg per h infusion.

5. Monitor
- Serum glucose hourly, alternating dextrostix and laboratory measurements.
- pH and electrolytes every 2 hours.
- Urine ketones.
- When the serum glucose falls to 12–15 mmol/L, change the replacement fluid to D5W one–half

normal saline. Continue the insulin infusion until the serum pH is normal and the urine ketones are negative. Maintain the serum glucose between 10–12 mmol/L by adjusting the glucose concentration in the replacement fluid.
• Once the pH is normalized, the insulin infusion may be discontinued and subcutaneous insulin started. The i.v. fluid infusion should be continued until the patient is alert and drinking well.

HYPOGLYCEMIA

Prolonged or recurrent hypoglycemia may cause irreversible brain damage. Early recognition and treatment is essential. The most common cause outside the neonatal period is in association with insulin treatment of diabetics. Hypoglycemia may accompany almost any illness which interferes with oral intake.

Diagnosis

• The signs and symptoms of hypoglycema are nonspecific and often overlooked, especially in the infant or young child.
• The patient is often pale, sweaty, tachycardic and "glassy–eyed".
• Secondary increased adrenergic stimulation is responsible for behavior changes (irritability, confusion, hyperactivity or anxiety), headaches and hunger.
• Neurological features may progress to convulsions and coma if untreated.

Laboratory diagnosis (hypoglycemia < 2.5 mmol/L)

• Any acutely ill child deserves a serum glucose determination.
• In a known diabetic, if unable to differentiate between a ketoacidotic and hypoglycemic coma, the patient should be treated with glucose as a clinical trial before the results are available.

Management

1. Oral therapy
If the patient is awake and able to swallow, juice or soft drinks should be given. If the patient is unable to swallow and intravenous or intramuscular therapy is not available, then dextrose solutions may be given by nasogastric tube.

2. Intramuscular therapy
Glucagon 0.03 mg i.m. (maximum 1 mg) should be used if i.v. access is not possible. This should be followed by oral or intravenous glucose. Glucagon will not work if the patient has no hepatic stores or a glycogen storage disease.

3. Intravenous therapy
1 mL/kg 50% glucose i.v. (0.5 g/kg), followed with i.v. glucose infusion of D10W.

ACUTE RENAL FAILURE

Acute renal failure can be defined as a sudden decline in renal function, resulting in retention

of nitrogenous wastes. The drop in glomerular filtration rate usually causes urine output to fall below 180 mL/m^2 per 24 h, however, in 10–20% of cases, the urine output remains above this level.
Treatment is directed toward the underlying etiology, which can generally be classified as prerenal, renal or postrenal. Emergency management of these patients should be directed toward correction of life threatening shock, electrolyte imbalance, acidosis and hypertension.

Management

- Ensure that there is no urinary obstruction. Catheterize infants if urethral valves are suspected.
- Fluids:
  Ensure the patient is not hypovolemic. Restore volume with normal saline 10 mL/kg bolus.
  If anuria persists, despite normal hydration, try lasix 1–2 mg/kg i.v.
  If no response, limit input to 10 mL/kg per d (250 mL/m^2 per d) plus measured losses.
- Electrolytes:
  Restrict sodium and potassium to 1 mEq/kg per d.
  If hyperkalemic (K > 7.0 mmol/L or symptomatic): discontinue all potassium intake, check for ECG abnormalities (tall T–waves, prolonged P–R interval, widened QRS), give kayexalate 1 g/kg as an enema in 20% sorbitol and also by nasogastric tube, calcium gluconate 0.5 mL/kg in 10% solution, NaHCO$_3$ 1–2 mEq/kg over 10 min.
  (Caution: incompatible with calcium gluconate).
- Nutrition: restrict protein to 1 g/kg per d. Calories should be provided as carbohydrate to spare tissue protein.
- Dialysis may be required for hyperkalemia, severe uremia, fluid overload or hypertension. Avoid all nephrotoxic drugs if possible.

ACUTE HYPERTENSIVE EMERGENCY

Act quickly. Neurological sequelae will be minimized by prompt recognition and control. Anticipate hypertensive problems in certain diseases. Some important conditions include acute glomerulonephritis, Henoch–Schönlein purpura, nephritis, hemolytic uremic syndrome, acute renal failure, postrenal transplantation or urological surgery, excess blood volume expansion and steroid use. Severe sustained hypertension is most often due to renal disease or renal vascular disease.

Diagnosis

Check the size of the BP cuff and the blood pressure. Too small a cuff will give a falsely high blood pressure. Hypertension exists if systolic or diastolic blood pressure is sustained over the 95th percentile for age as defined by the AAP standards. See chapter 24 (Appendix).

Management

1. Treatment
Urgent treatment should be instituted if:
- There are symptoms or signs of major organ involvement such as severe headache, seizures,

coma or cardiac decompensation.
- In a child < 4 years of age, BP > 130/90; in an older child, BP > 150/95. Higher levels may be acceptable in children with known chronic hypertension.

2. Drugs
- Nifedipine: in children 3–12 years of age, 5 mg sublingual or p.o.; in children > 12 years of age, 10 mg sublingual or p.o.; repeat in 15 min if necessary.
- Diazoxide: 3–5 mg/kg i.v. injection in < 30 s; repeat in 30 min if no effect.
- Furosemide: 1 mg/kg i.v. should be given as an adjunct to counteract the salt and water retention induced by diazoxide.
- Hydralazine: 0.1–0.2 mg/kg i.v. may be given as an alternative to diazoxide; repeat in 4–6 h if necessary.
- Sodium nitroprusside: 0.5 µg/kg per min i.v. (increasing rate up to 8 µg/kg per min) can be given for resistant or persistent hypertension, however, requires ICU monitoring.
- Propranolol: 0.5–1 mg/kg p.o. or 0.05–0.1 mg/kg i.v. slowly (caution: do not give to asthmatics).
If severe hypotension occurs, it should be treated vigorously. Blood pressure should be monitored every 2 minutes until stabilized and then every 30 minutes.

CHILD ABUSE

Child abuse commonly occurs in children < 3 years of age. Mortality is at least 3% and generally results from neurological or abdominal trauma.

1. Physical abuse
Any physical action which results in, or may result in, a nonaccidental injury to a child and which exceeds that which could be considered reasonable discipline.

2. Sexual abuse
Any sexual exploitation of a child whether consented to or not. It includes touching of a sexual nature, sexual intercourse and may include any behavior of a sexual nature towards a child. Sexual activity between children may constitute sexual abuse if the difference in age or power between children is significant.

3. Emotional abuse
Acts or omissions of those responsible for the care of a child which are likely to undermine a child's self–image, sense of worth and self–confidence.

4. Neglect
Failure of those responsible for the care of the child to meet the physical, emotional or medical needs to an extent that the child's health, development or safety is endangered.

Diagnosis

1. Suspicious clinical findings
- Multiple trauma of any form in the absence of a clear history.
- Fractures uncommonly produced by a single fall such as metaphyseal fractures, epiphyseal

separations and subperiosteal calcifications.
- Subdural hematomas.
- Retinal hemorrhages.
- Burns, usually cigarette or immersion burns (circumferential, no splash marks and sparing skin folds).
- Bites, welts, rope burns or multiple bruises (especially involving sides of face, ears, upper lip, buttocks, lower back and upper extremities).
- Poor hygiene and/or failure to thrive.
- Apathy, passivity, watchfulness, fearful expression, unquestioning reception of any caregiver.
- Abnormal perineal exam in the absence of a reasonable explanation.

2. Suspicious behavior patterns of abusive parents
- Aloof, angry or antagonistic.
- Unexplained delay in seeking medical attention.
- Inconsistent or vague accounts of the accident (history does not seem to fit either the injury pattern or the developmental age of the child).
- Inappropriate concern over the child's illness (either under or overconcerned).
- Repeated unfounded complaints of physical illness with frequent visits to various health authorities.
- History of the child being "accident prone".

3. Children at risk of abuse
- Premature babies.
- Mentally handicapped children.
- Developmentally delayed children.
- Physically handicapped children.
- Children who are recurrently "unwell".

Management

- If child abuse is suspected, a professional Child Protection Team should be notified, which usually includes a pediatrician and a Ministry social worker.
- Following a complete, well documented history and physical examination, workup may include CBC, coagulation screen, skeletal survey and medical photographs.
- If sexual abuse is considered, collection of specimens must be done, looking for evidence of sexually transmitted diseases and presence of semen.
- Experience has shown it is more important to foster confidence and trust in the hospital personnel than to start with an overly aggressive attempt to establish guilt.

POISONING

Pediatric poisonings tend to fall into two groups based on age and intent. The first group is the child < 5 years of age who accidentally ingests a single substance. The second group is the older child, usually an adolescent, who intentionally ingests a drug or poison as a suicide gesture. The physician should be aware that these children have often ingested more than one substance.

Home management

Often the first steps in management begin over the telephone. If the substance is clearly identified as nontoxic or the amount ingested is inconsequential, then nothing more than reassurance is necessary. Unfortunately, in most cases, the history is incomplete or the amount of poison ingested is unknown. These children should all be examined in the Emergency Room. Ensure that the parent brings the "poison's" container with the remaining contents to the hospital. Induction of vomiting with syrup of ipecac as a home therapy is generally not recommended.

Hospital management

Strict attention to the ABC's. Remember antidotes are uncommon. Focus should be on the general principles of physiological support, gut decontamination, seizure control and attentive neurological and cardiac monitoring. Once stabilized, psychiatric consultation should be obtained for all suicide attempts. Accidental ingestions are rarely true accidents and are frequently a sign of complete social disorder.

1. History
- All possible products ingested.
- Time of ingestion.
- Approximate amount ingested (a swallow for a 3 year old is 5 mL, a 10 year old is 10 mL and an adolescent is 15 mL). Remember that if the ingestion was intentional, this information should be very suspect.
- Current symptoms: the two systems most commonly affected by poisons are the neurological and gastrointestinal systems.

2. Examination
- Special attention to the vital signs, especially respiratory rate and temperature.
- Specific signs such as pupil size or odor of breath may be helpful in identifying the unknown ingestion.
- Full neurological evaluations, focusing especially on mental status.

3. Investigation
- General bloodwork to include CBC, electrolytes, BUN, creatinine, coagulation studies, liver function tests and arterial blood gases.
- Consider ECG or cardiac monitor.
- Chest X–ray: this may be helpful in identifying the presence or absence of radiopaque substances such as iron.
- Store plasma and urine for future analysis if necessary.

4. General principles of management
- Contact the local Poison Control Center or consult Poison Manual prior to initiating therapy.
- Gastric emptying procedures:
    Emesis:
    Recent studies are challenging the use of syrup of ipecac, both in the home and in the hospital setting. Although it does not appear to be as helpful as once thought, if the

ingestion has occurred within the hour, then it should be considered an option.
Dosage: 9–12 months, 10 mL; 1–2 years, 15 mL; > 12 years, 30 mL.
It should be given with 5 mL/kg fluid (usually juice) to a maximum of 300 mL.
Contraindications: decreased level of consciousness, caustic ingestion, hydrocarbon ingestion, seizures, recent hematemesis.
Lavage:
Recent research also questions the efficacy of gastric lavage.
If the patient presents within 1 hour of the ingestion (especially if massive amounts were taken and if the substance is known to be difficult or impossible to absorb), then lavage should be considered.

- Decreasing gut absorption:
  Adsorption of poison: activated charcoal 1 g/kg to a maximum of 50 g with sorbitol or dextrose may be given either orally or by nasogastric tube. It should not be given within 30 minutes of the syrup of ipecac as it will adsorb the emetic as well.
  Cathartics: sorbitol is generally recommended with the initial dose of activated charcoal, however, subsequent doses of charcoal should be given without sorbitol. Children may be particularly prone to diarrhea, possible electrolyte abnormalities and dehydration which may result from overly aggressive cathartic treatment.
  Whole bowel irrigation: this has been recently advocated as a useful decontamination procedure, especially in cases of substances that are not readily adsorbed. PEG solution 500 mL/h in toddlers and 1 L/h in adolescents; continue for approximately 3–4 hours or until the rectal effluent is the same as the influent.
  Enhancing elimination: dialysis or forced diuresis has limited but important roles in the management of poisoning patients. ICU support will be required.
- Antidotes (only a few poisons have specific antidotes):
  Acetaminophen: n–acetylcysteine.
  Anticoagulants: vitamin K.
  Benzodiazepines: flumazenil.
  Cholinergic syndrome (organophosphates): atropine.
  Cyanide: amyl nitrite or sodium thiosulphate.
  Digoxin: digibind.
  Iron: desferoxamine.
  Lead: EDTA.
  Methemoglobinemia: methylene blue.
  Methanol or ethylene glycol: ethanol.
  Narcotics: naloxone.
  Organophosphates: pralidoxine HCl.
  Phenothiazines: diphenhydramine.
  Details of use and dosage should be checked in specific formulary and references.

BURNS

Major and moderate burns

1. First 30 minutes
Immediate stabilization includes ABC's with particular attention to the airway and fluid status as

both may deteriorate suddenly.
- Airway/breathing:
    The best management is prevention, therefore, airway obstruction from inflammation should be anticipated early and intubation should be considered.
    Check for singed facial or nasal hair, hoarseness, stridor, wheezing or cough with carbonaceous sputum.
    Remember the patient who is already stridulous is not a candidate for paralysis and rapid sequence intubation. Gas induction by an experienced physician is the method of choice.
    Give humidified O_2 5–10 L/min as needed.
- Circulation:
    Insertion of two large bore i.v.'s with Ringer's lactate or normal saline bolus 10 mL/kg. The burn surface area should be calculated accurately and will determine fluid resuscitation.
    Parkland: 4 mL/kg × % burn over first 24 h.
    B. C.'s Children's Hospital: maintenance + (0.1 mL/kg per h × % burn) over first 24 h.
    A Foley catheter should be inserted. Ensure close monitoring of heart rate, blood pressure and urine output. See chapter 24 (Appendix) for chart to estimate burn surface area.

2. Secondary survey
- Careful inspection for further trauma as these patients will often have occult injuries sustained while trying to flee a burning building (i.e. falls).
- Insert nasogastric tube as these patients are likely to develop gastric dilatation.
- Cover the burn with a dry sterile dressing.
- Investigations may include:
    CBC, electrolytes, BUN, creatinine, glucose, cross–match, arterial blood gases.
    Urinalysis including myoglobin.
    Radiography if indicated.
- Subsequent management:
    Pain: morphine 0.1 mg/kg slow i.v. push followed by an infusion.
    Infection: tetanus prophylaxis.
    Routine use of systemic antibiotics is not indicated.
    Burn: use sterile technique to remove all burned clothing and foreign bodies. Debride dead epidermis and blisters which are opened. Wash the burn gently using antiseptic solution and cover with sterile dressing. Chemical burns should be flushed for a prolonged period of time (up to 2 hours with warm tap water). Tar may be removed with mineral oil.
    Eyes: irrigate any foreign body from the eyes and, if corneal abrasions or burns are suspected, apply antibiotic ointment and a patch. Ophthalmology consult.
    Plastic Surgery consultation.
- Admission criteria:
    Second degree burn > 25% BSA.
    Third degree burn > 5% BSA.
    Burns to hands, face, feet, perineum.
    Circumferential burns to limbs.
    Severe chemical burns requiring irrigation.
    Electrical burn.
    Poor social situation.
    Inhalational injury.

Minor burns

1. Minor first degree burns
Generally, a soothing moisturizing cream is all that is necessary.

2. Second and small third degree burns
- May require gentle cleansing and debridement with sterile saline solution. Leave intact blisters or those with only small puncture alone.
- Apply 1% silver sulfadiazine cream (flamazine). Dress with sterile mesh gauze and kling.
- Tetanus prophylaxis.

3. Special management
- Face and neck: burns may be treated with topical neosporin or polysporin ointment and dressings may be left off as they are difficult to anchor and quickly become macerated.
- Burned lips may be treated with a thin film of petrolatum.
- Ears are best protected from excessive pressure by topical flamazine and a fluff type occlusive head dressing.
- Eyes should be examined under fluorescein staining and, if corneal burns are present, should be treated with a broad spectrum topical antibiotic and patching. Ophthalmology should be consulted.
- Hands should be elevated for the first 48–72 hours to minimize swelling and a bulky, mitt–type dressing should be applied with the hand in the position of function.
- Lower extremities should be elevated for the first 48–72 hours or until any major swelling subsides. Thereafter, a loosely wrapped elastic bandage is best applied atop the sterile wound dressing.
- Follow–up care should be arranged and clearly explained to the parents. Many children may require daily dressing changes for the first few days.

CORTICOSTEROIDS

The major actions of corticosteroids are:
* Glucocorticoid action:
  Gluconeogenesis, immunosuppression, protein catabolism, membrane stabilization, fat redistribution, anti–inflammatory action, growth suppression and ACTH suppression.
* Mineralocorticoid action:
  Sodium and chloride retention, potassium excretion. Synthetic steroids were developed to modify the ratio of glucocorticoid to mineralocorticoid potency and allow for specific treatment with reduction in side effects.
* Cortisol secretory rate:
  Recent data suggest a lower basal cortisol secretory rate than previously reported. Basal rate is near 8–10 mg/m² per d rather than 10–15 mg/m² per d. Under stress, secretion may rise to 10 times basal secretory rate. Corticosteroid dosage in excess of basal secretory rate is suppressive.
* Mineralocorticoid requirements:
  The daily replacement requirements are reasonably constant and do not change so much with age as with salt intake and renal function. In infants with limited salt intake, salt supplementation is required. Usual dose: 0.05–0.2 mg/d fludrocortisone (florinef).

Table I lists biological half–life after i.v. or p.o. administration as short S (8–12 hours), intermediate I (12–36 hours), and L (36–72 hours). Many of the effects of corticosteroids continue after they have disappeared from the circulation as they function intracellularly.

Table I: Half–life and relative potency of commonly used steroids

Steroid potency	Glucocorticoid potency	Mineralocorticoid potency	Biological half–life
Betamethasone	25	Nil	L
Dexamethasone	40–80	Nil	L
Cortisol	1	1	S
Cortisone	0.8	0.8	S
Fludrocortisone	15	200	I
Prednisone	4	0.5	I
Prednisolone	4	0.5	I
Methyl prednisone	5	Nil	I
Triamcinolone	5	Nil	I

Steroid therapy and withdrawal

Steroid therapy must be tailored to the individual patient and the disease treated. In general, steroids with a high glucocorticoid to mineralocorticoid ratio and limited half–life should be used. Usually treatment is with prednisone because of its characteristics and relatively low price. Dexamethasone is usually avoided because, although it has a very favorable glucocorticoid to mineralocorticoid ratio, its half–life is very long and leads to marked suppression of growth. If possible, alternate day therapy should be used as this minimizes growth retardation.

In planning a schedule of steroid withdrawal, the two concerns are disease reactivation and symptoms related to steroid withdrawal and adrenal insufficiency. Steroid withdrawal symptoms consist of headache, lethargy, malaise and musculoskeletal symptoms similar to flu–like illnesses. When steroid dosage is below the basal secretory rate, signs of hypoadrenalism may develop. These may occur even at supraphysiological levels if the patient is under physical stress.

Steroids should be tapered slowly once the replacement dose is near the basal secretory rate. Adrenal suppression is likely to occur after someone has been on suppressive doses of steroids for more than 1 week or has had repeated shorter courses of steroids. Though the patient is able to maintain basal steroid production after steroid withdrawal, there may be a reduced ability to mount a stress response for as long as 1–2 years. This should be kept in mind for a patient under severe physical stress. When in doubt, patients should receive supplemental hydrocortisone until the physical stress has resolved.

DIABETES MELLITUS

The management of diabetic ketoacidosis is covered under chapter 3 (Emergencies).

1. Insulin choice
There are over 30 types of insulin produced in four general classes:
- Purified single peak mixtures:
    Mixtures of beef and pork insulin with most of the impurities (glucagon, enzymes, protein, VIP, proinsulin, etc.) removed. Concentration of proinsulin is used as a measure of purity and is usually 5–10 ppm. Older mixtures contained about 3,000 ppm and were associated with high rates of allergic reactions, insulin resistance and lipoatrophy.
- Monocomponent pork:
    Pure solution of pork insulin containing < 1 ppm of proinsulin. It varies by one amino acid from human insulin (beef varies by three).
- Semisynthetic human:
    Made from pork insulin by chemically altering its amino acid sequence to make it identical to human insulin. It contains < 1 ppm of proinsulin.
- Biosynthetic human:
    Recombinant DNA technology enables pure human insulin to be made by E. coli. It contains no proinsulin but is contaminated by very small amounts of E. coli proteins.

2. Insulin dose
- The starting dose is about 0.25 unit/kg per d of intermediate with a smaller dose of regular. The final dose necessary after the remission period is about 0.75–1 unit/kg per d.
- The usual ratio is two–thirds intermediate to one–third regular.

- Most children are managed on two divided doses a day; two–thirds of the dose is given in the morning and one–third at night.

SHORT STATURE

Short stature is a frequent presenting complaint. The key issue is to determine whether the child is showing a normal rate of growth; this requires careful serial measurements. Good health and nutrition are requirements for normal growth so any disorder affecting health or nutrition may alter the growth rate.

Children > 3 years of age can be measured standing if they can maintain a straight posture. Younger children should be measured supine. Accurate measurements are best done utilizing a stadiometer. A child's height should not be measured with marks on the child's bedsheet. Growth charts for both height and weight are given in chapter 24 (Appendix). Growth data should be plotted for age rounding off to the nearest month. Growth velocities should be measured at the midpoint of the time interval between the two measurement points.

Abnormalities influencing growth

- Genetic: familial short stature.
- Constitutional delay in growth: familial, sporadic, associated with delayed puberty.
- Chronic diseases: renal insufficiency, renal tubular acidosis, heart failure, malnutrition, gastrointestinal diseases, juvenile rheumatoid arthritis, miscellaneous diseases significantly affecting health, bone dysplasia (abnormal body proportions).
- Prenatal factors: maternal size, health, nutrition; drugs, alcohol, smoking; intrauterine growth retardation.
- Hormonal causes: hypothyroidism (slowing growth rate may be only sign), corticosteroid excess (exogenous and endogenous), growth hormone deficiency.
- Chromosomal abnormalities: Turner's syndrome, Down's syndrome, miscellaneous.

Clinical and laboratory evaluation

- Past growth data and pertinent personal, prenatal and family history.
- Accurate measurements.
- Body proportions.
- Evaluation of general health and nutritional status.
- Laboratory screening (be selective).
- Workup (guided by the history and physical examination): CBC and ESR, creatinine, urinalysis, nutritional assessment, malabsorption assessment, chromosomal analysis, assessment of thyroid function with both a measure of thyroid hormone and thyroid stimulating hormone (TSH), IGF1 (somatomedin) level.

Growth hormone testing

Because of the complexities in interpreting growth hormone levels, these should be performed only after discussion with an endocrinologist to determine which tests should be used. Growth hormone levels are often low on random sampling and provocative tests are necessary to rule out deficiency.

In general, two pharmacological and one physiological test are performed. Pharmacological tests are usually arginine and either clonidine or propranolol levodopa stimulation.

The physiological tests are either measuring growth hormone after 20 minutes of strenuous exercise or after patients have fallen asleep. Normal growth hormone responses are > 8 ng/mL. Interpretations of test results should be discussed with an endocrinologist as low levels do not always imply deficiency or need for treatment.

After a careful history, physical examination and assessment of bone age, patients will usually fall into three categories (Table II):

Table II: Clinical categories of children with short stature

Growth rate	Height	Bone age	Etiology
Normal	< 5 percentile	Usually within normal limits for chronological age	• Familial short stature, various causes of intrauterine growth retardation • Adult height is below average
Normal	< 5 percentile	Delayed in relation to chronological age but is similar to the degree of retardation in height	• Usually constitutional delay in growth • May be associated with delayed puberty • Adult height is usually within normal limits for the family but some patients do not achieve their predicted height
Slow	Dropping percentiles	Retarded; usually more than 2 standard deviations	• Multifactorial; may be endocrine or related to disease • Requires urgent further investigation

OBESITY

Definitions vary. A child who is more than 20% above the expected weight for height is considered obese medically. There are social and cosmetic concerns about the degree of body fat which lie outside this definition. A more accurate assessment of total body fat involves measuring skin–fold thickness. Normal values are included in chapter 24 (Appendix). Obesity is always caused by excessive caloric intake relative to expenditure. In most children, obesity is caused by an increased intake of calories rather than hormonal abnormalities. Extra nutrition usually stimulates growth and an overweight child with a slow rate of growth should always raise concern. Endocrine causes of obesity, such as hypothyroidism or steroid excess, are always characterized by slow growth rates.

The search for a metabolic defect in patients with obesity continues. Various theories, such as critical mass of adipose cells or different levels of basal energy requirements, remain to be proven. There does appear to be a familial tendency towards obesity but some of this may be caused by environmental factors. There is limited correlation between obesity in the first 2 years of life and adult obesity. Because of this, caloric restriction diets in this age should be approached with caution. The first 2 years of life are a period of rapid physical growth and maturation of the nervous system. Caloric restriction may lead to restriction of essential nutrients as well. The correlation between childhood and adolescent obesity and adult obesity is much greater. Approximately 85% of overweight adolescents will continue to adult obesity.

Evaluation

Assessment must include a detailed nutritional history. There should be a review of past growth data and family patterns of growth. The child's developmental history and exercise level should be reviewed. Assessment should include accurate measurements of height, weight and blood pressure. A careful history and physical examination will, in most cases, exclude organic causes of obesity. Endocrine workup should be reserved for patients showing growth retardation or other suspicious clinical signs. Marked obesity may cause disturbances in body homeostasis and this should be assessed. Testing should include a fasting blood sugar, insulin level, hemoglobin A_1C and lipid profile.

Treatment

Caloric restriction must be carefully supervised so that normal growth takes place. Caloric intake should be set at a level so that weight loss is no more than 1 kg/wk. The diet should be reviewed with a nutritionist to be certain that there is adequate provision for essential vitamins, minerals and protein. It may be necessary to supplement with a children's vitamin and iron preparation.

Behavior modification and an exercise program are necessary for successful weight loss. An ongoing relationship with one individual, usually outside the family, should be established; this individual will monitor the weight loss program. The child should be encouraged and praised for efforts at weight loss. Negative reinforcement is counterproductive and usually leads to stress within the family.

HYPOTHYROIDISM

Congenital hypothyroidism occurs in approximately 1:3,500–4,000 births. The provincial screening program takes blood on day 3 of life and measures TSH levels. This will detect disturbances in thyroid function but will not detect hypothalamic or pituitary causes of hypothyroidism. These are much rarer and unlikely to cause cretinism. They are associated with other signs of hypopituitarism. Hypothyroidism can occur at any age and should always be considered in children showing a slow growth rate, as this is usually the first manifestation of the condition. With early discharge and home births, it is essential to ensure that all newborns are appropriately screened.

Causes of hypothyroidism

- Anatomical: hypoplastic, ectopic or absent thyroid gland.
- Metabolic: inborn errors of thyroid hormone metabolism. These are inherited in an autosomal recessive pattern and are associated with goiters.
- Drugs: iodides, propylthiouracil, lithium. Certain foods are goitrogens. Excessive intake of cabbages or soya bean products may lead to goiter formation.
- Iatrogenic: surgical removal of the thyroid gland or radiation damage.
- Autoimmune thyroiditis: is more common in children with diabetes, Down's syndrome and Turner's syndrome. Patients with these conditions should be monitored regularly for thyroid dysfunction. There is often a strong family history of autoimmune thyroiditis, and children in

these families should also be regularly monitored.
- Secondary: pituitary or hypothalamic dysfunction.
- Intrauterine: maternal radioactive iodine or antithyroid medication.
- Miscellaneous: cystinosis, iodine deficiency.

Evaluation

The clinical picture may be subtle even in severe cases and patients may only manifest slow growth. The younger child with hypothyroidism will show delayed development and marked growth retardation.

Typical features

- Infant: cold, sluggish, large fontanelle, large tongue, coarse features, umbilical hernia, prolonged jaundice, poor suck, constipation, apneic spells, bradycardia, anemia.
- Child: growth retardation, constipation, anemia, dry skin, goiter.

Investigation

- Laboratory diagnosis is not difficult. TSH and either total or free thyroxine levels are usually sufficient. Thyroid microsomal antibody levels are usually positive in children with thyroiditis.
- Treatment is designed to normalize T_4 and TSH. Younger children require higher dosage per kilogram body weight. Full–term newborns are begun on 25–50 µg/d with regular monitoring of blood levels. Missed doses of medication should be given the following day. Up to 1 week's medication can be given on 1 day. Patients should be encouraged to use a weekly pill reminder system.

THYROID ENLARGEMENT

Smooth and symmetrical thyroid enlargement without particular hardness or nodularity may occur in a variety of conditions. Thyroid enlargement occurs in hypothyroidism. Thyroid enlargement may be sufficient to allow for compensation and maintenance of normal circulating thyroid hormone levels, or patients may have clinical hypothyroidism. Thyroid gland enlargement may also occur autonomously in hyperthyroidism.

In assessing the patient with thyroid enlargement, it is important to determine clinical status, that is euthyroid, hypothyroid or hyperthyroid. Initial laboratory tests should include a T_4 or free T_4, TSH and thyroid antibodies. Patients with normal T_4 and TSH may have compensated hypothyroidism. This can best be determined by testing TSH reserve with TRH stimulation. Suppressive therapy with thyroxine will usually lead to resolution of the goiter. Usual treatment doses in children are in the range of 2–3 µg/kg per d of thyroxine. Treatment should be monitored for the growth years with regular monitoring of T_4 and TSH levels. Depending on the etiology, it may be possible to discontinue therapy when the child's growth is completed. Causes of goiter may be familial and parents and siblings of the patient should be screened.

Unilateral thyroid enlargement or presence of a firm thyroid nodule raises concerns of malignancy. Nodularity will also occur in patients with benign thyroid tumors and in the occasional patient with thyroiditis. Because of the high incidence of malignancy in pediatric thyroid nodules, such patients should always be referred to specialists for further management. The initial approach may often include surgical removal of the nodule or lobe for a positive tissue diagnosis. Needle biopsies are not recommended as they may miss a focus of malignancy in a nodule. Occasionally, a child may be put on suppressive thyroxine therapy for several months to see if the nodule shrinks. Such patients must be followed closely to be certain that this indeed occurs; otherwise surgical removal is indicated. Children who have been exposed to radiation have an increased risk of thyroid nodularity and malignancy. Their thyroid glands should be carefully palpated on a yearly basis to be certain that no nodules have developed. If there is evidence of thyroid dysfunction on laboratory testing, thyroxine therapy should be implemented.

HYPERTHYROIDISM

Hyperthyroidism primarily affects children > 6 years of age. It can be seen in younger children and in the newborn period in infants of mothers with Graves' disease. Etiology includes Graves' disease and autoimmune thyroiditis and, in the newborn, transplacental passage of thyroid stimulating immunoglobulins. In children, presentation of hyperthyroidism is usually gradual. There may be a deterioration in school performance and handwriting, and patients often feel jumpy and nervous. As with adults, the disease is significantly more common in females than males, and there may be an increased family incidence.

On examination, patients will have tachycardia, widened pulse pressure and an enlarged thyroid gland. Testing for levels of T_4 or free T_4 will usually establish the diagnosis. TSH levels in hyperthyroidism are always fully suppressed. Thyroid ophthalmopathy is less common in children than in adults. There may be globe enlargement and some lid retraction but usually marked exophthalmos does not occur. The eyes should be examined carefully for signs of irritation and patients with eye findings of significance should always be referred to specialists for management. Most patients are managed initially on antithyroid medication (e.g. propylthiouracil) and in those with marked cardiac findings propranolol is given.

Approximately 50% of children with Graves' disease can be weaned off treatment after 2 years, and approximately 75% of all patients can be weaned off therapy after 3–4 years of treatment. Patients need to be monitored during therapy to be certain that their goiter is reducing and that they remain euthyroid.

Hypothyroidism can occur with overtreatment and hyperthyroidism may recur if compliance with therapy is poor. Suggested initial dosage for propylthiouracil is 5–10 mg/kg per d in 3 divided doses.

AMBIGUOUS GENITALIA

Male sexual differentiation initiated by the Y chromosome results in the transformation of the undifferentiated gonads into testes. The testes secrete testosterone from the Leydig cells which supports development of the internal male duct structures and masculinization of the external genitalia. The sertoli cells secrete Müllerian duct inhibitory factor, bringing about regression of Müllerian duct derivatives. In the absence of secretion of these testicular substances, female sexual differentiation occurs.

Exposure of the female fetus to androgens in utero from either maternal or fetal sources will result in virilization of the external genitalia. The internal reproductive structures remain female. The most common cause of virilization of the female fetus is congenital adrenal hyperplasia, and this condition should always be thought of in examining the child with ambiguous genitalia. Abnormalities in male sexual development may occur because of errors in one of the several steps involved in normal male development.

Causes of ambiguous genitalia in the male

- Genetic: mixed gonadal dysgenesis XO/XY, deletions of portions of the Y chromosome, true XX/XY mosaicism.
- Testicular agenesis: XY gonadal dysgenesis and agenesis (Swyer's syndrome) and anorchia (testicular regression syndrome).
- Defects in testosterone biosynthesis: defects in testosterone production leads to lack of virilization of the external genitalia. Some of these disorders will also have defects in cortisol synthesis and result in congenital adrenal hyperplasia. The testes continue to make Müllerian duct inhibitory factor and the internal structures are masculine. Absence of Müllerian duct inhibitory factor results in normal male genitalia but persistence of the uterus.
- Defects in androgen action: partial and complete androgen insensitivity results in patients who are phenotypically female but whose internal structures are male. Five–α reductase deficiency, in which testosterone cannot be converted to its active metabolite dihydrotestosterone, results in incomplete virilization in the newborn patients with full virilization at puberty.
- Miscellaneous: maternal exposure to synthetic sex steroids. Hypospadias and genital anomalies associated with urological and GI developmental anomalies; hypopituitarism with cryptorchidism and micropenis.

Evaluation

- Assessment in the newborn period is urgent.
- Always consider congenital adrenal hyperplasia, which requires urgent therapy.
- History should review maternal drug ingestion, family history of ambiguous genitalia, family history of infertility and unexplained fetal loss.
- Status of the genital structures and gonads should be determined. When gonads are palpable in the inguinal canal, they are almost always testes. The uterus may be palpated rectally or the presence of the uterus may be detected on pelvic ultrasound.
- Many referral centers have a gender assessment team, consisting of specialists in the fields related to sex determination. These include geneticists, endocrinologists, cytogeneticists and urologists. Because of the complexities and urgency in determining sex in the newborn period, patient referral to the team should be made as soon as abnormalities are noted.

Investigations

- Chromosomal studies to determine genetic sex.
- Pelvic ultrasound to determine internal structures.
- Measure of 17–hydroxyprogesterone level to determine the possibility of congenital adrenal hyperplasia (Table III). Urine and serum electrolytes should also be checked for salt loss.

There are milder forms of congenital adrenal hyperplasia which may present in childhood with mild virilization or premature pubic and axillary hair development.

Seventeen–hydroxyprogesterone levels are very high on day 1 of life. Testing on day 2 of life will show levels > 150 nmol/L in children with congenital adrenal hyperplasia. The occasional child with the disease may have levels somewhat lower than this and should be retested if the clinical situation is unclear. Normal levels of 17–hydroxyprogesterone after the first month of life are < 3 nmol/L.

Treatment for children with congenital adrenal hyperplasia is with hydrocortisone. Florinef and salt supplementation is needed for patients with salt loss. Hydrocortisone dosage must be significantly increased for illness, and physical stress and maintenance dosages must be adjusted as the child grows.

Table III: Clinical forms of congenital adrenal hyperplasia

Enzyme	Salt loss	Hypertension	Phenotype	Elevated steroid
21–hydroxylase	> 50%	No	Females virilized	17–hydroxyprogesterone
11–hydroxylase	No*	Yes	Females virilized	17–hydroxyprogesterone, 11–desoxycortisol
3–beta HSD	Yes	No	Ambiguous	17–hydroxyprogesterone, DHEAS
20–22 desmolase	Yes	No	Female	Cholesterol
17–hydroxylase	No	Yes	Female	Progesterone

May become a salt loser with treatment.
Approximately 90% of the patients with congenital adrenal hyperplasia have 21–hydroxylase deficiency.

PUBERTY

Clinical changes

The clinical stages of puberty are usually defined by Tanner's sexual maturation rating (Tables IV and V).

Table IV: Tanner's sexual maturation scale for boys

Stage	Pubic hair	Penis	Testes
1	None	Pre–adolescent	< 2.5 cm
2	Scanty, long, slightly pigmented	Slightly enlarged	Scrotum enlarged; skin pink and thinner; 2.5–3.2 cm
3	Darker, starts to curl	Longer	Larger; 3.3–4.0 cm
4	Coarse, curly, less than adult quantity	Length and breadth increased	Larger, scrotum darker; 4.0–4.5 cm
5	Adult distribution	Adult size	Adult size; > 4.5 cm

Table V: Tanner's sexual maturation scale for girls

Stage	Pubic hair	Breasts
1	Pre–adolescent	Pre–adolescent
2	Medial border of labia, sparse, light colored	Breast and papilla elevated; areolar diameter increased
3	Darker, beginning to curl	Breast and areola enlarged; no separation
4	Coarse and curly; less than adult amount	Areola and papilla form a second mound
5	Adult distribution	Adult form; nipple projects

Timing of pubertal events

Puberty begins about 6 months earlier in girls than in boys. The first signs of puberty are more noticeable in girls (breast development) than in boys (testicular enlargement). Girls have their growth spurt earlier in puberty than boys, and this increases the discrepancy between male and female puberty. Timing of puberty is often affected by familial patterns; early development is more common in girls while delayed development is more often seen in boys. The average onset of major pubertal events is given in Table VI. Normal values for testosterone and estradiol are given in Table VII and for luteinizing hormone (LH) and follicle stimulating hormones (FSH) in Table VIII.

Table VI: Average onset of major pubertal developments

Tanner stage	Female Mean	Female Range (yr)	Male Mean	Male Range (yr)
Breast (2)	11	8–13	–	–
Breast (5)	15	12–18	–	–
Testes (2)	–	–	11.5	9.5–13.5
Testes (5)	–	–	15	13.5–18
Pubic hair (2)	11.5	8–13	12	10–14
Pubic hair (5)	14	12–16	15	14–18
Peak height (3,4) velocity	12	9.5–14.5	14	10.5–16
Menarche (4)	13	10.5–15.5	–	–

Table VII: Normal values for testosterone and estradiol

	Testosterone (nmol/L)		Estradiol (pmol/L)	
Age	Female	Male	Female	Male
< 6 mo	< 0.6	< 0.6–10	< 40	< 40
6 mo to onset of puberty	< 0.6	< 0.6	< 40	< 40
Adult	0.7–2.8	13.9–41.6	110–1,650	55–165

Table VIII: Normal values for LH and FSH

	FSH (µIU/mL)			LH (µIU/mL)		
Age	Female		Male	Female		Male
0–1 yr	2–6		0.5–3	0.3		0.3
1 yr to onset of puberty	1–3		< 2	< 2		< 2
Adult	3–12	Follicular phase	1–14	2–14	Follicular phase	2–9
	8–22	Midcycle peak		16–80	Midcycle peak	
	2–12	Luteal phase		1–20	Luteal phase	
	> 35	Agonadal		> 20	Agonadal	

Normal variants

1. Premature thelarche

Precocious development of one or both breasts in a female infant without other signs of sexual development. Thelarche usually appears in the first 2 years of life and is transient. It is likely caused by transient hormone production from the ovaries stimulated by the pituitary. When assessed, LH and FSH are usually normal and estradiol may be slightly raised. Bone age is normal or mildly advanced. The condition is usually benign and self–limited, but the children need close follow–up to be certain they do not have true premature puberty.

2. Premature adrenarche

Precocious development of pubic and axillary hair or adult sweat characteristics without any other signs of sexual development. Girls are more commonly affected than boys and are often tall with slightly advanced bone age. The condition occurs commonly in children with cerebral damage. Gonadotropins are normal but the adrenal androgens DHEAS and androstenedione are slightly increased. Seventeen–hydroxyprogesterone and testosterone levels should also be assessed to rule out congenital adrenal hyperplasia or adrenal tumor.

3. Gynecomastia

Development of breast tissue in a male. This occurs commonly in about two–thirds of pubescent boys and is also seen in males in the newborn period, secondary to exposure to maternal hormones. Gynecomastia in adolescents usually regresses in 1–2 years, and levels of sex hormones and gonadotropins are normal for age. Testicular damage may result in increased production of estrogen in some patients and lead to gynecomastia. Clinical conditions with gynecomastia include Klinefelter's syndrome, hormonally active tumors in either the adrenal or testes, or underlying testicular damage with abnormal production of estrogen. Exposure to exogenous estrogen may also result in gynecomastia. The larger the breast size the less likely that full regression will take place. Plastic surgery should be considered as significant degrees of gynecomastia can cause significant emotional distress. Surgery should be offered early in the course, especially if the breasts are large and unlikely to regress.

PRECOCIOUS SEXUAL DEVELOPMENT

True precocious puberty

Defined as true puberty occurring before the age of 8 years in females and 9 years in males. True precocious puberty implies that there has been maturation of the hypothalamus and pituitary to produce pubertal levels of the gonadotropins, which stimulates the gonads. It is due to an identifiable lesion in about 10–20% in girls and 50–80% in boys.

Causes:
- Idiopathic: commoner in girls than boys, familial in some cases.
- CNS lesions: hydrocephalus, encephalitis, tumor, trauma, radiation.
- Skin and CNS: McCune–Albright's disease (pigmentation, precocity and fibrous dysplasia), tuberous sclerosis, neurofibromatosis.
- Others: prolonged hypothyroidism.

Pseudoprecocious puberty

This is the development of secondary sexual characteristics due to abnormal production or exposure of the child to sex hormones. Gonadotropin levels are low and the gonads are usually prepubertal in size. (If one testis is enlarged, suspect a tumor.) The precocious development may be isosexual or heterosexual. Congenital adrenal hyperplasia must always be ruled out.

1. Causes
- Masculinization: tumors of adrenal or testis, exposure to androgens, congenital adrenal hyperplasia.
- Feminization: tumors of ovary or adrenal, exposure to estrogens.

2. Evaluation
- Assess past growth data for determination of growth rate to see if it is in the pubertal range. Investigate family history and past medical history for possible causes of premature puberty. Neuroendocrine review of vision, headaches, seizures, polydipsia and polyuria. Review of exposure to sex steroids.
- Physical examination with accurate anthropometric measurements and Tanner's pubertal staging.
- Detailed CNS examination, including visual fields and fundoscopy. Palpation of the abdomen for masses and examination of the skin for café au lait spots and depigmented lesions.

3. Investigation
- FSH, LH, testosterone, estradiol.
- 17–hydroxyprogesterone, DHEAS.
- Abdominal ultrasound for assessment of uterus, ovaries and adrenal glands.
- Luteinizing hormone releasing factor study to determine if there has been maturation of the hypothalamus and pituitary into puberty.
- CT scan or MRI of the CNS if true precocious puberty has been diagnosed.
- Bone age.

4. Treatment
Treatment of the condition is determined by the underlying cause. For idiopathic premature puberty, treatment should be considered for younger children with advanced bone age, whose final adult height may be affected and who may have emotional and social problems because of premature sexual development. Preferred treatment is with analogues of luteinizing hormone releasing factor that can suppress gonadotropin production. Treatment is usually continued until pubertal development is appropriate for age. Early initiation of treatment will help preserve adult height potential.

DELAYED PUBERTY

Puberty is considered delayed if secondary sexual characteristics have not developed by 13 years of age in a girl or 14 years of age in a boy.

Causes

- Constitutional: commonest cause, often familial; more common in males.
- Systemic: any chronic disease or malnutrition (anorexia nervosa, cystic fibrosis, renal, etc.).
- Central (hypogonadotropic):
  Pituitary or hypothalamic damage (trauma, meningitis, radiation, tumor).
  Idiopathic isolated gonadotropin deficiency, Laurence–Moon–Biedl's syndrome, Prader Willi's syndrome, Kallmann's syndrome (hyposmia and gonadotropin deficiency).
- Gonadal (hypergonadotropic):
  Gonadal dysgenesis (male or female).
  Anorchia or removal of gonads.
  Damage to gonads (tumor, chemotherapy, trauma, radiation or surgery).

Evaluation

- Enquire about family history, particularly onset of puberty, as delayed puberty is commonly a familial problem. Timing of growth spurt in parents, aunts and uncles as well as age of menarche should be reviewed. As with premature puberty, growth parameters and Tanner's staging should be performed.
- Usual investigations include: LH, FSH, testosterone and estradiol, bone age. Further tests may include CT or MRI head scan and luteinizing hormone releasing factor study to assess gonadotropin status.

HYPOGLYCEMIA

Definitions of hypoglycemia (Table IX) vary, particularly for neonates, but values quoted in Nelson's are representative. This is only a guide and some children may be symptomatic above these levels.

Hypoglycemia is a common complication of many disease states, especially among neonates. It is also a marker of a wide range of metabolic diseases.

Table IX: Definition of hypoglycemia at different ages

Age	Serum (laboratory)	Whole blood (dextrostix)
Children	< 2.5 mmol/L	< 2.2 mmol/L
Full–term	< 2.0 mmol/L	< 1.7 mmol/L
Preterm	< 1.4 mmol/L	< 1.2 mmol/L

Causes

- Neonatal: IUGR, preterm, stress (sepsis, hypoxia, RDS, hypothermia).
- Endocrine: hypopituitary, growth hormone deficiency, hypoadrenalism, ACTH deficiency, congenital adrenal hyperplasia.
- Hyperinsulinism: beta cell tumor, Beckwith's syndrome, IDM, erythroblastosis, nesidioblastosis, insulin overdose.
- Drugs: ethyl alcohol, salicylates, propranolol, sulfonylurea.
- Decreased intake: malabsorption, malnutrition, ketotic hypoglycemia (children 1–5 years of age, often small for age; ketosis and hypoglycemia with fasting or illness).
- Hepatic: severe liver damage such as hepatitis, Reye's syndrome.
- Metabolic: fructose intolerance, galactosemia, branched chain amino acid abnormalities, glycogen storage diseases.

Evaluation

- Ask about presence of pallor, sweating, dizziness, tremor, drowsiness, confusion and seizures. Determine age of onset and frequency of attacks and also whether attacks occur during fasting or nonfasting state. Are symptoms associated with specific foods? Ask about family history.
- The examination will often be normal. If there is a history of significant hypoglycemia, perform a careful neurological exam as a baseline. Some clinical findings may suggest specific disease: micropenis or optic nerve hypoplasia (panhypopituitarism), ambiguous genitalia (congenital adrenal hyperplasia), cataracts (galactosemia), hepatomegaly (glycogen storage disease).

Investigation

There is no routine workup of hypoglycemia. The following tests are available but the choice depends on a careful history and physical examination.

The commonest presentations are: fasting attacks (most common is ketotic hypoglycemia), nonfasting attacks (hyperinsulinism), and hepatomegaly plus hypoglycemia (storage disorder).

- If an undiagnosed child has a hypoglycemic attack, take a heparinized tube of blood and send it for glucose, insulin, growth hormone and cortisol. Also send a urine sample for ketones. Normal, as opposed to low, insulin levels in the face of hypoglycemia is very suggestive of hyperinsulinism. Growth hormone and cortisol should both be high in the face of hypoglycemic stress.
- Fasting 12–24 hours: normal tables exist for the decrease of blood sugar with time during a controlled fast. A child with ketotic hypoglycemia will show an exaggerated fall.
- Glucagon test: a subcutaneous dose of 0.03 mg/kg fails to produce a rise in blood sugar in most cases of glycogen storage disease.
- Other tests: screening for galactosemia and fructose intolerance, toxic screens, liver function tests and serum NH_3 (Reye's syndrome), endocrine testing, serum amino acids and organic acids.

Treatment

See chapter 3 (Emergencies).

CUSHING'S SYNDROME

Cushing's syndrome is a rare disease in children and presents with marked slowing in growth rate and rapid weight gain. In children < 3 years of age, it is often caused by adrenal gland tumors. In older children, increased ACTH production leading to bilateral adrenal hyperplasia is more common. The commonest source of the elevated ACTH is a pituitary microadenoma. Clinically, most cases of Cushing's syndrome seen in childhood are caused by exposure to exogenous steroids used in the treatment of disease.

Causes

- Adrenal tumor: functioning carcinoma or adenoma.
- Adrenal hyperplasia: micro– or macroscopic pituitary adenomas (Cushing's disease); also abnormal hypothalamic pituitary adrenal feedback control.
- Ectopic ACTH: very rare in children. Occasionally found in Wilm's tumor, pheochromocytoma, neuroblastoma, leukemia and thymoma.
- Exogenous steroids: either systemic, inhaled or topical; by far the commonest cause.

Evaluation

- Ask about changes in mood, body shape, growth rate, spontaneous fractures, weakness and fatigue and drug exposure. The clinical signs that are commonly seen are facial plethora, pigmented striae and central obesity. The occasional patient will have signs of excess androgens including acne, pubic hair and genital enlargement; this occurs most commonly in patients with adrenal tumors.
- The differential diagnosis between Cushing's syndrome and spontaneous obesity is usually

simple. Obese children continue to grow normally whereas patients with Cushing's syndrome have growth failure.

Investigation

The investigation needs to cover two areas:
- Is there excess cortisol production?
- What is the cause: CNS, adrenal or ectopic ACTH?

1. Demonstrating excess cortisol
- 24 hour urine for free cortisol: very suggestive of Cushing's syndrome if elevated; levels above 250 nmol/d are clearly abnormal.
- Response to dexamethasone suppression: give 30 µg/kg p.o. (maximum 1 mg) at 23:00; 07:00 cortisol should be below 100 nmol/L. Obese children will respond with normal suppression.
- Loss of diurnal variation occurs but is not diagnostic on its own. Cortisol levels in the morning should be > 300 nmol/L at 07:00 and < 200 nmol/L at 23:00.

2. Demonstrating the origin of the excess cortisol
- ACTH levels are of limited use unless they are markedly elevated (normal levels are < 30 pmol/L). In most cases of Cushing's syndrome, ACTH levels are in the normal range and the high cortisol level is caused by lack of fluctuation of ACTH and constant maintenance of slightly elevated levels.
- High dose dexamethasone suppression test: if cortisol suppresses, then the likely diagnosis is pituitary dependent Cushing's disease.
- Further testing with petrosal sinus ACTH levels pre– and postcorticotrophin releasing factor may help localize a pituitary adenoma. Transphenoidal exploration may be appropriate even when there are no localizing findings as there is a high incidence of pituitary microadenoma as the cause of Cushing's syndrome in children.
- Lack of suppression of cortisol on high dose dexamethasone indicates a tumor. If ACTH levels are suppressed, an adrenal tumor should be suspected and CT scan performed. With high ACTH levels, the diagnosis is ectopic ACTH syndrome (this is often caused by carcinoids in children). Urine for 5–hydroxyindoleacetic acid and body MRI scans should be performed.

FLUIDS

Body fluid compartments, renal function and fluid requirements all vary with age. These changes must be appreciated when planning fluid management for a child.

Fluid compartments (Table I)

- Total body water (TBW): 75–80% of newborn's weight. Falls 5–7% in first few days then slowly down to adult levels by about 1 year of age. Adult levels are 60% of total body weight.
- Extracellular fluid (ECF): includes interstitial, transcellular and plasma fluid. 35–45% of newborn's weight falling to 20–25% by 1 year of age.
- Intracellular fluid (ICF): reasonably constant at 40% body weight throughout life.

Table I: Changes in fluid compartments with ages

Age	TBW	ECF	ICF
Newborn	75–80	35–45	35
1 wk	70–75	30–40	40
1 yr	60–65	20–25	40
> 5 yr	60	20	40

All values expressed as % body weight.

Renal function (Table II)

Renal function in infancy is not fully developed and does not reach adult values until 1.5–2.0 years of age. It is important to remember this when ordering fluids or drugs for infants.

Table II: Changes in renal function with age

Age	GFR (mL/min per m²)
Newborn	10–20
1–2 wk	20–35
2–4 mo	35–45
6–12 mo	45–60
1–3 yr	60–75

Fluid requirements

Fluid requirements increase with the patient's age and correlate well with surface area, caloric expenditure and body weight. These variables provide three methods for calculating fluid intake.

1. Surface area
Daily requirements correlate best with surface area (1,500 mL/m^2). The method does not work well for children < 1 year of age and requires a surface area chart.

2. Metabolic requirements
120–150 mL of fluid needed per 100 calories expended. Method requires a chart of caloric requirements against weight (Table III).

Table III: Calculating fluid requirements by surface area or energy consumption

Daily requirements	mL H$_2$O/m^2 per 24 h	mL H$_2$O/100 Cal per 24 h
Respiratory	200	15
Skin	550	40
Stool	100	5
Urine	875	65
Metabolic water	minus 250	minus 10–15

3. Body weight
This is the most widely used method since no tables are required and is easily memorized (Table IV).

Table IV: Calculating fluid requirements by body weight

Body weight	Fluids
0–10 kg	100 mL/kg
10–20 kg	1,000 mL + 50 mL/kg for each kg above 10 kg
> 20 kg	1,500 mL + 20 mL/kg for each kg above 20 kg

UNUSUAL FLUID REQUIREMENTS

Modifications of maintenance fluids may be necessary with general anesthesia, renal disease, central nervous system disease, morphine and other narcotic analgesics, and particularly in the neonatal period.

Neonatal period

Give approximately 70% of maintenance requirements in the first 2 days, increasing gradually to 100% by day 4–5. Low birth weight infants require relatively more water because of relatively greater insensible losses. Table V provides guidelines for fluid requirements in the neonate.

Table V: Neonatal fluid requirements

Birth weight (g)	Days 1–2	Day 3	Days 15–30
Term infant	70	80	90–100
1,751–2,000	80	110	130
1,501–1,750	80	110	130
1,251–1,500	90	120	130
1,001–1,250	100	130	140
751–1,000	105	140	150

All measurements are in mL/kg per d.

Average maintenance fluid requirements in neonates may require modification because of many factors, including radiant heaters, phototherapy, high ambient humidity, gestational age, fever and hypermetabolic state. Controversy exists with respect to fluid requirements in very low birth weight infants (< 1,500 grams) because of possible association of respiratory distress syndrome, patent ductus, bronchopulmonary dysplasia and necrotizing enterocolitis with high intravenous fluid volumes.

Increased requirements

The basic maintenance fluids must be increased in the following cases:
- Fever: increase 10% for each °C above 38 °C.
- Renal losses: diabetes insipidus or recovery phase of tubular necrosis.
- GI losses: nasogastric tube, ileostomy, pancreatic fistula. Replace GI losses volume for volume with a solution containing appropriate electrolytes (Table VI).

Table VI: Electrolyte contents of various GI fluids

GI fluids	H^+	Na	K	Cl	HCO_3
Gastric	80	40	20	150	0
Small bowel	0	130	20	120	30
Pancreatic	0	135	15	100	50
Diarrhea	0	40	40	40	40

All measurements are in mmol/L.

If replacing large losses, measure the electrolyte content of the fluid output for guidance.

Decreased requirements

A few situations require strict fluid restrictions and monitoring:
- Renal failure: severe restriction. In undialyzed patients, give 300 mL/m^2 or about 25 mL/kg.
- SIADH: caused by head injury, meningitis, surgery, etc. Cut back to two–thirds calculated maintenance. Follow serum sodium and clinical condition (may need further restriction). Only restrict water, not electrolytes.

ELECTROLYTES

Electrolyte requirements

Requirements vary with surface area and weight. Standard values are given in Table VII.

Table VII: Electrolyte requirements calculated by surface area and weight

Ion	Surface area mEq/m^2 per 24 h	Weight mEq/kg per 24 h
Na	40–60	2–4
K	20–50	1–3
Cl	60–100	3–5

Usual requirements are met by using the following standard solution:
- Fluid: D10W or D5W.
- Na: 2.5 mEq/100 mL.
- K: 2.0 mEq/100 mL.
- Ca gluconate: 200 mg/100 mL.

D10W is usually used in infancy for a few extra calories. D5W is used in older children since it is less irritating to the veins. Calcium is usually only added to infant solutions. It may cause a severe chemical burn if there is extravasation. High concentrations of calcium or glucose should only be given by central line.

Anion gap

The difference between the major measured plasma cations and anions is called the anion gap (AG):

$$AG = (Na + K) - (Cl + HCO_3)$$

The usual range is 15–20 mEq/L. This represents the difference between the remaining unmeasured cations (calcium, magnesium) and unmeasured anions (protein, organic acids, phosphate, sulfate).

Increased gap

• Endogenous acids: lactate, ketones, PO_4, SO_4, uremia, abnormal organic acids.
• Exogenous acids: salicylate, methanol, ethylene glycol.
• Decreased unmeasured cations: low Ca, low Mg.
• If chloride rises to balance HCO_3 loss, e.g. hyperchloremic acidosis of RTA, the anion gap will be normal. Hypokalemia and hyponatremia are usually balanced by hypochloremia so the anion gap remains normal.

Decreased gap

• Increased unmeasured cation: high Ca, high Mg.
• Decreased unmeasured anion: low albumin.

ABNORMAL FLUID AND ELECTROLYTE STATES

The fluid and electrolyte status of a patient is defined in two steps:
• The clinical assessment of the patient's fluid balance.
• The laboratory measurement of the electrolyte content of that fluid.

1. Fluid balance
A recent accurate weight or CVP monitoring line is helpful but frequently unavailable. Hydration is assessed by clinical signs, e.g. jugular venous pressure, heart failure, shock, urine output, signs of dehydration, edema, history and good charting. Serum sodium is a poor indicator of fluid balance. Hyponatremia may be found in gross fluid overload or in severe dehydration.

2. Electrolyte balance
Clinical signs like tetany and cardiac arrhythmias offer some clues but accurate electrolyte assessment depends on serum electrolyte measurements by the laboratory.

Dehydration

This is covered fully in chapter 3 (Emergencies). There are two aspects: fluid balance and electrolyte balance. The major aim is to prevent or treat circulatory collapse by preventing or replacing water and electrolyte losses.

1. Fluid balance
Assess volume status by clinical signs and weight loss:
• Mild:
    Up to 5% weight loss in infants and young children; 3% in the older child.
    Increased pulse rate.
    Dry mucous membranes.
    Slight decrease in urine output.
    Increased irritability due to thirst.
• Moderate:
    5–10% weight loss in infants and young children; 6% in the older child.

Increased severity of previously listed signs.
Reduced skin turgor.
Sunken fontanelle.
Sunken eyes; reduced eyeball tension.
Dusky skin.
- Severe:
    15% weight loss in infants and young children; 9–10% in the older child.
    Marked increase in severity of previously listed signs.
    Reduced blood pressure.
    Mottled skin.
    Cool extremities with poor capillary filling.
    Rapid thready pulse.
    Labored respiration, i.e. the patient is in circulatory shock.

2. Electrolyte balance
Assessed by measuring the serum sodium:
- Isotonic: sodium 135–145.
    Balanced loss of water and electrolytes.
- Hypotonic: sodium < 135.
    Danger of seizures if serum sodium declines rapidly or if sodium drops below 120 mEq/L.
- Hypertonic: sodium > 145.
    Dangerous condition if > 155.
    CNS damage and seizures may occur.
    CNS symptoms are also seen if patient is rehydrated too rapidly.

3. Treatment
- Rehydration using ad lib oral glucose–electrolyte solutions has been very successful in developing countries.
- The intravenous route is probably overused and should be reserved for patients with shock, coma, intractable vomiting or surgical patients.

Hypernatremia

- Increased sodium intake:
    Hyperosmolar feeds used to replace losses from diarrhea, excessive saline infusion.
    Hypernatremia seen in certain breast fed infants.
- Excessive water loss:
    Diabetes insipidus, renal tubular disorders, mannitol infusion, diarrhea.
    Other predisposing factors include fever, hyperventilation, obesity.
- Treatment:
    Intracellular fluid loss may occur. Rapid correction leads to large fluid shifts into cells and may cause cerebral edema, seizures and CNS damage.
    Calculate the fluid deficit and replace it over 2 days.
    Serum sodium should not fall by more than 10 mEq/d.
    If severe dehydration makes rapid fluid replacement necessary, use isotonic solutions like normal saline, albumin or plasma.

Once shock has been treated, change to D5W containing 30–50 mEq Na/L.

Hyponatremia

- Spurious: hyperglycemia, hyperlipemia.
- Water retention: SIADH (head injury, meningitis, asphyxia), renal failure, excess hypotonic fluids.
- Sodium loss: renal tubular disease, diuretics, Addison's disease, ileostomy, diarrhea, recovery of ATN.
- Treatment:
    Symptomatic hyponatremia (weakness, seizures and coma) should be treated, regardless of cause, with hypertonic saline; 3% saline contains 0.5 mEq Na/mL.
    Replacement = weight in kg × deficit in mEq × ½.
    Never try to correct to 140 mmol/L.
    125–130 mmol/L is usually adequate. Infuse over 1–2 h.
    As in hypernatremia, avoid rapid changes of fluids and electrolytes. Once the symptoms are corrected, treatment is continued usually by fluid restriction and is aimed at the cause.
    SIADH: urine sodium and osmolarity high, low volume output. Restrict fluids. Always associated with a serious systemic illness.
    Water retention: renal failure, water overload. Usually clinically obvious with edema hypertension, etc. Restrict fluids.
    Extrarenal sodium loss: nasogastric or ileostomy losses. Losses are usually clinically obvious. Replace with normal saline.
    Renal sodium loss: high urine output and high urine sodium. Increase sodium intake or treat with steroids if adrenal hyperplasia.

Hyperkalemia

- Spurious: bruised heel, hemolysis, difficult venepuncture.
- Potassium retention: renal failure, Addison's disease, adrenogenital syndrome.
- Potassium overload: increased intake p.o. or i.v., potassium salts, e.g. penicillin (usually with renal failure).
- Intracellular fluid–extracellular fluid shift: hemolysis, crush injury, burns, acidosis.
- Treatment:
    Oppose the effects of hypokalemia: calcium gluconate 0.5 mL/kg of 10% solution i.v.
    Shift potassium into the cells: 0.5 g/kg glucose plus 1 unit insulin/3 g glucose; sodium bicarbonate 1–2 mEq/kg.
    Remove potassium from the body: kayexalate 1 g/kg rectally or nasogastric tube dialysis.

Hypokalemia

- Potassium loss: diuretics, recovery phase of acute renal failure, renal tubular disorders, diarrhea and vomiting, nasogastric tube, ileostomy, Cushing's syndrome.
- Decreased potassium intake: malnutrition, inappropriate fluids.
- Extracellular fluid–intracellular fluid shifts: alkalosis, infusion of sodium, glucose plus insulin.

• Treatment:
   Rapid replacement of potassium is very dangerous and is only justified for treatment of cardiac arrhythmias, digitalis toxicity and respiratory muscle weakness.
   Replace losses over 2–3 days with oral solutions of potassium or fruit and tomato juices.
   Potassium is an intracellular ion so calculation of deficit is impossible based on serum levels. Use serum potassium as a guide.
   If replacing intravenously, then give by slow continuous infusion.
   Maximum daily dose = 3 mEq/kg per 24 h.
   Maximum rate = 0.5 mEq/kg per h.
   Correct alkalosis, if present, or potassium wasting will not stop.

Hypercalcemia

• Increased calcium intake: vitamin D overdose, p.o. or i.v. calcium.
• Endocrine: hyperparathyroidism, occasionally hyperthyroidism.
• Others: sarcoid, neoplasms, vitamin A overdose, thiazides.
• Treatment:
   Stop all calcium and vitamin D intake. Excretion of calcium is increased by normal saline at twice maintenance rate plus furosemide 1–2 mg/kg every 6 h. A close watch on serum electrolytes is necessary.
   Intravenous phosphate or sulfate are dangerous (ectopic calcification) and rarely used.
   Prednisone 1–2 mg/kg per d is effective in vitamin D toxicity and sarcoid.
   Mithramycin is used for metastatic tumor hypercalcemia (dose is 25 mg/kg per d).
   Calcitonin is occasionally used for resistant cases.

Hypocalcemia

• Decreased calcium intake: malabsorption, malnutrition, anticonvulsants.
• Hypoparathyroidism: newborn, DiGeorge's syndrome.
• Others: chronic renal failure, hypoproteinemia, vitamin D resistance, diuretics. Magnesium deficiency produces parathyroid hormone (PTH) resistance.
• Treatment: 0.5–1.0 mL/kg of calcium gluconate over 20 min i.v. Rapid infusion may cause bradyarrhythmias. If no response, suspect magnesium deficiency.

Hypermagnesemia

• Increased magnesum intake: magnesium containing enemas and laxatives. Newborns of mothers receiving magnesium sulfate for eclampsia.
• Others: renal failure, Addison's disease.
• Treatment: oppose the effects of hypermagnesemia (hypotonia, paralysis) by slow i.v. infusion of 0.5–1.0 mL/kg calcium gluconate. Stop all intake of magnesium.

Hypomagnesemia

• Decreased magnesium intake: malabsorption, malnutrition, prolonged TPN.
• Others: hypoparathyroidism, primary aldosteronism.

- Treatment: hypocalcemia may not respond to treatment until magnesium also increased. Daily requirement is 6 mg/kg per 24 h. If urgent, give 0.1 mL/kg of 50% magnesium sulfate slowly i.v. or i.m.

GASTROINTESTINAL BLEEDING

Definitions

1. Hematemesis
Refers to emesis of fresh blood (bright red) or old blood ("coffee grounds"; more than 2–3 minutes in gastric contents). It should be distinguished from nasal bleeding and hemoptysis, either of which may be swallowed and vomited or directly spat out. When the source of bleeding is in the GI tract, it is usually from a site proximal to the ligament of Treitz.

2. Hematochezia
Refers to the passage of fresh blood per rectum. The source of bleeding is usually in the colon although a large volume upper gastrointestinal (GI) bleed with rapid intestinal transit may present as hematochezia. In these circumstances, the blood may be bright red or slightly maroon.

3. Melena
Refers to the passage of shiny, black, tarry stools which are strongly positive on guaiac testing (Hemoccult).

Etiology

Table I classifies the causes of GI bleeding by age group and site of bleeding. There are several conditions that can mimic GI bleeding and they should be excluded:
• Swallowed blood from nasopharynx or lungs.
• Red colored candies, juices and foods.
• Black colored (Hemoccult negative) stools: Bismuth (Pepto–Bismol), iron preparations, licorice and blueberries.
• Normal color stools, false positive Hemoccult: spinach, meat fibers.
In some conditions, bleeding can be slow or "occult" with no overt bleeding episode. This may present as iron deficiency anemia.

Causes of occult GI bleeding (many of these disorders also cause overt GI bleeding):
• Inflammatory causes: duodenal ulcer, peptic esophagitis, gastric ulcer, Crohn's disease, ulcerative colitis, eosinophilic gastroenteritis.
• Infectious causes: *H. pylori* duodenal ulcer, *H. pylori* gastric ulcer, hookworm, strongyloidiasis, ascariasis, tuberculous enterocolitis, amebiasis.
• Vascular causes: gastroesophageal varices, portal hypertension gastropathy, angiodysplasia and vascular ectasias, hemangiomas.
• Drugs: nonsteroidal anti–inflammatory drugs.
• Extragastrointestinal causes: hemoptysis, epistaxis, oropharyngeal bleeding.
• Artefactual causes: hematuria, menstrual bleeding, false test positivity.
• Miscellaneous causes: long distance running, coagulopathies, factitions.

Table I: Common causes of gastrointestinal bleeding

Age group	Upper GI	Lower GI
Neonates (0–30 d)	Swallowed maternal blood Acute gastritis or gastric ulcer Duodenal ulcer	Milk allergy Swallowed maternal blood Necrotizing enterocolitis Midgut volvulus Coagulopathy
Infants (30 d–1 yr)	Esophagitis Acute gastritis or gastric ulcer Esophageal varices Duodenal ulcer	Anal fissure Milk allergy Intussusception Meckel's diverticulum Infectious diarrhea Midgut volvulus
Children (1–12 yr)	Duodenal ulcer Acute gastritis or gastric ulcer Esophagitis Esophageal varices Mallory–Weiss tear Nasopharyngeal bleeding	Juvenile polyps Anal fissure Infectious diarrhea Inflammatory bowel disease Meckel's diverticulum Nodular lymphoid hyperplasia
Adolescents (12–18 yr)	Duodenal ulcer Acute gastritis or gastric ulcer Esophagitis Esophageal varices Mallory–Weiss tear	Inflammatory bowel disease Infectious diarrhea Polyps Anal fissure Hemorrhoids

Evaluation and diagnosis

The management of acute GI bleeding should combine an "ABC" (airway, breathing, circulation) resuscitation approach while obtaining the history, performing physical examination and ordering laboratory tests.

Guidelines for the evaluation of GI bleeding are:
• History of past bleeding, quality and quantity of blood loss.
• Physical examination: resting heart rate, blood pressure lying and sitting, examine for ascites, hepatosplenomegaly and caput medusae.
• Tests: type and cross–match, complete blood count, platelet count, reticulocyte count, PT, PTT, alanine aminotransferase, aspartate aminotransferase, alkaline phosphatase, albumin, BUN; guiaic or Hemoccult stools at bedside.

1. History
• Upper GI bleeding:
    Ask about forceful vomiting (Mallory–Weiss tears) or abdominal pain (location, timing, nature), nonsteroidal anti–inflammatory drugs (especially aspirin–containing) and high dose steroids.
    Enquire about previous episodes of bleeding, liver disease, family history of GI bleeding.

- Lower GI bleeding:
  Streaks of blood coating the stools or a few drops after passage of stool suggest the presence of an anal fissure or a colonic polyp.

  Inflammatory bowel disease (IBD) or infectious colitis usually results in diarrheal stools mixed with blood or mucus, but mild or localized IBD may cause blood–streaking of formed stools.

  A large bleed with or without clots can be caused by IBD, infectious colitis, Meckel's diverticulum, Henoch–Schönlein purpura or hemolytic uremic syndrome. Bleeding from a Meckel's diverticulum usually presents with bright red blood with or without clots and no antecedent diarrhea or systemic illness. When bright red blood per rectum is from a Meckel's diverticulum, the hemoglobin virtually always falls significantly; minor bleeding is almost never due to a Meckel's diverticulum.

  Ask about abdominal pain (location, timing, nature), determine if the blood is on the surface or mixed in with the stools, melena or hematochezia.

  Enquire about infectious contacts, foreign travel, recent use of antibiotics (*Clostridium difficile*) and family history of IBD.

2. Examination
- The immediate priority is to evaluate for hypovolemia or imminent shock and the need for volume resuscitation. Tachycardia at rest is the first sign of hypovolemia (can be mild); low pulse pressure and orthostatic blood pressure are late signs in children.
- Examine the nasopharynx for evidence of bleeding.
- Look for clubbing, ascites, jaundice (liver disease) or pallor and signs of malnutrition (IBD).
- Purpura and petechiae may suggest hemolytic uremic syndrome or Henoch–Schönlein purpura, coagulation disorder or sepsis.
- Mucosal or skin vascular lesions may have gut involvement, although these are a rare cause for GI bleeding in children. Examine the abdomen for hepatosplenomegaly, peritonitis and masses.
- Epigastric tenderness may suggest acid peptic disease; right lower quadrant tenderness may suggest Crohn's disease or intussusception (usually < 2 years of age).
- Splenomegaly may signify portal hypertension.
- Perineal and rectal exam is mandatory. Anal fissures may be seen by spreading the buttocks apart and getting the child to bear down; do not use a test tube applied to the anal canal (it is misleading and dangerous). Small perineal skin tags may be seen with fissures but if tags are large or multiple, then Crohn's disease is likely. A hot, red perineum may be seen with perineal streptococcal infection. The rectal examination helps to document the nature of the stools, presence of blood or a polyp. Stool on the glove should be tested by Hemoccult test at the bedside.

3. Special tests
- Barium or other contrast studies are hardly ever indicated in the evaluation of acute GI bleeding. Gastric lavage with room temperature saline via a large bore nasogastric tube may help determine if bleeding was from upper GI tract. Do not use iced saline; large volume lavage may cause hypothermia in small or hypovolemic children.
- Upper GI endoscopy is the best diagnostic procedure for an upper GI bleeding as it allows definitive diagnosis and accurate location of the bleeding site as well as provides therapeutic options such as sclerotherapy and heat probe coagulation of active bleeding sites. In patients

with suspected peptic ulcer disease, upper GI endoscopy is mandatory for definitive diagnosis of the type of peptic ulcer and presence or absence of *H. pylori* antral gastritis; it therefore guides specific therapy.
- For lower GI bleeding, colonoscopy is the best diagnostic procedure as it allows localization of the bleeding source, tissue diagnosis for IBD, and diagnosis and removal of polyps. Barium enema is almost never indicated in the evaluation of GI bleeding in children because it is insensitive, nonspecific and exposes the gonads to irradiation.
- Upper and lower endoscopies are also essential in the detection and management of GI vascular lesions. Technetium scan is important to detect possible Meckel's diverticulum bleeding and should be done following a dose of H_2-receptor antagonist (so-called "enhanced" Meckel's scan). This should only be considered when blood loss was large enough to cause a 20–30 g/L drop in serum hemoglobin.
- In selected cases, a radiolabelled red blood cell scan or an angiography may help to identify a bleeding site, but this requires an active bleeding of more than 0.5 mL/min and is seldom required in children.

Management

1. The unstable child
- Follow "ABC" resuscitation guidelines:
    Give oxygen by mask, start two large bore intravenous lines and obtain tests as listed in Table II. A normal hemoglobin level does not rule out a severe acute bleed as hemodilution may not have yet occurred, and fluid resuscitation should be guided by resting heart rate. Give normal saline or Ringer's lactate 10 mL/kg boluses until the heart rate returns to normal for age. Packed red blood cells should be given to maintain oxygen carrying capacity. If more than 30% of blood volume is required, whole blood should be given and possibly platelet repletion. The commonest error in management of GI bleeding in children is inadequate volume repletion; be guided by the resting pulse.
- If upper GI bleed is confirmed or suspected by gastric lavage, the following steps are recommended:
    Start treatment with i.v. ranitidine or cimetidine.
    For children with liver disease or coagulopathy, give 1 mg vitamin K per year of age (maximum of 10 mg) i.v. or s.c. and fresh frozen plasma 5 mL/kg i.v. over 15–30 min.
    Very occasionally in children, vasopressin or somatostatin infusion may be used to reduce splanchnic blood flow in the event of an ongoing bleeding. Somatostatin may be preferred over vasopressin as it does not have cardiovascular side effects. Give either of these only under close expert supervision. Table II gives doses of commonly used drugs.
    Endoscopy should usually be performed once the child is in stable condition.

2. The stable child
- Verify actual bleeding and obtain history and physical examination.
- Laboratory tests as indicated under the guidelines for the evaluation of GI bleeding.
- Gastric lavage is usually unnecessary in children with minor bleeding.

Table II: Drugs used in the treatment of upper gastrointestinal bleeding

Drug	Dosage	Interval	Route	Comments
Ranitidine	1.25–1.9 mg/kg per dose 2.5–3.8 mg/kg per dose	q6–8h	i.v., p.o. or nasogastric tube	• Maximum i.v. dose 50 mg q6h • Reduce dosage in renal failure
Cimetidine	20–40 mg/kg per d	q6–8h	i.v., p.o. or nasogastric tube	• Maximum i.v. dose 300 mg q6h • Reduce dosage in renal failure
Antacid Maalox TC Amphogel	0.5 mL/kg per dose	Up to q2h	p.o. or nasogastric tube	• Can cause diarrhea • Aluminum or magnesium toxicity may occur in renal failure • Amphogel may cause hypophosphatemia
Vasopressin	Per 1.73 m² the dose is as follows: give 20 units in D5W over 10 min; then continuous infusion of 0.2 unit/min in D5W; double every 1–2 h if active bleeding persists, to a maximum of 0.8 unit/min		i.v.	• Adjust dose for child's size • Rapid i.v. push may cause bradycardia and hypotension • Vasopressin causes water retention and dilutional hyponatremia • Meticulous fluid balance is mandatory • Urinary catheter and CVP required if active bleeding continues for > 4–6h
Somatostatin	4 µg/kg (maximum 100 µg) in D5W i.v. or s.c. bolus followed by 4 µg/kg per h in D5W continuous infusion for 48 h		i.v. or s.c.	• Inspect for particulate matter and discoloration prior to administration • Monitor serum glucose levels

FAILURE TO THRIVE

Failure to thrive (FTT) is the term used to identify infants and children whose growth deviates > 2 standard deviations below that expected for age and sex. Failure to thrive is a physical sign, not a diagnosis, and when suspected, FTT is a prompt for further evaluation over a wide range of possible causes.

Differential diagnosis of failure to thrive:
• Cardiac disease: common with congestive failure.
• CNS abnormalities: cerebral palsy, diencephalic syndrome, increased intracranial pressure, neuromuscular disorders.
• Chronic Infections: tuberculosis, congenital syphilis, cytomegalic inclusion virus.
• Connective tissue disorders: juvenile rheumatoid arthritis.

- Endocrine: growth hormone deficiency, hypothyroidism, hypopituitarism, diabetes mellitus.
- Feeding disorders: occult neurological disorders, "difficult" breast feeder, improper formula mixing or administration, oropharyngeal disorders.
- GI diseases: postnecrotizing enterocolitis stricture, rumination, gastroesophageal reflux, pyloric stenosis, malrotation, Hirschsprung's disease, intractable diarrhea of infancy, postenteritis enteropathy, giardiasis, sucrase isomaltase deficiency, celiac disease, IBD, autoimmune enteropathy, chronic cholestasis.
- Genetic: "dwarfing" syndromes.
- Immunodeficiency: including HIV infection.
- Metabolic disorders: altered calcium, phosphorus metabolism (renal rickets), glycogen storage disease, mucopolysaccharidosis, mucolipidosis, sphingolipidosis, aminoaciduria, organic acidosis.
- Perinatal factors: fetal alcohol syndrome, intrauterine growth retardation, intrauterine infections.
- Psychosocial deprivation: maternal depression, emotional deprivation, maternal deprivation, reactive attachment disorder of infancy, psychosocial dwarfism.
- Pulmonary disease: bronchopulmonary dysplasia, cystic fibrosis.
- Renal disorders: renal dysplasia, renal tubular acidosis.

Evaluation

In the evaluation of FTT, it is helpful to think along the different factors that may affect growth: intake, digestion and absorption, losses, nutritional requirements, utilization (cellular level, genetics) and psychosocial factors. Depending on the community evaluated, about 50–80% of patients investigated for FTT will have an identified organic cause. When no organic cause is found, the problem may be attributable to psychosocial deprivation. In some of the cases, there is a mix of an organic cause and environmental factors.

1. History
- The most important aspect is an accurate growth curve for the child, consisting of sequential plotted values for height, weight and head circumference. This is the only way to make an objective determination of the presence or absence of FTT and may give important clues as to the underlying diagnosis. Children with FTT, secondary to malabsorption or inadequate calorie intake, initially will have normal linear growth rate and head circumference with decreased weight gain rate; this is the most commonly encountered situation.
- Children with endocrine disease will usually have stunted linear growth with normal weight. Some children are proportionally small and have normal growth rates; this may reflect constitutional growth delay or genetic or embryonal factors.
- Detailed perinatal history is important.
- Dietary history should include a 3 day calorie count, feeding patterns (breast or bottle, size of meal) and food selection by child or parents. Bizarre exclusion diets based on skin testing or a tenous history of "food allergies" often lead to FTT. Enquire about vomiting and diarrhea as possible causes for calorie losses.
- Enquire about other medical conditions or medications.
- Obtain growth data for the parents and siblings.

2. Physical examination

A global assessment of well being and activity is important.

- Look for signs of muscle wasting, loss of subcutaneous fat, evidence of specific vitamin or nutrient deficiencies, poor hygiene or neglect (flat occiput).
- Look for oral thrush, congenital malformations.
- Examine for hepatosplenomegaly or abdominal mass as well as for major systemic disease.

3. Laboratory tests

Basic laboratory tests can help in evaluating degree of malnutrition or identify specific nutrient deficiency. Tests for detection of possible etiology should be ordered as indicated by the history and physical examination:

- Basic screening tests: CBC, urinalysis, urea, creatinine, serum electrolytes, albumin, alanine aminotransferase, aspartate aminotransferase, alkaline phosphatase.
- Further tests (if needed): sweat chloride, IRT (immunoreactive trypsin), TSH, T_4, iron, zinc, vitamin D, stool cultures, pH, reducing substances, occult blood, endoscopy.

Management

- Most children with FTT do not require hospital admission for evaluation. In some cases a short admission for observation is the only way to secure a diagnosis (meticulous monitoring of intake/output, feeding pattern and weight gain). Children with significant malnutrition may also require admission to establish and monitor refeeding. If there is no significant diarrhea or vomiting, provide the child with full caloric requirements.
- The best estimate for caloric requirements at all ages is the total fluid requirement expressed in calories. Further adjustments will be dictated by the child's response.
- In cases where vomiting is significant, continuous nasogastric feeding may be tolerated and should start at a slow rate (25–30% of daily required volume) and advance as tolerated every 6–8 hours while pursuing a diagnosis for the vomiting.
- Patients who present with significant diarrhea may be kept n.p.o. for 12–24 hours to see if diarrhea resolves. They then can be fed with gradual increase of enteral nutrition while receiving the balance of their calories via i.v. catheter. Careful documentation of stool output (separated from urine), stool fat content, pH, reducing substances and electrolytes are important to understand the cause of diarrhea and can guide the refeeding process. Attention should be given to supplementation of trace metals and vitamins.

DIRECT HYPERBILIRUBINEMIA (CHOLESTASIS) IN INFANTS

A conjugated bilirubin level of > 2 µmol/L (laboratories may use different methodology with different references) or over 15% of the total bilirubin is abnormal and requires investigation. Jaundice becomes apparent when serum bilirubin exceeds 40 µmol/L (110 µg/L in the neonate). It is essential to differentiate conjugated hyperbilirubinemia from the far more common unconjugated hyperbilirubinemia of the neonate ("physiological jaundice") or that occasionally associated with breast feeding. While there are many causes for conjugated hyperbilirubinemia (cholestasis) in the newborn, in this age group four conditions account for the majority of the cases: extrahepatic biliary atresia (EHBA), idiopathic neonatal hepatitis (NH), alpha$_1$–antitrypsin deficiency and paucity of bile ducts. Early diagnosis of extrahepatic biliary atresia is essential, as early surgery (before 6–8 weeks) has a considerably better outcome.

Possible etiologies include:
- Neonatal hepatitis:
  Idiopathic viral (cytomegalovirus, rubella, reovirus type 3, herpes viruses such as simplex, zoster).
  Human herpes virus type 6, adenovirus, enteroviruses, hepatitis B, hepatitis C, parvovirus B19, human immunodeficiency virus, non A, non B, non C.
  Bacterial and parasitic (bacterial sepsis, syphilis, listeriosis, tuberculosis, toxoplasmosis).
- Bile duct obstruction:
  Cholangiopathies: extrahepatic biliary atresia, paucity of intrahepatic bile ducts, neonatal sclerosing cholangitis, choledochal cyst, spontaneous perforation of common bile duct, bile duct stenosis, Caroli's disease.
  Other: inspissated bile or mucous plug, cholelithiasis, tumors or masses (intrinsic and extrinsic).
- Idiopathic cholestatic syndromes:
  Arteriohepatic dysplasia (Alagille's syndrome), Byler's syndrome, hereditary cholestasis with lymphedema (Aagenaes' syndrome).
  Benign recurrent cholestasis, familial cholestasis of North American Indians.
- Metabolic diseases:
  Disorders of amino acid metabolism, tyrosinemia.
  Disorders of lipid metabolism: Wolman's disease, Niemann–Pick's disease, Gaucher's disease.
  Disorders of the urea cycle: arginase deficiency.
  Disorders of carbohydrate metabolism: galactosemia, fructosemia, type IV glycogenosis.
  Disorders of bile acid synthesis: peroxisomol disorders, Zellweger's syndrome.
  Disorders of oxidative phosphorylation.
  Other: $alpha_1$–antitrypsin deficiency, cystic fibrosis, hypopituitarism (septo–optic dysplasia), hypothyroidism, neonatal hemochromatosis.
- Toxic: drugs, parenteral nutrition.
- Miscellaneous associations: shock or hypoperfusion, histiocytosis X, intestinal obstruction, erythrophagocytic lymphohistiocytosis, Indian childhood cirrhosis, graft versus host disease, autosomal trisomies, neonatal lupus erythematosus, extracorporeal membrane oxygenation, veno–occlusive disease.

Evaluation of the cholestatic infant

1. History
- Idiopathic neonatal hepatitis (NNH) is more common in premature or low birth weight infants. In contrast, extrahepatic biliary atresia (EHBA) is more common in newborns of normal birth weight.
- White (acholic) stools are more common and observed earlier in the course of EHBA than in NNH.
- Neonatal hepatitis may have familial incidence of 10–15% but familial cases of EHBA are rare.

2. Physical examination
- In the first few weeks of life, infants with EHBA may appear remarkably well and thriving in contrast to the irritability, poor feeding and vomiting which may occur with infections or with metabolic disorders including galactosemia and tyrosinemia.
- Congenital infections may be associated with low birth weight, microcephaly, chorioretinitis and thrombocytopenia purpura.
- Syndromic intrahepatic paucity of bile ducts (Alagille's syndrome) is associated with dysmorphic features. Hepatomegaly is common in NNH and a midline liver may be palpable in the polysplenia syndrome (abdominal heterotaxia, malrotation, levocardia and EHBA). In EHBA, the liver may be enlarged and hard on palpation.
- Splenomegaly is seen with congenital infections or later as a result of advanced liver fibrosis and portal hypertension.
- Acholic stools are most commonly found in EHBA but can be seen occasionally when severe hepatocyte disease is present. Observation should be made of a cross–section of the stool as acholic stools may occasionally be covered by thin bile colored mucus layer from the intestine. Ascites, edema and coagulopathy may be present, but the presence of early coagulopathy, often in excess of that expected for the degree of jaundice, may indicate a metabolic disease. Hypotonia and other neurological abnormalities may be primary (peroxisomal disorders) or secondary (hypoglycemia). Dark urine in a jaundiced infant usually represents direct bilirubin pigment.

3. Laboratory tests
The initial evaluation should confirm the presence of cholestasis, provide an assessment of the severity of liver dysfunction and identify potentially treatable infections or metabolic diseases. A comprehensive investigation is necessary because of the lack of specific history or physical examination findings. Ideally, the evaluation should be concluded by day 35 of life to allow for timely surgery when indicated. Necessary tests include hepatobiliary scintigraphy (HIDA) which requires 5 days preparation with oral phenobarbital (5 mg/kg per d div. b.i.d.). Sonography is performed to determine gallbladder presence or size and presence of choledochal cyst but is often difficult to interpret at this age. Liver biopsy is diagnostic for the major causes of cholestasis in most cases and often provides important prognostic information.
- Initial evaluation:
  Fractionated serum bilirubin analysis.
  Serum tests for liver disease (AST, ALT, alkaline phosphatase, γGTP).
  Tests of liver function (PT, PTT, albumin, ammonia, cholesterol, blood glucose).
  Complete blood count, including platelet count.
  Bacterial cultures of blood, urine and other, if indicated.
  Urinalysis, including reducing sugars.
- Comprehensive evaluation (the following tests are selectively performed):
  Ultrasonography.
  Alpha$_1$–antitrypsin level and phenotype.
  Serologies (TORCH, VDRL, EB virus, parvovirus, herpes virus, HIV, other).
  Hepatobiliary scintigraphy (HIDA scan).
  Percutaneous liver biopsy (for light and electron microscopic examination, viral culture, enzymology, immunohistochemistry).
  Sweat test. Metabolic screen (serum amino acids).

Thyroid hormone, thyroid stimulating hormones (evaluation of hypopituitarism as indicated).
Red blood cell galactose–1–phosphate uridyl transferase.
Viral cultures. Serum iron and ferritin.
Urine and serum analysis of bile acids and bile precursors.
X–rays of long bones, skull for congenital infection, chest for lung and cardiac disease.
Bone marrow examination and skin fibroblast culture for suspected storage disease.
Exploratory laparotomy and intraoperative cholangiography.

Management

Although some cholestatic conditions can be successfully treated surgically or medically, many infants have chronic liver disease and will require careful follow–up and management for nutritional deficiencies and pruritus. Infants with cholestasis are at risk for developing fat soluble vitamin deficiencies (vitamins A, D, E, K) and steatorrhea with failure to thrive. With ongoing hepatic inflammation and fibrosis, they will likely develop portal hypertension with the attendant risk of variceal bleeding. When portal hypertension is present, parents and other physicians involved in the child's care should be given a list of aspirin–containing medications to be avoided. Proper choice of formula (high MCT, low LCT) and vitamin supplementation is important (Table III gives vitamin dosage guidelines). The treatment of pruritus includes nail clipping and drug therapy when indicated. Children with persistent cholestasis may also benefit from choleretic drugs.

Table III: Fat–soluble vitamin therapy for chronic cholestatic disorders

Vitamin	Deficiency	Drug	Dose	Monitoring
Vitamin A	Xerosis, night blindness	Emulsified vitamin A	5,000–15,000 IU/d	Serum level 400–500 μg/mL
Vitamin D	Rickets, osteoporosis	25–hydroxy vitamin D (Calderol) 1,25–dihydroxy vitamin D (Rocaltrol)	5–7 μg/kg per d 0.1–0.2 μg/kg per d	Physical examination, X–ray; serum level 25–30 ng/mL (can be higher), serum, urine calcium, inorganic phosphate and parathyroid hormone
Vitamin E	Peripheral neuropathy, ataxia, ophthalmoplegia	General D–α–tocopherol	150–300 IU/kg per d	Serum level > 5 mg/L; physical examination
Vitamin K	Coagulopathy	Vitamin K_3	5–15 mg/d	Prothrombin time, factor activities

VOMITING AND GASTROESOPHAGEAL REFLUX

Definitions

1. Vomiting or regurgitation
Refers to ejection of gastric contents through the mouth. The term "vomiting" is usually used when ejection of contents is forceful, whereas the term "regurgitation" is usually applied to effortless vomiting. To avoid confusion, it is always best to state whether vomiting is forceful or effortless, and if projectile, how far it is projected.

2. Gastroesophageal reflux (GER)
Refers to the backflow of gastric contents proximally into the esophagus, that is up to the cricopharyngeus muscle. GER may occasionally manifest as vomiting but also may be relatively "silent" (i.e. may not be felt or seen by the patient). Silent GER may lead to the same complications as those of overt vomiting (see GERD).

3. Gastroesophageal reflux disease (GERD)
Vomiting and GER are symptoms or signs and not diseases in of themselves. However, vomiting and GER (even when "silent") may lead to complications such as esophagitis, FTT or aspiration pneumonia. The presence of any of these complications is termed GE reflux disease or GERD. Esophagitis may be further complicated by anemia, poor feeding, esophageal stricture and neurological–like symptoms (e.g. Sandifer's syndrome).

Evaluation

Vomiting may be caused by a wide range of conditions, including mechanical obstruction, infections, metabolic disorders and food intolerance. It is helpful to further divide the etiology of vomiting by age groups (Table IV). Infants aged 4–12 months commonly have regurgitation ("physiological reflux") and only require extensive evaluation if they have signs or symptoms suggestive of GERD such as FTT, anemia, irritability with feeds (suggestive of esophagitis), cough, wheezing or apnea. New onset of vomiting beyond age of 8–12 months or persistent vomiting beyond 18–21 months always should be investigated. The following approach refers to chronic vomiting and therefore excludes vomiting due to acute abdominal emergencies.

1. History
- Vomiting soon after meals may suggest hiatal hernia, incompetent LES, peptic ulcer disease, gastritis; esophagitis itself may lead to vomiting. Vomiting may also be due to partial intestinal obstruction or gallbladder disease as well as nongastrointestinal causes; neurological disorders are an important cause of vomiting, as are UTI and renal disorders. Vomiting of undigested food several hours after meals may indicate delayed gastric emptying. It is important to obtain a detailed description of the vomitus, e.g. blood, coffee grounds, bile and whether it was forceful or projectile (e.g. pyloric stenosis).
- Enquire about nausea, diarrhea, constipation and jaundice as possible clues to etiology.
- Enquire about signs of GERD, including choking, cough, dysphagia (difficulty swallowing) and odynophagia (painful swallowing).
- Rule out poisoning, enquire about neurological and urinary symptoms, and about medications

with GI side effects.

Table IV: Causes of vomiting in infancy and childhood

Digestive tract disorders		Infective disorders	
Functional and Psychogenic		Gastroenteritis	1,2,3
Idiopathic neonatal vomiting	1	Food poisoning	2,3
Idiopathic infantile vomiting		Urinary tract infection	1,2,3
("pylorospasm")	1,2	Respiratory tract infection (including	
Feeding problems ("rumination", that is		otitis)	1,2,3
abnormal mother–child relationship)	1,2	Appendicitis (and other surgical	
Cyclic vomiting	3	emergencies)	2,3
Self–induced vomiting	3		
Hiatal hernia and gastroesophageal reflux	1,2,3	**Neurological disorders**	
Gastric outlet malformation	1,2,3		
Acquired gastric outlet obstructions,		Meningitis and encephalitis	1,2,3
e.g. corrosive gastritis, CGD IBD	1,2,3	Intracranial birth injury	1
Hypertrophic pyloric stenosis	2,3	Migraine	3
Volvulus: gastric or intestinal	1	Motion sickness	3
Malrotation and partial obstructions	1,2		
Atresias	1,2,3	*Increased intracranial pressure*	
Meconium ileus	1,2,3	Hydrocephalus	1,2,3
Ménétrier's disease	1	Subdural hematoma	1,2
Meconium ileus equivalent	3	Tumor, including diencephalic syndrome	2,3
Inspissated milk syndrome and		Hypertension, including renal causes	2,3
lactobezoar	1	Kernicterus	1,2
Duplications	1		
Intussusception	1,2,3	**Toxic or metabolic disorders**	
Hirschsprung's disease	2,3		
Malformation and obstruction	1,2	Adrenal hyperplasia	1,2
Peptic ulcer	1,2	Aminoacidopathies and organic	
Trichobezoar	3	acidurias	1
		Galactosemia	1
Food intolerances		Hypercalcemia	1,2,3
Celiac disease	3	Uremia	1,2,3
Milk protein intolerance	1,2	Drugs, e.g., digoxin, cytotoxic agents,	
Other food intolerances	2	anticonvulsants	1,2,3
		Vitamin A excess	2
		Diabetes mellitus (ketoacidosis)	3
		Poisons (many)	3
		Hepatic disorders	
		Hepatitis	1,2
		Cardiac failure	1,2
		Reye's syndrome	3

Key: 1 = < 3 mo; 2 = 3 mo–1 yr; 3 = > 1 yr.

2. Examination
- Evaluate for dehydration and jaundice and for altered growth pattern.
- Examine for systemic disease, especially that of the central nervous system.
- Look for abdominal distention or visible peristalsis and for alteration of bowel sounds.

- Palpate for organomegaly and masses.
- Pyloric stenosis presents as an olive–sized mass in the right upper quadrant (with active peristalsis postfeed and nonbilious vomiting).
- A lower quadrant mass may represent Crohn's disease or intussusception.

3. Tests
- Urinalysis should be routinely performed.
- Serum amino acid and organic acid analysis is indicated when a metabolic disorder is suspected; abnormal liver tests with elevated ammonia levels may suggest liver disease or Reye's syndrome.
- In the vomiting child, there are some indications for pH probe testing (which can quantify acid GER). Scintigraphy (so-called "reflux scan") is only indicated if pulmonary aspiration is suspected; scintigraphy is not useful for detection or quantitation of GE reflux.
- Barium swallow is important to evaluate anatomical abnormalities but is not helpful in detection or quantification of GER. Children often will show physiological reflux on a barium study or show reflux due to crying or struggling during the study when no pathological reflux is present; conversely, barium study is insensitive and often will not show reflux when pathological reflux is, in fact, present. Upper GI series has limitations because the study is unphysiological. Barium does not contain the food components that influence GI motility, and reflux is examined at only a "snapshot" segment of a 24 hour period. However, barium study is important as a "road map" for detection of anatomical abnormalities such as malrotation and hiatal hernia. Barium study also has a high false–positive and false–negative rate for peptic ulcer disease.
- An upper GI endoscopy may be required to evaluate for esophagitis and for other possible causes for vomiting such as peptic ulcer disease, many types of gastritis, celiac disease and food allergy.
- Laboratory evaluation for vomiting: (* = for specific indication only)
    Urine: urinalysis, culture, organic acids*.
    Blood: electrolytes, glucose, urea, calcium, phosphorus, venous pH, lactate, amylase, ALT, AST, alkaline phosphatase, albumin, amino acids* and ammonia*.
    Radiology: flat film of the abdomen, barium swallow, ultrasound*.
    Upper GI endoscopy*.
    Esophageal motility*, 24 hour intraesophageal pH study*.

Management

Vomiting is a symptom or sign of an underlying disorder and therefore the management should be directed at the specific cause of the vomiting; only very seldom is treatment directed at the vomiting itself. Correction of acidosis, abnormalities of fluid and electrolyte balance take priority. In some cases, correction of hydration may terminate the vomiting. When nausea is a significant complaint and especially in the presence of abdominal distention with or without bowel obstruction, intermittent suction via nasogastric tube can be helpful. Prokinetic medications (such as cisapride, Prepulsid) may be of help but should be used selectively and only prescribed for long–term use in conjunction with a full evaluation. Note that metoclopramide (Reglan) has been rendered virtually obsolete for GER by its short–term and long–term side effects and by the advent of cisapride. The treatment of GERD must be carefully individualized and is best done in consultation with the gastroenterologist. In children with epigastric or retrosternal "burning pain" and vomiting, H_2–receptor antagonists (H_2–RA) may be used empirically for 1–2 weeks for symptomatic relief, but endoscopy should be performed before long–term therapy is considered as acid suppression may partially or wholly mask an underlying diagnosis. Proton pump inhibitors (e.g. omeprazole, brand name Losec) should not be used without specific endoscopically documented indications as they will even more effectively mask underlying disease, making definitive diagnosis difficult. In addition, proton pump inhibitors are, as yet, not approved for use in children. Surgical management of GERD should be reserved for carefully selected children who have failed a carefully prescribed, optimized medical regimen as antireflux surgery is associated with high failure and morbidity rates and, in some cases, mortality (especially in the neurologically impaired child).

Empiric treatment with antibiotics for suspected peptic ulcer disease in children should never be undertaken. In the majority of cases, an ulcer is not present; the antibiotic courses required to eradicate *H. pylori* require good compliance and are not without side effects and complications. Furthermore, even when an ulcer is present, about 15–20% of duodenal ulcers in children are not related to *H. pylori* and the treatment indicated is different. Similarly, Pepto–Bismol should not be used as empiric antacid therapy as it will partially treat *H. pylori*, making definitive diagnosis and treatment difficult. Definitive diagnosis of peptic ulcer is important, as > 60–70% of ulcers in children may be complicated by bleeding or perforation.

CHILDREN POSTLIVER TRANSPLANT

The main medical concerns that are specific to children post–transplantation include acute and chronic rejection, increased risk for infections (chickenpox, measles, etc.) and lymphoproliferative disease (often associated with Epstein–Barr virus). In addition, these children may suffer from side effects associated with immunosuppressive medications. Any fever over 37.8 °C, lasting more than 24 hours, should be investigated. Similar precautions are required for generalized or localized areas of redness or tenderness, sore throats or ears, persistent cough or rashes. Routine monitoring of liver and renal function is indicated and the physical examination should include blood pressure measurements.

Acute rejection

Elevated alanine aminotransferase (ALT), aspartate aminotransferase (AST) and alkaline phosphatase (alk phos) are early markers of acute liver rejection. Hyperbilirubinemia and jaundice become apparent in later stages and with chronic rejection. These laboratory tests are not specific for rejection and therefore are indications for further evaluation of hepatitis and liver injury. It is important to verify that the child was properly medicated and to exclude possible causes of low drug levels (diarrhea, vomiting).

A full physical examination to evaluate for infections and lymphadenopathy is indicated:
• Liver biopsy for histology.
• Virology and bacterial cultures for diagnosis prior to initiation of treatment.
• Once acute rejection is present on biopsy, the treatment for an acute liver rejection should be confirmed with the Gastroenterology service, but current guidelines for children < 30 kg are: (for children > 30 kg, all doses are doubled)
  Methylprednisolone (SoluMedrol) 25 mg i.v. q6h × 4 doses.

Methylprednisolone (SoluMedrol) 20 mg i.v. q6h × 4 doses.
Methylprednisolone (SoluMedrol) 15 mg i.v. q6h × 4 doses.
Methylprednisolone (SoluMedrol) 20 mg i.v. q12h × 2 doses.
Methylprednisolone (SoluMedrol) 20 mg i.v. o.d. × 1, then discontinue SoluMedrol and start
prednisone 1–2 mg/kg per d (may be given orally if the child has good enteral absorption).

Chickenpox

An infected person may spread the virus 2 days before and 5 days after the start of the rash.
Children receiving immunosuppressive drugs may spread the virus as long as new lesions are
appearing. Post–transplant children should be given varicella zoster immunoglobulin (VZIg) within
4 days following contact with chickenpox. If lesions appear, then the child should be treated with
i.v. acyclovir (Avirax, Zovirax) until no more new lesions appear. The dose of immunosuppressive
medications may be reduced with an increased risk of acute rejection requiring careful monitoring
of liver function tests. Children may become immunized to chickenpox with decreased risk of
infection in subsequent exposures. Children who had chickenpox prior to transplant and those
who demonstrated antibodies may be followed clinically for appearance of lesions without giving
VZIg.

ACUTE DIARRHEA

Acute diarrhea is usually due to viral gastroenteritis. Extraintestinal infections often cause
diarrhea in infants and toddlers. Serious abdominal pathology such as appendicitis, inflammatory
bowel disease and poisoning should always be considered. The complications of acute diarrhea
include dehydration, electrolyte and acid–base disturbance, sepsis, protein–calorie malnutrition
and chronicity. Enteritis means small bowel inflammation and colitis refers to large bowel
inflammation. Most infectious diarrhea is due to "gastroenteritis" or "enterocolitis".

Common causes of acute diarrhea:
• Infectious enteritis: viral, bacterial, parasitic.
• Cow/soy milk intolerance (< 6–8 months).
• Extraintestinal diseases: otitis, pneumonia, urinary tract infection.
• Antibiotic related diarrhea.
• Inflammatory bowel disease.
• Hemolytic uremic syndrome, Henoch–Schönlein purpura.

Evaluation

1. History
• Determine the duration of illness, diet, infectious contacts (including pets and travel) and
  medications (antibiotics).
• Ask about vomiting and obtain a description of stool frequency, volume, consistency, urgency
  and presence of blood or mucus.
• Ask about weight loss and enquire about urinary signs and symptoms such as frequency,
  urgency and dysuria.
• In most cases, infectious gastroenteritis presents with vomiting and diarrhea of rapid onset.

Fever and headache are common, and abdominal pain is generally periumbilical or diffuse and crampy.
- Dysentery (the passage of blood and mucus in the stools) means that colitis is present. Infectious dysentery is usually bacterial, although infants and toddlers infected with rotavirus may also have blood and mucus in the stools.

2. Examination
- Examine the abdomen for masses, tenderness and peritonism.
- Look for signs of acute dehydration and hypovolemia such as tachycardia, dry mucous membranes, postural hypotension and sunken eyes.
- Document that diarrhea is in fact present: perform a rectal examination and obtain stool for investigation.
- The presence of a purpuric skin rash suggests vasculitis due to Henoch–Schönlein purpura, hemolytic uremic syndrome or, rarely, sepsis.
- The diarrhea associated with these disorders is often bloody.
- Consider the diagnosis of bacteremia in the ill patient.

3. Laboratory tests
- Stool studies:
    In the majority of patients who are well with a brief history of uncomplicated, nonbloody diarrhea, dietary management without stool studies is acceptable. Gross examination of the stool for color, consistency, odor, blood and purulent exudate is helpful. The presence of mucus and blood suggests colitis from any cause.
    In children with complicated, bloody or prolonged diarrhea, the following stool studies are needed:
    Culture of fresh stool for bacterial enteropathogens including *Escherichia coli, Yersinia enterocolitica, Campylobacter jejuni, Clostridium difficile, Salmonella* and *Shigella. Aeromonas hydrophila* and *Vibrio parahaemolyticus* are rarer bacterial pathogens. Send a specimen for determination of *C. difficile* toxin.
    Obtain a specimen to be used for microscopic examination for ova and parasites and for ELISA testing for rotavirus (Rotazyme).
    In *C. jejuni* infection, a dark field examination performed within 2 hours may show the typical "darting gull wing" appearance.
    Test stool for pH and reducing substances. If the stool pH < 6, the child may have carbohydrate malabsorption. Mix 5 drops of stool water wrung out from the diaper or drawn up in a dropper with 10 drops of water and add a Clinitest tablet. In general, the presence of more than 1% reducing substance is abnormal (healthy breast fed infants may have over 2% reducing substances). Carbohydrate malabsorption may be due to carbohydrate overload or disaccharidase deficiency.
    Test for occult blood using Hemoccult cards.
    Smear stool on a slide, apply methylene blue and look for polymorphonuclear leukocytes (their presence suggests colitis).
- Other studies:
    Send a urine sample for urinalysis and culture. In children with high fever, toxicity or other risk factors for bacteremia, obtain a blood sample for culture.
    CBC, differential count, platelet count, BUN and measurements of creatinine and

electrolytes should be ordered in children who require admission.

4. Specific disorders
- Food poisoning: exposure to toxins produced by *Staphylococcus aureus*, *Salmonella* or *Clostridium perfringens* can result in acute onset of diarrhea, vomiting and abdominal pain. Symptoms tend to occur within hours of ingestion and are usually of short duration (< 24 hours).
- Viral causes of diarrhea: in North America, viruses account for 70–80% of cases of acute diarrhea. Common pathogens are rotavirus, Norwalk agent, enteroviruses and adenoviruses. Viral infections decrease the absorptive surface of the small bowel; this type of lesion takes 3–6 days to heal.
  Rotavirus infection: is especially common in infants, causing over 60% of cases of acute infectious diarrhea in this age group during the winter months. Infection with rotavirus presents with repeated vomiting and profuse, watery, foul–smelling stools for 5–7 days. Occasionally, rotavirus infection may result in enterocolitis with blood and mucus in the stool.
  Norwalk virus infection: occurs in school age children, typically causing "winter vomiting" illness. It usually lasts 1–2 days; myalgia and malaise are commonly associated.
- Bacterial causes of diarrhea: in North America, the common bacterial enteropathogens are *C. jejuni*, *E. coli*, *Shigella*, *Salmonella* and *Yersinia*. Bacterial enterocolitis often causes dysentery characterized by the passage of blood, mucus and polymorphonuclear leukocytes in the stools. Vomiting is less common than in viral infection. The diagnosis is made by stool culture, although there are certain features particular to the various pathogens:
  C. jejuni is often seen in children under 5 years of age.
  E. coli is associated with travel and ingestion of undercooked hamburgers. It may precede the onset of hemolytic uremic syndrome.
  Vibrio infection is more common in patients exposed to raw seafood or sea water.
  Shigella infection can result in high fever and seizures, especially in children < 5 years of age.
- Risk factors for development of bacteremia in children with bacterial diarrhea include < 1 year of age, immunodeficiency or immunosuppression, sickle cell disease (especially *Salmonella* infection) and pre–existing malnutrition; rarely, bacterial pathogens result in extraintestinal infection such as pneumonia and osteomyelitis.
- Antibiotic associated diarrhea: antibiotics may cause transient diarrhea that resolves after the antibiotic is stopped.
  Rarely, *C. difficile* colitis can occur spontaneously in the absence of antibiotic administration, though it is usually seen during or after treatment with antimicrobials (all antibiotics other than rifampicin and parenteral aminoglycosides have been implicated). Onset may occur up to 6 weeks following antibiotic administration. The clinical presentation can vary from mild diarrhea to severe disease with bloody stools, fever, toxicity, abdominal pain and distension. The diagnosis is made by the presence of *C. difficile* toxin and by a positive culture of *C. difficile* in fresh stool. Occasionally, the diagnosis must be made by colonoscopy, which reveals pseudomembranous colitis. Treatment is with vancomycin 1 g/1.73 m^2 per d p.o. div. q.i.d. for 14 d. Vancomycin is expensive. Metronidazole is also expensive but it may be less effective and associated with a higher relapse rate. It is a reasonable initial therapy in a patient who is not severely ill.

* Parasites:
    Giardia lamblia: this small bowel parasite is the most common parasitic cause of diarrhea in North America. Children may be asymptomatic or have diarrhea, flatulence, bloating, abdominal pain or weight loss. Vomiting is infrequent and there is no dysentery. Stools examined for ova and parasites are negative for trophozoites in up to 50% of cases. If *Giardia* is strongly suspected (if patient is from an endemic area or has been exposed to inland lake water or a camping trip, if there is *Giardia* in the household, or if signs and symptoms are of recent onset), the child may be treated empirically with quinacrine, metronidazole or furazolidone. Children with recurrent or persistent symptoms should be referred to a gastroenterologist.

    Entamoeba histolytica: although most severe cases are subacute, this parasite can cause severe dysentery with blood and mucus in stools. The most common extraintestinal manifestation is liver abscess. The diagnosis is made by serological and stool examinations and by the presence of fecal monocytes on a stool smear (in contrast to polymorphonuclear leukocytes in bacterial colitis or IBD). All stages of amebiasis, including asymptomatic carriers, require treatment with diiodohydroxyquin or metronidazole.

    Dientamoeba coli and *Blastocystis hominis*: these are parasites with an unclear correlation to symptoms. They are probably commensals rather than pathogens. If they are present in a concentration of > 5 per high power field in a child with recent onset of diarrhea, a course of treatment with metronidazole may be warranted.

    Cryptosporidium: this is a parasite of veterinary origin that primarily infests the small bowel but may also involve the colon. It causes acute, large volume, watery diarrhea that is self–limited in hosts with normal immunity. Suspect immunocompromise in the child with severe intractable disease; death may occur in these children due to fluid, electrolyte and nutritional deficiency. There is no known effective treatment. *Cryptosporidium* is a leading cause of morbidity and mortality in patients with AIDS.

Management

Most cases of acute diarrhea are self–limited. Symptomatic therapy and adequate hydration are often all that are required. Specific medications for infectious diarrhea are outlined in Table V.

1. Intravenous fluids
The first priority is assessment and treatment of dehydration. Admission and intravenous fluid therapy are usually indicated for patients who fulfill any of the following criteria:
* Under 3 months of age with bacterial diarrhea.
* Toxic or presence of underlying systemic illness.
* Severely dehydrated or cannot be rehydrated orally.
* Large volume, grossly bloody stools or significant abdominal pain.
* Compromised by chronic debilitating diseases, immunodeficiency or malnutrition.

2. Oral rehydration
Most children can be successfully rehydrated via the oral route. In the child < 2 years of age, use commercially prepared oral rehydration solutions (ORS) such as Gastrolyte, Lytren, Pedialyte RS or Ricelyte. In the child > 2 years of age, use an ORS if tolerated or clear fluids such as Gatorade

or quarter strength apple juice.
- The breast fed infant should continue to breast feed. ORS may be added as a supplement if there is significant dehydration.
- In formula fed infants and older children, calculate the volume of fluid required for rehydration, maintenance and replacement and divide into small aliquots given every 30–60 minutes. If this is tolerated and the hydration status is adequate, the child should be reweighed and may then be discharged home. Arrange for follow–up within 24 hours.
- Instruct the parents to continue administration of ORS or clear fluids for no longer than 24 hours. After 24 hours they should begin feeding with a diet low in lactose, high in starch and low in fat (BRAT diet, consisting of bananas, rice cereal, apple sauce and dry toast or crackers) and then onto a full regular diet, as tolerated. In formula fed children, formula should be reintroduced in reduced strength (one–half or one–fourth), increasing to full strength over 2 days. Diarrhea often continues or recurs. If the patient remains well hydrated and is gaining weight, advise the parents to persist with a gradual return to a regular diet.
- Parents should be instructed to return with the child if oral intake is not tolerated or if symptoms become worse.

Table V: Treatment of infectious diarrhea

Infection	Indication for treatment	Medications
Campylobacter jejuni	Systemically ill, severe pain, duration > 3 d	Erythromycin 40 mg/kg per d p.o. div. q6h for 5–7 d
Enteropathogenic *E. coli*	Always treat if patient is symptomatic; if systemically ill or toxic, use i.v. therapy	TMP–SMX 10 mg/kg per d as TMP p.o. b.i.d. (i.v. use: ampicillin 100 mg/kg per d div. q6h and gentamicin 5 mg/kg per d div. q8h)
Shigella	Always treat if patient is symptomatic	TMP–SMX 10 mg/kg per d as TMP p.o. b.i.d. or i.v. div. q12h or ampicillin 100 mg/kg per d p.o. or i.v. div. q6h
Salmonella	Treat if patient is systemically ill, < 1 yr old, has metastic disease or sickle cell disease, or is immunocompromised; do not treat chronic carriers	Ampicillin 100 mg/kg per d p.o. or i.v. div. q6h or amoxicillin 50 mg/kg per d p.o. div. q8h
Clostridium difficile Toxin positive	Watery or bloody diarrhea, pseudomembranes seen on colonoscopy	Metronidazole 15–25 mg/kg per d p.o. div. b.i.d. or t.i.d. (maximum dose 250 mg t.i.d.) or vancomycin 1 g/1.73 m^2 per d p.o. div. q.i.d. for 14 d
Aeromonas		TMP–SMX 10 mg/kg per d as TMP p.o. div. q12h for 5 d
Giardia lamblia	Always treat if patient is symptomatic or for epidemiological reason (e.g. child is in daycare)	Furazolidone 8 mg/kg per d p.o. div. q.i.d. for 7–10 d or quinacrine 6 mg/kg per d p.o. div. t.i.d. for 7 d or metronidazole 15 mg/kg per d p.o. div. t.i.d. for 5 d

TMP–SMX = trimethoprim–sulfamethoxazole

3. Medications
• Antidiarrheal and antinauseant medications should not be used in children with diarrhea or vomiting. They may mask symptoms and promote bacteremia, fluid loss and complications such as toxic megacolon.
  Drugs that should be avoided in children with acute diarrhea: diphenoxylate (Lomotil), loperamide (Imodium), paregoric, morphine, codeine, belladonna alkaloids (Donnagel, Donnatol, Diban), Pomalin, kaolin with pectin (Kaopectate).
• In general, antibiotic therapy should be withheld until culture results are available, unless the child appears ill. For treatment guidelines, see treatment of infectious diarrhea.

Key points

• In infants, consider extraintestinal causes of diarrhea such as UTI or otitis media.
• Bacteremia is common in infants < 3 months of age with bacterial colitis.
• Most children with acute infectious diarrhea can be orally rehydrated.
• Do not use antidiarrheal medications in children with acute diarrhea.

LIVER FAILURE

Liver failure occurs when the synthetic and excretory functions of the liver decline, compromising the clinical status of the child. Table VI outlines the common causes. Failure of synthetic function is reflected by a prolonged prothrombin time and decreased serum albumin; failure of excretory function is manifested by increased serum bilirubin and ammonia levels.

The clinical and biochemical manifestations of liver failure:
• Jaundice.
• GI bleeding due to portal hypertension.
• Ascites.
• Hepatic encephalopathy.
• Palmar erythema or spider angiomas.
• Hypoalbuminemia.
• Coagulopathy.
• Raised transaminases (AST, ALT) and alkaline phosphatase.
• Hyperammonemia.
Not all of these features are required to diagnose liver failure. Abnormal liver function tests (raised AST, ALT) may reflect liver damage but do not indicate liver failure per se. Similarly, portal hypertension may be seen in the absence of liver disease.

Evaluation

1. History
• In children with acute onset of liver failure, enquire about exposure to infectious agents or persons, blood products (including gamma globulin), tattoos, ear piercing, drugs and toxins (including anesthetic agents).
• Ask about travel and a family history of jaundice or liver disease.
• In the infant, ask about the pregnancy, birth weight, feeding history (inborn errors of

metabolism, galactosemia, hereditary fructose intolerance—HFI), hemolysis, anemia or maternal history of hepatitis.
- In children with known liver disease, determine if there are precipitating factors such as intercurrent infection (UTI, sepsis, primary bacterial peritonitis), dehydration, hypokalemic alkalosis (often due to overdiuresis), GI bleeding, high dietary protein intake or recent high volume paracentesis of ascitic fluid.

Table VI: Causes of liver failure

Type	All ages	Onset more common in newborn
Idiopathic	Cryptogenic cirrhosis	Idiopathic neonatal hepatitis
Infectious	Hepatitis B, hepatitis C; rarely hepatitis A, cytomegalovirus, Epstein–Barr virus, adenovirus, coxsackievirus, disseminated herpes, rubella, bacterial sepsis, leptospirosis	Hepatitis B, TORCH, syphilis
Vascular	Shock, hypoxemia, ischemia, veno–occlusive disease, acute Budd–Chiari's syndrome	
Toxic	Drugs (acetaminophen, salicylates, ketoconazole, phenytoin, valproic acid, iron, antineoplastic drugs); ethanol, CCl_4, halothane, penthrane, mushrooms (*Amanita phalloides*)	Parenteral nutrition
Metabolic	Alpha$_1$–antitrypsin deficiency, Reye's syndrome, Wilson's disease, hemochromatosis	Alpha$_1$–antitrypsin deficiency, tyrosinemia, galactosemia, GSD, Wolman's disease, HFI
Other		Biliary atresia, polycystic disease, congenital hepatic fibrosis

2. Examination
- Look for signs of liver failure.
- Examine the abdomen and determine liver size, consistency and tenderness.
- Perform a full neurological examination.
- Measure vital signs and look for orthostatic changes that may indicate acute or chronic blood loss.
- Perform a rectal examination to identify the presence of melena or fresh blood in the stool and test the stool specimen for occult blood (using a Hemoccult card).
- Children requiring emergency treatment for liver failure are invariably jaundiced, with the exception of patients with Reye's syndrome.
- There may be evidence of coagulopathy, including purpura, bleeding or oozing from areas subjected to trauma (gums, venepuncture sites).
- The initial signs of hepatic encephalopathy are confusion and vomiting, with progression to irritability, stupor, hyperreflexia and asterixis (liver flap). Obtundation, coma, areflexia, apnea and seizures are signs of end–stage encephalopathy.

3. Laboratory tests
- To assess severity of liver failure:
  Obtain blood for CBC, differential and platelet counts, PT, PTT, reticulocyte count and measurements of AST (SGOT), ALT (SPGT), alkaline phosphatase, bilirubin, total protein, albumin, ammonia, electrolytes, serum osmolality, BUN, creatinine, blood gases and glucose.
  Send a urine specimen for measurement of sodium, specific gravity and osmolatity.
- To determine etiology of liver failure:
  When the cause is unknown, send specimens of blood for hepatitis serological examination (hepatitis A IgM, B–surface antigen, B–surface antibody, B–core antibody and C–antibody) and blood culture. Send urine samples for urinalysis and culture in all cases.
  Other investigations that may be ordered as indicated include: toxic screen, measurements of serum iron, ferritin, copper, ceruloplasmin, alpha$_1$–antitrypsin, syphilis serological examination, TORCH titers and acute viral titers for coxsackievirus, adenovirus and reovirus. Measurements of urine reducing substances, organic acids, amino acids and a 24 hour urine specimen for copper measurement may also be ordered as indicated.
  Obtain a specimen of ascitic fluid for culture when peritonitis is suspected and perform an eye examination (including slit–lamp examination) to look for Kayser–Fleischer rings as evidence of Wilson's disease.

Management

1. Principles of emergency treatment
- Reverse hepatic encephalopathy by treating the metabolic disturbances and any precipitating factors.
- Stop GI bleeding.
- Prevent onset of hepatorenal syndrome by careful fluid management and early recognition of decreased renal function (as shown by oliguria or increased serum creatinine level).
- Rule out and treat sepsis and hypoglycemia.
- Institute careful nutritional management.

2. The unstable child
The following steps are recommended for the acutely ill child with encephalopathy or bleeding (consult a gastroenterologist when possible):
- Assess and maintain airway, breathing and circulation: give oxygen by mask, start a large bore intravenous line, check blood sugar level by dextrostix and send blood specimens for investigations. Infuse 10% with maintenance Na and K dextrose at a rate according to the patient's fluid status.
- If there is suspicion of sepsis: begin therapy with ampicillin 200 mg/kg per d i.v. div. q6h and gentamicin 5 mg/kg per d i.v. div. q8h after cultures have been obtained.
- Insert the largest nasogastric tube the child will tolerate and perform lavage with 5 mL/kg of room temperature normal saline.
  If there is bleeding, treat aggressively with antacids, H$_2$–blockers (cimetidine, ranitidine) or vasopressin.
  If the PT is prolonged > 3 seconds over control values, give vitamin K, 1–5 mL i.v. or s.c. daily, whether the patient is bleeding or not.

If PT and PTT are markedly prolonged, give fresh frozen plasma (FFP) 5–10 mL/kg i.v. over 30–60 min.
- Treat encephalopathy by decreasing ammonia production as follows:
  Give lactulose through a nasogastric tube, 1–2 mL/kg q4h, until profuse, watery diarrhea occurs. When stools are watery and clear, decrease the amount and frequency of lactulose. Lactulose may cause abdominal distention or discomfort.
  If lactulose is not tolerated, give neomycin 50 mg/kg per d through a nasogastric tube div. q6h. Lactulose and neomycin do not need to be given concurrently.
  If the child is constipated and is not receiving lactulose, treat with an enema or magnesium citrate 4 mL/kg via nasogastric tube.
- Carefully monitor fluid status with strict intake and output measurements. Children with hepatic failure may have oliguria due to the hepatorenal syndrome or established acute tubular necrosis.
  Diagnosis of hepatorenal syndrome: chronic liver disease with ascites, slow onset azotemia, good renal tubular function (urine osmolality greater than that of serum, urine sodium concentration very low [< 10 mmol/L or 10 mEq/L], urine to serum creatinine ratio > 30), no sustained benefit from intravascular volume infusion.
  Intravenous albumin is indicated in children with oliguria due to poor renal perfusion or respiratory embarrassment secondary to ascites. The dose is 1 g/kg (4 mL/kg of 25% solution) infused over 1–2 h i.v. and repeated p.r.n. or q12h.
  Diuretics may be indicated for the treatment of the child with ascites or oliguria. Frequently monitor and maintain serum electrolyte levels as near to normal as possible. The total body sodium is usually high and potassium low; use low sodium or sodium free i.v. fluids (10% dextrose in water with or without one–fourth normal saline) and, if potassium losing diuretics are used, add potassium to the i.v. fluid and give spironolactone.
- Nutrition must be maintained:
  Branched–chain amino acid solutions, given i.v. (Hepatamine) or p.o. (Hepatic Aid), or special enteral formulas (Portagen or Pregestemil) are often required.
- Monitor the following laboratory values:
  Every 12 hours initially: CBC, platelet count, PT, PTT, ammonia, glucose, serum osmolality, electrolytes, BUN, creatinine, and urine electrolytes and osmolality.
  Daily: bilirubin, AST, ALT, alkaline phosphatase, albumin levels, and blood and urine cultures.
  Many children with acute liver failure require urinary catheter and central venous pressure (CVP) line placement to monitor fluid status accurately.

3. The stable child
- The child with mild chronic encephalopathy from liver failure can be managed as follows:
  Lactulose: 1–2 mL/kg per dose via nasogastric tube q4–6h in patients in hepatic coma; decrease dose and frequency when encephalopathy resolves.
  Neomycin: 50 mg/kg per d p.o. or nasogastric tube div. q6–8h.
  Albumin: 1 g/kg per dose i.v. over 15–30 min.
  Furosemide: 1.0 mg/kg i.v. or p.o.
  Chlorothiazide: 20–40 mg/kg per d p.o. div. q12h.
  Hydrochlorothiazide: 2–5 mg/kg per d p.o. div. q12h.
  Spironolactone: 1–3 mg/kg per d p.o. div. q12h.

Ranitidine, cimetidine, vasopressin: see upper GI bleeding.
- Admit the patient and place him/her on a high carbohydrate diet with a largely vegetable protein intake, the quantity of which will vary with the degree of encephalopathy and the serum ammonia level. Do not routinely give a low protein diet because malnutrition may result.
- Prescribe lactulose to give 1–2 soft stools daily (10–30 mL/d in the older child and 2.5 mL b.i.d. in children < 1 year of age).
- Diuretics may be given to the patient with ascites. Always include a potassium sparing diuretic such as spironolactone.

Disposition

Admit all children with acute liver failure. Patients with encephalopathy or GI bleeding should be managed in the ICU.

Key points

- The initial management of the child with liver failure includes diagnosis and treatment of sepsis, hypoglycemia, encephalopathy and GI bleeding.
- Decreased urine output in the patient with liver failure may be due to acute tubular necrosis or hepatorenal syndrome.

GENERAL SURGERY
Geoffrey Blair and Grant Miller

CHAPTER 7

INTRODUCTION

Pediatric general surgery deals with the unique physiology and surgical diseases of children. This involves a broad spectrum of conditions, both congenital and acquired, including soft tissue lesions, thoracic noncardiac conditions, abdominal pathology (particularly gastrointestinal) and the management of multisystem trauma. There is some overlap with urology, orthopedics and otolaryngology, plastic and reconstructive surgery.

Many conditions are congenital, and the understanding and recognition of these conditions requires a knowledge of their embryological origin. Some surgical diseases occur within certain narrow age ranges which allow for a limited differential diagnosis. The diagnosis can be made, in most cases, by the clinical history and physical examination, with often only simple investigations required for confirmation.

PREOPERATIVE CONSIDERATIONS

Anesthesia

All complex cases should be discussed with the anesthetist involved. It is unusual that the pathology is such that you cannot take a little time to correct fluid and electrolyte disorders.

Preoperative teaching

- When reasonable, it is worthwhile to prepare and comfort children in advance of what to expect postoperatively. Such things as management of patient controlled analgesia (PCA) is best taught preoperatively.
- Therapists involved in postoperative chest physiotherapy appreciate the opportunity to see and teach patients preoperatively.
- Psychologists may be available to assist with postoperative pain management.
- Nursing staff should be made aware of the types of tubes or drains that may be used and any special nursing requirements for postoperative care so that they can adequately prepare the child.

Bowel preparation

1. Washout
- Indicated for elective colon and rectal procedures (e.g. anorectoplasty, colostomy closure, pullthrough for Hirschsprung's disease, etc.). Not indicated for small bowel surgery.
- "Golytely" 30 mL/kg per h given by small nasogastric tube for 6 h; continue for 2 more hours if the effluent is not clear.
- Maxeran may help if nausea or vomiting occurs.
- In the presence of a colostomy, the mucous fistula or rectum should be washed out with saline enemas of 150 mL × 3.

2. Antimicrobial preparation
• Use an antibiotic with broad enteric coverage (e.g. cefoxitin 40 mg/kg).
• A single dose given on induction of anesthesia may be adequate.

Prophylactic antibiotics

• There have been no adequate studies of surgical antimicrobial prophylaxis in children. If given
  for clean cases that involve the insertion of a foreign body or for clean contaminated cases,
  the antibiotic should be administered intravenously within the hour preceding the start of the
  operation.
• Clean cases and upper gastrointestinal tract or biliary tract: cefazolin 25 mg/kg.
• Clean or contaminated cases of the GI tract (i.e. large bowel or rectum): cefoxitin 40 mg/kg.
• For neonates: ampicillin 25 mg/kg plus gentamicin 2.5 mg/kg.
• Contaminated cases require a full course of antibiotics.

Endocarditis prophylaxis

• Indicated for any child with a congenital cardiac lesion. Recommended by the American Heart
  Association.
• Oral or respiratory tract procedures: ampicillin 50 mg/kg (or clindamycin 10 mg/kg) i.v. on
  induction of anesthesia and half the dose 6 h postoperative.
• Genitourinary or gastrointestinal procedures:
  Ampicillin 50 mg/kg plus gentamicin 2 mg/kg on induction of anesthesia and half the dose
  of ampicillin 6 h postoperative.
  Or, vancomycin 20 mg/kg plus gentamicin 1.5 mg/kg (maximum 50 mg) on induction; repeat
  vancomycin 8 h postoperative.

Laboratory tests

• There are no routine tests. Bloodwork should only be done when clinically indicated.
• Blood should be typed and cross–matched for any case in which you anticipate that blood loss
  could exceed 10% of blood volume (i.e. blood loss of ~10 mL/kg).

NPO orders

• < 1 yr old: may have breast milk until 6 h preoperative and clear fluids until 3 h preoperative.
• 1–5 yr old: may have solids until 8 h preoperative and clear fluids until 6 h preoperative.
• < 5 yr old: n.p.o. 8 h preoperative.

POSTOPERATIVE CONSIDERATIONS

"AIDS" mnemonic to postoperative orders:
    4 **A**'s: analgesics, antiemetics, antibiotics, activity.
    2 **I**'s: intravenous fluids, investigations.
    3 **D**'s: dressings, drugs, drains.
    1 **S**: signs to be observed.

Transfusion of blood products

- Always discuss with the surgeon and the parents where appropriate.
- Transfusion of 10 mL/kg increases Hgb 25–30 g/L.
- Unnecessary to transfuse if Hgb > 80 g/L and not actively bleeding.

Feeding protocol

- Bowel sounds are not reliable.
- Small intestine ileus resolves within hours postoperatively.
- Gastric emptying returns approximately 24 hours postoperative and is heralded by decreased and clearer gastric drainage.
- Colonic ileus takes 3–4 days to resolve and is heralded by the passage of flatus or stool.
- In general, if the abdomen is soft and not distended and the patient is hungry and has passed gas, then (s)he is ready to eat.
- There is no evidence that a graduated diet is of any benefit.
- If you are unsure if the child will tolerate feeds, try clear fluids first and if tolerated, then feed ad lib.
- If vomiting or retching occurs, then do not hesitate to reinsert a nasogastric tube as it is most likely the ileus has not resolved.

Activity

There are very few indications to restrict a child's activity postoperatively and this should be done only in exceptional circumstances. If in doubt, check with the surgeon.

SURGICAL DRAINS AND TUBES

Nasogastric tubes

- Used for decompression of the stomach and upper GI tract.
- Essential in any bowel obstruction (relief of aerophagia).
- Single lumen tubes must be on intermittent low suction.
- Sump type tubes work on either intermittent or continuous low suction.
- All tubes need to be irrigated frequently (i.e. q2–4h) and air should be injected into the sump port q2–4h. If not working, check the position.
- Size guideline: infant, 8–10 Fr.; child, 10–14 Fr.

Gastrostomy and jejunostomy tubes

- Used primarily for feeding, except some gastrostomy tubes are used for decompression of gas bloat symptoms.
- Infections of the site are unusual.
- Skin irritation is common and usually responds to local wound care with regular cleansing (water and mild soap).
- Avoid cleansing with hydrogen peroxide and avoid dressings, both of which tend to promote

skin irritation.
- A paste of sulcrate and desitin applied b.i.d. may be beneficial for skin irritation.
- Troublesome skin irritation may be a sign that the tube is leaking or is an inappropriate size.
- Avoid latex catheters except for temporary replacements.
- If the catheter falls out, an attempt should be made at reinserting the same catheter or inserting another catheter posthaste. A Foley catheter will do when necessary. Aspiration of gastric juice from the catheter is an adequate check for placement of gastrostomy tubes. Replaced jejunostomy tubes should ideally be checked by contrast radiography prior to using (except for chronic, well established sites).
- If using a balloon catheter to replace a jejunostomy, do not inflate the balloon (causes a bowel obstruction).

Wound drains

- Several drains are used and are usually dictated by surgeon preference (e.g. Penrose, Davol, JP, Jackson Pratt, Hemovac, etc.).
- Usually used to drain unwanted fluid collections such as pus or lymph or occasionally after a bowel or urinary tract anastomosis.
- Drainage of < 30 mL/24 h of serous fluid indicates that the drain can be removed (usually 3–4 days postop), but always check with the surgeon first.

Chest tubes

- Size guideline: infant, 10–12 Fr.; preschool, 12–16 Fr.; child, 16–20 Fr.; adolescent, 20–28 Fr.
- Use one size larger if draining an exudate.
- It must be to underwater seal and suction should usually be used.
- The tube (for a pneumothorax) can be removed when there is radiological evidence of resolution of the pneumothorax and there has been no further bubbling in the bottle system while deep breathing or coughing for 24–48 hours while on underwater seal and off suction.
- The tube is preferably removed during expiration. It should be removed rapidly and the wound dressed with petrolatum gauze to prevent air from entering the chest. Repeat a chest X–ray in approximately 4 hours.

WOUND CARE

- A primarily closed wound is sealed within 24 hours and a dressing is not required after that time except for patient preference.
- Shower and sponge bathing may begin after 24 hours postoperative.
- Wounds left open require frequent dressing changes with saline moistened gauze. These wounds may be secondarily closed after 3–5 days if granulation tissue formed is healthy.
- Saline is the only safe solution for open wounds; antiseptic solutions tend to cause tissue injury.
- In an otherwise healthy wound, the timing of suture or staple removal depends on the location and tissue tension: head and neck, 3 days; thorax, 7–10 days; extremity, 10–14 days.
- Adhesive strips used for wound closure can be allowed to simply fall off on their own or removed after 1–2 weeks.

PAIN MANAGEMENT

- Pain management is a significant problem for the surgical patient.
- Intravenous morphine can be given as a continuous infusion or as a bolus therapy.
- Check with the hospital pharmacist as most hospitals have guidelines for the use of narcotics in children.
- In general, a continuous infusion of 10–40 µg/kg per h of morphine is safe in monitored children > 6 months of age.
- Patient controlled analgesia is very useful and, in general terms, if the child can play video games, (s)he can be taught to use PCA.
- Oral acetaminophen, in combination with codeine, is very effective when oral intake is allowed.
- Most hospitals now have pain management teams, who can be very useful and involve psychologists, nurses, surgeons and anesthetists.

COMMON POSTOPERATIVE PROBLEMS

Fever

- Think of the 4 W's: wind, water, wound, "w" (v)eins.
- Atelectasis is the most common cause of fever in the first 24–48 hours postoperative.
- Urinary tract infections are usually associated with indwelling urinary catheters and usually occur around day 3 postop.
- Wound infections occur 3–5 days postop. Leaving the dressing off after 24 hours allows for earlier pickup of wound infections,
- If temperature > 38.5 °C, draw blood for CBC and blood cultures; obtain urine for routine and microscopic analysis; obtain a chest X–ray.
- Peripheral i.v. sites and central i.v. catheters are often the site of infection in children.

Low urine output

- After a major procedure and particularly if i.v. narcotics or epidural morphine are used, a child may not be able to void. In/out catheterize the bladder q6h p.r.n.
- Urine output is considered low if < 0.5 mL/kg per h.
- Assess volume status and urine specific gravity.
- Usually due to volume deficit or a blocked catheter. If the catheter is patent, give an i.v. bolus of crystalloid (0.9% NaCl) 10 mL/kg given over 15 min and reassess.

Hyponatremia

- In an otherwise normal postoperative child, this is almost always due to inadequate sodium intake, excessive losses (i.e. nasogastric losses) or excess hypotonic fluid. This is potentially a serious problem and should be addressed early. The sodium level can drop to dangerous levels in only a few hours following surgery.
- Electrolytes should be checked q2–3 d in a fasting child.
- Rule out hyperglycemia (pseudohyponatremia).
- Assess volume status, replace ongoing losses (i.e. normal saline for nasogastric losses), and

restrict fluid if appropriate.

Ileus (postlaparotomy)

- In the absence of ongoing significant intra–abdominal pathology, a small bowel ileus resolves within hours of surgery.
- A gastric ileus will last for 24–48 hours (heralded by the return of hunger).
- A colonic ileus will last for 3–4 days and is heralded by the passage of flatus or stool.
- Prolonged ileus may occur in a variety of situations (i.e. gastroschisis, following repair of intestinal atresia or malrotation, ongoing inflammation such as pancreatitis, etc.).

Small bowel obstruction

- Suspect obstruction if the patient has had a period of return of bowel function postoperatively, followed by the onset of bilious green emesis, abdominal distension and obstipation.
- Confirm by physical examination and abdominal X–rays; in addition, check electrolytes.
- Suck and drip (intravenous and nasogastric tube); consider laparotomy especially if there are signs of peritonitis, elevated WBC or metabolic acidosis.

Bleeding

- Suspect in the patient with postoperative tachycardia or hypotension.
- Remove dressings and check wound for signs of bleeding.
- Apply direct pressure to visible bleeding or wound hematoma (minimum 10 minutes).
- Check CBC, coagulation profile and family history.
- Cross–match if concealed bleeding (i.e. intra–abdominal, intrathoracic, etc.).
- Transfuse if Hgb < 70 and hemorrhage is not controlled.

Sepsis

- Presentation of sepsis may be very subtle in neonates.
- Beware of the surgical neonate reported by an experienced nurse to "not look right".
- Irritability, hypothermia, tachycardia, apnea and bradycardia can all be signs of sepsis.
- CBC, blood cultures, urinalysis, urine culture, chest X–ray.
- Monitor carefully.
- Err on the side of caution and start empiric broad spectrum antibiotic coverage early.
- Check intravenous sites for signs of sepsis.

SURGICAL EMERGENCIES IN THE NEWBORN

Externally visible anomalies

- Imperforate anus
- Gastroschisis
- Omphalocele

1. Imperforate anus
- Entails a wide spectrum of anorectal anomalies (simple or complex) and includes: covered anus, absent anus, cloaca, etc.
- Arises as a result of faulty development and partitioning of the original primitive cloaca into discrete urinary, genital and anorectal passages.
- In most cases of imperforate anus, there is a fistula which may be externally visible on the perineum, vaginal fourchette or scrotum, or into the urethra, bladder neck or vagina.
- An "anterior ectopic anus" is actually an imperforate anus with a wide short fistula to the perineum. Undertake a careful examination of the perineum.
- Passage of meconium in the urine of a male indicates a fistula to the urethra or bladder neck.
- In females, meconium from the vagina indicates a rectovaginal fistula.
- Consider the VACTERL (vertebra, anorectum, cardiac, trachea, esophagus, renal, limb) association of anomalies in these children.
- A spinal ultrasound will help to exclude an associated spinal cord defect (i.e. tethered cord, anterior lipomeningocele, etc.).
- Initial care includes nasogastric decompression and intravenous fluids.
- Almost all of these children need a colostomy in the first few days of life, with planned reconstruction of the anorectum at approximately 6 months of age and, later, closure of the colostomy.

2. Omphalocele
- It is an opening of variable size, sometimes with only a few loops of bowel within the base of the umbilical cord, or it may be a huge defect containing the liver and most of the gut.
- The contents are enclosed within a translucent membrane, which is the expanded base of the umbilical cord (this sac may be ruptured at birth but usually remains intact).
- The viscera appear normal but the intestine is malrotated.
- The presence of a herniated liver is considered a "giant omphalocele", the closure of which is usually extremely difficult.
- Large omphaloceles are associated with hypoplasia of the abdominal wall. The viscera may not be reducible, preventing primary closure.
- Cardiac anomalies are seen in 25%; pulmonary hypoplasia is sometimes seen in association with "giant omphaloceles"; 50% of omphaloceles will have significant congenital problems in other systems.

3. Gastroschisis
- This is a defect of the abdominal wall, almost always to the right of the umbilicus with the umbilical cord inserted on the left edge of it. There is no covering and only the intestine is eviscerated.
- Exposure to the amniotic fluid results in inflammation, thickening and foreshortening of the bowel.
- There is a higher incidence of intestinal atresia but other anomalies are no more common than in otherwise normal newborns.

Management of gastroschisis/omphalocele

- Intravenous fluids (large third space losses especially in gastroschisis).

- Nasogastric tube.
- Cover the exposed viscera with saline gauze and plastic wrap or a plastic bowel bag.
- Prevent hypothermia.
- Ampicillin and gentamicin.
- Abdominal wall closure or application of a synthetic pouch should be done within the first 24 hours of life.
- Those that cannot be closed primarily are usually managed with a pouch of synthetic material (silo), which is sutured to the fascia edges and is made smaller each day (over 4–7 days) to gradually reduce the viscera.
- Complications include: respiratory failure, sepsis, splanchnic ischemia.
- TPN is usually required as there is often a prolonged ileus, especially in gastroschisis where it may be 3 weeks or more before enteral feeds are tolerated.

Surgical causes of respiratory distress

- Signs of respiratory distress: respiratory rate > 40/min; chest wall retractions, tracheal tug, nasal flaring, cyanosis, choking, episodic apnea and stridor.
- Surgically correctable causes include: choanal atresia, Pierre Robin's syndrome, laryngeal obstructions, congenital lobar emphysema, congenital diaphragmatic hernia, chylothorax, tracheoesophageal fistula.

1. Tracheal obstruction
- Vascular rings and mediastinal masses can compress and obstruct the trachea.
- Usually present with expiratory and inspiratory wheeze or stridor.
- Chest X–ray may show compression of the airway and/or the tumor.
- Other investigations that may be necessary include: esophagogram, esophagoscopy, bronchoscopy, arteriogram.
- Treatment is based on the findings.

2. Congenital lobar emphysema
- A check type valve obstruction of an upper lobe or middle lobe bronchus results in critical overexpansion of the affected lobe.
- Respiratory distress may take several days to weeks to develop.
- The emphysematous lobe compresses normal lung and causes mediastinal shift.
- Diagnosis is confirmed by chest X–ray.
- Bronchoscopy may successfully remove an obstructing mucous plug or foreign body.
- Immediate thoracotomy and lobectomy is often required.
- Asymptomatic patients can be observed carefully as a small number will resolve.

3. Congenital diaphragmatic hernia
- Usually a left–sided posteriolateral defect with herniation of the intestine and spleen into the chest. Liver and stomach may also be herniated.
- It is associated with pulmonary hypertension and respiratory distress due to pulmonary hypoplasia.
- A vicious cycle may occur, caused by hypoxia and acidosis which worsens the pulmonary hypertension and right to left shunt, resulting in rapid deterioration.

- The baby usually has some degree of respiratory distress, a cardiac apex displaced to the right and a scaphoid abdomen.
- Treatment is aimed at preventing this vicious cycle.
- Supplemental oxygen, nasogastric decompression, normothermia and acid–base balance are important.
- Intubation and aggressive ventilation management are often required.
- Overall mortality rate is 50%.
- Operative repair is most often delayed until the baby is stabilized; this can take days.

4. Other lesions
- Cystic adenomatoid malformation, pulmonary cysts and lung sequestrations can cause respiratory distress.
- These lesions should be excised even if asymptomatic as they can be complicated by infection or malignancy (pleuropulmonary blastoma).

5. Pneumothorax or pneumomediastinum
- Alveolar rupture is usually caused by excessive intratracheal pressure, often during resuscitation.
- Air tracks along the bronchovascular plane, producing pulmonary interstitial emphysema (PIE).
- Further dissection of air can lead to pneumomediastinum or pneumothorax.
- Pneumomediastinum can be associated with airway compression, but it is unusual to require decompressive skin incisions above the clavicles.
- Pneumothorax should be treated by chest tube insertion and underwater seal drainage.

GI tract obstruction

- Cardinal signs are: bilious green emesis, abdominal distension, failure to pass meconium.
- Causes: esophageal atresia (± tracheoesophageal fistula), malrotation with volvulus, duodenal atresia, intestinal atresia, meconium ileus, enteric duplication cyst, Hirschsprung's disease, necrotizing enterocolitis (NEC).
- As you progress down the GI tract, vomiting yields to abdominal distension and then to failure to pass meconium as the first presenting or dominant sign.
- Emesis is small and immediate if due to an esophageal obstruction, forceful (with some delay) if due to gastric outlet obstruction, and voluminous and green with more distal obstructions.
- Nonbilious emesis suggests an obstruction above the level of the Vater's ampulla or a nonobstructive cause such as gastroesophageal reflux.
- Beware of the child who vomits green material; bilious emesis is due to a surgically correctable cause until proved otherwise; this is distal to the Vater's ampulla.
- Abdominal distension is more prominent with a more distal obstruction (i.e. large intestine or distal small intestine).
- A maternal history of polyhydramnios should raise the suspicion of a proximal GI tract obstruction (i.e. esophageal or duodenal atresia).
- Rectal bleeding may indicate intestinal vascular compromise in such conditions as NEC and volvulus.
- Sepsis may manifest as a pale, grey, cyanotic infant with hypothermia, bradycardia, hypoglycemia, acidosis and apnea.

1. Emergency management
- Fluid resuscitation plus ventilatory support.
- Correction of electrolyte and metabolic disorders.
- Nasogastric decompression (8–10 Fr. tube).
- Emergency cross–match.
- Antibiotics (i.e. ampicillin and gentamicin).
- Prevent hypothermia.

2. Investigations
- Rectal examination and plain abdominal X–ray.
- Double bubble = duodenal atresia (consider volvulus if the child is very ill or if there is a small amount of gas distal to the duodenum).
- Pneumatosis intestinalis or portal vein gas = NEC or volvulus.
- On a cross table, prone lateral abdominal X–ray:
  Rectum diameter < colon diameter = Hirschsprung's disease.
- A contrast enema X–ray may help to rule out Hirschsprung's disease, meconium ileus, malrotation, intestinal atresia (microcolon).

3. Specific conditions
- Esophageal atresia:
  Usually (85%) associated with tracheoesophageal fistula (usually distal TEF).
  May be associated with the VACTERL association of anomalies.
  It is a defect in the normal separation and partitioning of the primitive foregut into esophagus and trachea. May be suspected on a prenatal ultrasound if polyhydramnios present and the stomach is not visualized.
  Newborn is unable to swallow his/her saliva and appears very mucousy. May aspirate, causing choking, coughing and respiratory distress.
  If a distal TEF is present, the stomach can become very distended and cause respiratory embarrassment. Reflux of acid may cause chemical pneumonitis.
  Diagnosis is confirmed by the inability to pass a nasogastric tube (8 or 10 Fr.)—passed approximately 11 cm from the nare. A tube of too small a caliber will curl and give a false finding.
  Chest or abdominal X–ray will confirm the presence of the catheter tip in a proximal esophageal pouch (a small volume of air injected at the time of the X–ray makes an excellent and safe contrast medium). Air in the stomach = distal TEF.
  Assess the vertebral bodies and cardiac silhouette for defects and lung parenchyma for pneumonitis.
  Echocardiogram (cardiac defect and aortic arch position) and abdominal ultrasound (renal defect) preoperatively.
  High risk TEF:
  Birth weight < 1,500 grams or major cardiac anomaly.
  Emergency gastrostomy tube ± thoracotomy to ligate TEF.
  Delay repair of esophageal atresia.
  Low risk TEF:
  Thoracotomy day 1 or 2 of life.
  Ligation of fistula and repair of esophageal atresia.

Esophageal atresia without a TEF:
Usually not amenable to early primary repair (gap is too long).
Continuous suction on the pouch and gastrostomy feeds allow the baby to grow, and repair is often achieved by 3–4 months of age.
TEF without esophageal atresia:
So called H–type TEF occurs in the neck and not the thorax.
Usually delayed diagnosis in a child with variable choking spells following feeds or with aspiration pneumonitis.
Diagnosis is usually confirmed by cineradiography and/or endoscopy.
Repair is via a cervical approach.
- Duodenal atresia:
An embryological error in recanalization of the primitive duodenum in the region of the Vater's ampulla.
Usually vomit bile.
Abdominal X–ray demonstrates a "double bubble" sign.
May be a maternal history of polyhydramnios.
30% have Down's syndrome.
May be a membranous web or complete atresia with a narrow or wide gap ± an annular pancreas.
Treatment is by duodenoduodenostomy or duodenojejunostomy.
- Intestinal atresia (jejunoileal atresia):
In most cases due to an intrauterine vascular accident.
May be single or multiple atresias.
May be loss of a large portion of intestine (short gut syndrome).
Usually have a microcolon on contrast enema.
Treatment is by resection or tapering of the proximal, very dilated and atonic segment with either an anastomosis or enterostomy.
- Malrotation and volvulus:
An error in the normal 270° counterclockwise rotation of the intestine around the superior mesenteric artery (SMA) axis results in the absence of the broad fixation of the small intestine mesentery along a line from the ligament of Treitz to the ileocecal junction in the right iliac fossa.
The resulting narrow base of the mesentery puts the intestine at risk for twisting around the SMA axis, resulting in vascular compromise (volvulus). This causes luminal obstruction and intestinal ischemia.
Emergency surgery is necessary to prevent intestinal infarction.
May be associated with Ladd's bands, which are peritoneal bands running from the right posterolateral abdominal wall across the duodenum to the abnormally located cecum.
Volvulus usually occurs in the first week of life. Presents with signs of intestinal obstruction as well as shock ± bloody stools.
Abdominal X–rays are nonspecific with signs of obstruction.
A contrast upper GI study or enema should be done if the child is hemodynamically stable, otherwise the clinical picture with plain X–ray signs of obstruction are sufficient grounds for an emergency laparotomy.
Correction is by division of Ladd's bands and placing the intestine in a nonrotated position, with the large bowel on the left and the small bowel on the right. This results in widening

of the base of the mesentery.
- Meconium ileus:
  Mechanical obstruction of the small intestine due to inspissated meconium, which is usually early manifestation of cystic fibrosis.
  Presentation similar to intestinal atresia.
  Plain X–rays reveal: dilated loops of small bowel of varying size, relative absence of air–fluid levels, ground–glass or stippled effect (usually on the right side) and/or random areas of eggshell calcifications.
  Calcifications usually indicate prenatal perforation, resulting in sterile meconium peritonitis. If perforation is suspected, then laparotomy is indicated.
  If no perforation is suspected, then the diagnosis is confirmed by water soluble contrast enema which will reveal a microcolon and inspissated meconium in the terminal ileum.
  This may be therapeutic in relieving the obstruction due to the osmotic effect of the contrast. Adequate hydration is necessary to prevent hypovolemia.
  If this is unsuccessful, then laparotomy is required with enterotomy and irrigation of the intestine with saline or acetylcysteine.
  A temporary ileostomy may be required and can be used to facilitate further washouts p.r.n.
  Cystic fibrosis must be ruled out.
- Enteric duplication:
  Error in recanalization of the solid stage of the primitive gut results in a double lumen. May occur anywhere along the GI tract but most commonly it is a local phenomenon at the ileocecal region.
  Usually a closed cyst but it may be tubular and communicating forms exist. It occurs on the mesenteric side and shares a common blood supply with the adjacent bowel.
  Occasionally it may be lined with gastric mucosa, which can be detected by Meckel's scan and can lead to bleeding or perforation. The commonest manifestation is obstruction due to compression by an enlarging cyst or intussusception of a small cyst.
  Usually not diagnosed until laparotomy but sometimes an ultrasound may be diagnostic.
  Treatment is by resection of the affected portion of the intestine.
- Hirschsprung's disease (aganglionosis):
  Absence of myenteric and submucosal plexus ganglion cells. Involves the rectum and/or varying amount of the adjacent large bowel.
  Involvement of the small intestine, including total intestinal aganglionosis, is rare. Usually only the rectum and lower sigmoid colon are involved.
  There is failure of receptive relaxation of the affected bowel, stopping peristalsis and causing obstruction. The intestine proximal to the aganglionic segment becomes dilated with hypertrophy of the muscularis propria and impaction by stool. The commonest presentation is neonatal intestinal obstruction; sometimes it presents later with severe constipation and failure to thrive.
  All have delayed passage of meconium as a newborn. Fecal stasis can lead to a life threatening enterocolitis, requiring fluid resuscitation, antibiotics, colonic irrigations and emergency colostomy.
  X–ray may reveal: multiple dilated loops of bowel with air–fluid levels consistent with a distal obstruction, absence of rectal gas, rectal diameter < colonic diameter on a prone cross table abdominal X–ray. Contrast enema may show an empty rectum which is tapered plus delayed (> 24 hours) emptying of contrast.

Diagnosis is confirmed by rectal biopsy.

Treatment is by defunctioning colostomy (in ganglionated portion of bowel).

At approximately 3 months of age, a pullthrough procedure is done to anastomose ganglionated bowel to the sphincters just above the dentate line.

- Small left colon, meconium plug syndrome, immature left colon:

  Poorly understood conditions which may mimic Hirschsprung's disease.

  All are probably a form of transient motility disorder of the colon.

  Not associated with cystic fibrosis.

  May be a maternal history of diabetes.

  Their natural history is spontaneous resolution.

  Rule out Hirschsprung's disease by rectal biopsy.

- Necrotizing enterocolitis:

  Most common surgical emergency in the newborn. The cause is unclear but ICU acquired bacteria colonize the gut and breach the intestinal mucosa and the immature gut barrier defenses. The bowel is damaged by the products of inflammation, allowing further bacteria invasion and bowel injury.

  Most common site is the terminal ileum, followed by the colon.

  Most common physical findings are: abdominal distension, vomiting or gastric retention, gross or occult blood per rectum, physiological instability.

  Laboratory findings are nonspecific but include: low WBC, thrombocytopenia (< 150,000), metabolic acidosis.

  Radiology is the cornerstone of the diagnosis and the plain X–ray findings are: bowel distension, pneumotosis intestinalis, portal vein gas, pneumoperitoneum, fixed dilated intestinal loops.

  Treatment is nonoperative unless there is evidence of intestinal necrosis, intestinal perforation, or obstruction due to stricture.

  Nonoperative treatment is supportive and includes: fluid and electrolyte correction, gut rest with nasogastric decompression, systemic antibiotics aimed at enteric organisms and coagulase negative *Staphylococcus* (cefotaxime and vancomycin), close observation and serial abdominal X–rays for 24–48 hours, gut rest and antibiotics times 7 days.

  Perforation is treated by resection of necrotic bowel and exteriorization of both ends of the intestine. Intestinal continuity re–established when the baby is fully recovered and gaining weight.

OTHER PEDIATRIC SURGICAL CONDITIONS

Mediastinal masses

- Relatively common in infants and children.
- Most are asymptomatic.
- Can be classified based on whether it is cystic or solid and its location (Table I).
- Ultrasound, CT scan and MRI are important adjuvant studies.
- Serum alpha$_1$–fetoprotein and beta hCG may also be useful.
- Most benign or congenital mediastinal masses are asymptomatic.
- Neoplasms are more likely to present with cough, esophageal obstruction or airway obstruction.

• With the exception of lymphoma and Hodgkin's disease, most of these masses should be excised to confirm the pathology and to prevent complications from infection or tumor growth.

Table I: Classification of mediastinal masses

Location	Cystic	Solid
Anterior	Dermoid cyst, thymic cyst, cystic hygroma	Germ cell tumor, teratoma, lymphoma, Hodgkin's disease, thymoma
Middle	Bronchogenic cyst	Lymphoma, Hodgkin's disease
Posterior	Enterogenous cyst	Neurogenic tumor

1. Superior mediastinal syndrome
• Includes superior vena cava obstruction and airway obstruction. The children can deteriorate or obstruct rapidly.
• Presents as: cough, hoarseness, dyspnea, orthopnea and chest pain.
• Signs include: head/neck swelling, suffusion and conjunctival edema, wheezing and stridor.
• Chest X–ray demonstrates a mediastinal mass, often anterior, pericardial effusion and/or pleural effusion.
• Rule out iatrogenic causes. Rule out infection (fungal, tuberculosis).
• Serum AFP and beta hCG.
• Echocardiogram to rule out pericardial effusion.
• Thoracocentesis for pleural effusion and examine for malignant cells.
• Peripheral blood smear (leukemia or lymphoma); bone marrow aspiration or biopsy (may have to be done sitting); biopsy of suspicious peripheral lymph nodes.
• CT scan of chest if possible but it may be too dangerous to lie down.
• Mediastinal biopsy requires general anesthesia.
• General anesthesia should be avoided in SMS unless the child is asymptomatic and has no compromise of airway or great vessels on imaging.
• Consider emergency systemic steroid treatment and/or radiotherapy with delayed biopsy.
• Differential diagnosis:
    Primary causes: malignant tumors (Hodgkin's disease and lymphoma, germ cell tumor), granuloma (histoplasmosis, tuberculosis).
    Secondary causes (thrombosis): postcardiac surgery, venous access device.

Congenital lung anomalies

1. Congenital lobar emphysema
• Area of hyperinflated lung. Usually confined to a single lobe.
• Some present in neonatal period because of acute air trapping and should be removed surgically.
• Others cause no trouble and may be found as an incidental finding on chest X–ray in an adult.

2. Congenital adenomatoid malformation
• Intrapulmonary mass that communicates with the tracheobronchial tree.
• There are three types: large cysts; small, multiple bronchial–like cysts; micro–, compact cysts

fetal lung–like appearance.
- Often asymptomatic. A large cyst in a newborn may cause respiratory distress.
- Investigate with chest X–ray, ultrasound and CT scan.
- Treatment is excision to confirm the pathology; rule out associated malignancy and prevent complications.

3. Pulmonary sequestration
- Usually asymptomatic at birth but later may cause recurrent pulmonary infections.
- 90% are intralobar; 10% are extralobar.
- Blood supply is systemic and there is no normal communication with the tracheobronchial tree.
- Investigations include: chest X–ray, dynamic CT scan (delineate lesion and blood supply), MRI (delineate lesion and blood supply), aortogram (delineate blood supply).
- Treat by excision to confirm pathology, rule out associated pleuropulmonary blastoma and prevent recurrent infections.

Neck masses, cysts, sinuses

Simple classification divides these into lateral and midline:
- Midline: ranula, lymphadenopathy, thyroglossal duct cyst, epidermoid cyst, ectopic thyroid.
- Lateral: lymphadenopathy, lymphangioma (cystic hygroma), sternomastoid tumor, branchial remnant (i.e. cyst or fistula).

1. Midline lesions
- Ranula: this cystic dilation of a sublingual gland bulges into the floor of the mouth and resembles the distended throat of a croaking frog (RANA). It is treated by drainage into the floor of the mouth by wide unroofing and marsupialization.
- Lymphadenopathy: any pathological process that affects lymph nodes (e.g. inflammation, infection, malignancy) can present as a midline neck swelling, but more commonly it is in a lateral position.
- Thyroglossal duct cyst: as the thyroid develops from a diverticulum in the midline at the base of the tongue, it descends downward to its eventual position low in the neck. A tract may be left behind with a cyst forming, usually below the hyoid bone and in communication with the foramen cecum. This cyst may become infected or may simply increase in size over time as mucous accumulates. It usually presents at 2–3 years of age. It most commonly becomes infected by *H. influenzae*. Drainage, either spontaneous or surgical, is usually glairy and may become chronic (the cyst is congenital but a thyroglossal duct fistula is acquired). Antibiotics are given if it is infected. Excision is performed when the infection has resolved. This involves excision of the cyst, the tract up to the foramen cecum and the middle one–third of the hyoid bone (Sistrunk procedure).
- Epidermoid cyst: are often referred to as "dermoids". They are portions of epidermis trapped under the skin. Its wall contains all skin appendages (sebaceous cysts are only keratinizing epithelium without appendages). There may be a small sinus. They tend to occur at cervical midline (sternal notch, submental, prehyoid), supraciliary (lateral angular dermoid), scalp away from midline. Cysts can be simply excised. Dermoid sinuses may occur along the midline from the nose up along the cranium and down to the spine and sacrum (some of these have an internal opening into the meninges and a neurosurgeon should be consulted).

2. Lateral lesions
- Lymphadenopathy: most commonly viral but occasionally bacterial causing lymphadenitis. Usually *Streptococcus* or *Staphylococcus*. Those that develop into an abscess require incision and drainage. A firm node more than 3 cm and present for over 3 weeks should raise suspicion of malignancy and should be considered for biopsy.
- Lymphangioma (cystic hygroma): soft, mobile, lobulated, fluctuant, subcutaneous mass which is variable in size and may suddenly enlarge. May not be evident at birth. It is invasive and may be intimate with nerves and blood vessels. They are at risk for enlargement, infection or hemorrhage. They may compromise the airway at birth or when they suddenly enlarge. They rarely resolve spontaneously. Surgical excision may be challenging and early surgical evaluation is important.
- Sternomastoid tumor: idiopathic benign fibromatosis of the sternomastoid muscle causes a firm, large, ovoid, unilateral neck tumor in a newborn. It is associated with torticollis (head is flexed toward the affected side and the chin rotated to the opposite side of the lesion). Early diagnosis and nonoperative treatment by aggressive physiotherapy can prevent a fixed contracture which requires surgical release (myotomy). May cause facial asymmetry.
- Branchial remnants (fistula or cyst)
  First branchial cleft remnants are akin to a duplication of the eustachian tube. They present as a swelling behind the ear lobe and run parallel to the eustachian tube. They may also present as a swelling near the angle of the mandible and then course upwards to the external auditory canal. Either may form an abscess or sinus. Treatment is by excision of the entire fistula.
  Second branchial fistula presents as a tiny opening along the anterior border of the middle one–third of the sternomastoid muscle and drains clear fluid. The internal opening is at the tonsillar fossa. Treatment is by excision of the entire fistula.
  Branchial cyst (lymphoepithelial cyst) presents as a lateral neck cyst usually in adolescents or young adults. They are usually deep to the middle one–third of the sternomastoid muscle, often following an upper respiratory infection. They do not communicate with the skin or the pharynx. Treatment is by excision.
  Third and fourth branchial fistulae are rare and usually present as a deep neck abscess or suppurative thyroiditis.

Ingested foreign body

- This is a common occurrence and most are benign and pass easily through the GI tract with no difficulty.
- As a general guideline, most foreign bodies that pass the cricopharyngeus will pass through the GI tract.
- Foreign bodies that impact usually do so at the cricopharyngeus or the gastroesophageal junction.
- These can usually be easily removed but should be done with maximum protection against aspiration. This is best accomplished in the Operating Room with general endotracheal anesthesia.
- A rigid esophagoscope is the most effective technique.
- Those that go into the stomach will pass and intervention is usually unnecessary unless a reasonable period of time has passed (i.e. 3 weeks) and the foreign body remains impacted.

- Other areas where foreign bodies may impact include the duodenum, duodenojejunal flexure, terminal ileum, cecum and appendix.
- These should be dealt with on an individual basis (i.e. operative intervention or observation).
- Obstruction or perforation require operative intervention.

Caustic ingestion

"Accidental" ingestions are rarely true accidents and are frequently a marker of poor social conditions.

There are two populations at risk for caustic ingestion:
- Young children (< 5 years of age): accidental ingestion.
- Older child or adolescent: intentional ingestion (suicide).

1. Agents ingested
- Alkali, 90%; acid, 10%.
- Most commonly ingested substances are household cleaners (potassium hydroxide, sodium hydroxide, sulfuric acid).
- Bleach and liquid detergents are rarely a problem.

2. Alkalis
- Cause the severest injuries.
- Produce liquefactive necrosis.
- Have a high risk of esophageal perforation.

3. Acids
- Produce coagulative necrosis.
- Gastric antrum may be most severely injured.

4. Symptoms (may be absent or include the following)
- Drooling, dysphagia, vomiting, fever and chest pain.
- Wheezing or stridor may be present if there is associated laryngeal spasm.

5. Evaluation
- There is a high correlation between esophageal injury and burns of the lips, tongue and mouth.
- All suspected ingestions should be evaluated carefully.
- Serial plain X–rays of chest and abdomen rule out perforation.
- Endoscopy is the key to diagnosis; evaluation of the extent and severity of injury should be done within 24 hours.
- A contrast swallow done within 48 hours will evaluate: stomach and esophagus, esophageal motility (rigid esophagus = high risk of stricture), serial studies to assess for stricture.

6. Treatment
- Goal of treatment is to prevent sepsis and stricture formation.
- Treatment is based on the severity of injury at endoscopy.
- Antibiotics (ampicillin and gentamicin) for 1 week.

- Steroids to decrease stricture formation are controversial.
- Mild injuries can be given a liquid diet and observed for 48–72 hours.
- Moderate to severe injuries require esophageal stenting with a feeding tube ± gastrostomy.
- After 3 weeks, if there is no stricture, the child can be discharged; if the esophagus is strictured, then aggressive frequent esophageal dilations are begun.
- One–third of lye ingestions develop strictures but only 5% are resistant to esophageal dilation therapy.
- Esophageal replacement (gastric tube, gastric pull–up, jejunal or colon graft) is considered if 1 year of aggressive frequent dilations fail to resolve the stricture.
- Long–term follow–up is necessary for strictured esophagus left in situ for risk of carcinoma.

Emesis

1. Bilious (green) emesis
- Beware the child who vomits "green" for (s)he has a surgical lesion until proved otherwise. This is a surgical emergency; treatment and investigations should proceed quickly.
- Causes in children beyond the neonatal period include: adhesive small bowel obstruction, intestinal volvulus, paralytic ileus.
- All require fluid resuscitation, correction of electrolytes and nasogastric decompression.
- Physical examination must rule out signs of peritonitis which mandate emergency laparotomy.
- Abdominal X–rays (AP supine and upright) provide the next step in the investigation.
- Warning signs of possible vascular compromise of the intestine are: persistent or worsening pain and tenderness, elevated WBC after fluid resuscitation and metabolic acidosis.
- Nonoperative treatment in adhesive small bowel obstruction is often unsuccessful and should be limited to those who show definite and rapid improvement following nasogastric decompression.

2. Nonbilious emesis
- Not usually a surgical cause.
- Causes: intussusception (colicky abdominal pain), gastroenteritis, gastroesophageal reflux, hypertrophic pyloric stenosis.
- Hypertrophic pyloric stenosis:
    Peaks at 6 weeks of age; the incidence drops off rapidly thereafter.
    Suspect in the 6 week old hungry, otherwise healthy baby, who has forceful (projectile), nonbilious emesis.
    Vomitus may be coffee ground due to an associated gastritis or esophagitis.
    The child may also be jaundiced.
    Peristaltic gastric waves may be visible.
    A pyloric tumor may be palpated in the quiet infant with an empty stomach.
    The tumor is the size and shape of a mobile "olive" and is usually felt in the epigastrium or right upper quadrant under the rectus muscle. If unsure about the presence of a pyloric tumor, confirm by ultrasound or GI contrast study.
    Check electrolytes for hypokalemic, hypochloremic, metabolic alkalosis.
    When the diagnosis is confirmed, rehydrate and correct electrolytes preoperatively; this is not a surgical emergency.
    Correction is by pyloromyotomy, widely splitting the hypertrophied pyloric muscularis

propria longitudinally, thereby relieving the obstruction. Most babies start to feed 12–24 hours postop and are discharged home 24–48 hours postop.

- Gastroesophageal reflux (GER):

    It is not unusual for infants to spit up or vomit but not all have GER.

    Complicated GER should be suspected if the child who vomits is failing to thrive, chokes or aspirates, has blood–streaked emesis, has persistent nondietary related iron deficiency anemia, or has recurrent, persistent or chronic lung disease.

    Children with neurodevelopmental disabilities are particularly prone to severe GER.

    Principles of investigation are: upper GI contrast study, pH probe study, endoscopy and esophageal biopsy.

    Treatment is nonoperative for most patients.

    Operative therapy is controversial but, in general, is reserved for those children who fail to improve with nonoperative treatment or develop complications such as an esophageal stricture or life threatening aspiration.

    Various surgical options include:

    Feeding jejunostomy; feeding or decompression gastrostomy.

    Antireflux procedures (fundoplication) such as: Nissen (falling out of favor with pediatric surgeons), Thal, Toupet, Boix Ochoa, others.

    The number and variety of procedures reflects the satisfaction with the results of any one procedure.

- Gastroenteritis:

    "Gastro" should not be an automatic diagnosis whenever you are presented with a vomiting child. When considering the diagnosis, there are a few signs and symptoms to be especially cautious of: severe colic (especially with a periodic pattern), gross abdominal distension, vomiting without diarrhea, bilious vomiting, abdominal tenderness which is localized or lateralized, involuntary guarding, bloody stools, abdominal surgical scar or a hernia.

Abdominal pain

1. Intussusception
- Crampy, severe, intermittent pain is the predominant early symptom of intussusception.
- This is caused by the intestine telescoping in on itself, resulting in obstruction. Usually it involves the terminal ileum and right colon to the midtransverse colon.
- It may be idiopathic (thought to be due to hypertrophied Peyer's patches) or secondary to a lesion such as a Meckel's diverticulum.
- Typically presents with colicky severe abdominal pain. The child will look pale and lethargic.
- Initially vomiting is on a reflex basis and is nonbilious. It becomes bilious as the obstruction worsens.
- Passage of "currant jelly" stools is indicative of the mucosal congestion and slough caused by the obstruction and veno–occlusion.
- A sausage–shaped mass may be palpable in the right upper quadrant or epigastrium. Abdominal X–rays reveal a distal small bowel obstruction.
- In the absence of peritonitis, the diagnosis is confirmed by contrast (air or radiopaque material) enema. The enema can be used therapeutically to reduce the intussusception in this situation.
- If there is peritonitis or if the therapeutic enema is unsuccessful, laparotomy is required to

either reduce or, rarely, resect the affected bowel.
- Recurrence is < 10%.

2. Appendicitis
- This is a common cause of pain and is the most common surgical emergency in children.
- Consider appendicitis in all ages but most commonly between 4 and 15 years of age.
- Fifty percent of patients do not have a typical history.
- Vague, central abdominal pain is the earliest symptom, followed by anorexia and the onset of nausea and vomiting.
- Pain eventually shifts to the right iliac fossa as local parietal peritoneal inflammation develops.
- Fever is usually low (< 39 °C) or absent (high fever suggests other pathology or perforated appendicitis).
- Key to the diagnosis is a physical examination. Suspicious signs to observe include: lying very still on one side and/or knees flexed; movement or cough worsens pain.
- A careful and complete examination is necessary to rule out other causes (e.g. pneumonia, hepatitis).
- Localized tenderness in the right iliac fossa (McBurney's point) is very suspicious.
- If the pain is worsened by jumping up and down, this suggests peritonitis; especially useful in retrocecal appendicitis.
- A rectal examination should be done to assess for: rectal vault tenderness, pelvic abscess, uterine or adnexal pathology.
- Laboratory tests are nonspecific: WBC is usually normal or mildly elevated (it may be high in perforated appendicitis).
- Urinalysis may be abnormal due to urinary tract pathology or due to an inflamed appendix in contact with the ureter or bladder.
- Plain X–rays are nonspecific but may help with other diagnoses (e.g. pneumonia, urolithiasis, intussusception).
- Abdominal or pelvic ultrasound may be useful in equivocal cases or in suspected gynecological pathology.
- The differential diagnosis of appendicitis is extensive:
    GI: gastroenteritis, mesenteric adenitis, constipation.
    GU: urolithiasis, cystitis or pyelonephritis, ovarian cyst rupture or torsion, mittelschmerz.
    Other: Henoch–Schönlein purpura, HUS, primary peritonitis, pneumonia, measles, diabetic ketoacidosis.
- Patients can be placed into one of three diagnostic groupings based on the history, physical examination and investigations:
    Highly suspicious: operate.
    Moderately suspicious: admit and observe with serial physical examinations; consider an ultrasound.
    Low suspicion: management is determined by the differential diagnosis.
- For nonperforated appendicitis:
    A single dose of preoperative antibiotics is adequate.
    Diet is resumed 24 hours postop.
    Discharged home in 48–72 hours.
- For perforated appendicitis:
    Bowel rest until bowel function returns.

Parenteral antibiotics × 5 days (ampicillin, gentamicin, flagyl).
- Complications:
  Wound infection: nonperforated cases, 1%; perforated cases, 5–20%; pelvic abscess, 5%; adhesive small bowel obstruction, 5%.

Rectal bleeding

1. Causes
- Causes are best categorized by age group:
  Neonate: swallowed maternal blood, hemorrhagic disease, NEC, volvulus, gastroenteritis, anal fissure.
  Infant: gastroenteritis, anal fissure, volvulus, intestinal duplication.
  Preschool: gastroenteritis, anal fissure, rectal prolapse, Meckel's diverticulum, juvenile polyp.
  School age: anal fissure, gastroenteritis, colitis, colorectal polyps, Meckel's diverticulum.
- In an ill child with an acute abdominal condition consider: intussusception, gastroenteritis, Henoch–Schönlein purpura.
- A small amount of blood in an otherwise well child: anal fissure, fistula in ano, rectal polyp, rectal prolapse, AV malformation, idiopathic.
- Major bleed in an otherwise healthy child: Meckel's diverticulum, intestinal duplication, upper GI pathology (i.e. esophageal varices or peptic ulcer).

2. Management
- Depends on the age group and suspected pathology.
- All patients should have a hemoglobin measurement, PT, PTT and platelet count.
- Careful physical examination, including the anorectum.
- If bleeding is profuse: monitor vitals carefully, pass a nasogastric or orogastric tube to rule out upper GI source; type and cross–match blood (10 mL/kg); establish reliable i.v. access.
- Neonate: an Apt test can help for swallowed maternal blood, abdominal X–rays to rule out NEC or midgut volvulus.
- Infant: abdominal X–rays to rule out midgut volvulus or intussusception, contrast radiology as indicated.
- Preschool: proctosigmoidoscopy to rule out polyps or prolapse, nuclear medicine scan for Meckel's diverticulum, upper and lower endoscopy as indicated.
- School age: abdominal X–rays to rule out colitis, Meckel's nuclear medicine scan, endoscopy as indicated.
- Other tests such as tagged RBC nuclear medicine scans and arteriography are used in select cases.
- Management of the bleeding is dependent on the cause. Most are managed nonoperatively.
- Meckel's diverticulum requires urgent resection once the diagnosis is confirmed (Meckel's scan sensitivity 40–90%).
- Intestinal duplication can give a false positive Meckel's scan but treatment is still excision.
- Bleeding polyps should be excised, usually endoscopically.
- Most fissures are managed nonoperatively with stool softeners.

Abdominal mass

• Consider: patient age, location of mass, signs and symptoms.
• Begin with the least invasive investigations (i.e. plain X–rays and ultrasound) to confirm: presence of the mass, site of the mass, extent of the mass (may require CT or MRI).
• Causes categorized by age group:
  Neonatal:
  Seventy percent are renal lesions, 30% are nonrenal lesions.
  Renal (70%): multicystic dysplastic syndrome, hydronephrosis, ureteropelvic junction obstruction, posterior uretheral valves, ureteral duplication and ectopy complex, polycystic kidney, Wilm's tumor, renal vein thrombosis.
  Nonrenal (30%): adrenal neuroblastoma (25% of nonrenal lesions), GI duplication cyst, liver, spleen, biliary masses, hydrometrocolpos, ovarian tumor.
  Infant:
  Renal (50%): see neonatal list of causes.
  Nonrenal (50%): retroperitoneum, adrenal tumor, teratoma; gastrointestinal (appendix abscess, duplication, intussusception, choledochal cyst, liver tumor); genital (ovarian tumor; most common nonrenal cause of a cystic abdominal mass in children).
  Child (> 2 years of age):
  Visceromegaly (infection, leukemia or lymphoma, portal hypertension), Wilm's tumor, neuroblastoma, appendix abscess, intussusception, pregnancy (most common pelvic mass in girls > 9 years of age).
• Further management of abdominal masses is guided by: age, signs and symptoms, site and extent on imaging studies.
• Suspected neoplasms usually require open biopsy to obtain adequate tissue for cytogenetics, special stains and electron microscopy.

Jaundice

Differential diagnosis:
• Obstructive: spontaneous perforation of bile duct, biliary atresia, choledochal cyst, inspissated bile syndrome.
• Nonobstructive:
  Infectious: TORCH, viral, other.
  Metabolic: $alpha_1$–antitrypsin deficiency, glycogen storage disease, cystic fibrosis, other.
  Cholestasis: cystic fibrosis, congenital hepatic fibrosis, arteriohepatic dysplasia (Alagille's syndrome), Byler's disease, parenteral alimentation.
  Other: hemolytic disease, drugs, physiological, others.

1. Biliary atresia
• Healthy child often with a history of onset of jaundice after birth.
• Consider if direct hyperbilirubinemia and jaundice persisting > 2 weeks.
• Rule out other causes: liver enzymes, TORCH screen, $alpha_1$–antitrypsin level.
• Percutaneous liver biopsy.
• Abdominal ultrasound.

- Hepatobiliary nuclear medicine imaging:
  Excretion of radioisotope into the intestine excludes biliary atresia.
  No excretion of radioisotope is an indication for laparotomy, operative cholangiogram and open liver biopsy.
  Portoenterostomy (Kasai procedure) is most successful when done before 8 weeks of age.
- Outcome is difficult to predict:
  One–third have resolution of jaundice.
  One–third have persistent or worsening jaundice and require liver transplantation.
  One–third have resolution of jaundice but later relapse and require liver transplantation.

2. Choledochal cyst
- This cystic abnormality results in the cystic dilation of the biliary tree and may be intrahepatic, extrahepatic or both.
- Theories of etiology are varied but the currently accepted one is an anomalous arrangement of the pancreaticobiliary duct system; allows pancreatic enzyme reflux into the biliary ducts; causes inflammation and injury.
- These present as either: infant (< 6 months) with jaundice; child (> 2 years) with any or all of abdominal pain, jaundice, abdominal mass. Direct hyperbilirubinemia and elevated alkaline phosphatase are usually present. Amylase may be mildly elevated.
- Diagnosis is confirmed by ultrasound ± hepatobiliary nuclear imaging. In select cases, ERCP or transhepatic cholangiography may be useful.
- At risk for the development of biliary cirrhosis, recurrent cholangitis and possible malignant degeneration.
- Preferred treatment is cyst excision with Roux–en–Y hepatojejunostomy.

3. Gallbladder disease
With increasing frequency, infants and children are being diagnosed with: acute hydrops of the gallbladder, acalculous cholecystitis, cholelithiasis or cholecystitis.
- Acute hydrops of the gallbladder:
  This is severe edema around the gallbladder and biliary tree, usually in septic neonates.
  Diagnosed by ultrasound.
  Treated by bowel rest and antibiotics.
  Cholecystostomy may be necessary.
  Cholecystectomy is indicated if there is evidence of cystic duct obstruction or gangrenous changes of the gallbladder wall.
- Acalculous cholecystitis:
  Infants or older children.
  Associated with severe systemic diseases such as: severe burns, multisystem trauma, severe sepsis and Kawasaki's disease.
  Present as nausea, vomiting, fever, right upper quadrant pain and tenderness.
  Possibly leukocytosis and jaundice.
  Diagnosis is confirmed by ultrasound and/or hepatobiliary nuclear imaging.
  Initial treatment is supportive with bowel rest and antibiotics.
  If improvement is not rapid, then cholecystectomy is indicated (high incidence of ischemic necrosis of the gallbladder).
  Cholecystostomy is an alternative to cholecystectomy unless gangrenous changes are

present.
- Gallstones:
  Increasing incidence of gallstones in children.
  Three types of gallstones: cholesterol stones, pigment stones (black—hemolytic disease, brown—calcium bilirubinate) and duct stones (associated with cholangitis or bile duct stricture).
  All are at risk for complications such as: cholangitis, obstructive jaundice, pancreatitis, pericholecystic abscess.
  Most accurate diagnostic test is an ultrasound.
  All symptomatic patients should be treated by cholecystectomy to prevent the complications of gallstones.
  Lithotripsy and urodeoxycholic acid therapy are of limited usefulness. They have low success rates and high recurrence rates.

Drainage from the umbilicus

Causes of umbilical drainage include: umbilical granuloma, omphalitis, vitelline duct remnant, urachal sinus.

1. Umbilical granuloma
- This common lesion is granulation tissue, which can develop after separation of the cord.
- It is easily treated by local application of silver nitrate.
- Large granulomas may require excision.
- Can cause cellulitis or omphalitis.

2. Omphalitis
- Localized form is usually due to poor hygiene.
- May be associated with vestigial remnants.
- May progress rapidly.
- Can cause a necrotizing soft tissue infection: requires aggressive debridement, high mortality.
- Can cause portal vein thrombosis and portal hypertension.

3. Vitelline duct remnant
These include:
- Umbilical polyps: mucosal rests.
- Vitelline duct sinus: mucosa lined cyst that communicates with the umbilicus.
- Vitelline duct fistula: mucosa lined tract from umbilicus to distal small intestine.
- Vitelline duct cyst: mucosa lined cyst along the tract of the vitelline duct.
- Vitelline duct band: obliterated duct forming a band from the distal intestine to the umbilicus; can cause intestinal obstruction or volvulus.
All these can cause infection. All are treated by excision.

4. Urachal sinus, fistula, cyst
- Along the course of the primitive allantois.
- From the dome of the bladder to the umbilicus.
- Can cause an enlarging suprapubic mass and is at risk for abscess formation.

- Obtain a voiding cystourethrogram to rule out an associated bladder outlet obstruction.
- Abscesses are treated by antibiotics, drainage and delayed excision.
- Cyst, fistula and sinus are treated by excision.

Scrotal mass

Differential diagnosis:
- Testicular.
- Nontesticular.

1. Testicular
- Varicocele, granuloma, epididymoorchitis, orchitis, cysts.
- Tumors: benign (teratoma), malignant (primary), germ cell tumor, nongerm cell tumor (Leydig cell tumor), secondary (leukemia, lymphoma).

2. Nontesticular
- Epididymis, cord, supporting stoma (benign, malignant).
- Paratesticular tumors (rhabdomyosarcomas, mesotheliomas, fibromas, lipomas, adenomatoid growths).

Acute scrotal conditions

   Testicular torsion, torsion of the appendage, epididymitis, orchitis, tumor, trauma.

1. Testicular torsion
- Three types: intravaginal (occurs in older children; testicle is freely suspended within the tunica vaginalis), extravaginal (occurs perinatally), mesorchial.
- Typically presents with very sudden onset of pain, particularly during physical activity such as playing sports.
- Affected testicle: has a transverse orientation; epididymis lies anterior, is enlarged, tender and elevated.
- Suspected diagnosis can be confirmed by Doppler ultrasound.
- In most cases, the diagnosis is apparent and should be confirmed by prompt surgical exploration.
- Contralateral orchidopexy should be performed at the same time.

2. Torsion of testicular appendages
- Torsion of appendix testis or appendix epididymis.
- Scrotal examination may reveal a "blue dot" sign.
- Usually a very tender localized nodule.
- Often obscured by a reactive hydrocele.
- Treatment is rest and analgesia or scrotal exploration and excision of the appendage.

3. Testicular and paratesticular tumors
- A solid scrotal mass requires prompt evaluation.
- Most common tumors are: germ cell tumors (teratoma, yolk sac tumor), secondary (leukemia

or non–Hodgkin's lymphoma), rhabdomyosarcoma.
- Chest X–ray and serum alpha$_1$–fetoprotein preoperative.
- Explore through an inguinal incision unless suspected secondary (these can be approached through a scrotal incision).
- Isolate cord structures and perform a high inguinal orchiectomy.

Soft tissue tumors

- Most are benign and of vascular origin.
- Can be classified (Table II) based on the mature tissue they resemble (not necessarily the tissue they arise from).

Table II: Benign and malignant tumors of soft tissue

Tissue	Benign tumors	Malignant tumors
Adipose	Lipoma, lipoblastoma	Liposarcoma (rare)
Fibrous	Fibroma, fibromatosis	Fibrosarcoma
Muscle	Myofibromatosis	Rhabdomyosarcoma
Vascular	Hemangioma, lymphangioma	Hemangioendothelioma
Neural	Neurofibroma	Neurofibromatosis
Miscellaneous	Inflammatory pseudotumor	Synovial sarcoma

- These tumors require careful clinical evaluation to determine appropriate management.
- Plain X–rays and ultrasound (Doppler) are appropriate first line investigations.
- CT or MRI may further delineate suspected malignant neoplasms.
- Suspected malignancy must be ruled out by incisional biopsy.
- Further treatment is based on the pathology and may include any or all of the following: wide local excision (possible amputation), chemotherapy, radiotherapy.

1. Hemangioma
This is a hamartoma rather than a neoplasm. Often not noticeable at birth and for several days to months.
- Approximately 5% are:
    Large.
    Involve vital organs.
    Cause life threatening complications, e.g. hemorrhage, airway obstruction, platelet trapping (Kasabach–Merritt's syndrome), congestive heart failure.
- Classification is based on cell kinetics:
    AV malformation: usually present at birth; do not grow; may be multiple.
    Hemangioma: usually not noticeable at birth; enlarge rapidly by cell proliferation; most common are capillary, cavernous, mixed.
- Investigations can include:
    CBC, platelet count, PT, PTT, plain X–rays, ultrasound, technetium labelled RBC scan, CT,

MRI, angiogram.
- There are many treatment options available:
   Observation: most will involute partially or completely.
   Compression therapy: continuous or intermittent.
   Sclerotherapy: requires multiple treatments.
   Chemotherapy: some success reported with cyclophosphamide.
   Steroids: mechanism of action is possibly modulation of endothelial proliferation; may be given systemically or intralesionally.
   Embolization: useful in cardiac failure, Kasabach–Merritt's syndrome and hemorrhage.
   Excision: for AV malformations and for small lesions persisting > 4 years; large lesions are often not resectable for physiological or cosmetic reasons. If complications develop, consider excision; consider embolization prior to excision.

2. Lymphangioma
- Can be classified as: capillary, cavernous, cystic hygroma, lymphangioendothelioma.
- Two–thirds are present at birth.
- Spontaneous resolution is rare.
- Complications include:
   Airway obstruction: due to local infiltration or compression from rapid enlargement.
   Infection: can cause rapid enlargement.
   Infiltration of surrounding tissues making excision difficult.
   Hemorrhage.
   Erosion of skin.
   Dental malocclusion or other skeletal deformity.
- Treatment of choice is excision but vital structures should be preserved; 5–15% recurrence.
- For unresectable or recurrent disease, intralesional injection (bleomycin or OK–432) may be tried.
- Laser and dry ice are useful for cutaneous capillary lymphangioma.

Undescended testes

This is a very common complaint. An empty scrotum may be due to rectractile testes, ectopic testes, absent testes or true undescended testes.

1. Retractile testes
- Due to active cremaster muscle.
- May be a history of the testicle having been felt in the scrotum.
- Descends when relaxed or asleep. Testicle is usually normal.

2. Ectopic testes
An otherwise normal testicle is drawn into an abnormal location (thigh, groin, suprapubic) by the gubernaculum.

3. Absent testes
- Most often due to perinatal torsion.
- Diagnosis is established by laparoscopy to rule out an intra–abdominal testis.

4. True undescended testes
- These are at risk for malignant degeneration and for inadequate spermatogenesis.
- They are usually unilateral.
- Bilateral ones should raise the suspicion of an endocrinological disturbance.
- Most will descend by 9 months of age.
- An orchidopexy should be performed before 2 years of age on all testes not descended by one year of age.
- Orchidopexy may have to be done earlier if there is an associated symptomatic hernia.
- Orchidopexy decreases the histological dysgenetic changes.
- Maintains adequate spermatogenesis?
- It does not decrease the risk of malignancy but makes malignancy easier to detect.

Inguinal hernias/hydroceles

- These are common.
- Occur mostly in boys and mostly right–sided.
- Incidence correlates with prematurity.
- Due to a patent processus vaginalis.
- Increase in intra–abdominal pressure forces abdominal contents into the patent processus vaginalis, creating a hernia.
- Hydroceles are fluid filled remnants of the processus vaginalis and may be in communication with the peritoneal cavity, in which case the cyst will vary in size from time to time. These are treated as an inguinal hernia.
- Noncommunicating hydroceles are persistent in their size, usually present since birth and will often resolve.
- Hernias are at risk for incarceration and subsequent ischemic injury to the bowel, ovary or testicle.
- Inguinal hernias in females often present as herniation of an ovary which often incarcerates.
- Inguinal hernias do not resolve spontaneously.
- Repair is by high ligation of the patent processus vaginalis sac.

HISTORY OF HEALTH CARE ETHICS

The term "bioethics" was first introduced by the American physician, Van Rensselaer Potter, in 1971 in his book, *Bioethics: Bridge to the Future.* In this book, Potter used the term to emphasize the importance of developing new biological knowledge in combination with an understanding of human values. The study of health care ethics arises out of attempts to address the ethical issues caused by developments in the biological sciences and their application to medical practice.

Medical ethics, or the study of physician morality, has a much longer history and in Western history can be said to have developed its lasting foundation in the era of Hippocrates (b:460, d:377?). The Hippocratic Oath, which may actually have been previously constructed by Pythagoras, lays down the foundations for the virtuous physician.

The oath has four distinct parts consisting of:
- The actual oath.
- A covenant outlining the duties of medical students to their teachers and their obligations regarding the transmission of medical knowledge to others.
- The ethical code involving, among other things, prohibitions against giving poisons, performing abortions, having sexual relations with patients and revealing to others details of a patient's private life.
- A prayer expressing hope for reward upon keeping the oath.

This oath, influenced by Platonic, Aristotelian and Stoic philosophy represented the ideal of the time. Noticeably absent was the concept of patient autonomy. A physician of the time was expected to have developed both technical skills and the skill of phronesis, which consisted of recognizing the right thing to do in a particular situation.

Between 500 and 1500 AD, the Hippocratic corpus was adopted and modified by the major religions. The virtue of phronesis was a gift of God imbuing the physician with God's authority, further reinforcing the paternalistic nature of the physician–patient relationship. This was not purely an issue of power but was considered necessary for ensuring that the patient had faith in the cure since this was seen as coming from God. In the West, the arrival of the Reformation and subsequently the Age of Enlightenment allowed physicians to move away from religious influence and develop their own rules of professional conduct. Professional guilds were organized (such as the Royal College of Physicians, 1518) which developed standards of competence and behavior for their members. Thomas Percival's book, *Medical Ethics (1803)*, gave an interpretation of medical morality from the physician perspective and served as the basis for a professional code of ethics. Descartes' dualistic theory moves medicine into the field of science and the body and further from theology and faith.

Interestingly, the Age of Enlightenment ushered in an era of patient consumerism or autonomy, at least among those with discretionary income. Orthodox medicine was competing with many other "healers" who claimed a scientific or religious basis to their methods. At this time, it was the reputation of the individual, whether orthodox or not, which tended to influence consumer choice.

As orthodox medicine became more scientifically based and as it developed a greater understanding of the body in health and disease, it gained a professional ascendancy and redeveloped its paternalistic roots. Science now substituted for faith.

Modern bioethics can be said to be a revolt against this physician–centered ethical construct. This change took place from the mid–60's and was stimulated both by technological and societal factors.

1. Technological
- The development of effective drugs gave rise to many benefits (contraceptives, vaccines, antibiotics) but occasionally some disasters (thalidomide). Many such drugs required human safety trials, spotlighting the potential for abuse in research on humans.
- Many new technologies were in short supply, meaning that not all those in need could receive life prolonging therapy. Choices had to be made (dialysis machines, transplantation). How should those choices be made and who should make them?
- Transplantation technology required a new definition of death since adhering to the old definition would render the donor organs unsuitable.
- Cardiorespiratory support capable of maintaining life in order to allow for recovery could also prolong life when this might not be considered desirable.

2. Societal
- The increasing acceptance and codifying of the concept of individual rights has brought us back to the model of the patient as sceptical consumer of health care goods. The paternalistic model of medical care was challenged by patients asserting their right to make choices for themselves.
- An increasing moral pluralism made it difficult to maintain a singular moral paradigm and gave rise to an examination both within and without the profession as to what ought to be done in particular situations and whether certain duties were obligatory.
- Other factors include a distrust of institutions and authority and the increasing influence of feminism.

The above and other factors have caused an evaluation of the ethics of health care encounters and relationships, the structure of health care and the goals of medicine from within and without the medical profession. It is no longer just "our thing".

PHYSICIAN–PATIENT/PARENT RELATIONSHIPS

The goal of medicine is "right and good healing action taken in the interests of a particular patient" (Pellegrino). In complying with the goal, the physician–patient relationship carries a significant moral component, with reciprocal rights and obligations recognized by the parties concerned.

The nature of the physician–patient relationship has changed greatly over the last few decades:
- Move from paternalistic prescriptive medical advice to one of information sharing and respect for patient autonomy, as alluded to in the introductory section.
- While in the primary care ambulatory setting, the physician–patient relationship may be a long–term one–to–one relationship. The complexity of modern medical care frequently gives

rise to situations where the physician comes to the patient as a stranger. The patient may also encounter teams of caregivers, a situation which may complicate and diffuse the relationship.

In the pediatric setting, the relationship is further complicated by the presence of a third party, the parent or guardian, in the physician–patient relationship. The parents have moral, social and legal responsibility for the well–being of the child and are allowed a significant degree of discretion as to how this well–being may be brought about. This is not an absolute authority as the child has interests which should not be infringed upon, even by the parents. The physician therefore has a relationship with both the child, as a moral being, and the parents, who are charged with furthering the best interests of the child within the context of the family.

This equation becomes modified as the child develops and becomes capable of expressing his/her own interests and choices. (This will be explored more under consent and confidentiality.)

In a multicultural society, attitudes toward health care practices may vary significantly. There may be an expectation of physician paternalism. There may be a feeling of vulnerability with concomitant suspicion. The family relationships may be hierarchial with one autocratic decision maker (usually male). Community or religious leaders may have a significant or dominant role in decisions made within a family. It is therefore important for the physician to recognize that there is potential for cultural conflict and that there may be a need to search for common ground.

Models of physician–patient relationships

1. Paternalistic model (authoritarian)
In this model, the physician makes decisions in the patient's best interests and acts accordingly. Paternalism can be classified as weak, which allows the physician to act paternalistically when the patient is incapable of making an informed decision (encumbered), or strong when the physician makes decision on unencumbered patients. In the pediatric setting, the physician is abrogating the role of the parent of the noncompetent child when adopting either approach. Paternalism denies patient or parent autonomy and creates a dependency situation. As such, it is an affront to human dignity and denies the need for patient or patient to maintain control in moments of great vulnerability.

2. Consumer model
Here, the physician is provider of information with respect to medical benefit and harm. The patient or parent then decides which intervention is most desirable to them. Frequently, the information transmitted and acted upon is purely technical, and this model allows no opportunity for an exploration of common values. This model also encourages commodification of medical technology.

3. Interpretative (negotiation) model
The physician provides necessary technical information but also assists the patient and/or parent in making choices consistent with their values and their perception of the child's best interests. This model respects the autonomy of the patient and/or surrogate decision maker. The physician's value system is downplayed in this model.

4. Deliberative or interactive model
The physician provides information about medical interventions and explains the values related

to the various interventions. The patient and/or parent is thereby encouraged to examine and appraise their own values in order to select the intervention most suited to their value system. This model requires very significant ethical sophistication on the part of the physician and might be considered an ideal model toward which one might aim.

It is important to realize that any model of physician–patient relationship cannot be a construct developed purely by the profession. Basic principles will guide what society determines are the professional duties of a physician. The development of the relationship between physician and patient is based on this prior "contact" and clarifies specific obligations inherent in each physician–patient relationship.

The physician–patient relationship should have four fundamental characteristics according to Fried:
- Humanity: the acceptance that each person is a unique individual with individual needs, weaknesses and strengths.
- Autonomy (self–determination): the need and capacity to think about personal goals and the freedom to act accordingly.
- Lucidity: honest open communication, with the physician imparting all information relevant to allowing another to make an appropriate choice for himself/herself. This quality dictates the necessary prerequisite for informed consent.
- Fidelity: faithfulness in responding to justified expectations. The patient justifiably expects that the physician will have the necessary skill and commitment to good care, and that the physician is not using him/her as a means to a personal end.

The sum of the above creates an ethic of personal care.

ISSUES IN MEDICAL EDUCATION

Students within the health care system have several relationships which have ethical obligations.

In medicine in Canada, there are three categories of student physician:
- Undergraduate medical students: are not yet doctors. They carry out medical responsibilities under close supervision.
- Interns and junior residents: have received medical degrees but require further general or specialist training before being licensed to practice outside an educational setting. Supervision is required but may be distanced.
- Senior residents and fellows: often capable of receiving full licensure to practice generally. They are mainly in training for subspecialty.

Supervision for all of the above is provided by staff physicians, who have the responsibility to direct patient care, educate and evaluate students with whom they are involved. From this, it can be seen that students have the following relationships:

1. Student physician–patient relationships
- If the student is involved in caregiving, then the characteristics of humanity, respect for

autonomy, lucidity and fidelity apply. With respect to lucidity and fidelity, students should be honest about their level of training and skill. This may be facilitated by the educational institution providing information about its educational role. The attending physician also has a duty to provide information about student involvement to parents and patient.
- At times, the student may not be involved in providing care but is performing a medical task such as history taking or patient examination in order to learn or improve such skills. Here, both student and supervisor should provide appropriate information and be prepared to accept a reasonable refusal.
- Confidentiality should be respected. Information contained in the chart should not be accessed by those not involved in caregiving without the express permission of patients or parents. This may be done at time of admission or shortly thereafter. Should this information be imparted to others for educational purposes, patient anonymity should be maintained.

2. Peer relationships
- Professional practice requires that high standards of competence be maintained. Therefore, if a student observes incompetent or unethical behavior by a colleague, it is professionally incumbent on him/her to report this. It is important that a mechanism exists to allow this, and subsequent investigation should be in a nonprejudicial manner to both parties. Clear guidelines should be available within the educational program to facilitate this process.
- As students move up the hierarchy, they will usually be involved in teaching and evaluating "junior" colleagues. In order that this be done properly, clear guidelines as to expectations should be available and the evaluation process be rendered as objective and constructive as possible.

3. Student–staff relationships
- From the educational viewpoint, the staff physician serves as an evaluator of the student's progress. As above, it is incumbent on the evaluator to be as objective and constructive as possible.
- The educator is also responsible for acting as an appropriate role model for the student. Dilemmas may arise when the trainee physician disagrees with the staff physician about the clinical care of a particular patient, hence, there is a conflict between duties owed to the patient and duties owed to one's superiors. It is necessary to have a mechanism for arbitrating such disputes so that the best interests of the patient are respected and the student–staff relationship not harmed.

In summary, a medical trainee has duties to patients (and parents), peers and teachers, and is owed duties by peers and teachers. The prime duty is to the patient, as laid out in the physician–patient relationships. This duty takes place in the context of interprofessional duties demanding mutual respect.

CONSENT IN PEDIATRICS

The term "consent" may be interpreted in many ways. It may be acquiescence, compliance, permission, agreement, approval or collaboration. These terms reflect a spectrum ranging from passive acceptance of what is ordered to joint decision making. The patient should be an active participant in the decision making process as dictated by the assessment of the physician–patient

relationship and the moral principles of respect for persons. There is legal support for this
relationship; the only qualifier is that the patient should be deemed competent to make such a
decision. In order to make an informed decision, the adult patient needs to have sufficient
information about the medical situation and the likely outcomes or harms weighted appropriately.
There is debate about how all embracing the information given should be, paticularly with respect
to harm. It should certainly be sufficient to allow the patient to make a reasonable and objective
decision. The combination of information delivered and patient comprehension gives rise to
informed consent. Since there are two components to informed consent, that is, the delivery of
appropriate information and the ability of the patient to understand this information and make
appropriate decision about his or her care, there is room for considerable misunderstanding and
debate.

In the past, children under a certain age were deemed legally to lack the competence to make
decisions for themselves. Most recently in several jurisdictions, this legal presumption of
incompetence has been rescinded. In British Columbia, the new Infant Act makes no legislative
age of consent. This requires that consent in the pediatric age group be obtained by first
determining whether the child is legally competent to consent. Should this not be the case, we are
left with the problems of who should decide and how should that decision be made.

Determining competency

The child is a developing human being. While it would be ludicrous to assume that a newborn
could make decisions for himself/herself, it would be presumptive to assume that a teenager
cannot. For a child to be deemed incompetent to decide for himself/herself, it must be shown that
the child lacks the capacity to understand the relevant information, weigh it against personal values
and indicate a rational preference for treatment.

Some generalizations can be made. An awareness of the cognitive developmental stages of
childhood allows one to state fairly clearly that children under 7 years of age are not capable of
receiving information and providing true informed consent. Between 7 and 11 years, children
develop the ability to perform mental operations and consider two aspects of a problem. From 11
years onwards, they develop the ability to think in abstract form and hypothesize. These are
generalizations, however, and in specific instances over the age of 7 years, it is incumbent on the
physician to determine whether or not the child has the capacity to make an informed decision in
the particular medical situation. The situation itself is another variable factor. In a noncomplex
"yes or no" situation, with great benefit and minimal harm, a relatively young child may well be
capable of giving true consent after receiving the appropriate information.

How do we decide whether an individual, child or not, is capable of giving informed consent?
First they need to have the medical situation described to them with possible interventions and
recommendations as to the best options. Ideally, they should be able to demonstrate that they
have understood this by reiteration of the explanation and should also demonstrate general
understanding by asking questions about the situation and options. The more complex the
situation, the more important it is to determine understanding. This also presupposes that the
physician can communicate well so that situation and options are clearly laid out before the
patient.

Should a child not meet the standards of competence to consent, this does not mean that
(s)he should not be involved in the process. Assent, defined as "to agree voluntarily in the
absence of full comprehension to the action or suggestion of another", should be sought from

those children capable of what Piaget terms "concrete operations" (7 years and over).

Decision making for the noncompetent child

Our society charges parents with the care and protection of their children. As such, they may, with constraint, direct the form of their children's upbringing and development to autonomous beings. They are, therefore, presumed to be the surrogate decision makers most capable of making decisions in the best interests of their noncompetent children. This, in a functional family, is likely to be true although parents may make decisions in the perceived best interests of the family as a whole. This might be opposed by a deontological ethic but would likely be supported by a consequentialist viewpoint.

Specific problems with parental consent arise when the parents hold particular religious views and when they espouse alternate health approaches. These situations, while recognized in law for the parents themselves, require careful consideration. It would be reasonable to assume that if the child is incapable of assent or consent to medical intervention, (s)he is also incapable of assent or consent of the parents' views. The presumption that parents are the best decision makers for the noncompetent may also be challenged and overridden if there is strong evidence that the parents have brought harm to the child, such as evidence of child abuse or neglect. In this situation, the physician may make best interest decisions for the child, the child being temporarily or permanently apprehended by the state.

On occasion, situations may arise when rapid and/or critical decisions may occur in the care of children in the absence of somebody recognized as qualified to give consent. Here it would be reasonable to assume that life supportive decisions by any party should be implemented until reflection upon variable outcomes can be made.

In summary, consent issues in children should be first based on a respect for autonomy. If that autonomy cannot be exercised, then decisions for the noncompetent child should be made by those who best know the child, in partnership with the caregivers acting in the best interest of the child. Best interests should be calculated by examining the benefits and harms offered by the proposed interventions.

CONFIDENTIALITY

- "The adult social practice of designating certain information as confidential has a two–fold aim. On the one hand, it seeks to facilitate communications about intimate or other sensitive matters between persons standing in special relationships to each other. On the other hand, the practice is designed to exclude unauthorized persons from access to such information."
- Historically, the health profession's respect for confidentiality has always been considered a major value. "Whatsoever I shall see or hear in the course of my profession...I will never divulge holding such things to be holy secrets." (Hippocratic Oath)
- "An ethical physician will keep in confidence information derived from a patient and divulge it only with the permission of the patient except when otherwise required by law." (CMA Code of Ethics)

Respect for confidentiality is rooted in several aspects of the physician–patient relationship. Respect for the humanity of others would lead one to preserve their privacy in the intimate medical setting. Respect for autonomy would acknowledge that information about an individual belongs to that indivdual and should not be divulged to others without his/her consent. Finally, the primary basis of a patient's relationship to caregivers is one of trust. In order to receive appropriate health care, patients have to reveal information about themselves to physicians who may be total strangers to them. They may not want anyone else to know about this information. They must have good reason to trust their caregivers not to divulge this information. A caregiver's duty of fidelity to the patient would support that this trust be respected.

While confidentiality is an important duty, it cannot be an absolute duty. In the modern health care system, any individual may require access to part or all of the information received from a patient in order to play his/her role in the delivery of care to that patient. In a multicultural setting, interpreters may be privy to information about another, and in small linguistic communities this may raise difficulties in the maintenance of confidentiality. Some considerations, e.g. sexually transmitted diseases and genetic abnormalities, may affect others who may have a right to the information obtained.

In pediatrics, issues also arise as to whether or not information obtained from the competent child should be disclosed to the parents. In this case, the physician has a primary obligation to respect the confidence of the competent patient, but (s)he needs to weigh this against whether or not appropriate and needed health care will be received by the patient in the absence of parental knowledge or can only best be delivered if the parents are aware. It is important to note that in British Columbia, there is no legal compulsion to inform parents of a competent child. In the case of noncompetent children, the same duty of confidentiality is owed to those who provide information on the part of the children.

Disclosure of information

Once a patient has given information to a physician, both verbally and by submitting to a physical examination and appropriate investigations, the physician is in a position to give information (diagnosis, management options) back to the patient. For a competent patient, such information is necessary for him/her to make informed decisons about his/her care (see consent). Problems arise if the physician or parents, having been informed before the child, feel that some information should be withheld from the patient, such as poor prognosis. Here, a determination should be made as to whether disclosure will pose a significant risk of harm to the patient due to a substantial adverse effect on the patient's physical, mental or emotional health.

Disclosure to others may be mandated in law, such as child abuse or neglect. It may also be justifiable to disclose information to a third party when there is strong risk of harm to that third party. When such breaches of confidentiality are deemed necessary, only such information as is required should be shared and only to those who have a need for such information. The child or parents should be asked to agree to the sharing of such information even though refusal will not necessarily prevent the information from being transmitted.

In summary, the physician has a strong duty to maintain confidentiality in the physician–patient relationship based on respect for patient humanity and autonomy and the patient's expectations in trust in the relationship. This transfers duty to the decison makers in the case of the noncompetent child. This duty may be overridden if there is a countervailing strong prospect of significant harm to the patient or to a third party arising out of the maintenance of confidentiality.

WITHHOLDING/WITHDRAWING TREATMENT

Preamble

This section is confined to issues surrounding the provision or nonprovision of life sustaining therapy in the case of patients who are likely to die should such therapy not be provided. It is recognized that issues of withholding treatment, which the patient wishes but does not need, occur in other settings (e.g. antibiotics for a "cold"), but these issues are best explored in the section on physician–patient relationships (q.v.).

In considering the physician's involvement in activities related to the care of patients at the end of life, several fundamental questions arise. What is it to be a human being? What should our attitudes as persons and physicians be towards death, which is after all the inevitable end–point of life for us all? What are our obligations as persons and physicians to patients facing mortal illness? If sustaining life requires scarce or expensive technological resources, how should this be considered in making a clinical decision as to their use?

Until the mid–20th Century, life threatening illness and trauma most often resulted in death, with physicians being powerless to prevent it. However, a burgeoning of knowledge and technology has resulted in the ability to sustain life in previously fatal situations. Most often this allows for ultimate recovery of a life that is judged by the patient and others to have value. On occasion, the perceived life may be thought to be burdensome (lacking in quality) and in other circumstances the institution of life sustaining measures may be considered either a futile or excessively burdensome form of treatment.

Decision making in this arena may also give rise to a situation where physician and patient or proxy decision makers disagree as to the best course of action. There may also be disagreements within the health care team in a clinical setting where the multidisciplinary team approach is more the norm than the intimate long–term single physician–patient relationship.

Treatment withholding/withdrawal issues in pediatrics are also complicated by the fact that the patient is frequently incapable of expressing a preference in this matter. If the child in question is deemed noncompetent to decide, it is usually assumed that the parents should make decisions for the child. Some would argue that this is an excessive burden for the parents and that some form of shared decision making process be adopted. Should this be a consensus decision or depend on the majority opinion? Can we, and how do we, determine when death would seem preferable to continued life?

Definitions

1. Withholding treatment
The decison not to institute a treatment which may sustain life (either because it is refused by the competent patient or because it is deemed not to be in the best interests of the noncompetent patient).

2. Withdrawing treatment
The act of removing previously instituted life sustaining treatment (either at the request of the competent patient or because it is deemed not to have proven effective in providing for the best interests of the noncompetent patient).

3. Euthanasia
The deliberate, rapid and painless termination of life of a person afflicted with incurable and progressive disease. This may be voluntary or nonvoluntary and, if voluntary, may take the form of assisting the patient in the taking of his/her own life (assisted suicide).

4. Palliative care
Health care directed towards the relief of suffering caused by a disease process which in itself may or may not be treated with curative intent. Most often applied when the underlying disease is considered incurable.

5. Terminal care
Health care directed towards the relief of suffering in a patient who has clearly embarked on the process of dying.

6. Double–effect
This rule or principle arose out of a deontological base (Catholic doctrine) and serves to justify acts which have two foreseen effects: beneficial and intended or harmful and unintended.
- The act itself must be good or, at the least, morally neutral.
- The intention of the agent must be to seek the good effect. The bad effect can be foreseen and tolerated but not intended.
- The bad effect must not be the means to achieve the good effect.
- The good effect must outweigh the bad effect.

7. Futility
The concept that physicians are not obliged to offer and patients are not obliged to undergo treatments that are futile. There are two aspects to this concept:
- Quantitative futility: the treatment is useless for the purpose intended based on empiric data; as such, it need not be offered.
- Qualitative futility: the treatment may have some effect for a specific aspect of the patient's condition but is unlikely to produce a benefit for the patient as a whole.

8. Do not resuscitate (DNR) orders
Orders not to resuscitate a patient, should that person cease cardiorespiratory function, represent one of the few situations in an institutional setting where a medical intervention with a patient is asked not to occur. It must have been specifically ordered and agreed to by patient (or proxy) and physician. Much debate about futility surrounds the exercise of cardiopulmonary resuscitation and its likely outcomes in different medical situations. Ideally, CPR should be assessed as any other treatment modality with an analysis of benefits and burdens and incorporated into management plans accordingly.

CONTENT/ETHICAL PROBLEMS

Are withholding and withdrawing treatment equivalent moral acts?

The physical difference between withholding treatment not yet started and withdrawing treatment already commenced would seem to be clear: the first is an act of omission while the second is an act of commission. Many physicians feel that the legal interpretation of such types of act would suggest that it is better not to initiate treatment than to discontinue treatment already started. The US Presidents Commission has suggested that little, if any, legal significance attaches to the physical distinction between withholding and withdrawing. Indeed they note that not starting treatment that might be in a patient's best interests is more likely to be held a civil or criminal wrong than stopping such treatment when it has proved unavailing.

This points to where the equivalence lies. If, in making decisions about whether to treat or whether to discontinue an already commenced treatment, it can be concluded that the treatment is not in the patient's best interests, then either act is appropriate. If doubt exists, then treatment should be instituted but may be withdrawn should it prove excessively burdensome and/or unavailing.

Under what circumstances should treatment be withheld/withdrawn?

The American Academy of Pediatrics states that the following principles should be honored:
- There should be a presumption in favor of treatment.
- Decision makers should have a right to adequate information about treatment, options and likely outcomes.
- The competent patient has the right to refuse offered treatment. There is a limited right for parents or guardians to refuse treatment for their noncompetent children, subject to demonstrating that they are acting in the child's best interests.
- The decision to limit treatment applies specifically to treatments discussed by the physician and patient and/or parents or guardians.
- There must be ongoing respect for the patient and continuing assurance of effort to maintain the patient's comfort.

The 1987 Canadian Pediatric Society statement likewise accepts that in the noncompetent child, judgment should be made on a best interest standard with the base assumption that the child has a justified claim to life.

The statement concludes that life sustaining therapy can reasonably be considered unacceptable when:
- There is irreversible progression to imminent death (terminal illness).
- The treatment in question is clearly ineffective (futile) or harmful (burdensome).
- The cure is one in which life would be severely shortened regardless of therapy and where nontreatment will allow a greater degree of caring and comfort (palliative care).

Emphasis should be placed on the concept that withholding or withdrawing is not an abandonment of all treatments received by the patient. Each treatment offered should be examined for its intent, efficacy and the burdens that it brings. This approach to withholding or withdrawing is a rejection of approaches which emphasize a treat at all costs mentality (do whatever can be done; do whatever prolongs life—vitalism; do whatever is medically indicated for the disease—technical solution to a moral problem). There is likewise no recourse in these statements to a substituted judgment standard. The emphasis on a child's best interests allows caregivers to focus on what is the aggregate sum of benefits and burdens for the child, relegating other interests (family, physician, societal) to contextual background. Benefits and burdens should be considered as those direct effects brought about by the treatment and those effects brought about by continued life.

Should active euthanasia be considered an option in the context of withholding or withdrawing treatment?

Active euthanasia is a criminal offense in Canada, whereas the Canadian courts in the main have accepted that the decisions to withhold or withdraw treatment are decisions to be made within the physician–patient relationship without fear of criminal repercussion. Nonetheless, some would argue that the intent involved in not using life sustaining therapy and the intent involved in active euthanasia are one and the same, an end to a life involving suffering. All that is different is the action taken. Opponents of active euthanasia would suggest that the intent is indeed different, withholding being intended to allow the patient to die a "natural" death whereas there is nothing natural about killing in this situation.

Euthanasia supporters might also point out that palliative care procedures may give rise to an earlier death than would otherwise occur, e.g. the use of pain suppressing drugs giving rise to respiratory failure. Some responses to this utilize the principle of double–effect, stating that the good intention and effect are that of providing relief from suffering, while the bad effect (by no means certain) is an earlier death. This argument cannot be used by proponents of euthanasia where the good effect (relief from suffering) is achieved through the bad effect (killing).

Other arguments against euthanasia rest on the effects it would have on the physician–patient relationship and the principle of trust that arises from this. Others feel that a great social harm will arise from sanctioning active euthanasia.

The pediatric concern with this issue is related to whether or not a slippery slope effect would occur should competent patients be allowed to request and receive active euthanasia. The feeling is that such action would eventually be applied to patients incapable of direct consent or refusal. At least one Dutch commentator feels that this situation has already developed in Holland where voluntary active euthanasia is tolerated legally.

"Futility" in decisions involving withholding/withdrawing treatment

The concept of futile treatment has been widely debated in recent years.

As the definition shows, treatment futility can exist in two forms:
- A treatment is quantitatively futile if it will not produce a desired physiological effect in the patient. In other words, it is ineffective and therefore does not need to be offered.
- Qualitative futility exists when a treatment will produce a predicted effect but this effect is of no real benefit to the clinical goals for the patient. In this situation, therefore, the treatment can only be appropriately defined once the needs of the patient have been thoroughly explored and defined. Qualitative futility can therefore be considered to be a value statement.

DNR as a futile treatment

The issue of CPR is an area where the futility debate has been most active in the adult sphere. CPR was developed as a means of attempting to resuscitate those who die a sudden unexplained death. It is now, in an institutional setting, the only intervention which requires a negative order to prevent its implementation. There are many conditions, e.g. terminal cancer, where CPR would be both quantitatively and qualitatively futile, i.e. ineffective and not being in the patient's best interests.

CPR needs in childhood are somewhat different from adult CPR needs, being more often than not related to primary respiratory arrest. Rather than a global DNR order, it would seem much more appropriate to delineate levels of care from aggressive to terminal, in consultation with patients and parents/guardians. This approach is superficially attractive but is difficult to implement in practice.

Who makes the decision to withhold or withdraw therapy?

1. The child
The basis for decision making in competent patients is the provision of all the information necessary by the physician in order that the patient may make informed decisions. In pediatrics, there is a graduation from demonstrably noncompetent patients to demonstrably competent patients, with the determination of competence or capacity to decide, depending on the developmental level of the child, the state of the child and the circumstances to be decided upon. Given that the nonuse or withdrawal of life sustaining treatment is a high stakes decision, the competence of a child to decide should be rigorously established. With respect to assessing competence in this situation, it has been suggested that the child is capable of foregoing such treatment if (s)he has experienced an illness for some time, understands the illness and the benefits and burdens of its treatment, has the ability to reason about the illness and treatment, has previously been involved in treatment decisions and, most importantly, understands the personal meaning and finality of death. Some adolescents have these abilities but may still need to share the decision making with parents because of personal vulnerability.

2. The parents/guardians
If the patient is deemed noncompetent, it is usually assumed that the parents are the next most appropriate decision makers. This position has been accepted by the Canadian Pediatric Society (CPS). The basis for the assumption is that the parents best know the child and are most likely to consider the child's best interests. They have a legal duty in law to provide for the necessities of life for the child. At the same time, leaving this decision solely to the parents is likely to give rise to considerable distress which may interfere with their rational assessment of the benefits and burdens of proposed intervention or nonintervention. There are also exceptions to the role of parents as decison makers. The CPS statement excepts parents as decision makers when:
- They are incompetent to make decisions for themselves.
- There are unresolvable differences between the parents.
- They have clearly relinquished responsibility for the child. This may be because they no longer wish to care for the child or have already ceded the care of the child to others. At other times, it may be, because in the judgment of others, they have abused the child emotionally or physically.

3. Others
Weir has suggested that there are four qualifications needed by the decision maker: relevant knowledge and information, impartiality, emotional stability and consistency.
Based on this, he has listed the decision makers in the following order:

- Parents or other family members.
- Attending physician.
- Ethics Committee.
- Courts.

It could be suggested that decison makers should actually be a group of people who know the child and have obligations to the child by dint of special relationship. Accordingly, as Bartholome suggests, the decision making group should involve parents and other involved family, physicians, nurses and/or other therapists acting together to share information and deciding in the best interests of the child. Should they come to no consensus, particularly if the ethical issues are perplexing or complex, then subsequent recourse to an institutional Ethics Committee could be made. Recourse to the courts could be considered when the family is deadlocked.

JUSTICE AND WITHHOLDING OR WITHDRAWING LIFE SUSTAINING TREATMENT

General

It is recognized that these days there is an increasing demand for health care resources. Such resources are also becoming more costly as technology advances.

Life sustaining treatment seems to hold a special place when medical care and technology are evaluated. The US Presidents Commission states that "the level of care deemed adequate should reflect a reasoned judgment not only about the impact of the conditon on the welfare of the individual but also of the efficacy and costs of care itself in relation to other conditions and the efficacy and costs of care available for them". This is essentially a utilitarian argument. However, in a life threatening situation, there is a strong imperative to rescue endangered life. As such, there has been a tendency to allocate funds to provide for the availability of life sustaining treatments, perhaps at the expense of denying adequate funding for the management of chronic but not life threatening disease. It would seem important, therefore, that life sustaining treatment be carefully evaluated as to the feasibility of achieving the patient's goals. In this regard, aggressive life sustaining treatment of the terminally ill, or others whose interests are not served by such life prolongation, is not only unethical with respect to the patient but is an unethical use of a precious resource.

Issues at the microallocation level

Institutions which provide health care have a finite budget and must make allocations to multiple health care resources within this budget. Such institutions may have a specific mandate, such as cancer care for children, and therefore may allocate funds towards specific target population needs. As part of the allocation, they may elect to apportion resources to provide for life sustaining therapy. These resources will be both human and technological. In certain circumstances, the availability of one or both may become limited. In this situation, how can it be decided who will benefit from or who has least claim to these resources?

Should utilization issues be considered in decision to withhold or withdraw when such treatment is available?

If the discussion over burdens and benefits has indicated that active life sustaining treatment is likely to be in the best interest of the child, then such treatment should be offered.

What should be done when there is competition for a scarce resource (e.g. the last ventilator in ICU)?

The issue hearkens back to the days of committees deciding on hemodialysis allocation. Factors which were then considered included age (life yet to be lived), likely benefit to society, past worthiness, likelihood of a good outcome, present medical need and time of presentation (first come first served). A lottery system has also been suggested. Most of these have been considered socially judgmental and discriminatory and some, in the case of children, are irrelevant. Presently, most decision makers base their choices on a combination of medical need and a first come first serve criteria. Others still have concern about ignoring social considerations.

Making these decisions creates a conflict between the physician's role as advocate for the patient and the physician's duty to others. A just distribution of such resources can be achieved either by a cooperative arrangement among physicians to determine those most in need or a set of policies outlining a process for allocation within the institution.

Such policies should delineate the criteria to be used for selection or deselection of patients and should be based on clinical information. Such hospital policies stand in the shadow of the law and while prescriptive cannot be considered to be absolute.

Can a patient be removed from life sustaining therapy to allow for this to be used for another patient with a better chance of recovery or better ultimate prognosis?

A utilitarian argument would suggest that this is an appropriate act and might suggest that any argument to the contrary is merely the assertion of a property right. However, there would seem to be a strong assault on the principle of trust in such an act. Most would feel that such a decision should only be made if the goals of treatment for the first patient have demonstrably not been achieved.

RESEARCH

For some 1,500 years, the practice of medicine was empiric and dogmatic, resting on the authority of Galen (138–201 AD). From the 17th Century on, medicine developed scientific principles and medicines moved from empiricism towards scientific research. As stated by Claude Bernard, the recognized father of experimental medicine, this means "methodically organized experimentation that will allow physicians to prove that their interventions, and not nature on its own or some other factors, have brought about the prevention and cure they claim to have achieved" (1865).

The aim of research, therefore, is to produce improvement in clinical practice. Such research may be nontherapeutic where the aim of the inquiry is not likely to provide direct benefits to the research subject (e.g. phase one drug trials) or they may be therapeutic in which there is a foreseeable likelihood that there will be direct benefit to the research subject (e.g. phase three drug trials).

Since research is aimed at bringing about greater knowledge and improvement in the delivery of clinical care, it would seem that it is an ethical imperative or at least ethically desirable. However, evidence of past abuses (Tuskegee, Willowbrook) demonstrate that it is important to respect the humanity and autonomy of the research subject. Arising out of such abuses in the past, all grant dependent protocols in Canada are subject to the prior approval of an institutional review process. Ideally, unfunded research protocols should receive similar reviews. The review includes consideration of the scientific adequacy of the proposal, the credentials of the researcher, the research environment and steps taken to avoid or reveal conflicts of interest on the part of the researcher if (s)he also fills a clinical care role with the research subjects. Also included are considerations of the consent/assent process, of the harm/benefit ratio, of attention to confidentiality issues and the equity in selection of research subjects. This process is broadened in the case of children as research subjects.

Children as research subjects

Given that we have established the values of research to the improvement and refinement of clinical care, it would be reasonable to assume that the clinical care of children would be benefited by research on child subjects. One could argue that the results of research on adults could be extrapolated to guide the use of validated adult interventions in children. However, this would be an empiric approach and could be harmful rather than beneficial. It would, therefore, appear that if we are to improve our ability to provide good clinical care for children, then there must be research on child subjects. It could be deemed an inequity if a total ban on children as research subjects were enforced, as this would deprive a whole group of a benefit that is offered to others.

Having established the need for such research, it is important to ensure that only such research that requires child subjects should utilize such subjects. If research with adults can answer the questions and the answer will be applicable to children, then such research should be done with adults. If this is not the case, then a careful assessment of the risk of harm and the possibility of benefit should next be undertaken. Here, the risk of harm applies to the individual, but there is debate about whether the benefit should be to the individual child or to children in society as a whole. The parents and child should then receive all relevant information about the research project in order that they may provide informed consent. They should be aware that the prime goal of the research is to improve our knowledge.

Other issues arise when the researcher is the individual providing clinical care for the child–patient. Here, the physican needs to give assurances to the parents and child that should research and treatment goals come into conflict, the physician will respect the clinical care needs of the individual child. Secondly, when a physician involved in the clinical care of a child invites the child to be part of a research venture, the parents and child may be reluctant to refuse because of the past relationship or out of fear that the clinical care may be compromised by a refusal. Again, the physician needs to reassure the child and parents that the delivery of clinical care is not contingent upon agreeing to participate in a research protocol.

Canadian guidelines, about the use of children in reasearch, have been laid out by the National Council on Bioethics and Human Research. In addition to looking at the nature of research and researcher as previously mentioned, it also recommends the inclusion of someone with a knowledge of pediatrics on the review panel, in addition to a patient/parent advocate and a representative of an agency who represents the health care of children in general.

It can be accepted that the competent child may consent to research. Can the parents of a noncompetent child enroll such a child in a research protocol? Some would argue that they should only do so if there is expectation of direct benefit to the child. Others would argue that so long as there is a minimum risk of harm to the child they may do so even when there is no expectation of direct benefit but a chance of future benefit to children. Should parents wish to involve a child in research but the child expresses dissent, then researchers should respect the humanity of the subject and not include such a child. It is also important not to deceive the child subject even if noncompetent, as this may undermine any trust the child has in parents and physicians.

Innovative therapy

This can be defined as the use of a new or nonstandard, nonevaluated intervention for the purpose of direct patient benefit. Accordingly, it differs from research in its focus on individual therapeutic benefit rather than being directed towards an increase in medical knowledge. Such therapy is usually offered when other standard therapies have been unsuccessful. This therapy should be peer reviewed (Ethics Committee) and continued use of such therapy should not be maintained without a proper clinical trial protocol.

To summarize, ethical research is a beneficent activity designed to increase knowledge and improve medical care. A properly designed study will minimize the risk of harm and will be offered to subjects honestly and openly, respecting the humanity and autonomy of those persons.

Refusal of parents or subjects to participate should not result in any penalty with regard to their clinical care.

This chapter was prepared with the help of the pediatric ethics network (Pedethnet), funded by SSHRC and AMS. Special credit goes to the following committee members: S. Tallett, M. Rowell, M. Sidarous, J. Hellmann, A. Lynch, N. Kenny and R. Hilliard.

Hematological disorders may be divided into disorders of red blood cells (RBC's), white blood cells (WBC's), platelets and coagulation.

DISORDERS OF RED BLOOD CELLS

Anemia

May be due to:
- Decreased production of RBC's: dietary deficiency (iron deficiency is most common), bone marrow failure or infiltration, dyshematopoiesis (abnormal RBC formation).
- Blood loss: acute, chronic.
- Increased destruction (hemolysis) of RBC's: hemoglobin (e.g. thalassemia and sickle cell disease), congenital abnormalities of membrane (e.g. spherocytosis), enzymes (e.g. G6PD, PK deficiency), immune hemolysis, nonimmune hemolysis.

1. Diagnosis of anemia
- History (key points):
    Duration of symptoms and pallor.
    Previous history of anemia, blood disorders, transfusions.
    Blood loss (epistaxis, GI bleeding, menstruation).
    Detailed dietary history (include volume of milk consumed, amount of meat and green vegetables, history of pica).
    History of jaundice and dark urine.
    Recent infections, particularly viral infection.
    GI symptoms, diarrhea, abdominal pain, GI blood loss.
    History of chronic illness.
    Medication history and history of ingestion of fava beans (important in G6PD deficiency).
    Family history of anemia, gallstones, transfusions.
- Physical examination (key points): cardiovascular stability (heart rate, blood pressure, postural hypotension, congestive cardiac failure), nutritional status, jaundice, lymphadenopathy, hepatosplenomegaly, petechiae, bruises.
- Investigations: the choice of investigations should be guided by the history and physical examination. Preliminary tests may include:
    Cross–match (for unstable patients only).
    CBC should include hemoglobin, mean cell volume (MCV), morphology, white blood count and differential, platelet count.
    WBC and platelet count will show whether this is an isolated anemia. Decrease in other cell lines indicates bone marrow failure or infiltration.
    MCV: if low, usually due to iron deficiency or thalassemia; if high, usually due to increased RBC production (blood loss, hemolysis) or may be due to dyserythropoiesis or bone marrow failure.
    Morphology: specific abnormalities may indicate the diagnosis.

Reticulocytes: if low, poor RBC production; if high, increased RBC loss or destruction.
Direct antiglobulin (Coombs') test for immune hemolytic anemia.
LDH and bilirubin: increased levels are indicative of hemolysis.
Stools for occult blood.
Other tests: iron studies (ferritin, serum iron, TIBC, free erythrocyte protoporphyrin), coagulation screen (PT, PTT, fibrinogen), bone marrow aspirate and biopsy, specific tests for abnormalities of RBC membrane, enzyme, hemoglobin.

2. Management of anemia
This depends on the cause, but there are a few general principles.
Admit to hospital for:
- Cardiovascular compromise, acute onset of severe anemia, significant bleeding, suspicion of severe underlying disease.
- Transfusion: avoid transfusion if possible as there are significant risks. Transfuse for cardiovascular compromise or uncontrollable bleeding.

It is beyond the scope of this chapter to discuss management of all causes of childhood anemia. However, the more common and clinically significant causes of anemia will be discussed.

3. Iron deficiency anemia
Iron deficiency is the most common nutritional deficiency in children. The incidence is up to 5% in school age children and up to 25% in pregnant teenage girls.
- Causes of iron deficiency:
  Deficient intake:
  Normal dietary requirement is 1 mg/kg per d (maximum 15 mg/d). Preterm and low birth weight infants require 2 mg/kg per d. Cows milk and human milk contain equal amounts of iron (0.5–1.5 mg/L) but breast fed babies absorb 49% of the iron in contrast to 10% absorbed from cows milk.
  Infants and children at risk for dietary iron deficiency include: low birth weight infants, infants fed unsupplemented cows milk from birth, delayed introduction of solid foods (after 6 months), excess milk intake at the expense of other foods (usually > 1 L/d during the second year of life).
  Increased demand:
  Excessive growth: low birth weight infants, multiple births, adolescence, pregnancy.
  Cyanotic congenital heart disease.
  Blood loss:
  Perinatal: any cause of perinatal blood loss results in low iron stores at birth.
  GI: most common site for chronic blood loss. Hypersensitivity to heat labile cows milk protein causes blood loss and exudative enteropathy.
  Anatomical lesions such as Meckel's diverticulum, gastritis, parasites.
  Other sites: e.g. nose, uterus, kidney, lung.
  Impaired absorption:
  Celiac disease, prolonged diarrhea, inflammatory bowel disease.
  Impaired utilization:
  Lead poisoning, sideroblastic anemia.
- Diagnosis:
  Hemoglobin – low.

MCV – low; mean cell hemoglobin (MCH) – low; mean cell hemoglobin concentration (MCHC) – low; red cell distribution width (RDW) – widened.
Morphology: hypochromic, microcytic.
Reticulocytes: usually normal but may be increased if iron deficiency is due to bleeding.
Serum ferritin (reflects body iron store) – low; usually a reliable test but may be falsely elevated in infection or inflammation.
Serum iron (reflects the balance between iron absorbed and iron used or stored) – low; can fluctuate quite markedly.
Total iron binding capacity – high. Percent saturation – low. As the serum iron falls, the iron binding capacity increases and the percent saturation falls.
Free erythrocyte protoporphyrin (FEP) – high. These are heme precursors which accumulate as iron availability decreases.
Therapeutic trial of oral iron; in iron deficiency, an increase in reticulocytes is usually seen within 3–4 days and an increase in hemoglobin in 5–10 days.
• Differential diagnosis (iron deficiency should be differentiated from other causes of microcytic, hypochromic anemia):
    Hemoglobinopathy: thalassemia (α and β), hemoglobin E.
    Lead poisoning.
    Chronic inflammation or infection (usually normochromic, serum iron and TIBC reduced).
• Treatment:
    Diet: use breast milk or iron fortified formula until 12 months. Restrict milk to ≤ 500 mL/d. If there is evidence of GI blood loss and protein loss, then use formula, evaporated milk or boiled milk.
    Oral iron: use ferrous iron preparation (ferric iron is poorly absorbed). Ferrous sulfate contains 20% elemental iron. Dose: 6 mg/kg per d elemental iron (usually divided into 3 doses); give between meals.
    Parenteral iron: iron–dextran complex can be given safely intramuscularly but its use should be restricted to patients who are noncompliant with oral iron or are truly intolerant of oral iron (rare) or patients with severe bowel disease and malabsorption.
    Blood transfusion: only used for severe iron deficiency anemia associated with cardiac failure (hemoglobin usually < 40 g/L) or when rapid correction is necessary such as presurgery. Transfusion should be given slowly when there is cardiac compromise and in several aliquots of 2–3 mL/kg over 4 h each. Give lasix 0.5 mg/kg between aliquots and check for congestive cardiac failure. Limit donor exposures by giving all aliquots of blood from a single donor unit.

4. Folic acid deficiency anemia
Folate deficiency is rare. The most common causes are: chronic hemolytic anemia, goats milk feeding, GI disease causing poor ileal absorption and severe malnutrition.
• Diagnosis:
    Hemoglobin – low.
    MCV – high. MCHC – normal.
    Neutrophils – hypersegmented.
    Red cell and serum folate levels – low.
• Treatment:
    Folic acid orally. Dose 100–200 μg/d. The elixir is usually 1 mg/mL.

5. B$_{12}$ deficiency anemia

B$_{12}$ deficiency is rare. The most common causes are: dietary (vegan diet in the child or mother, if breast feeding), congenital abnormalities in vitamin B$_{12}$ absorption, transport or metabolism, failure to secrete intrinsic factor (pernicious anemia), failure to absorb B$_{12}$ in the terminal ileum (inflammatory bowel disease).

- Diagnosis:
    Hemoglobin – low. MCV – high. MCHC – normal.
    Serum B$_{12}$ levels: low.
    Detailed tests may be required to determine the cause of B$_{12}$ deficiency.
- Treatment: vitamin B$_{12}$ is usually given intramuscularly initially. Dose depends on the cause of deficiency.

Bone marrow failure

This may be a failure of all three cell lines (aplastic anemia, hypoplastic anemia) or an isolated failure of a single cell line (RBC's, WBC's or platelets).

1. Aplastic anemia (AA)

Bone marrow failure causing decreased or absent production of red cells, white cells and platelets.

- Severe AA is defined as:
    Granulocyte count < 0.5×10^9 /L.
    Platelet count < 20×10^9 /L.
    Reticulocyte count < 20×10^9 /L.
    Bone marrow aspirate and biopsy showing < 25% hematopoietic cells remaining.
- Causes:
    Congenital:
    Fanconi's anemia (FA): autosomal recessive. Associated with congenital anomalies, short stature, skeletal abnormalities (especially thumbs), renal and cardiac abnormalities, deafness. Pancytopenia usually occurs after 4 years of age. Chromosomes show increased breakages and structural changes.
    Dyskeratosis congenita (DC): usually sex linked recessive. Associated with increased skin pigmentation, mucosal leukoplakia and nail atrophy.
    Acquired aplastic anemia:
    Idiopathic: 70% of cases have no identifiable cause.
    Drugs: usually reversible, dose dependent (chemotherapy drugs) or unpredictable, dose independent (antibiotics—chloramphenicol; anticonvulsants—phenytoin; antirheumatics—phenylbutazone and gold); antidiabetics—tolbutamide and chlorpropamide; antimalarial—quinacrine).
    Insecticides: DDT, parathion, chlordane.
    Toxins: benzene, carbon tetrachloride, glue, toluene.
    Irradiation.
    Infection: viral hepatitis A, B, C (usually associated with the most severe form of AA); HIV, EBV, chronic parvovirus, other viral infections.
    Pregnancy.
    Paroxysmal nocturnal hemoglobinuria (PNH).

Thymoma.
- Clinical presentation (key points):
    History must include exposure to known causes as above and family history of FA and DC.
    Physical findings are usually related to pancytopenia, i.e. pallor, petechiae and bruises, signs of infection.
    Check for skeletal abnormalities (particularly short stature and abnormal thumbs), skin changes, dysmorphic features and leukoplakia.
- Diagnosis (investigations):
    CBC, differential, morphology, reticulocytes. All cell lines are low in AA.
    Fetal hemoglobin. Usually increased in AA.
    Bone marrow aspirate and biopsy, including immunophenotyping and cytogenetics.
    Hematopoietic cells are decreased or absent and replaced by fat. Erythroid precursors are often megaloblastic.
    Chromosomal analysis of peripheral blood, including tests for chromosome breakages.
    Acidified serum lysis test or sugar water test to exclude PNH.
    Chest X–ray to exclude thymoma.
    Viral serology for hepatitis A, B, C, EBV, parvovirus, HIV.
    Pregnancy test.
    Group and screen including complete RBC phenotype.
- Treatment:
    Supportive care: this is essential for all patients. Remove cause if possible, e.g. exposure to drugs and toxins.
    Prevent infection:
    Avoid exposure (do not admit to hospital if avoidable).
    Careful handwashing and skin hygiene.
    Good oral hygiene: chlorhexidene mouthwash, dental care with soft toothbrush, mycostatin oral prophylaxis (2–5 mL t.i.d.).
    Avoid rectal trauma (no rectal thermometers or suppositories) and keep stools soft.
    Treat infection aggressively.
    Bleeding:
    Prevent bleeding, if possible, by avoiding trauma, sports, etc. (avoid aspirin, nonsteroidal anti–inflammatory drugs).
    Prevent menstruation with oral contraceptives (a high dose may be necessary initially to stop menstruation and the patient may then be maintained on a normal daily dose of Min–Ovral).
    Platelet transfusion may be necessary to maintain the platelet count > 10×10^9 /L but transfusion should be avoided if possible (platelets should be irradiated, filtered, CMV negative if patient seronegative for CMV).
    Anemia:
    Red blood cell transfusion may be necessary to maintain the hemoglobin at a safe level but the patient should not be transfused unless clinically indicated. RBC's should be irradiated, filtered and CMV negative (if patient CMV seronegative).
    Transfusion should be avoided if possible. Transfusion may sensitize the patient to HLA antigens, which can cause poor response to platelet transfusion in the future and reduce the success rate with allogeneic bone marrow transplant.
    Growth factors: GCSF may be helpful but their exact role has not yet been established in

aplastic anemia.
- Specific treatments:
  Bone marrow transplant: this is currently the treatment of choice for patients who have an HLA matched sibling donor. Long–term survival after bone marrow transplant is 70% for transfused patients and 85% for nontransfused patients.
  Immunosuppressive therapy: this has been used successfully for patients with moderate aplastic anemia or those who do not have a bone marrow donor. It does not improve the outcome in patients with congenital aplastic anemia. The most successful regimen has been a combination of prednisone, antithymocyte globulin and cyclosporine.

2. Anemia due to isolated failure of RBC formation
- Diamond Blackfan anemia (DBA):
  This is a rare congenital disorder manifested by failure to produce RBC precursors in an otherwise healthy bone marrow. Autosomal dominant or recessive.
  Clinical features: anemia presenting in first year of life; 25% have short stature, skeletal anomalies or facial dysmorphism.
  Laboratory features:
  Hemoglobin – low. MCV – high (> 90). Reticulocytes – low. WBC and platelets – normal. Fetal hemoglobin – increased. Chromosomes – normal.
  Bone marrow: marked reduction in erythroid precursors.
  Differential diagnosis:
  Transient erythroblastopenia of childhood.
  Late hyperegenerative anemia from Rh or ABO hemolytic anemia of the newborn.
  Treatment:
  Steroids: 85–90% respond to prednisone 2–4 mg/kg per d with reticulocytosis in 1–3 wk. The dose of prednisone should then be reduced to the minimum to maintain a reasonable hemoglobin; 20% of patients will eventually improve and become steroid independent.
  Transfusion: chronic transfusion therapy is necessary for patients who fail to respond to prednisone. RBC's should be filtered and CMV negative.
  Bone marrow transplant has been used successfully for steroid resistant patients.
- Transient erythroblastopenia of childhood (TEC):
  This is a severe reversible anemia which occurs in previously healthy children between ages 6 months to 5 years.
  Clinical features:
  Slow onset of anemia (1–2 month history) in an otherwise healthy child.
  History of viral illness in preceding 1–2 months.
  Laboratory features:
  Hemoglobin – low. MCV – normal. Reticulocytes – low.
  WBC: 10% have neutropenia.
  Platelets: 5% have thrombocytopenia.
  Fetal hemoglobin – normal.
  Bone marrow: decrease in erythroid precursors.
  Viral studies may have evidence of recent parvovirus infection.
  Treatment:
  Spontaneous recovery occurs usually within 4–8 weeks.
  Transfusions: may be necessary for cardiovascular compromise. Transfuse slowly and

minimize donor exposure by giving several small aliquots from 1 unit of blood.

3. Congenital dyshematopoietic anemia (CDA)
This is a group of disorders in which there is ineffective and abnormal erythropoiesis. Most patients have mild anemia but a minority have severe anemia and may become transfusion dependent. Red cell survival is short and the patient may have chronic or intermittent jaundice.
• Diagnosis: bone marrow shows characteristic changes with abnormal erythropoietic precursors.
• Treatment: usually none required as the anemia is mild; chronic transfusions and chelation therapy may be necessary for severe anemia. Splenectomy may reduce transfusion requirement.

4. Anemia due to bone marrow infiltration
• Bone marrow infiltration may be due to malignant disease (e.g. leukemia, lymphoma, neuroblastoma) or nonmalignant disease (e.g. Gaucher's disease, cystinosis, osteopetrosis or other metabolic disorders).
• All three cell lines will eventually be affected but anemia may be the initial presentation. Peripheral blood may show a leukoerythroblastic picture with early myeloid and erythroid precursors present in peripheral blood. Normal peripheral blood examination does not exclude bone marrow infiltration and if there is clinical suspicion, a bone marrow should always be performed.

5. Anemia of chronic infection and inflammation
Anemia complicates many chronic systemic diseases associated with infection or inflammation such as chronic pyogenic infections and rheumatoid arthritis.
• Mechanism of anemia:
    Decreased RBC survival due to increased activity of reticuloendothelial system.
    Decreased bone marrow response to anemia.
    Impaired iron metabolism with defective release of iron from tissue into the plasma.
    Chronic blood loss may contribute (inflammatory bowel disease or aspirin).
• Laboratory findings:
    Hemoglobin – usually 60–90.
    MCV – normal (occasionally low). MCH – normal (occasionally low). RDW – normal.
    Reticulocytes – normal to low. WBC – increased.
    Iron studies: serum iron – low. Iron binding capacity – low. Percent saturation – normal to low. Ferritin – high (acute phase reactant). FEP – moderately high.
    Bone marrow – normal to hypercellular.
• Treatment:
    Treatment of underlying disease is the most important.
    RBC transfusion for severe anemia if symptomatic.
    Iron supplements only if a child has associated iron deficiency.

6. Anemia of chronic renal disease
Renal insufficiency is usually associated with chronic anemia and sometimes pancytopenia.
• Mechanism of anemia:
    Erythropoietin deficiency (90% is produced by the kidney) causing impaired bone marrow

response to anemia. Uremia also contributes to impaired bone marrow function.
Decreased RBC survival due to the toxic effect of urea and microangiopathic hemolytic anemia.
Blood loss (uremia causes impaired platelet function).
Folate deficiency (folate is dialyzable).
- Laboratory findings:
    Hemoglobin – low (40–50). MCV, MCH – normal. Reticulocytes – low.
    WBC – often high. Platelets – normal.
    Bone marrow – hypercellular.
- Treatment:
    Erythropoietin (recombinant human – rHuEPO) 50–100 unit/kg t.i.d. i.v. or s.c. The dose may need to be adjusted according to the response. Hypertension occurs in 30% of patients (secondary to hyperviscosity) and blood pressure needs to be monitored closely.
    Folic acid: 1 mg/d if on dialysis.
    Iron supplements: 6 mg/kg per d elemental iron, if iron deficient.

7. Anemia of liver disease
Patients with chronic liver disease may also be anemic.
- Mechanism:
    Decreased RBC survival due to fragmentation in cirrhosis.
    Hypersplenism with sequestration.
    Blood loss from varices causing iron deficiency.
    Folate deficiency and poor nutrition.
- Laboratory findings:
    Hemoglobin – low. MCV – moderately high.
    Morphology: spur cells, target cells.
    Nutritional supplements.
- Treatment:
    Splenectomy for hypersplenism.
    Transfuse as clinically indicated.

8. Physiological anemia of infancy
The normal neonate has a higher hemoglobin than older children (Hgb 160–180). Within the first week of life, the hemoglobin starts to decrease to a nadir of approximately 90 at 6–8 weeks.
- Mechanism of "physiological anemia":
    Decreased production of erythropoietin. Sudden cessation of erythropoietic production occurs with the onset of respiration when the arterial oxygen saturation rises.
    Decreased survival of fetal RBC's.
    Expansion of blood volume concomitant with rapid weight gain in the first 3 months causes "dilution" of hemoglobin.
    Dietary factors may aggravate physiological anemia: vitamin E deficiency (premature infants, fat malabsorption—cystic fibrosis), folate deficiency, iron deficiency (rare in the first 3 months unless there has been significant blood loss).
    Physiological anemia is exaggerated in the premature infant.
- Treatment:
    No treatment is required for normal physiological anemia as the hemoglobin will

spontaneously rise after 8–12 weeks.
Erythropoietin: used for preterm infants to reduce the need for transfusion.
Transfusion: may be needed if physiological anemia is exacerbated by other factors such as chronic blood loss (bleeding or blood tests), infection, complications of prematurity. Use small aliquots, CMV negative, filtered RBC's. Try to avoid donor exposure by using several aliquots from one donor.

Hemolytic anemias (HA)

The characteristic feature of hemolytic anemia is decreased RBC survival. RBC's usually remain in the circulation for 100–120 days and about 1% are removed from circulation and replaced every day. In response to shortened RBC's, survival hematopoiesis increases.
Hemolytic anemia may be due to: defects of RBC's (membranes, enzymes, hemoglobin), immune destruction of RBC's or nonimmune hemolysis.

* Characteristic features of hemolytic anemia:
  Anemia:
  Hemoglobin – normal to low. MCV – high (because of high proportion of young RBC's). Reticulocytes – high. The bone marrow can increase its output 6–8 fold in response to anemia so, theoretically, the RBC's survival could be reduced to 15–20 days with no reduction in hemoglobin. However, most children with increased hemolysis do have a mild reduction in hemoglobin. Chronic hemolysis results in expansion of the medullary (bone marrow) spaces.
  Aplastic crises:
  Children with any type of chronic hemolytic anemia are at risk for an aplastic crisis. With a short RBC survival time, cessation of RBC production causes rapid, life threatening development of anemia. Parvovirus infection is the most common cause of aplastic crisis. *Laboratory findings:* hemoglobin – low. MCV – normal to high. Reticulocytes – low.
  Elevation of unconjugated bilirubin with or without jaundice. Accelerated destruction of RBC's increases the biliary excretion of heme pigments.
  Plasma hemoglobin – increased.
  Serum haptoglobin – decreased. Free hemoglobin usually combines with haptoglobin and is then removed from the circulation by the reticuloendothelial system. In hemolytic anemia, the free hemoglobin exceeds the amount of haptoglobin (produced by the liver) and hence haptoglobin level is decreased or absent. Depletion of haptoglobin is most severe in intravascular hemolysis.
  Pigmented gallstones (calcium bilirubinate).
* Screening laboratory investigations:
  CBC, MCV, morphology, reticulocytes.
  Bilirubin, LDH (elevated because of RBC destruction).
  Haptoglobin, plasma hemoglobin.
  Fecal and urine urobilinogen – increased.

1. Membrane defects
* Hereditary spherocytosis (HS):
  Caused by an abnormality (either dysfunction or deficiency) of a membrane protein (most

commonly spectrin) which results in membrane instability.

RBC's become very permeable to sodium with an influx into the cell. This, combined with loss of part of the membrane, results in the characteristic spherocytic shape.

Spherocytes become sequestrated and destroyed in the spleen because of decreased deformability.

- Clinical features (key points):

  Autosomal dominant inheritance; 20% have no known family history. Severity may vary within a family.

  Race: usually northern European.

  Onset from birth; 50% present in the newborn period with anemia and jaundice. The majority present before puberty.

  Anemia and jaundice. Severity depends on the rate of hemolysis.

  Gallstones.

  Splenomegaly.

- Laboratory investigation:

  CBC and morphology.

  Hemoglobin – low to normal. MCV – normal. MCHC – high.

  Morphology shows microspherocytes and polychromasia.

  Reticulocytes – high.

  Direct antiglobulin test – negative.

  Bilirubin, LDH – high.

  Osmotic fragility – increased. This is performed by placing RBC's in hypotonic saline. Sodium and water then enter the RBC's. A normal RBC can swell but a spherocyte is already swollen and further increase in cell volume causes rupture of the cell.

  Abdominal ultrasound for presence of gallstones.

- Treatment:

  Folic acid supplement (folate is not "recycled" after hemolysis in contrast to iron which is recycled).

  Transfusion of RBC's for aplastic crisis.

  Splenectomy produces clinical "cure". Spherocytes are removed by the spleen and, after splenectomy, RBC survival increases to almost normal.

  Splenectomy should be considered for all patients with evidence of significant hemolysis (consistently low hemoglobin, high reticulocytes, history of aplastic crisis, gallstones) but, if possible, should be delayed until at least 5 years old, preferably older.

  Cholecystectomy: if the patient has gallstones, a cholecystectomy should be considered at the same time as splenectomy.

  Infection prophylaxis before and after splenectomy.

  Immunize with pneumococcal vaccine and *Haemophilus influenzae* B vaccine 4–6 weeks prior to splenectomy.

  Prophylactic penicillin should be continued throughout life. If < 5 years of age, penicillin 125 mg p.o. b.i.d.; if > 5 years of age, penicillin 250 mg p.o. b.i.d.

  If a splenectomized patient becomes febrile, obtain blood culture. Treat with i.v. ceftriaxone until cultures are negative. If blood cultures are positive, treat with appropriate intravenous antibiotic.

- Hereditary elliptocytosis:

  Clinical presentation and treatment is very similar to hereditary spherocytosis.

2. Hemolytic anemia due to RBC enzyme defects
- Glucose 6 phosphate dehydrogenase (G6PD) deficiency:
  G6PD is the first enzyme of the pentose phosphate pathway of glucose metabolism. Deficiency affects the cells ability to inactivate (reduce) oxidant compounds in the cell and may result in hemolysis. Three percent of the world's population (over 100 million people) have G6PD deficiency.
  Genetics: sex linked recessive inheritance (gene is on the X chromosome). Heterozygous females show intermediate expression because of random X inactivation (Lyon hypothesis).
  Race: most common in people of Mediterranean ancestry, Africans and Chinese. Over 100 different variants of G6PD exist. The most clinically significant are: type Mediterranean (associated with the most severe hemolysis in Caucasians), type Canton (associated with severe hemolysis in Southeast Asians); type A (found in Africans) causes less severe hemolysis.
  Precipitating causes of significant hemolysis in G6PD deficiency:
  Drugs: analgesics—acetanilid, acetylsalicylic acid in large doses; antimalarial—pentaquine, pamaquine, primaquine, quinocide; sulfonamides—sulphanilamide, n–acetylsulfanilamide, sulfapyridine, sulfamethoxypyridazine, salicylazosulfapyridine; sulfones—thiazolsulfone, diaminodiphenylsulfone (DDS and dapsone); nitrofurans; miscellaneous—naphthalene (may be absorbed through the skin in newborns when clothes have been stored in moth balls), phenylhydrazine, toluidine blue, nalidixic acid.
  Fava beans (broad bean): is a Mediterranean dietary staple. Ingestion of the bean or inhalation of its pollen can cause severe hemolysis in G6PD deficiency.
  Infection or diabetic ketoacidosis can precipitate hemolysis in severely affected individuals.
  Clinical features: intermittent, self–limited episodes of hemolysis causing pallor, jaundice and splenomegaly (usually occurring 48–96 hours after drug or fava bean ingestion or during infections). Neonatal jaundice is common in the Mediterranean and Canton variants. Often there is no history of drug exposure. Exposure to moth balls (naphthalene) may be a precipitating factor.
  Laboratory features (during episodes of hemolysis):
  Anemia: hemoglobin may fall to life threatening levels.
  Morphology: fragmented RBC's and spherocytes.
  Heinz bodies (precipitated hemoglobin) present in RBC's.
  Reticulocytes – high. Bilirubin, LDH – high.
  Diagnosis: measure G6PD level in RBC's (may be < 10% of normal). Immediately after an episode of hemolysis, reticulocytes and young RBC's predominate so G6PD may be falsely high. Repeat test 4 weeks later or do test on reticulocyte depleted sample.
  Treatment (prevention): avoid precipitating factors. Increase awareness of G6PD deficiency in appropriate ethnic groups.
  Supportive care: transfusion may be necessary during severe hemolytic episodes. Splenectomy may be beneficial for severely affected patients.
- Pyruvate kinase deficiency (PK):
  PK is the last enzyme in the Embden–Meyerhof pathway (anaerobic metabolism).
  Deficiency affects the ability of the cells to generate energy. As a result, potassium leaks from the cell and hemolysis occurs.
  PK deficiency is much less common than G6PD deficiency.
  Genetics: autosomal recessive inheritance. Race is predominantly Northern European.

Several variants described.

Clinical features: anemia varies from severe HA presenting at birth to mild, well compensated hemolytic anemia presenting in adulthood. Hemolysis is not drug related but may be exacerbated by infection. Neonatal jaundice is common. Splenomegaly, gallstones. Aplastic crisis (usually precipitated by parvovirus) may occur.

Laboratory features:

RBC morphology (macrocytosis and chromatophilia due to high reticulocytes). Spiculated pyknocytes.

RBC PK level decreased to 5% of normal. PK level and reticulocytes are high. Therefore, the measured PK level may need to be adjusted for the reticulocyte count.

Treatment:

Intermittent or chronic transfusion may be necessary for severely affected patients.

Neonatal exchange transfusion may be necessary for anemia or severe jaundice in the neonatal period.

Splenectomy decreases transfusion requirement. Avoid until > 5 years of age if possible.

• Many other enzyme deficiencies causing hemolytic anemia have been described but most of these are extremely rare.

3. Structural hemoglobin defects
• Normal hemoglobin: tetrameric molecules containing pairs of α and β globin subunits.
• Normal postnatal hemoglobins: Hb A – $\alpha_2 \beta_2$, Hb F – $\alpha_2 \gamma_2$, HbA$_2$ – $\alpha_2 \delta_2$.
• Genes for α chains located on chromosome 16.
• Genes for β chains located on chromosome 11.
• Sickle cell disease (SCD):
   Sickle hemoglobin is identical to hemoglobin A with the exception of a single amino acid substitution (valine for glutamic acid) in the β chain.
   Hemoglobin S – $\alpha_2 \beta^s_2$: in the oxygenated state, hemoglobin S functions normally. In the deoxygenated state, hemoglobin S forms molecular polymers which elongate into rigid crystal–like rods, which distort the RBC's into the characteristic sickle shape. Sickle cells are destroyed prematurely. Sickle cells cause increased blood viscosity and impaired blood flow.
   Ameliorating factors: persistent elevated production of hemoglobin F. Coinheritance of α–thal.
   Clinical features:
   Anemia is not present at birth but develops by 4 months as hemoglobin F is replaced by hemoglobin S.
   Moderate to severe anemia, hemoglobin 50–90. Normocytic, normochromic. Morphology shows irreversibly sickled cells.
   Howell–Jolly bodies may indicate hyposplenism.
   Sickle cell test may be needed to demonstrate sickle cells.
   Reticulocytes – high.
   Neutrophils and platelets – often elevated.
   ESR – low (sickle cells cannot form rouleau).
   Anemic crises:
   Splenic sequestration may occur between ages 6 months to 6 years.
   Sudden pooling of blood in the spleen causes severe abdominal pain and hypovolemia.

May be rapidly fatal.

Aplastic crisis: may follow viral infection, usually parvovirus. Cessation of hematopoiesis with ongoing hemolysis causing rapid development of anemia.

Megaloblastic crisis: folate deficiency may occur because of high cell turnover.

Hyperhemolysis:

May occur in children with a combination of sickle cell disease and G6PD deficiency. Rapid destruction of RBC's may follow viral infection or ingestion of oxidant drugs.

Vaso occlusive episodes: acute painful vaso occlusive episodes represent the most frequent and prominent manifestation of sickle cell disease. Decreased deformability of red cells results in occlusion of the microvasculature, causing tissue infarction. Most patients experience some pain on a daily basis.

Bone pain: dactylitis ("hand–foot syndrome"): due to ischemic necrosis of the small bones; it is often seen in toddlers and results in painful, symmetric swelling of the hands and feet. Older children experience pain in the long bones and in the back. Severe episodes cause aseptic necrosis of bone. Abdominal crisis is due to vaso occlusion and infarction of the liver, spleen, mesentery or abdominal lymph nodes. Recurrent splenic infarcts eventually cause "autosplenectomy".

CNS crisis: vaso occlusion in the brain may result in seizure, stroke or blindness.

Pulmonary crisis: pulmonary infarction is often associated with pneumonitis and causes chest pain and dyspnea.

Priapism: vaso occlusion in the corpora cavernosa causes obstruction of venous outflow.

Infection: children with sickle cell disease have an increased risk of infection due to pneumococcus, meningococcus, *H. influenzae* type B, *Staphylococcus* and *Salmonella*. This increased susceptibility to infection is largely because of impaired splenic function. *Salmonella osteomyelitis* may be due in part to bone necrosis.

Gallstones: secondary to hemolysis.

Genitourinary problems: papillary necrosis causes renal colic and hematuria. An acquired tubular absorption defect may result in inability to concentrate urine. Priapism causes severe pain and eventually impotence.

Diagnosis (prenatal):

May be diagnosed on amniocentesis or chorionic villus biopsy.

Hemoglobin electrophoresis will demonstrate Hb S.

Management:

Anemia: transfusion is indicated for patients with extensive pulmonary infarction, CVA, sequestration or severe anemia (< 40). Use washed or filtered packed red cells whenever possible. A complete RBC phenotype should be performed prior to transfusion and, if possible, the transfused blood should be closely phenotypically matched.

Vaso occlusive crisis: avoid anoxia, e.g. anesthesia, if possible. Hydration is essential. Due to inability to concentrate urine, patients require 1–1½ times the normal maintenance fluids. If acidotic, patients may need bicarbonate 0.5 mEq/kg i.v. Adequate analgesia is important; morphine is often required. Partial exchange transfusion if the vaso occlusive crisis continues for several days. Aim to reduce Hb S to < 40%.

Infection: prophylaxis (oral penicillin from 3 months of age).

< 1 year: 62.5 mg p.o. b.i.d.

1–3 years: 125 mg p.o. b.i.d.

3–6 years: 250 mg p.o. b.i.d.

Pneumococcal vaccine at age 2 years. *H. influenzae* vaccine in the first year.
Management of fever:
Detailed history and physical examination.
Investigations (CBC, reticulocytes; culture of blood, urine and stool—if diarrhea; CSF if under 1 year of age or any signs of meningitis; chest X–ray, bone X–ray—if signs of osteomyelitis).
For unidentified focus: cefotaxime 150 mg/kg per d i.v. div. q8h.
For chest infection: cefotaxime plus erythromycin (if *Mycoplasma* suspected) 50 mg/kg per 24 h div. q6h.
For osteomyelitis: cefotaxime (200 mg/kg per 24 h div. q6h).
When antibiotic sensitivity is known, make appropriate changes to treatment.
Antisickling therapy: agents which stimulate production of hemoglobin F can reduce sickling tendency; 5–azacytidine, hydroxyurea, recombinant human erythropoietin and butyric acid analogues have all shown beneficial effect.
Bone marrow transplant: has been used successfully for severe sickle cell disease.
• Thalassemias:
The thalassemias are a group of disorders in which there is impaired production or total absence of one or more of the hemoglobin polypeptide chains. Clinically significant disease occurs when there is an impaired production of β chains (β thalassemia) or α chains (α thalassemia). Thalassemia genes are found in people originating from Mediterranean countries, Africa, Middle East, India and Southeast Asia. Thalassemia is one of the most prevalent human genetic disease.
β thalassemia:
Genetics: there are two genes for β globin synthesis. β thalassemia is usually due to a point mutation in one or both genes. Normal β–β. Homozygous β thalassemia (major) occurs when there are two abnormal β chain genes, β°/β°. Heterozygous β thalassemia (minor, trait) occurs when there is one normal and one abnormal gene, β/β°. An intermediate form of thalassemia (thalassemia intermedia) occurs when the abnormal β globin gene causes reduced, but not absent, production of β globin chains. Thalassemia intermedia β+/β+.
Homozygous β thalassemia (major):
Clinical features (in untreated or inadequately treated patients): anemia (progressive severe hemolytic anemia is usually clinically apparent after 6 months of age). Failure to thrive in infancy, growth retardation, delayed puberty, hepatosplenomegaly, hypersplenism; abnormal facies (due to bone marrow expansion), maxillary hyperplasia, frontal bossing; osteoporosis and pathological fracture (due to bone marrow expansion and cortical thinning); jaundice (not severe), gallstones. Death is within the first few years of life.
Laboratory features:
Anemia: hemoglobin – low. MCV – very low (< 55), hypochromia. Reticulocytes – high. RBC morphology: fragmented poikilocytes, target cells, extreme anisocytosis, nucleated RBC's.
Hemoglobin electrophoresis: Hb A – absent. Hb F – very high (> 90%). HbA$_2$ – increased. Bilirubin, LDH – high.
Management:
Regular transfusions to maintain Hgb > 100 "hypertransfusion".
Usual requirement is 15 mL/kg PRBC every 4 wk. Use washed or filtered PRBC to remove

WBC and avoid febrile reactions due to antileukocyte antibodies. Use phenotypically matched blood if possible. Hypertransfusion permits normal activity and growth, reduces bone marrow expansion and hepatosplenomegaly.

Chelation therapy:
Iron overload (hemosiderosis) occurs secondary to transfusion therapy. Each 500 mL of blood delivers 200 mg of iron which cannot be excreted. Iron accumulation in the heart and other organs is the major cause of death in adequately transfused patients.

Deferoxamine is an iron chelating drug which should be used for all patients receiving regular transfusions when the serum ferritin is > 1,500 mg. A sustained high blood level of deferoxamine is necessary; 20–80 mg/kg deferoxamine given via subcutaneous infusion over 8–10 h five times per week. Usually given at home via a subcutaneous pump at night. Complications of deferoxamine include local reactions at the infusion site; decrease the concentration of infusion or add hydrocortisone 2 mg/mL of deferoxamine.

Toxicity: eye cataracts, impaired vision; usually reversible; hearing impairment with high dose; increased infection (*Yersinia*). Oral chelators are currently being investigated and may be available in the future.

Splenectomy: reduces transfusion requirement and should be considered for patients who have evidence of hypersplenism (thrombocytopenia, leukopenia) or who have an annual transfusion required of > 250 mL/kg. If possible, splenectomy should be delayed until the child is > 5 years of age. The provision of Pneumovax and *H. influenzae* vaccines plus prophylactic penicillin is vital.

Bone marrow transplant: allogeneic bone marrow transplant from a matched sibling donor can be curative and is performed more frequently for β thalassemia. The risks of BMT must be weighed against the risks of lifelong transfusion.

Complications of adequately treated β thalassemia:
Hemosiderosis: iron accumulation in the heart causing cardiac failure and in the liver causing cirrhosis are the most common causes of death. Pancreatic hemosiderosis causes diabetes.

Endocrine abnormalities: short stature, delayed puberty and hypothyroidism are due to a combination of anemia and iron overload.

Risks of transfusion:
Infection (hepatitis, HIV), transfusion reactions, etc.

Prognosis: with adequate transfusion and chelation life expectancy, at present, is about 25–30 years.

Heterozygous β thalassemia (β-thal minor, trait):
Mild anemia, usually asymptomatic. MCV – low. RDW – normal. Hypochromia.
RBC morphology shows target cells, anisocytosis, basophilic stippling. Often misdiagnosed as iron deficiency. Genetic counselling important.

α thalassemia:
Genetics: there are four genes for α globin synthesis. Most α thalassemia syndromes are caused by deletion of one or more genes.

Normal	αα/αα
α silent carrier	-α/αα
α trait	-α/-α or --/α
Hb H disease	-α/--
α hydrops fetalis	--/--

α silent carrier: no clinical manifestations; mild microcytosis only.

α trait: mild microcytic anemia; Hb barts (γ_4) present in minute quantities at birth.

Hb H disease, i.e. deletion of three α genes: moderate to severe anemia Hgb 60–100; may need occasional transfusion; RBC morphology (microcytosis, inclusion bodies); hemoglobin electrophoresis (newborn, Hb barts—γ_4, 20–30%; child or adult, Hb H—β_4, 4–20%).

α hydrops fetalis, i.e. deletion of four α genes: this results in absent α chain production and is a lethal disease. Most infants are stillborn or live for only a few hours. Hemoglobin electrophoresis shows Hb barts γ_4, Hb Portland $\zeta_2 \gamma_2$.

4. Immune hemolytic anemias
- Alloimmune: hemolytic disease of the newborn. Blood transfusion reaction (immediate or delayed).
- Autoimmune:
  "Warm" antibodies: IgG (rarely IgM).
  "Cold" antibodies: IgM.
  Warm/cold Donath Landsteiner: paroxysmal cold hemoglobinuria (PCH).
- Hemolytic disease of the newborn: this occurs when there is a blood group incompatibility between the mother and fetus. Maternal antibodies directed against fetal red cells cross the placenta and cause destruction of fetal red cells. The most common RBC antigens eliciting this response are D antigen of the Rhesus group and A and B antigens of the ABO system.
- Rhesus isoimmunization:
  Pathogenesis: mother Rh negative. Mother becomes "sensitized" to Rh antigens by either fetal blood entering the maternal circulation or incompatible blood transfusion. Fetus Rh positive. Rarely occurs during first pregnancy as "sensitization" usually occurs at the end of pregnancy or during delivery. ABO incompatibility reduces the severity of disease as fetal cells are rapidly removed from the maternal circulation before Rh sensitization can occur.
  Clinical features:
  Anemia: very variable; mild anemia to extremely severe anemia such as hydrops fetalis which may cause death in utero or shortly after birth.
  Jaundice: unconjugated bilirubin; rises rapidly during the first 24 hours and may cause kernicterus; hepatosplenomegaly; late hyporegenerative anemia with absent reticulocytes may continue for several weeks after birth; exchange transfusion may be necessary.
  Laboratory diagnosis (infant): direct antibody test (direct Coombs') positive, that is, antibodies are present on surface of RBC's.
  Hemoglobin – low. Reticulocytes – high.
  Morphology: nucleated red blood cells, polychromasia, anisocytosis, platelets and white blood cells may be low. Bilirubin – high.
  Laboratory diagnosis (mother): indirect antibody test (indirect Coombs') positive, that is, antibodies are present in the mother's serum.
  Management:
  Prenatal: all pregnant women should be screened early in pregnancy for Rh status and presence of antibodies. If mother is Rh negative, the father's Rh status and zygosity (homozygous or heterozygous) should be determined. Maternal antibody titer should be monitored throughout pregnancy. Amniocentesis may be required to assess fetal

hemolysis. Maternal plasmapheresis (to reduce Rh antibody level), intrauterine fetal transfusion or premature delivery should be considered if there is evidence of severe fetal hemolysis.

Postnatal: phototherapy for mild hemolysis. Exchange transfusion for rapidly increasing bilirubin.

Prevention of rhesus hemolytic disease: for unimmunized Rh negative women, sensitization can be prevented by giving Rh immunoglobulin at times that Rh positive cells may enter the maternal circulation. This achieves removal of Rh positive cells from the maternal circulation before an antibody response is elicited. Rh immunoglobulin should therefore be administered at 28 weeks gestation and within 72 hours of delivery, after any fetal loss and after any intervention during pregnancy, e.g. chorionic villous sampling.

- ABO isoimmunization:
  Pathogenesis:
  Most common: mother – group O, baby – group A or B.
  Less common: mother – group A, baby – group B or mother – group B, baby – group A.
  Hemolysis is much less severe than Rh hemolytic disease.
  Clinical features:
  Infant not significantly affected at birth; does not cause hydrops fetalis.
  Anemia and jaundice occur within the first 24 hours. Jaundice may be severe enough to cause kernicterus.
  Laboratory diagnosis (infant):
  Direct antibody test: positive.
  Indirect antibody test: positive (i.e. free antibody in infant's serum).
  Hemoglobin – low; reticulocytes – high.
  Morphology: polychromasia, spherocytes, bilirubin high.
  Demonstration of incompatible blood groups between mother and baby.
  Management: phototherapy, exchange transfusion for severe hemolysis.

- Autoimmune hemolytic anemia – warm autoimmune hemolytic anemia:
  Pathogenesis:
  Usually due to IgG antibodies (rarely IgM).
  Antibody usually directed against an Rh antigen.
  Maximal activity at 37 °C.
  Precipitating factors:
  Idiopathic.
  Secondary: infection; viral (e.g. EBV, CMV, hepatitis) or bacterial (e.g. *E. coli, Mycoplasma pneumoniae*); drugs and chemicals (antibiotics—penicillin and cephalosporins, phenacetin, quinidine); hematological disorders (leukemia, lymphoma, ITP); immunological disorders (SLE and other autoimmune diseases).
  Clinical features:
  Sudden onset of anemia.
  Hemolysis may progress rapidly and can be life threatening within hours (do not underestimate); jaundice; splenomegaly; fever often associated with hemolysis.
  Laboratory features:
  Anemia: hemoglobin may be profoundly low. Reticulocytes – high.
  Morphology (spherocytes, polychromasia, nucleated RBC's).
  Direct antiglobulin test (positive).

Bilirubin – increased. LDH – increased. Haptoglobin – decreased.
Hemoglobinuria.
Management (acute immune hemolytic anemia is an emergency):
Transfusion: will only provide temporary benefit but is indicated for severe anemia.
Cross–match is difficult as the autoantibody usually behaves as a panagglutinin. Use the
most compatible blood available. RBC's should be washed.
Steroids: should be started as soon as the diagnosis has been made. Prednisone 2–6
mg/kg per d. Continue steroids until hemolysis decreases and then slowly taper.
Plasmapheresis: may help temporarily.
IVIg: in high doses; 5 g/kg may be beneficial.
Splenectomy: should be considered for severe cases unresponsive to steroids.
Prognosis:
Most patients have an acute presentation with a complete recovery within 3 months.
A small percentage go on to develop chronic hemolytic anemia which may last months to
years.
Treatment for chronic disease is steroids and splenectomy.
- Autoimmune hemolytic anemia – cold autoimmune hemolytic anemia:
  This is caused by IgM antibodies that are more active at a low temperature. Antibody has
  specificity for the i antigen (when precipitated by EBV, specificity may be anti–i). Cold
  agglutinin disease is usually precipitated by viral infection (EBV, CMV) or *Mycoplasma
  pneumoniae*. May cause severe hemolysis which can be intermittent. Often precipitated
  by cold exposure.
  Treatment:
  Transfusion (cross–match may be difficult; if possible, the blood should be warmed).
  Plasmapheresis is more beneficial than in warm hemolytic anemia.
  Cytotoxic therapy for severe disease, e.g. cyclophosphamide.
  Steroids, splenectomy (usually not effective).
- Paroxysmal cold hemoglobinuria (Donath Landsteiner):
  This is usually precipitated by viral infection in children and is due to an IgG antibody with
  anti–P specificity which causes complement activation.
  Treatment is with transfusion and steroids.
- Nonimmune hemolytic anemia may be due to a variety of causes:
  Infection: e.g. *Clostridium perfringens*, malaria.
  Drugs: e.g. vitamin K.
  Hematological disorders: e.g. leukemia, lymphoma, microangiopathic hemolytic anemia.
- Microangiopathic hemolytic anemia:
  This is due to a variety of causes which produce intravascular hemolysis due to mechanical
  damage to red blood cells.
  Laboratory features:
  Hemoglobin low. Platelets often low.
  Red cell morphology: fragmented cells, burr cells, schistocytes, microspherocytes, helmet
  cells.
  Causes:
  Renal disease: e.g. HUS, renal transplant rejection.
  Cardiac disease: e.g. SBE, intracardiac prostheses.
  Liver disease, hematological disease (e.g. TTP, DIC), burns, hemangioma.

Polcythemia

1. Neonatal polycythemia
- Venous hematocrit > 65% or venous hemoglobin > 220 g/L.
- Causes:
    Hypoxia, hypertransfusion, congenital abnormalities.
- Complications:
    CNS: intracranial hemorrhage, seizures.
    Necrotizing enterocolitis.
    Renal failure.
    Congestive cardiac failure.
- Treatment: symptomatic infants should be treated by partial exchange transfusion.

2. Polycythemia in childhood
- That is, an increase in the circulating RBC mass which exceeds the upper limits of normal.
- Laboratory features:
    Hgb > 170 g/L, hematocrit > 50%.
    Primary polycythemia: polycythemia rubra vera, benign familial polycythemia.
    Secondary polycythemia: due to insufficient oxygenation; due to increased erythropoiesis caused by renal, adrenal, liver disease or administration of testosterone or growth hormone.
- Clinical symptoms: headache, blurred vision, thrombosis (particularly in the central nervous system), myeloproliferative disease (associated with PCV).

DISORDERS OF WHITE CELLS AND IMMUNITY

An intact immune system is essential for host defense. Major deficiencies of neutrophils, T and B lymphocytes, or complement predispose to the development of significant infections, autoimmune disorders and cancer. Varying degrees of deficiency can be significant in young children due to their immune immaturity. Roughly 80% of cases concern deficiencies of antibody production, 10–20% are mixed T and B lymphocyte diseases, about 5% are pure defects of polymorphs and only 1% are single deficiencies of complement. As usual, a detailed history and physical examination are the most important part of an immune evaluation.

Diagnosis of immunodeficiencies

1. History (key points)
- Type and frequency of infections (normal toddlers may have a new URTI every month).
- Age at onset (ask about neonatal problems, e.g. hypocalcemia, delayed cord separation).
- Family history, including sex of affected relatives and presence of consanguinity.
- Medical history (immunizations, malignancy, drugs, diabetes, etc.).
- Presence of risk factors for acquired immunodeficiency.

2. Physical examination
Some immune disorders have associated abnormalities that may give useful clues to the diagnosis:

- Congenital heart disease (aortic arch abnormalities or truncus arteriosus are associated with DiGeorge's syndrome).
- Down's syndrome (variable degrees of immunodeficiency).
- Progressive neurological deterioration (ataxia telangiectasia).
- Lymphadenopathy and skin lesions (chronic granulomatous disease).
- Thrush, dermatitis or severe eczema (consider severe combined deficiencies).
- Look for evidence of B cell tissue (lymph nodes, tonsils).
- Height and weight.

3. Investigations
The choice of investigation should be guided by the history and physical examination.
- Basic evaluation:
    CBC, differential, platelet count, white blood cell morphology, relevant cultures and immunoglobulin levels. The results from these basic investigations will guide subsequent testing.
- Tests of specific areas of the immune system will include:
    Complement: total hemolytic complement CH_{50}, with individual component assays in some cases.
    T cell: T cell subsets, T cell mitogen proliferation test, delayed hypersensitivity skin test (Candida, tetanus and mumps).
    Neutrophils/spleen: peripheral smear for Howell–Jolly bodies, NBT test, myeloperoxidase stain, test for neutrophil chemotaxis.
    Antibodies: some patients are able to make immunoglobulins that do not have any clinical antibody activity. Consequently, it is better to measure specific antibodies rather than general IgG (isohemagglutinins and antibodies to tetanus and diphtheria, also B cell subsets).

4. Management
- General measures include the following:
    Live vaccines should only be given if there are neutrophil or complement disorders. They should be avoided in T cell and B cell disorders.
    Passive immunizations should be given to all patients with a severe immunodeficiency, following exposure to varicella.
    Pure IgA deficiency is the commonest of the antibody deficiencies. Washed and packed red cells should be given if a transfusion is necessary to avoid the chance of anaphylaxis.
    Patients with T cell defects are at risk of graft versus host reaction following transfusion of blood products. Consequently, all transfusions should be irradiated and CMV free.
    Prophylactic antibiotics following splenectomy and TMP–SMX should be used in patients with neutropenia to avoid PCP.
- Specific therapies:
    Although SCID, due to adenosine deaminase deficiency, has attracted a lot of attention through the use of transfection of blood lymphocytes with genetic material, in practical terms, there are only two specific therapies:
    Gamma globulin replacement for antibody defects.
    Bone marrow transplantation for combined defects.

Classification of immunodeficiencies

1. Immunoglobulin deficiency
• Transient hypogammaglobulinemia of infancy: prolongation of natural immunoglobulin dip at 6 months. Immunoglobulin levels are variable but rarely absent. Recovery occurs between 1–4 years of age.
• IgA deficiency: commonest deficiency, incidence 1:500; 25% have associated connective tissue disease. Recurrent infections in 50%. Danger of sensitization and the short half–life of IgA make replacement impractical.
• Hypogammaglobulinemia syndromes: diagnosis, treatment and complications are the same but it is worth distinguishing X–linked from other types for genetic counselling.
• Common variable immunodeficiency syndrome: the name says it all; this is a collection of diseases that may present with congenital or acquired antibody deficiencies that do not fit into any other classification. Together, they are the second commonest type of immunodeficiency.
• Selective immunoglobulin subclass deficiencies: these are all very rare.
• Immunodeficiency with high IgM: the IgM does not have any clinical activity so the patients present as hypogammaglobulinemia.

2. Defects of cell mediated immunity
• Predominantly T cell defects: chronic mucocutaneous candidiasis and thymic hypoplasia (DiGeorge's syndrome); a mixture of absent thymus, absent parathyroid glands and major cardiac abnormalities (typically truncus arteriosus). The condition should always be considered before transfusing a neonate who has congenital heart disease (truncus or total anomalous venous drainage). The blood should be irradiated if DiGeorge's syndrome is suspected.
• Combined B and T cell disorders: severe combined immunodeficiency (SCID). This term covers a range of conditions that have, in common, a combination of deficient B and T cell function such as ADA deficiency, PNP deficiency and Nezelof's syndrome.
• Other combined disorders: Wiskott–Aldrich's syndrome, ataxia telangiectasia and chronic mucocutaneous candidiasis.

3. Neutrophil defects
• Deficient chemotaxis: Chédiak–Higashi's syndrome, impaired chemotaxis with hyper IgE (Job's syndrome).
• Bacterial killing defects: several intracellular abnormalities reduce the ability of neutrophils to kill bacteria (chronic granulomatous disease, leukocyte G6PD deficiency and glutathione dehydrogenase deficiency).
• Leukocyte adhesion defect: LFA1 deficiency, Mac–1 deficiency.
• Defective neutrophil production: cyclic neutropenia, Kostmann's syndrome, Schwachman–Diamond's syndrome.

4. Complement disorders
Several very rare deficiencies of complement components exist, usually on an autosomal recessive basis. They are associated either with recurrent bacterial infections (particularly *Neisseria*) or immune complex disorders such as SLE.

5. Secondary immunodeficiency
Immunodeficiency syndromes, secondary to a wide range of pediatric illnesses, are common. Treatment is more usually aimed at the cause of the immunodeficiency:
- Immunoglobulin loss: protein losing enteropathy, nephrotic syndrome, severe burns.
- Severe malnutrition: impairs the function of all parts of the immune system.
- Immunosuppression: steroids and chemotherapy.
- Infections: apart from HIV, several viruses have a depressing effect on the immune system (EBV, CMV, measles, hepatitis).

PLATELET DISORDERS

Thrombocytopenia

Thrombocytopenia (platelets $< 100 \times 10^9$ /L) may be due to:
- Decreased or abnormal platelet production.
- Abnormal distribution of platelets.
- Increased platelet destruction.

Effect of thrombocytopenia on bleeding:
- Platelets $< 20 \times 10^9$ /L: spontaneous bleeding may occur.
- Platelets $20–50 \times 10^9$ /L: increased bleeding and bruising with trauma; spontaneous bleeding rare.
- Platelets $50–100 \times 10^9$ /L: increased bleeding with major trauma only.

Decreased or abnormal platelet production

1. Thrombocytopenia absent radii syndrome (TAR)
- Thrombocytopenia associated with bilateral absent radii. Often have congenital heart disease.
- Genetics: autosomal recessive. Platelet count $10–30 \times 10^9$ /L in the neonatal period. May increase after the first year of life.
- Bone marrow: megakaryocytes absent or significantly reduced. Myeloid hyperplasia.
- Treatment: supportive; transfuse as necessary. Bone marrow transplant may be curative.

2. Wiskott–Aldrich's syndrome
- Thrombocytopenia associated with eczema and defective cell mediated immunity.
- Genetics: X–linked. Males only affected. Often presents with melena in the neonatal period. Thrombocytopenia due to impaired production and shortened survival of platelets.
- Laboratory features:
    Small platelets (MPV < 7.1 fl).
    Bone marrow shows normal or increased megakaryocytes.
    Isohemagglutinins often absent. IgM decreased. IgA and IgG increased.
- Treatment:
    Supportive: platelet transfusions. Aggressive treatment of infections.
    Splenectomy: contraindicated because of increased risk of postsplenectomy sepsis.
    Steroids: may improve eczema and slight improvement in platelet count but increased risk of infection.

IV gamma globulin infusions may reduce risk of infection.
Bone marrow transplant may be curative.

3. Other hereditary platelet disorders
- May–Hegglin anomaly, Bernard Soulier's syndrome.
- Thrombocytopenia due to ineffective production of abnormal platelets.

4. Congenital rubella syndrome
- Thrombocytopenia associated with cardiac defects, cataracts, deafness, hepatosplenomegaly.
- Bone marrow shows decreased megakaryocytes.

5. Metabolic disorders
- Hyperglycinemia with ketosis.
- Methylmalonic acidemia may cause thrombocytopenia in infancy.

6. Acquired disorders
- Bone marrow aplasia (congenital or acquired).
- Bone marrow infiltration (benign or malignant).

Abnormal platelet distribution

1. Hypersplenism
- Usually one–third of the platelets are in the spleen and two–thirds in the bloodstream.
- Any condition causing splenomegaly can cause increased sequestration and destruction of platelets in the spleen.
- Usually associated with anemia and leukopenia.

2. Cyanotic heart disease
- May result in thrombocytopenia due to margination of platelets in the small blood vessels.
- Platelet function may also be impaired.

Increased platelet destruction

1. Immune thrombocytopenia
Idiopathic thrombocytopenia purpura (ITP): this is an autoimmune disorder characterized by development of an antiplatelet antibody. It is the most common cause of thrombocytopenia.
- Clinical presentation:
    Age: any age but most common between 2 and 6 years. Both male and female equally affected.
    Abrupt onset of petechiae, purpura and bleeding in an otherwise well child. Bleeding is usually in the skin and mucous membranes.
    Preceding history of viral infection in most cases.
    Absent systemic symptoms.
    Physical examination shows petechiae and purpura. Occasionally mild splenomegaly.
    Liver and lymph nodes not enlarged.
    Muscle bleeds and hemarthroses do not occur.

- Key point: evidence of mucous membrane bleeding (buccal mucosa, gums, retina and conjunctiva) is suggestive of a more severe bleeding tendency.
- Laboratory evaluation:
  Platelet count: significantly decreased, often < 20×10^9 /L.
  MPV increased (indicative of "young" platelets).
  CBC: normal except thrombocytopenia.
  Antiplatelet antibodies: usually positive.
  Bone marrow aspirate and biopsy show increased megakaryocytes, otherwise normal. Bone marrow should be performed if there is any suspicion of other underlying disease, e.g. ALL; also essential if steroids are to be used for treatment to avoid later diagnostic confusion.
  Coagulation profile: normal.
  ANA, anti–DNA: to exclude other autoimmune diseases.
  Coombs' test: to exclude immune hemolytic anemia, group and screen (in case life threatening bleeding occurs).
  Viral serology: HIV.
- Differential diagnosis:
  Leukemia or other causes of bone marrow infiltration should be excluded by bone marrow aspirate and biopsy if there is any clinical or laboratory suspicion. The use of steroids may mask the diagnosis of ALL so bone marrow is usually recommended prior to treatment with steroids (except in emergency cases).
  Other autoimmune diseases, such as SLE, should be excluded by clinical findings, ANA, anti–DNA.
  Consumption coagulopathy: exclude by checking coagulation profile.
- Natural history of ITP:
  60% of children recover spontaneously within 1 month and 80–90% recover within 6 months.
  10–20% continue to have ITP beyond 6 months and are then said to have chronic ITP. Of these, 50% will eventually recover.
  Treatment with steroids, IVIg or anti–Rh(D) does not alter the chances of eventual recovery.
- Treatment:
  The aim of treatment in acute ITP is to reduce the risk of serious hemorrhage while waiting for spontaneous recovery.
  Indications for treatment: platelet count < 20×10^9 /L. Children with platelet > 20×10^9 /L do not usually need treatment.
  Mucous membrane bleeding, GI bleeding, menorrhagia or evidence of other significant bleeding. Trauma or prior to surgery when platelets < 50×10^9 /L.
- Treatment guidelines:
  IVIg and steroids both produce a rapid increase in the platelet count in the majority of patients.
  For patients who are not actively bleeding: prednisone (ensure bone marrow is performed if there is any clinical or laboratory suspicion of ALL)—4 mg/kg per d × 6 d, then 2 mg/kg per d × 5 d, then 1 mg/kg per d × 5 d, then taper and discontinue by day 21. Side effects are rare with a short course of prednisone (e.g. hypertension, hyperglycemia, weight gain, gastritis or peptic ulcer).

High dose intravenous gamma globulin: use for patients who develop recurrent thrombocytopenia after prednisone or who do not respond within 3–4 days of prednisone treatment (0.8 g/kg i.v. × 1 dose).
Side effects: severe headache may occur in 20% of patients. Anaphylaxis may occur in IgA deficient patients.
Anti–Rh (D) therapy: use for patients who are Rh (D) positive and who have failed or relapsed following treatment with prednisone or IVIg (25 µg/kg per d × 2 d).
Side effects: mild hemolytic anemia, shaking, chills.
For actively bleeding patients: intravenous methylprednisolone 30 mg/kg per d × 3 d plus IVIg 0.8 g/kg per d × 1 dose.
For life threatening hemorrhage such as intracranial hemorrhage: splenectomy as soon as possible plus i.v. methylprednisolone 30 mg/kg plus IVIg 0.8 g/kg plus continuous platelet transfusion (while waiting for splenectomy); plasmapheresis, if fails.
For chronic ITP (treatment depends on severity of thrombocytopenia): anti–Rh(D) 25 µg/kg per d × 2 d; may be given every 4–6 wk. IVIg 0.8 g/kg × 1 may be given every 4–6 wk.
Low dose prednisone 0.5 mg/kg on alternate days may help maintain capillary integrity. Alternate day regimen causes minimal side effects. Short pulses of prednisone (2 mg/kg per d × 3 d) may be used for relapsing patients. Avoid giving pulses more frequently than once per month.
Splenectomy: approximately 50% of patients have a complete, long lasting response to splenectomy. It should be considered for patients with severe ITP, not controlled with other methods, or for chronic ITP lasting several years, or patients whose lifestyle is impaired by thrombocytopenia. Patients should be immunized with Pneumovax and *H. influenzae* vaccines prior to splenectomy and should take life long penicillin prophylaxis to prevent overwhelming postsplenectomy infection.
Supportive care: avoid contact sports, intramuscular injections and vaccinations. Advise that toddlers wear a soft helmet. Avoid aspirin or other nonsteroidal anti–inflammatory drugs. Prevent or treat menorrhagia with oral contraceptives.

2. Neonatal immune thrombocytopenia
The neonate is at risk for autoimmune thrombocytopenia or isoimmune thrombocytopenia.
• Autoimmune thrombocytopenia (NITP):
  This occurs in infants born to mothers with ITP and is due to passive transfer of antibody across the placenta.
  Diagnostic evaluation: history of ITP in mother, thrombocytopenia in mother, antiplatelet antibody present in mother.
  Treatment:
  Prenatal: IVIg 1 g/kg weekly from 34 wk.
  Postnatal to infant: IVIg 1 g/kg daily × 2. Prednisone 2 mg/kg per d. Platelet transfusion for bleeding. Monitor closely over the first week of life. Severe bleeding is rare in this disorder.
• Isoimmune (alloimmune) thrombocytopenia (NATP):
  This occurs when the mother and fetus have incompatible platelet antigens. It is analogous to Rhesus disease, i.e. the mother actively makes antibodies against the fetal platelets. The usual platelet antigenic system involved is the PL^{A1} system where the mother is PL^{A1} negative and the fetus PL^{A1} positive. Bleeding manifestations are more frequent and more

severe than in NITP and intrauterine intracranial hemorrhage can occur.

Diagnostic evaluation:

Platelet antigens: demonstration of incompatible platelet groups between the mother and infant. CBC in mother shows normal platelets. Antiplatelet antibody in mother - positive.

Treatment:

Antenatal (if the infant is known to be at risk, i.e. previously affected infant): IVIg 1 g/kg weekly from 20 wk. Cesarean section recommended. Have maternal platelets available for delivery.

Postnatal: transfuse 1 unit of mother's platelets suspended in normal plasma. The platelets should be washed and irradiated.

If the mother's platelets are not available, transfuse PL^{A1} negative platelets from the blood bank. IVIg 1 g/kg i.v. daily × 3 d. Prednisone 2 mg/kg per d × 1 wk.

3. Other causes of immune thrombocytopenia
- Infection: associated with viral infection (HIV, CMV, EBV, parvovirus and bacterial infection, e.g. TB).
- Drugs: many drugs can cause immune thrombocytopenia (antibiotics, heparin and cimetidine, analgesics, anticonvulsants).
- Collagen vascular disease: SLE.
- Evans' syndrome: autoimmune hemolytic anemia and thrombocytopenia.

4. Nonimmune causes of increased platelet consumption or loss
- Disseminated intravascular coagulation (DIC):
  Acute DIC (usually associated with overwhelming infection) will result in thrombocytopenia due to excess consumption.
- Hemolytic uremic syndrome:
  Increased platelet activation results in aggregation of platelets in small blood vessels which subsequently trap and damage RBC's. The resulting RBC morphology of fragmented red cells is known as microangiopathic hemolytic anemia. Thrombocytopenia is rarely severe and platelet transfusions are only used for life threatening hemorrhage.
- Thrombotic thrombocytopenic purpura (TTP):
  Associated with microangiopathic hemolytic anemia and platelet consumption.
  Microthrombi cause extensive tissue damage. Bleeding is rare.
  Treatment: plasmapheresis removes the platelet aggregating substances in the majority of cases.
- Kasabach–Merritt's syndrome (giant hemangioma):
  Platelet trapping and localized intravascular coagulation results in thrombocytopenia and depletion of other coagulation proteins. Bleeding can be severe.
  Treatment: many modalities of treatment are available but none is universally successful. Treatment methods include: surgical resection, external compression, corticosteroids, antifibrinolytic therapy (aminocaproic acid, tranexamic acid), interferon α 2a (inhibits angiogenesis).

5. Thrombocytosis
- Platelet counts of over 750×10^9 /L may be associated with a hematological disease (iron deficiency anemia, hemolytic anemia, primary myeloproliferative disease), hemorrhage, acute

and chronic inflammatory conditions, Kawasaki's disease, postsplenectomy (often associated with extremely high platelet counts of > 1,000 × 10⁹ /L).

- Thrombocytosis in children is rarely associated with thrombosis, however, if the platelet count is > $1,000 × 10^9$ /L, treatment with aspirin (80–160 mg/d p.o.) or dipyridamole (3–6 mg/kg per 24 h div. t.i.d.) should be considered.

Platelet function defects

Disorders of platelet function in children are rare. Symptoms consist of skin and mucous membrane bleeding as in thrombocytopenia.

1. Laboratory evaluation
- CBC and platelet count.
- Platelet morphology.
- Bleeding time: this is a difficult test to perform reliably in young children. It is always prolonged in functional platelet disorders.
- Platelet aggregation.

2. Congenital platelet function disorders
- Bernard Soulier's syndrome.
- Glanzmann's thrombasthenia.
- Storage pool disease.
- May–Hegglin anomaly.

3. Acquired platelet function disorders
- Drugs: aspirin, nonsteroidal anti–inflammatory drugs, penicillin, heparin.
- Uremia.
- Liver disease.

4. Treatment
- Remove cause of platelet dysfunction if possible, e.g. drugs.
- Platelet transfusion for bleeding or surgery.
- DDAVP may shorten bleeding time in uremia.

DISORDERS OF HEMOSTASIS

Normal hemostatis consists of:
- Primary hemostasis: this process involves the vascular response to injury and formation of the platelet plug.
- Secondary hemostasis: this process involves activation of the coagulation cascade and formation of a stable fibrin clot.

1. Clinical evaluation of a coagulation disorder
- History (key points):
    Bleeding: site, severity, duration, preceding trauma, menorrhagia, previous episodes of bleeding, epistaxis, menorrhagia, umbilical stump bleeding.

Bruising: spontaneous or with trauma, superficial or deep joint or muscle bleed.

Petechiae: skin, mucous membranes, spontaneous or with trauma.

Age of onset: bruising or bleeding at birth, as a toddler, melena in infancy. Bleeding with dental extraction, venepuncture, immunizations.

Drugs: including aspirin, nonsteroidal anti–inflammatory drugs, antibiotics.

Family history of easy bruising or bleeding, transfusion after surgery or childbirth.

General health, including renal or liver disease.

Symptoms suggestive of a primary (platelet) disorder: petechiae, small bruises, mucous membrane bleeding (including epistaxis and menorrhagia).

Symptoms suggestive of a secondary (hemostatic) disorder: deep bleeding into joints and muscles, large bruises.

2. Laboratory evaluation (if platelet dysfunction is suspected)
- CBC, platelet count.
- Bleeding time: this is performed by making a standard incision on the forearm and measuring the time taken to stop bleeding. A blood pressure cuff is inflated to 40 mm Hg to ensure standard capillary pressure. This test evaluates the primary hemostatic mechanism but is a difficult and traumatic test to perform in small children.
- Platelet aggregation: platelet function can be assessed in vitro using a series of platelet activating factors.
- Prothrombin time: this measures the time required for plasma to clot after the addition of exogenous thromboplastin and calcium. Prolonged PT indicates deficiency of factor II (prothrombin), V, VII or X. Normal 15–20 seconds. (screens extrinsic and common pathways)
- International normalized ratio: since thromboplastin can vary greatly in potency, the value of the PT can differ between laboratories. To adjust for this variability, the PT is modified by a factor that reflects the sensitivity of the thromboplastin. The resulting "adjusted" PT is termed the international normalized ratio (INR) and should be used in preference to the PT.
- Activated partial thromboplastin time (APTT): measures the time for plasma to clot after activation of factor XII with an inert activator and calcium. Prolonged PTT indicates an abnormality of factor XII, XI, IX, VIII, X, V or II. Normal PTT 25–40 seconds. (screens intrinsic and common pathways)
- PTT mixing study: in this study, normal plasma is added to the patient's plasma to determine whether prolonged PTT is due to deficiency of factor VIII, IX, XI or XII (mixing study will correct PTT) or due to an inhibitor against factor VIII, IX or XI (mixing study will not correct PTT).
- Thrombin time: measures time for plasma to clot after addition of thrombin. Measures fibrinogen and ability of fibrin to polymerize.
- Factor assays: coagulation factors can be measured individually once screening tests have been performed.
- For von Willebrand's disease: von Willebrand's factor antigen, ristocetin cofactor.
- Fibrinogen level.
- Fibrinogen degradation products or D–dimers if DIC is suspected.

Congenital coagulation disorders

1. Hemophilia A (factor VIII deficiency)
- Genetics: X–linked (males only affected). 80% have positive family history; 20% represent

a new mutation. Prenatal detection available. Accounts for 85% of hemophilia.
- Clinical symptoms: severity of symptoms related to the level of factor VIII.
    Severe: factor VIII < 1% of normal.
    Moderate: factor VIII 1–5% of normal.
    Mild: factor VIII 6–25% of normal.
    Large bruises: often not apparent until infant starts to crawl or walk.
    Bleeding: from mouth, circumcision, injections.
    Hemarthrosis: may occur in any joint but most frequent in knees, ankles and elbows.
    Pain: soft tissue and joint bleeding is extremely painful. Infants may present with crying or refusal to move a limb, unexplained irritability.
- Laboratory diagnosis:
    PTT: prolonged.
    PTT mixing studies: correction of PTT.
    Factor VIII: significantly reduced.
    Platelet count, PT, bleeding time. TT – normal.
- Treatment:
    Supportive care: avoid trauma if possible. Teach parents to recognize symptoms. Avoid aspirin and nonsteroidal anti–inflammatory drugs. Physiotherapy to affected joints. Hepatitis B vaccine. Adequate analgesia.
    Home therapy: i.v. infusion of factor VIII is usually given at home by the patient or parent. This enables treatment to be given earlier and more frequently.
    Factor replacement: factor VIII replacement may be achieved by using fresh frozen plasma, cryoprecipitate or concentrates from plasma pools. However, over the last couple of years, recombinant factor VIII has become commercially available and is now recommended in preference to blood derived factor VIII to avoid the risk of viral transmission.
    Recommended doses of factor VIII:
    Hemarthrosis: 25 unit/kg b.i.d. for 2–3 d.
    Epistaxis/oral bleeding: 25 unit/kg (1 dose usually sufficient); aminocaproic acid 50 mg/kg q.i.d. for 5–7 d or tranexamic acid 25 mg/kg t.i.d. for 5–7 d.
    GI bleeding: admit; 50 unit/kg b.i.d. until bleeding resolved, then daily × 4 d.
    CNS bleed: admit; 75 unit/kg t.i.d. (monitor factor VIII levels to maintain level > 50%); continue treatment for at least 2 wk.
    Retroperitoneal or retropharyngeal bleed: admit; 50 unit/kg b.i.d. until bleeding resolved.
    Prophylactic treatment: there is an increasing trend towards prophylactic factor VIII infusion prior to sports or towards regular treatment (3 times per week) for patients with chronic joint bleeds.
    DDAVP (desmopressin): can increase factor VIII levels in patients with mild hemophilia to 25–50% of normal. Can be used for mild bleeding. Dose 0.3 µg/kg i.v. given over 30 min; may be given daily for 2 d.

2. Hemophila B (factor IX deficiency, Christmas' disease)
- Genetics: X–linked (males only affected). Prenatal detection available. Accounts for 15% of hemophilia.
- Symptoms: identical to factor VIII deficiency.
- Laboratory diagnosis:
    PTT: prolonged. Mixing studies show correction of PTT.

Factor IX: significantly reduced.
Other tests: normal.
- Treatment:
  Supportive care as for factor VIII deficiency.
  Replacement therapy: factor IX can be replaced with fresh frozen plasma or factor IX concentrates. The usual recommendation is to use highly purified factor IX concentrates. Recombinant product is not yet commercially available.
  Recommended doses of factor IX: as per factor VIII.

3. Von Willebrand's disease
- Genetics: autosomal dominant; rarely autosomal recessive. It is due to deficiency or abnormal synthesis of von Willebrand's protein, which is responsible for activating platelet adhesion and carrying factor VIII in the plasma.
- Clinical symptoms: symptoms are very variable depending on severity. Bleeding manifestations are not usually as severe as factor VIII or factor IX deficiency. Symptoms include mucous membrane bleeding (epistaxis, gum bleeding, bleeding after dental extraction), menorrhagia, bleeding after trauma, surgery or childbirth. Hemarthroses are rare.
- Laboratory evaluation: platelet count normal, PT normal, PTT usually prolonged, bleeding time prolonged, von Willebrand's factor antigen reduced, von Willebrand's multimers abnormal, ristocetin cofactor reduced.
- Treatment:
  DDAVP: dose 0.3 µg/kg i.v. over 30 min. Can increase the level of von Willebrand's factor in most types of von Willebrand's disease.
  Severe bleeding episodes may need treatment with fresh frozen plasma, cryoprecipitate or von Willebrand's factor concentrate (Humate P).

4. Afibrinoginemia and dysfibrinoginemia
- These are rare disorders associated with severe bleeding following trauma or surgery but not usually with spontaneous bleeding.
- Laboratory evaluation: thrombin time significantly prolonged.
- Treatment: cryoprecipitate.

5. Factor XIII deficiency
- This is a rare disease usually associated with delayed bleeding.
- Diagnosis: factor XIII assay.
- Treatment: fresh frozen plasma or cryoprecipitate

6. Acquired coagulation disorders
- Vitamin K deficiency:
  The vitamin K dependent factors are II, VII, IX and X and the anticoagulants protein C and protein S.
  Hemorrhagic disease of the newborn: the normal infant is born with low levels of factors II, VII, IX and X and these fall within the first few days of birth because of low initial stores of vitamin K. Premature and low birth weight infants have even lower initial stores. Vitamin K deficiency may result in bleeding from the GI tract, umbilicus or other sites (usually between days 2–4 of life). Vitamin K 1 mg i.m. is therefore given routinely to newborn

infants.
Laboratory diagnosis: PTT prolonged. PT prolonged. Factors II, VII, IX, X reduced; red cell morphology, fibrin split products, platelets normal.
Treat with vitamin K 1–5 mg i.m. or i.v.; for serious bleeding, fresh frozen plasma.
- Vitamin K deficiency in older children:
  This may be seen in children with fat malabsorption, prolonged administration of broad spectrum antibiotics, cystic fibrosis and biliary atresia.
  Treatment: vitamin K p.o. or i.v.
- Liver disease:
  Almost all coagulation factors are produced exclusively in the liver with the exception of factor VIII and von Willebrand's factor. Severe liver impairment, therefore, results in generalized reduction in factor levels.
  Laboratory evaluation: PT, PTT prolonged. Factors I, II, V, VII, IX, X reduced. Red cell morphology may show target cells.
  Treatment: Vitamin K p.o. or i.v. may increase levels of factors II, VII, IX and X. Fresh frozen plasma will increase levels of all coagulation factors. Cryoprecipitate to increase fibrinogen.
- Disseminated intravascular coagulation:
  Intravascular coagulation may be precipitated by many disorders including widespread tissue injury from massive trauma or burns, severe infection, malignancy (particularly promyelocytic leukemia), incompatible blood transfusion. The intravascular coagulation results in mechanical injury to red cells causing red cell fragmentation. Consumption of platelets and coagulation factors eventually results in a hemorrhagic state.
  Clinical manifestations: tissue infarction particularly affecting skin and kidneys; severe bleeding and ecchymosis.
  Laboratory diagnosis: PT, PTT prolonged. Fibrin split products markedly increased. Red cell morphology shows fragmented red blood cells and decreased platelets. Factors I, II, V, VIII, XIII reduced.
  Treatment: treat underlying disease. Replace blood components with platelets, fresh frozen plasma and cryoprecipitate.

7. Inhibitors of hemostasis
- Lupus anticoagulant (antiphospholipid syndrome):
  The lupus anticoagulant is an acquired circulating immunoglobulin, which is not usually associated with SLE. It occurs most frequently following viral infection in children.
  Clinical manifestations: this anticoagulant does not produce bleeding but may be associated with increased thrombosis.
  Laboratory evaluation: PTT prolonged. PTT mixing studies not corrected. Specific tests include dilute Russell's viper venom (DRVVT) and tissue thromboplastin inhibition (TTI). Antiphopholipid antibodies.

THROMBOTIC DISORDERS

Thrombotic disease (both arterial and venous thrombosis) is rare in children compared with adults.

1. Venous thrombosis
- Occurs under conditions of slow blood flow associated with activation of the coagulation system or impairment of the fibrinolytic system with or without vascular damage.
- Clinical manifestations: DVT, phlebitis, renal vein thrombosis, pulmonary embolus.

2. Arterial thrombosis
- Usually occurs under conditions of rapid blood flow associated with vascular damage and platelet activation.
- Clinical manifestations: stroke, ischemic limb, myocardial infarction.

3. Predisposing conditions associated with thrombosis of arteries or veins
- Vascular injury: trauma, burns, vasculitis.
- Decreased blood flow: dehydration, shock, hyperviscosity.
- Obstructed blood flow: immobilization, pregnancy, cardiac disease.
- Drugs: L. asparaginase, oral contraceptives.
- Nephrotic syndrome.
- Inherited thrombotic disorders: antithrombin III deficiency, protein C deficiency, protein S deficiency.
- Investigation of a suspected thrombosis:
    Ultrasound with Doppler studies.
    Ventilation perfusion scan (for pulmonary embolus).
    Radiological contrast studies.
- Laboratory investigations:
    PT, PTT, fibrinogen, fibrin split products, red blood cell morphology (for DIC).
    Antithrombin III, protein C, protein S (for inherited thrombotic disorders).
    Tests for lupus anticoagulant: DRVVT.

Antithrombin III deficiency (AT III)

AT III inhibits the vitamin K dependent factors (II, VII, IX and X). Therefore, reduction of AT III permits increased coagulation activity. Normal neonates have lower levels of antithrombin III but this is balanced by low levels of vitamin K dependent factors.

- Inheritance is autosomal dominant. AT III deficient patients have 20–60% of normal levels. AT III deficiency is associated with recurrent venous thrombosis. This usually begins in late childhood.
- Treatment (acute): infusion of AT III concentrates or FFP; warfarin (long–term).

Protein C deficiency

- Protein C inhibits clot formation and enhances fibrinolysis. Therefore, a reduction in protein C permits uninhibited clot formation.
- Homozygous protein C deficiency may present in the neonate with widespread thrombosis (purpura fulminans neonatalis).
- Heterozygous protein C deficiency is associated with recurrent venous thrombosis starting in adolescence.

ANTICOAGULANT THERAPY

1. Heparin
- Heparin enhances the rate at which AT III causes inhibition of the vitamin K dependent factors.
- May be given i.v. or s.c. (not i.m. or p.o.). Onset of action is rapid. Half–life 30–60 minutes.
- Monitoring (see Table I).
- Indications: acute and short–term management of venous thrombosis.
- Protocol for heparin therapy (for patients > 1 mo of age):
    Loading dose: 75 unit/kg (maximum: 5,000 unit/dose). Order initial loading dose STAT.
    Dilute loading dose to 5–10 mL (total) and give over 10–15 min i.v. Use heparin drip
    solution for subsequent boluses.
    Initial maintenance dose: > 1 yr of age, 20 unit/kg per h; < 1 yr of age, 25 unit/kg per h.
    Obtain APTT 4 hours after loading dose and adjust dose according to nomogram.
    If APTT is stable and therapeutic 4 hours apart, check daily APTT.
- Usual concentration for maintenance heparin:
    50 unit/mL for majority of patients.
    100 unit/mL for patients who are severely fluid restricted.
    Use D5W (but also compatible with saline).
    Double check written orders for heparin therapy.
- Remarks:
    Always obtain baseline PT, APTT and fibrinogen before starting treatment.
    Dedicated i.v. for heparin infusion; not to be interrupted by other medications.
    Blood for APTT should not be drawn on extremity where heparin drip is infusing.
    Follow daily platelet count. Risk of heparin induced thrombocytopenia is greater after the
    first 5 days.
    Heparin level is indicated if APTT is unreliable (e.g. presence of lupus anticoagulant) or if
    patient's heparin requirement is unusually high (> 40 unit/kg per h).
    Therapeutic heparin range: 0.35–0.60 anti–Xa unit/mL.

2. Warfarin
- Warfarin decreases the rate of synthesis of the vitamin K dependent factors.
- Administration: p.o. It takes 4–5 days to achieve adequate anticoagulation.
- Indications: long–term management of thrombotic disease.

Table I: Monitoring heparin infusion

APTT (s)	Bolus (unit/kg)	Hold time (min)	Rate change	Repeat APTT
< 50	50	0	↑ 20%	4 h
50–59	0	0	↑ 10%	4 h
60–85	0	0	0	4 h then q24h
86–95	0	0	↓ 10%	4 h
96–105	0	30	↓ 10%	4 h
> 105	0	60	↓ 15%	4 h

- Protocol for warfarin therapy:
    Loading dose for day 1:
    Usual loading dose: 0.2 mg/kg for 1 d. Maximum initial dose limit: 10 mg/dose.
    Consider not giving bolus dose in patients with poor liver function, congenital heart disease with heart failure, etc.
    Loading dose for days 2–7:
    Once daily evening dose; round dose off to nearest 0.25 mg.
    INR
    1.1–1.4: 0.2 mg/kg
    1.5–1.9: 0.1 mg/kg
    2.0–3.0: 0.1 mg/kg
    3.1–4.0: 0.05 mg/kg
    > 4.0: hold until INR < 4.0, then restart at 25% of loading dose
    Usual maintenance dose about 0.1 mg/kg per d.
    Long–term maintenance dosage guidelines:
    Remember INR value reflects dosage given 2 days ago.
    INR
    1.1–1.4: ↑ dose by 20%
    1.5–1.9: ↑ dose by 10%
    2.0–3.0: no change
    3.1–4.0: ↓ dose by 10%
    4.1–4.5: ↓ dose by 20%
    4.6–5.0: hold 1 dose, then restart at 20% less
    > 5.0: hold until INR < 4.5, restart at 20% less
- Antidote for warfarin:
    No bleeding (reversal for invasive procedures):
    Patient may require warfarin again in the near future: 0.5–2 mg Vitamin K_1 s.c.
    Patient may require warfarin again: 2–5 mg Vitamin K_1 s.c.
    Significant bleeding:
    Non–life threatening: 0.5–2.0 mg Vitamin K_1 s.c. and consider 20 mL/kg of FFP.
    Life threatening and will cause significant morbidity: 5 mg Vitamin K_1 by slow i.v. infusion over 10–20 min (risk of anaphylaxis).
    20 mL/kg of FFP. Consider giving factor IX concentrate (contains factors II, VIII, IX, X).
- Remarks:
    Always obtain baseline PT, international normalized ratio (INR), APTT, fibrinogen before starting treatment. Aim at INR between 2.0–3.0 for vast majority of patients. Try to give warfarin as an evening dose.
    For patients with deep vein thrombosis (DVT), start warfarin day 1 or 2 of heparin; continue heparin for at least 5 days. For postoperative cardiac patients, start warfarin when patients tolerate p.o. and as ordered by surgeons.
    When INR is > 2.0, heparin can be discontinued. INR usually decreased by a small percentage the following day.
    Duration of warfarin therapy depends on the underlying problem.
    Children with uncomplicated DVT will receive warfarin for 3 months.
    Hematology consultation for follow–up and monitoring of nonsurgical patients is encouraged.

INFECTIOUS DISEASES
Jack Forbes and Simon Dobson

CHAPTER 10

PEDIATRIC ANTIBIOTICS

Table I: Dose range of common pediatric antibiotics

Name	Route	Dosage (mg/kg per d)	Interval	Comments
Cephalosporins – 1st generation				
Cefazolin (Ancef)	i.m., i.v.	50–100	q8h	Prophylaxis and therapy *S. aureus*; useful in penicillin allergy (< 5% cross react)
Cephalexin (Keflex)	p.o.	25–50	q6h	Prophylaxis and therapy *S. aureus*, especially sequential therapy in skeletal infections
Cephalosporins – 2nd generation				
Cefaclor (Ceclor)	p.o.	40	q8h, q12h otitis media	Expensive; covers Gram positive and *H. influenzae*; otitis media, sinusitis and mild pneumonia; serum sickness 2–3% patients
Cefoxitin (Mefoxin)	i.v., i.m.	80–160	q4–6h	Gram negative and anaerobe coverage but not enterobacteriaceae or enterococci; combination therapy in intra–abdominal sepsis
Cefuroxime (Zinacef)	i.v.	100–150	q8h	Epiglottitis in immunocompetent children, pneumonia, skeletal infections, cellulitis; not neonates, nosocomial infections, meningitis or compromised host
Cefuroxime axetil (Ceftin)	p.o.	30	q12h	Not available in liquid form
Cephalosporins – 3rd generation				
Cefixime	p.o.	8	q12–24h	Oral antibiotic with broad spectrum including enterobacteriaceae; resistant species include penicillin resistant pneumococcus, staph. spp, *Listeria* and enterococcus
Cefotaxime (Claforan)	i.v.	100–150 (200 meningitis)	q6–8h, q6h	Gram negative sepsis or meningitis (infants < 3 mo, in combination with ampicillin)

Name	Route	Dosage (mg/kg per d)	Interval	Comments
Ceftazidime (Fortaz)	i.v.	100–150 (225 meningitis)	q8h	Therapy for *P. aeruginosa* and resistant enterobacteriaceae; poor antistaphylococcus activity; combination therapy in compromised hosts
Ceftriaxone (Rocephin)	i.v., i.m.	50–100 (100 meningitis)	q24h, q12h	Initial single therapy for meningitis beyond neonatal period; high incidence of diarrhea; biliary pseudolithiasis
Penicillins				
Amoxicillin (Amoxil)	p.o.	40	q8h	Similar to ampicillin but better absorbed; otitis media, sinusitis and UTI
Amoxicillin and Clavulanate (Clavulin or Augmentin)	p.o.	40 mg amox component	q8h	β–lactamase producing organisms; useful after animal bites
Ampicillin	p.o., iv., i.m.	50–100, 100–200 (meningitis 200–400)	q6h, q6h	Gram positive and negative cover; resistance 25% in *H. influenzae*, *M. catarrhalis* and most hospital staph.; combination therapy for meningitis in infants < 3 mo
Carbenicillin (Geopen)	i.v.	500	q4–6h	Ampicillin spectrum plus *P. aeruginosa*
Cloxacillin (Tegopen)	i.v.	50–100 (severe infections 150–200)	q6h	Nephrotoxic and myelosuppressive in prolonged high dose; cephalexin better tasting alternative to p.o. cloxacillin
Penicillin G (Sodium)	i.v.	100,000–250,000 (meningitis 250,000) unit/kg per d	q4–6h	Pneumococcal and meningococcal disease
Penicillin V	p.o.	25–50	q6–8h	
Piperacillin (Pipracil)	i.v.	200–300	q4–6h	Gram positive (not resistant staph.); Gram negative (includes *Klebsiella*, enterobacteriaceae and pseudomads); anaerobes include *B. fragitis*
Pivampicillin	p.o.	40–60	q12h	Similar to ampicillin
Ticarcillin (Ticar)	i.v.	200–300	q4–6h	Ampicillin spectrum plus *P. aeruginosa*

Table 1: (cont.) Dose range of common pediatric antibiotics

Name	Route	Dosage (mg/kg per d)	Interval	Comments
Ticarcillin and Clavulanate (Timentin)	i.v.	200–300	q4–6h	Not for children < 12 yr; extends spectrum to cover penicillinase producing strains; expensive
Aminoglycosides				
Amikacin (Amikin)	i.m., i.v.	15–22.5	q8h	Covers most Gram negatives; not anaerobes; nephro– and ototoxic; postlevel 20–30 mg/L; prelevel < 10 mg/L; maximum 1–2 g/24 h
Gentamicin (Garamicin)	i.m., i.v.	6–7.5 (7–10 cystics)	q8h	See amikacin; postlevel 6–10 mg/L (CF 10–20); prelevel < 2.0 mg/L; maximum 300 mg/24 h
Tobramycin (Nebcin)	i.m., i.v.	6–7.5 (7–10 cystics)	q8h	See amikacin above; postlevel 6–10 µg/mL; predose < 2 mg/L; maximum 300 mg/24 h
Macrolides, chloro– and vanco–				
Chloramphenicol (Chloromycetin)	i.v., p.o.	50–70 (meningitis 75–100)	q6h	Bone marrow depression; postlevel 15–25 mg/L
Clindamycin (Cleocin)	i.v., p.o.	25–40, 20–30	q6–8h, q6h	Covers *S. aureus* and anaerobes
Erythromycin (Ery C)	p.o.	40	q6h	Community acquired pneumonitis and *Mycoplasma*, bacteroides, *Legionella*, *Chlamydia*, *Campylobacter*; lower GI irritation given after meals
Erythromycin estolote (Ilosone)	p.o.	40	q8–12h	As above
Erythromycin ethylsuccinate (EES)	p.o.	40	q6h	As above
Erythromycin and Sulfisoxazole (Pediazole)	p.o.	40 erythro 1 mL/kg per d	q6–8h	As above
Erythromycin gluceptate or Pactobionate	i.v.	20–40	q6h	1–2 h infusion; as above
Trimethoprim (TMP) and Sulfamethoxazole (SMX) (Bactrim or Septra)	p.o. / i.v.	8–12 TMP, 40–60 SMX / as above	q12h / q6h	Side effects as per sulfas; overall 10–33%; *Pneumocystis* prophylaxis 5 mg TMP/25 mg SMX per kg per d in 2 doses; *Pneumocystis* therapy 20 mg TMP/100 mg SMX per kg per d

Name	Route	Dosage (mg/kg per d)	Interval	Comments
Vancomycin	i.v.	40, (60 meningitis)	q6–8h	All staph. and strep. spp; nephro– and ototoxicity; red–man syndrome with rapid infusion; postlevel 25–40 mg/L; prelevel 5–10 mg/L
Other antibiotics				
Aztreonam (Azactam)	i.v., i.m.	90–120	q6–8h	Same activity as aminoglycosides; not Gram positive or anaerobes; not yet approved in children < 12 yr
Ciprofloxacin	p.o., i.v.	20–30	q12h	Not approved in children < 18 yr; may be used in special cases; maximum 500 mg b.i.d.
Clarithromycin	p.o.	15	q12h	Not available in liquid form; approval for use in children < 12 yr is pending
Doxycycline (Vibramycin)	p.o., i.v.	2–4	q12–24h	Should not be used in children < 9 yr
Imipenem–Cilastatin (Primaxin)	i.v., i.m.	60–100	q6h	Broad spectrum; does not cover *P. maltophilia* or *P. cepacia*; not used in children < 12 yr; not used for therapy of meningitis; maximum dose 2 g/d
Tetracycline	p.o.	25–50	q6h	Should not be used in children < 9 yr

ANTIBIOTIC CHOICE

Many situations occur in which antibiotics must be started before bacterial cultures are available. Table II gives some best bets for various clinical cases. See the formulary for drug doses.

Table II: Antibiotic choice for specific clinical situations

Indication	Comments	Antibiotic
Febrile, septic child		
Infants < 3 mo	Onset < 7 d usually maternal origin: group B *Streptococcus*, *E. coli*, *Listeria*; > 7 d usually hospital origin: *S. aureus*, *S. epi*, group B *Streptococcus*, *Listeria*, *E. coli* and other Gram negatives	Ampicillin and gentamicin; cephalosporins have poor *Listeria* cover so not used alone if no cultures; an alternative is ampicillin plus cefotaxime
Infants > 3 mo	Roughly 5% of infants with high fever and high WBC are bacteremic; *S. pneumoniae*, *H. influenzae*, *N. meningitidis*	Cefotaxime or ceftriaxone

Table II: (cont.) Antibiotic choice for specific clinical situations

Indication	Comments	Antibiotic
Child	Be guided by the underlying disease such as osteomyelitis or pneumonia; if nothing obvious clinically, always check the urine	Cefotaxime plus cloxacillin
Immunocompromised or asplenic	*S. aureus, S. epidermidis, S. pneumococcus*, Gram negatives to include *Pseudomonas*	Ampicillin (or piperacillin in high risk patients) plus cloxacillin plus tobramycin; for a patient with penicillin allergy, give vancomycin plus ceftazidime
Pneumonia		
Newborn	Congenital: torch infections and *Listeria*; < 7 d: group B *Streptococcus, E. coli, Listeria*, Gram negatives; > 7 d: respiratory viruses, *Chlamydia, S. aureus, Pneumocystis*, group B *Streptococcus, E. coli, Listeria*	Ampicillin and gentamicin; add cloxacillin for *S. aureus* cover in older babies
Child (mild)	Usually in children < 5 yr: viral (RSV, parvovirus flu, adenovirus flu, etc.); other pathogens include *S. pneumoniae, S. aureus*, group A *Streptococcus, Mycoplasma, H. influenzae*)	Amoxicillin or erythromycin; cefixime or cefaclor or TMP–SMX as alternatives
Child (severe)	Rarely tuberculosis, Legionnaires' disease, *Chlamydia*; *S. pneumoniae, S. aureus*, group A *Streptococcus, Mycoplasma, H. influenzae*	Cefuroxime i.v.; erythromycin for atypical pneumonias
Cystic fibrosis	*Pseudomonas* and *S. aureus*; *H. influenzae* in young child	Cloxacillin and cefotaxime for young child; tobramycin and ticarcillin for older child
Immunocompromised	Any organism, but particularly *Pneumocystis*, CMV, Gram negatives, *S. aureus* or fungi	Cloxacillin and gentamicin plus septra; BAL or lung biopsy often necessary for diagnosis
Lung abscess	Anaerobic oral flora, occasionally *S. aureus* and *Klebsiella*	Clindamycin, cloxacillin or cefuroxime
CNS infection		
Infants < 3 mo	Group B *Streptococcus, E. coli, Listeria*, other Gram negatives	Ampicillin and gentamicin (neonates); ampicillin and cefotaxime (infants 1–3 mo)

Indication	Comments	Antibiotic
Children > 3 mo–18 yr	*H. influenzae, N. meningitidis, S. pneumoniae,* rarely *Streptococcus* and Gram negatives; if *S. aureus,* consider SBE as an underlying cause	Cefotaxime or ceftriaxone (adjust antibiotic when organism is known)
Brain abscess	Mixed oral organisms—aerobic and anaerobic *S. aureus, S. pneumoniae*	Vancomycin, cefotaxime and metronidazole (not clindamycin since no CSF penetration) until organism is known
Bowel infections		
Peritonitis	Gram negatives, anaerobes	Gentamicin and clindamycin
Necrotizing enterocolitis	*S. epidermidis,* Gram negatives, anaerobes	Vancomycin and cefotaxime
Bone and joint		
Neonates	Group B *Streptococcus, S. aureus,* Gram negatives	Cloxacillin and cefotaxime
Infants	*H. influenzae,* group A *Streptococcus* or *Staphylococcus*	Cefuroxime or cefotaxime or cloxacillin
Children (> 4 yr)	*S. aureus,* group A *Streptococcus* and pneumococci	Cloxacillin; alternative is β–lactamase or clindamycin
Miscellaneous		
Cellulitis	Group A *Streptococcus, S. aureus, H. influenza* in young children	Cefuroxime or ceftriaxone
Otitis media	Pneumococcus, *H. influenza,* group A *Streptococcus, B. catarrhalis, S. epidermidis*	Amoxicillin or erythromycin plus sulfa, or TMP–SMX or cefaclor or cefixime or oral cefuroxime
Pharyngitis	Usually viral; group A *Streptococcus,* rarely *Candida, C. diphtheria*	Penicillin or erythromycin
Sinusitis	*H. influenzae,* pneumococcus and anaerobes	See otitis media
Urinary tract infections	*E. coli* then other Gram negatives: *Proteus, Pseudomonas, Klebsiella, S. fecalis* and *S. aureus; S. epidermidis* if catheterized	Amoxicillin or TMP–SMX or sulfisoxazole or tetracycline (< 8 yr); ampicillin and gentamicin for pyelonephritis

COMMON INFECTIOUS DISEASE PROBLEMS

Pediatric diarrhea

Diarrhea is a common pediatric problem. Table III lists some of the major infectious causes and their treatment.

Table III: Common causes of pediatric diarrhea

Organism	Comments	Treatment
Campylobacter spp. (Gram negative rod)	Commonest bacterial gastroenteritis; food and water source; usually self–limiting gastroenteritis; rarely septicemia in neonates or immunocompromised	Usually not treated; oral erythromycin or tetracycline for high risk patients; gentamicin for septicemia
Crypotosporidium (protozoan)	Widespread among animals; usually mild gastroenteritis but chronic and severe if immunocompromised, especially AIDS, lymphoma leukemia, etc.; need to request modified AFB stain to diagnose	Spiramycin possibly effective
Escherichia coli (Gram negative rod)	Large inoculum required; food and water spread; type of disease not correlated well with serotype; enteropathogenic, toxogenic and invasive types; usually self–limiting gastroenteritis with watery diarrhea; rarely invasive in infancy; hemolytic uremic syndrome with type 0157	Only consider treating if bloody diarrhea; ampicillin or TMP–SMX may be considered with toxogenic or invasive types
Entamoeba histolytica (protozoan)	Food and water borne; often asymptomatic carrier; also acute gastroenteritis with bloody diarrhea; rarely invasive with systemic abscesses (often hepatic)	Lumen amebicide: diloxanide furoate or iodoquinol for carriers and gastroenteritis; tissue amebicides: metronidazole, chloroquine plus iodoquinol
Giardia lamblia (protozoan)	Water most important source; small inoculum; often asymptomatic; also acute gastroenteritis; may produce chronic diarrhea or malabsorption, especially if immunocompromised	Metronidazole or furazolidone
Rotavirus (reovirus)	Commonest cause of gastroenteritis in children; often preceded by flu–like illness; possibly respiratory spread; mostly winter; not food borne; many other viral causes of gastroenteritis such as enterovirus, adenovirus, etc.	Supportive treatment only

Organism	Comments	Treatment
Salmonella spp. (Gram negative rod)	Meat, poultry and human carriers; about 2,000 serotypes, only 20 important; usually self–limiting gastroenteritis but septicemic illnesses occur, particularly in immunocompromised and neonates	Gastroenteritis untreated except in infants < 3 mo or immuno–suppressed patients; ampicillin or TMP–SMX for patient at risk; ampicillin or cefotaxime or ceftriaxone for invasive disease
Shigella (Gram negative rod)	Man only reservoir; small inoculum needed; invades bowel wall; toxin produced; sick child, high fever, seizures in 10%; blood, pus and mucus in stool; rarely a septicemic illness	Ampicillin or TMP–SMX; resistance is common
Yersinia enterocolitica (Gram negative rod)	Milk, water, food and human carrier; usually acute gastroenteritis; may mimic appendicitis or ulcerative colitis and cause a reactive arthritis (Reiter's syndrome); very rarely a septicemic illness	Gastroenteritis untreated; i.v. gentamicin for septicemia or adenitis; TMP–SMX for oral treatment

Fever in children < 3 years

Common final diagnoses in this age group are:
- Otitis media: 37%
- Nonspecific illness: 25%
- Pneumonia: 15%
- Recognizable viral illness: 13% (exanthem, croup, gastroenteritis, aseptic meningitis).
- Recognizable bacterial illness: 10% (cellulitis, meningitis, bacteremia, urinary tract infections).

Several serious bacterial illnesses have their highest occurrence in this age group: bacteremia is most frequent in children with higher temperatures. The bacteria most often isolated from blood of children with fever, without a source for the fever, are *S. pneumoniae*, *H. influenzae*, *Neisseria meningitidis*, *S. aureus*, *S. pyogenes* and *Salmonella* spp. Since the immunization of infants with *H. influenzae* type B vaccine, the proportion of children with invasive disease caused by this pathogen has diminished significantly.

Likelihood of serious disease increases with the presence of fever (especially > 40 °C), petechiae, toxic–looking child, age < 3 months, abnormal investigations (e.g. increased white blood count > 15,000/mm^3).

1. History
- Child's well being (irritability, alertness, appetite).
- Characteristics of fever (duration, severity).
- Associated symptoms.
- Past history (immunizations, previous illness or fever, medications).
- Social history (infectious source, e.g. daycare, school friends, recent travel).
- Family history (any ill family members or visitors).

2. Examination
- Record temperature.
- Vital signs (pulse, respiratory rate) and general status (responsiveness, position).
- Rash (describe and locate).
- Lymphadenopathy (local or generalized).
- ENT (remove wax if necessary).
- Respiratory (unequal air entry, adventitious sounds).
- Cardiovascular (presence of murmurs).
- Abdomen (rectal examination if indicated).
- Musculoskeletal (swellings, joint movements, focal tenderness).
- CNS (meningism frequently not present, fontanelles, sensorium).

3. Investigations
- Indicated if: clinical risk factors present, no specific cause of fever evident, degree of illness inappropriate for proposed diagnosis.
- Initial workup: CBC (leukocytosis, thrombocytopenia), urinalysis.
- Subsequent workup: lumbar puncture (unless decreased level of consciousness), blood cultures (if leukocytosis present); urine if urinalysis abnormal; CSF examination if lumbar puncture done; throat swab (usually insensitive); viral (stool, urine, CSF, nasopharyngeal washing).
- Antigen analysis: urine and CSF may be helpful, especially if prior treatment given.
- Chest X–ray: more important for children < 3 months or indicated with respiratory symptoms in children with fever > 40 °C or WBC > 15,000/mm^3.

4. Management
- Febrile child with focus: investigate and treat as appropriate.
- Febrile child without focus:
     Since there is no completely reliable indicator of sepsis other than positive blood cultures, most people treat cautiously. All febrile children < 3 months of age should be admitted, investigated and treated. Those > 3 months of age with a temperature > 39 °C and WBC > 15,000/mm^3 should probably be observed in hospital for 24 hours while waiting for results of cultures. The use of antibiotics in this group depends on the physician's subjective impression of the child's condition and cannot be expressed in a protocol. Children discharged from the Emergency Room should be reviewed within 24 hours.

Fever of unknown origin (FUO)

1. Definition
Children with a documented fever of > 38.5 °C for > 7 days and who have been adequately evaluated for the more common causes of fever.

2. Etiology
- About one–third are unusual etiologies, one–third are atypical presentations of common disorders and one–third remain undiagnosed. Principle causes of FUO in children are infectious, collagen vascular diseases and malignancy in ± 10%. The younger the child, the more likely there is an infective cause.

- Unusual presentations of common diseases: UTI, upper respiratory infection (sinusitis, otitis, tonsillitis), pneumonia, chronic mastoiditis, CMV, EBV (infectious mononucleosis), meningitis, allergic disorders, dehydration, rheumatic fever.
- Infectious diseases: osteomyelitis, septic arthritis, occult abscesses (dental, liver, pelvic, abdominal), pyelonephritis, hepatitis (chronic active), endocarditis, tuberculosis, salmonellosis, brucellosis, spirochetes (leptospirosis, relapsing fever, syphilis, Lyme's disease), malaria, rickettsial infections (Q, RMSF).
- Collagen vascular diseases: juvenile rheumatoid arthritis, SLE.
- Malignancies: leukemia, lymphoma, neuroblastoma.
- Miscellaneous: Crohn's disease, drug fever, serum sickness, factitious fever, sarcoidosis, ectodermal dysplasia.

3. Prognosis
- Generally better than adults but still has a 5–10% mortality.

4. Approach
The diagnostic evaluation is largely dependent on a meticulous history and physical examination (see p. 177, "Fever in children < 3 years"):
- History:
    Complete travel history (any prophylactic treatment).
    Contacts with ill individuals (especially TB) or animals (pets and wild).
    Insect contact (ticks and mosquitos).
    Diet (unpasteurized milk, water supply, raw fish or game).
    Medications (including topical or nonprescription drugs).
    Ethnic or genetic background.
- Examination:
    Growth parameters.
    Anomalous dentition or alopecia.
    Ophthalmological anomalies.
    Nasal discharge, sinus tenderness, sinus transillumination.
    Repeated skin examination.
    Careful examination of bones and muscles.
    Rectal examination imperative in all ages.
    Pelvic examination in sexually active adolescents.
- Investigations (guided by history and physical examination and prior screening data):
    Suggested workup in two phases, where phase 1 is a broad screen for all patients and phase 2 includes invasive procedures which are done sequentially as indicated.
    Phase 1: CBC, ESR, urinalysis and culture, chest X–ray, blood culture, ASOT, ANA, EBV serology, TB skin test (test also for anergy), lumbar puncture (young infant).
    Phase 2: hospitalize, repeat blood cultures, sinus and mastoid X–rays, ophthalmological examination, serology (CMV, toxoplasmosis, hepatitis, brucella, leptospirosis), liver enzymes, abdominal ultrasound or CT scan, upper GI with follow through, bone scan, gallium scan, biopsy (lymph node, liver where indicated), bone marrow (histology and cultures—bacteria, tuberculosis and fungal—where indicated).

Lower respiratory tract infections

Lower respiratory infections are frequent problems (240 episodes per 1,000 infants < 1 year) and grouped pathologically as bronchiolitis, acute bronchitis and pneumonia.

1. Bronchiolitis
Bronchiolitis is a major cause of morbidity in the first 2 years. The most common etiological agent is respiratory syncytial virus (RSV) in winter and early spring. Bronchiolitis is more severe in premature infants and in children with bronchopulmonary dysplasia or congenital heart disease.
• Diagnosis: results obtained within hours by sending fresh nasopharyngeal secretions for immunofluorescent stain to virology laboratory.
• Treatment:
    Support with oxygen, hydration and appropriate nutrition. Bronchial narrowing may sometimes be reversible with smooth muscle relaxants and a trial dose of β–mimetic is worth administering. Antibiotics may be indicated for otitis media or pneumonia.
    Specific antiviral therapy with ribavirin may be indicated in some infants such as those with significant congenital heart disease, significant lung disease (e.g. bronchopulmonary dysplasia, etc.), immunocompromised from disease or therapy, certain metabolic or neurological diseases. Because treatment is expensive (Can. $1,550/dose), it is reserved for patients with a positive screening test for RSV. Patients infected with other respiratory viruses are less likely to benefit. Recent studies have shown no benefit from the drug.
    Ribavirin is given as an aerosol, administered 20 h/d for 5–7 d by mask or head box (not croup tent), using a special aerosol generator. It should be given with caution to patients on a ventilator because precipitated drug can block expiratory valves. Adverse effects are limited to chemical conjunctivitis and face rash.

2. Pneumonia
The causative agent in pneumonia depends on several variables:
• Age group: *Mycoplasma* is increasingly common above 5 years of age, while group B *Streptococcus* and *Listeria* are usually seen in young infants.
• Season: respiratory viruses are more common in fall to early spring, while *Mycoplasma* is endemic year round.
• Underlying diseases: *Pneumocystis*, CMV or fungus are common agents in patients with immunosuppression.
• Geographic: large variations exist in causative agents around the world. Neonatal *Chlamydia* is much rarer in Europe than in USA. TB is still common in many countries.
• Approach: unfortunately, there is no easy way to distinguish viral from bacterial infections. Clinical features such as wheeze, rash, arthralgia, cough and crepitations may occur frequently in viral or bacterial illness. Laboratory investigations such as C–reactive protein, ESR, white count and differential are also of little help.
• History: age, season, hospital (nosocomial) or community acquired, associated features (otitis, sinusitis, cough, sputum), underlying illness (anatomical abnormality, neurological disorders, cystic fibrosis, malnutrition, asthma, aspiration of foreign body), social history (including possible infectious source, animal or bird exposure), family history (family or visitors, TB contacts), travel history (histoplasmosis, blastomycosis in USA).
• Examination: general status (cyanosis, respiratory rate, distress), lymphadenopathy, pulse

rate, blood pressure and fever, skin, ENT, use of accessory muscles, auscultation (sensitivity of diagnosing pneumonia low).
- Investigations:
    Chest X–ray.
    CBC, electrolytes, blood gas if indicated.
    Blood culture (pleural fluid tap if present).
    Nasopharyngeal washing for RSV and viral culture.
    Throat culture and sputum cultures (both have a poor correlation with etiological agent; a Gram stain of sputum may be helpful).
    Antigen detection: urine (poor sensitivity unless bacteremia present).
    Cold agglutinins or *Mycoplasma* serology.
- Treatment:
    Supportive care consists of close attention to hydration and oxygenation. Particularly in the younger age groups, it may be necessary to ventilate some children through the worst part of the illness.
    Specific treatment is guided by the most likely organism (see Table II). Consider additional coverage for *S. aureus* in sicker children. Because of the difficulty in differentiating viral and bacterial disease, all children with an initial diagnosis of pneumonia should be started on antibiotics. These may need to be changed as test results, such as blood cultures and nasopharyngeal washings, are returned.

Infectious exanthems

The differential diagnosis of infectious exanthems is based on: past history of infectious disease and immunization, incubation period (period of exposure to illness), type of prodromal period (long, short, absent, illness prior to rash), features of the rash (character, distribution and duration), presence of pathognomonic or other diagnostic signs, laboratory diagnostic tests. The pattern of the rash gives some guidance to the etiology (Tables IV and V). The collection of suitable samples is covered in Table VI.

Table IV: Differential diagnosis of fever and rash

Lesion	Pathogen or associated factor
Maculopapular or macular rash	• Viruses: measles, rubella, roseola, fifth disease (parvovirus), Epstein–Barr virus, enteroviruses, hepatitis B virus (papular acrodermatitis or Gianotti–Crosti's syndrome) • Bacteria: rheumatic fever (group A *Streptococcus*), scarlet fever, *Corynebacterium haemolyticum*, secondary syphilis, leptospirosis, *Pseudomonas*, meningococcal infection (early), *Salmonella*, Lyme's disease • Rickettsia: Early Rocky Mountain spotted fever, typhus (scrub, endemic) • Other: Kawasaki's disease
Diffuse erythroderma	• Bacteria: scarlet fever (group A *Streptococcus*), toxic shock syndrome (*S. aureus*) • Fungi: *Candida albicans*
Urticarial rash	• Viruses: Epstein–Barr virus, hepatitis B • Bacteria: *Mycoplasma pneumoniae*, group A *Streptococcus*
Vesicular, bullous, pustular	• Viruses: herpes simplex, varicella zoster, coxsackievirus • Bacteria: staphylococcal scalded skin syndrome, staphylococcal bullous impetigo, group A streptococcal crusted impetigo • Other: toxic epidermal necrolysis, erythema multiforme (Stevens–Johnson's syndrome), rickettsial pox
Petechial purpuric	• Viruses: atypical measles, congenital rubella, CMV and enterovirus infection • Bacteria: sepsis (meningococcal, gonococcal), endocarditis • Rickettsia: Early Rocky Mountain spotted fever, epidemic typhus • Other: vasculitis, thrombocytopenia, Henoch–Schönlein purpura
Erythema nodosum	• Viruses: Epstein–Barr virus, hepatitis B • Bacteria: group A *Streptococcus*, tuberculosis, *Yersinia*, cat–scratch disease • Fungi: coccidioidomycosis, histoplasmosis • Other: sarcoidosis, inflammatory bowel disease, estrogen containing oral contraceptives
Distinctive rashes (Ecthyma gangrenosum, erythema chronicum migrans, necrotic eschar)	• *Pseudomonas aeruginosa*, Lyme's disease, aspergillosis, mucormycosis

Table V: Patterns of rash with some common pediatric diseases

Disease	Prodrome	Rash	Typical feature	Laboratory
Maculopapular eruptions				
Atypical measles	2–4 d fever, cough, headache, myalgia	Mainly limbs; may be vesicular	Frequent pleural effusion	As in measles
Drug eruptions	None	Variable; usually widespread, pruritic, sudden onset ± systemic effects	Circumstantial	None
Enteroviral infectious	Variable	Rubella–like; hand, foot, mouth disease; discrete and nonpruritic	Summer and fall months; may have aseptic meningitis	Viral culture; stool, CSF, nasopharyngeal washing
Erythema infectiosum (Parvovirus B16)	None	Slapped cheek; lace pattern; evanescent; lasts ± 2 wk	Typical rash in well child; may be pruritic	None
Erythema subitum (Herpes 6)	3–4 d high fever with rapid resolution and then rash	Discrete rose–red; trunk to face and limbs; disappears in 1–2 d	Rash after fever	None
Infectious mononucleosis	1–2 d	Triad: tonsillitis, lymphadenopathy, hepatosplenomegaly ± enanthem 50%; exanthem 15%	Incubation period 30–50 d; exanthem with ampicillin 80%	Atypical lymphocytes; monospot; serology
Kawasaki's disease	4–6 d fever, sore throat, lymphadenopathy	Generalized rash; palms and soles swelling to desquamation; cracked red lips, strawberry tongue, conjunctivitis	Constellation of features	None
Measles	3–4 d fever, conjunctivitis, coryza, cough	Reddish brown; face to trunk to limbs; confluent on trunk; fades day 5 brawny desquamation	Koplik spots; incubation period 10–12 d	Serology culture in special circumstances
Meningococcemia	Variable but usually < 24 h; fever, irritable, ± meningism	Transient mac–pap rash to petechial, purpuric rash; no regular distribution	Irregular distribution petechiae; short incubation period	Cultures: blood, CSF or petechiae

Table V: (cont.) Patterns of rash with some common pediatric diseases

Disease	Prodrome	Rash	Typical feature	Laboratory
Rubella	0–4 d malaise, low fever, lymphadenopathy (occipital)	Pink; face to limbs within 48 h; discrete; disappears day 3–4; no desquamation	Postauric or occipital nodes; incubation period 14–21 d	As in measles
Scarlet fever	12 h to 2 d fever, sore throat, vomiting	Erythematous and blanches "sandpaper"; oral pallor; flexor surfaces to generalized 24 h; desquamation in 1–2 wk	Strawberry tongue, membranous tonsillitis	Culture; ASOT
Staphylococcal toxic shock (*S. aureus*)	None; fever, headaches, confusion, vomiting and diarrhea, shock	Scarlatiniform mainly on trunk and limbs; edema face; desquamation	Fever, toxicity, shock	Culture; phage typing
Papulovesicular lesions				
Coxsackievirus	Variable	Hand, foot, mouth disease	Summer and fall months; may have aseptic meningitis	Viral culture: stool, CSF, nasopharyngeal washing
Herpes simplex	None	1°: mostly subclinical; may be generalized; reactivation: localized, thin walled vesicle which rupture or heal in 10 d	Skin or genitalia (usually HSV2); incubation period 6 d	Same as varicella
Herpes zoster	None	Unilateral and along dermatome; vesicles grouped together and become confluent	Dermatome distribution	Same as varicella
Impetigo	None	Vesicles become confluent and rapidly progress to pustulo and crust; not in crops and not on mucus membrane	Yellow crusting; contagious	Culture (group A *Streptococcus*); *S. aureus* 2° agent

Disease	Prodrome	Rash	Typical feature	Laboratory
Papular urticaria (Insect bites)	None	Hypersensitivity reaction; urticarial eruption ± vesicles; may later form persistent papules	Preceeding insect exposure; exposed areas; pruritic	None
Pediculosis (Lice)	None	Scalp, body and pubic lice; pruritic excoriation	Nits on hair shaft	Nit microscopy
Scabies (Sarcoptes scabiei)	None	Discrete "burrows" ± vesicle or excoriated papule which may become generalized	Pruritic; contagious	Burrow scraping microscopy
S. aureus toxic shock	None; fever and irritability with rash	Generalized; tender; bullae 1–2 d to moist desquamation	Nikolsky's sign	Cultures
Varicella	1–2 d fever, malaise	Rapid evolution macules → papules → vesicles → crusted lesions; central; crops; mucus membranes; all stages present	Incubation period 14–21 d; "tear–drop" vesicles	Vesicle scraping for immuno–fluorescence; serolgy

Table VI: Laboratory diagnosis of common pediatric viral diseases

Virus suspected	Clinical disease commonly associated with virus	Clinical specimens*
Adenovirus	Acute respiratory disease, pneumonia, pharyngoconjunctival fever, keratoconjunctivitis, etc.	Throat swab, rectal swab, stool, eye swab
Cytomegalovirus	Mononucleosis, hepatitis, pneumonia	Buffy coat, urine, throat swab, serology
Enterovirus	Aseptic meningitis, pleurodynia, myocarditis, pericarditis, herpangina, poliomyelitis	Stool, rectal swab, throat swab, CSF
Epstein–Barr virus	Mononucleosis, chronic mononucleosis syndrome	Serology
Hepatitis A virus	Jaundice	Serology
Herpes simplex virus	Gingivostomatitis, keratoconjunctivitis, herpes labialis, genital herpes, encephalitis	Vesicle fluid, throat swab or mouthwashing, vaginal swab, brain biopsy, serology
Influenza and parainfluenza viruses	Pharyngitis, croup, bronchiolitis, pneumonia, urinary tract infection	Nasopharyngeal washing, nasal swab, throat swab, blood, urine
Measles virus	Measles, SSPE, encephalitis	Throat swab, CSF, serology, urine
Mumps virus	Parotitis, orchitis, aseptic meningitis	Throat swab, serology, urine, CSF
Respiratory syncytial virus	Croup, bronchiolitis, pneumonia	Nasopharyngeal aspirate
Rhinovirus	Nonspecific febrile illness, common cold	Nasopharyngeal washing
Rotavirus	Gastroenteritis	Stool
Rubella virus	Congenital rubella rash, lymphadenopathy	Throat swab, rectal swab, urine, serology
Varicella zoster virus	Chickenpox, herpes zoster	Vesicle fluid, lesion swab, serology

* For antibody determinations, acute phase serum should be collected immediately after onset; convalescent serum should be collected 10–14 days later

PARASITIC DISEASES

Air travel and increasing numbers of immunosuppressed patients have markedly increased the incidence of exotic parasitic diseases in nontropical countries. Table VII provides information on the commoner parasites plus drug treatment and dosage.

Table VII: Common parasitic diseases

Organism	Comments	Treatment
Amebiasis (*Entamoeba histolytica*)	Asymptomatic carrier, gastroenteritis or systemic invasion with hepatic abscesses; cysts and trophs in fresh stool, serology	• Carrier: iodoquinol 40 mg/kg per d div. 3 for 20 d; maximum 2 g/d or diloxanide furoate 20 mg/kg per d div. 3 for 10 d • Dysentery: metronidazole 35 mg kg/d div. 3 for 10 d plus iodoquinol as above • Invasive: as for dysentery above, followed by chloroquine phosphate 10 mg base/kg per d for 14–21 d; needle aspiration of large abscesses may be considered
Ascariasis (*Ascaris lumbricoides*)	Common, usually asymptomatic; rare lumen obstruction by worms; eggs in feces	• Mebendazole 100 mg b.i.d. for 3 d or pyrantel pamoate 11 mg/kg (one dose); maximum dose 1 g
Beef tapeworm (*T. saginata*)	Symptomless; proglottids in feces	• Niclosamide or praziquantel (see pork tapeworm)
Cutaneous larva migrans (*A. braziliense* and others)	Serpiginous skin lesions; larvae die in a few weeks without treatment	• As for visceral larva migrans • Ethylene chloride spray externally may be effective but painful and may damage tissue
Dwarf tapeworm (*Hymenolepis nana*)	Usually asymptomatic	• Praziquantel 25 mg/kg (1 dose) or niclosamide as for pork tapeworm but treat for 6 d
Echinococcosis (*Echinococcosis multilocularis*)	Symptoms from slow growing space occupying cysts, usually lung and liver; rarely anaphylaxis from cyst leak; clinical diagnosis (Casoni test and serology of some use)	• Surgical treatment when indicated; albendazole 15 mg/kg per d p.o. div. q12h × 28 d • May be given for extended periods if inoperable • *E. granulosus* relatively benign; may resolve without treatment
Fish tapeworm (*Diphyllobothrium latum*)	Rare disease but present around Great Lakes; usually asymptomatic; 1% have B12 deficiency anemia; eggs in feces	• As for pork tapeworm
Giardiasis (*Giardia lamblia*)	Asymptomatic, acute gastroenteritis or chronic disease with malabsorption; cysts and trophs in fresh stool or duodenal aspirate	• Metronidazole 15 mg/kg per d div. 3 for 5–7 d • Furazolidone 5 mg/kg per d div. 4 for 7–10 d; maximum 400 mg/d

Table VII: (cont.) Common parasitic diseases

Organism	Comments	Treatment
Hookworm (*Necator americanus, Ancylostoma duodenale*)	Often asymptomatic; anemia with large worm loads; eggs in feces	• Mebendazole 100 mg b.i.d. for 3 d or pyrantel pamoate 11 mg/kg for 3 d; maximum dose 1 g
Malaria (*Plasmodium falciparum, P. malariae, P. vivax, P. ovale*)	*P. falciparum* most serious: hemolysis, shock, cerebral malaria; widespread drug resistance, especially SE Asia, against chloroquine and fansidar (pyrimethamine and sulfadoxine); *P. falciparum* has no hepatic cycle *P. malariae, P. ovale*, and *P. vivax*: less severe, no drug resistance; hepatic cycle present so must follow chloroquine with primaquine for eradication	
	Treatment of *P. ovale, P. vivax, P. malariae* and sensitive *P. falciparum*	• Chloroquine base 10 mg/kg p.o. stat, then 5 mg/kg at 6, 24 and 48 h after initial dose; i.v. dosing dangerous but available for unconscious patient: quinidine 10 mg/kg i.v. in 1 h infusion, then 0.02 mg/kg per min for maximum 3 d
	Treatment of resistant *P. falciparum*	• Quinine sulphate 25 mg/kg per d div. 3 for 3 d; maximum 2 g/d plus pyrimethamine–sulfadoxine (fansidar); < 1 yr, ¼ tablet; 1–3 yr, ½ tablet; 4–8 yr, 1 tablet; 9–14 yr, 2 tablets • Other regimes are available, e.g. quinine plus tetracycline or quinine plus clindamycin • Parenteral therapy as above
	Prevention of relapse *P. ovale, P. malariae, P. vivax*	• Primaquine base 0.3 mg/kg per d p.o. for 14 d; maximum 15 mg/d; check G6PD status
	Prophylaxis for *P. ovale, P. vivax, P. malariae* and sensitive *P. falciparum*	• Chloroquine base 5 mg/kg once weekly p.o.; 1 wk before to 4 wk after exposure
	Prophylaxis for resistant *P. falciparum*	• Mefloquine: (per wk) 15–19 kg, ¼ tablet; 20–30 kg, ½ tablet; 31–45 kg, ¾ tablet; > 45 kg, 1 tablet; start 1 wk before to 4 wk after exposure • Chloroquine as above plus carry fansidar to use if fever develops; fansidar associated with severe erythema multiforme reactions; also does not cover *P. vivax*; check for recommendations before travel • Doxycycline: > 8 yr, 2 mg/kg per d p.o. daily (maximum 100 g/d)
Pinworm (*Enterobius vermicularis*)	Common, usually asymptomatic; pruritus, vulvitis and vaginitis; treat whole household; scotch tape swab for eggs	• As for hookworm; pyrantel pamoate or mebendazole

Organism	Comments	Treatment
Pneumocystis (*Pneumocystis carinii*)	Pneumonia in immuno– compromised or newborns; occasionally in sputum but usually needs lung biopsy	• Septra (TMP 20 mg/kg per d + SMX 100 mg/kg per d) div. 4 i.v. for 14–21 d or pentamidine i.v. • Oral septra reserved for mild disease or when pneumonitis resolving: same dose or pentamidine 4 mg/kg per d i.v. for 14–21 d
Pork tapeworm (*Taenia solium*)	Adult worms symptomless; autoinfection with eggs leads to cysts in tissues including CNS (cysticercosis); proglottids and eggs in feces	• Praziquantel: 10–20 mg/kg (1 dose) • Niclosamide: 11–34 kg, 2 tablets (1 g); > 34 kg, 3 tablets (1.5 g) then 1 g/d for 6 d
Schistosomiasis (Bilharzia) (*S. mansoni, S. hematobium, S. japonicum*)	Very common in people from Asia and Africa; often asymptomatic; hepatospleno– megaly, cystitis hematuria, portal hypertension; eggs in feces, urine and rectal biopsy	• Praziquantel 40 mg/kg (2 doses) in 1 d (60 mg/kg div. 3 in 1 d for *S. japonicum*)
Strongyloidiasis (*Strongyloides stercoralis*)	Usually asymptomatic; occasionally large loads from re–infection; rarely fatal in immunocompromised	• Thiabendazole 50 mg/kg per d div. 2 for 2 d; longer for compromised patients; maximum dose 3 g/d
Toxoplasmosis (*Toxoplasma gondii*)	Usually mild illness; severe CNS damage with congenital or immunocompromised host; serological diagnosis	• No controlled trials of treatment and outcome; following drugs are used: pyrimethamine 2 mg/kg per d for 3 d, then 1 mg/kg per d for 4 wk (maximum 25 mg/d) plus sulfadiazine 120 mg/kg per d div. 4 for 4 wk (maximum 3 g) or spiramycin 50–100 mg/kg per d div. 4 for 4 wk
Trichinosis (*Trichinella spiralis*)	Often asymptomatic: large loads produce fever, muscle pain, periorbital edema; rarely encephalitis and myocarditis; serology or deltoid biopsy	• Mebendazole 200–400 mg t.i.d. × 3 d, then 400–500 mg t.i.d. × 10 d
Visceral larva migrans (*Toxocara canis, T. cati*)	Fever, cough, hepatosplenomegaly; rarely ocular involvement; gamma globulin and eosinophils increased; clinical diagnosis	• Thiabendazole 50 mg/kg per d div. 2 for 5 d; steroids for severe cases and ocular involvement.
Whipworm (*Trichuris trichiura*)	Common, usually asymptomatic; large loads may produce anemia, bloody stools and rectal prolapse; eggs in feces	• Mebendazole 100 mg b.i.d. for 3 d

ACTIVE IMMUNIZATION

The following list provides notes on the vaccines commonly given to children in Canada. Tables VIII, IX and X give Canadian immunization schedules.

Diphtheria

- Cell free toxoid.
- No protection against infection, only against diphtheria toxin.
- Immunity is long lasting but titers decline with time and can be boosted by additional doses.
- Febrile and local reactions increase in severity with age so a smaller dose is used in patients > 7 years.
- Available alone or in combination with pertussis and tetanus designated DPT.
- "Adult" preparation is mixed with tetanus toxoid designated (Td) since a smaller amount of diphtheria toxoid is present. It is used in patients ≥ 7 years of age.

Tetanus

- Cell free toxoid providing protection against tetanus toxin.
- Long lasting immunity but booster doses every 10 years are recommended (administered as Td).
- Adverse reactions are rare unless boosters are given too frequently.
- Available alone or in combination with pertussis and/or diphtheria toxoid.

Pertussis

- A suspension of killed bacteria containing the common serotypes.
- Immunity is not perfect (about 60–85% protection).
- Adverse effects cause controversy. Fever and local reactions are very common (approximately 50%).
- If pertussis occurs in infants and children who have received 3 or more doses of vaccine, it is usually mild.

Persistent screaming within 48 h	1:1,000
Hypotonic/hyporesponsive	1:2,000 (staring spell, convulsions and floppiness)
Febrile convulsion within 3 d	1:2,000
Encephalopathy within 7 d	1:100,000
Permanent brain damage	no proven association

- Reactions increase with age while disease severity decreases with age so pertussis vaccine is not recommended if > 7 years of age.

Contraindications to pertussis vaccine:
- Absolute: anaphylaxis.
- Relative: hypotonic/hyporesponsive episodes (no long–term sequelae).
- Deferred: consider if progressive, evolving or unstable neurological condition (to prevent confusion with adverse reaction), e.g. tuberous sclerosis, CNS malformations, degenerative conditions, poorly controlled convulsions. Continue other vaccine components as per schedule.

Give pertussis component alone later, once neurological condition is stable.

The following are not contraindications to pertussis vaccine:
- High fever within 48 hours of previous dose.
- Febrile convulsions.
- Afebrile convulsions.
- Family history of convulsions.
- Persistent crying.

Measles

- Live attenuated measles virus.
- Provides good long–term immunity after one dose. It will also prevent or attenuate measles if given within 72 hours of exposure.
- Adverse reactions are usually not serious.

Fever and rash (noncontagious)	5–15%
Encephalitis	1 in 1 million
SSPE	very rare

- It is a live virus so do not give to immunocompromised patients (although it is recommended for children with HIV infection).
- Grown on chick embryo cells and contains neomycin so contraindicated in patients with extreme hypersensitivity to eggs or neomycin.
- Available alone or in combination with mumps and rubella.

Mumps

- Live attenuated virus.
- Provides good long–term immunity after 1 dose.
- Usually few adverse reactions.
- Grown on chick embryo cells and contains neomycin so contraindicated if hypersensitivity to eggs or neomycin.
- Available alone or in combination with measles and rubella. Contraindicated in pregnancy or immunocompromised patient (except HIV infected children).

Rubella

- Mild disease. Vaccination to prevent congenital rubella syndrome.
- Live attenuated virus grown on human diploid cells.
- One dose provides good long–term protection.
- Adverse reactions unusual, e.g. rash, lymphadenopathy plus transient arthritis. Side effects may be more severe in older adolescents and adults.
- Contraindicated in pregnancy or immunocompromised patient (except HIV infected children).

Polio

- Two types of trivalent polio vaccine available (live and killed). Both provide good long–term

immunity. Boosters are only recommended for adults at high risk.
    Killed virus vaccine (Salk): s.c. or i.m. when given with combined vaccines (tetanus or diphtheria toxoids). Very few adverse reactions.
    Live attenuated virus (Sabin): given p.o. Thought to provide greater protection against wild strains of polio.
- Close contacts also immunized from fecal–oral spread. Very rare incidence of paralytic polio in recipients and close contacts. Oral polio vaccine is contraindicated in immunocompromised or hospital inpatients.

HIB

- *H. influenzae* type B (HIB) conjugate vaccines are licensed. There is one combination HIB conjugate with DPT IPV vaccine (PENTA). Currently, 3 doses are given at 2, 4 and 6 months and a booster at 18 months.
- Administered at the same time as DPT at separate site.
- Children > 5 years of age are not immunized unless at increased risk of invasive disease. No severe side effects: local reaction, 7%; irritability, 16%; fever > 39 °C, <1%.

Others

    Several other vaccines are useful in certain clinical situations, e.g. pneumococcal, influenza, hepatitis B, meningococcal.

Routine immunization schedules

General precautions for immunizations:
- Only defer immunization for febrile illnesses, not mild respiratory tract infections.
- Severe anaphylaxis induced by eggs or neomycin is a contraindication to the use of measles and mumps vaccines.
- Live virus vaccines, particularly rubella, are contraindicated in pregnancy.
- Live virus vaccines are contraindicated in immunosuppressed patients, except MMR in HIV infected children. Inactive vaccines such as DPT can be used but may not induce a good response. Oral polio should not be given to hospital inpatients or in immunocompromised children.
- Preterm infants can be immunized by their postnatal age, not corrected age. Full doses of vaccine should be used.
- Eczema is not a contraindication to vaccination.
- Live virus vaccines should not be given for at least 3 months following infusion of blood or gamma globulin.
- Vaccines should always be given in a setting in which anaphylactic reactions can be readily treated.

PASSIVE IMMUNIZATION

    Gamma globulin solutions are available for prophylaxis and treatment of a variety of conditions. Most are now of human origin and are reasonably safe. If animal globulins are used, great care must be taken to test for sensitivity before full doses are given.

Human immunoglobulin (Ig)

* Ig is obtained from pooled human donors and contains specific antibodies in proportion to infections and immunization experience of the donor population.
* Ig is recommended for intramuscular administration.
* Used for replacement therapy in antibody deficiency disorders, hepatitis A prophylaxis and measles prophylaxis.
* Consists primarily of 95% IgG and trace amounts of IgA and IgM.

Table VIII: Routine immunization schedule for infants and children

Age at vaccination	DPT	Polio	HIB[a]	MMR	Td[b]
2 mo	X	X	X		
4 mo	X	X	X		
6 mo	X	(X)[c]	X		
12 mo				X	
18 mo	X	X	X		
4–6 yr	X	X			
14–16 yr		(X)[c]			X

Notes refer to Tables VIII, IX and X:
DPT = diphtheria, pertussis and tetanus vaccine
HIB = Haemophilus B conjugate vaccine
MMR = measles, mumps and rubella vaccine
Td = tetanus and diphtheria toxoid, "adult type"
a. HIB schedule shown is for HbOC or PRP–T vaccines.
   If PRP–OMP is used, give at 2, 4 and 12 mo of age.
b. Td (tetanus and diphtheria toxoid), a combined adsorbed "adult type" preparation for use in patients $\geq$ 7 yr of age, contains less diphtheria toxoid than preparations given to younger children and is less likely to cause reactions in older patients; repeat every 10 yr throughout life.
c. Omit this dose if OPV is used exclusively.
d. Delay until subsequent visit if child is < 12 mo of age.
e. Recommended schedule and number of doses depend on the product used and the age of the child when vaccination is begun. Not required past age 5 yr.
f. Omit these doses if the previous doses of DPT and polio were given after the fourth birthday.

Table IX: Routine immunization schedule for unimmunized children < 7 years of age

Timing	DPT	Polio	HIB	MMR	Td[b]
First visit	X	X	X	(X)[d]	
2 mo later	X	X	(X)[e]		
2 mo later	X	(X)[c]			
6–12 mo later	X	X	(X)[e]		
4–6 yr[f]	X	X			
14–16 yr		(X)[c]			X

Table X: Routine immunization schedule for unimmunized children ≥ 7 years of age

Timing	Td[b]	Polio	MMR
First visit	X	X	X
2 mo later	X	X	
6–12 mo later	X	X	
10 yr later	X		

Intravenous human immunoglobulin (IVIg)

- IVIg is used in replacement therapy in antibody deficiency disorders, Kawasaki's disease, pediatric AIDS (controversial), bone marrow transplantation (controversial), very low birth weight infants (controversial).

Hepatitis B immunoglobulin (HBIg)

- Specific immunoglobulin from pooled human donors who have high levels of antibody to HBV.
- HBIg is used in the following situations: needlestick or mucosal exposure to blood, newborn of hepatitis B carrier (give HBIg soon after delivery and start hepatitis B vaccine—at the same time—while in the nursery), sexual contact of hepatitis B patient (give HBIg and consider vaccination).

Zoster immunoglobulin (VZIg)

- From pooled human plasma.
- Give within 96 hours of exposure.
- Protection lasts 3–4 weeks.
- VZIg may prolong the incubation period of chickenpox to 28 days.
- The following patients should be treated with VZIg after close contact with chickenpox: immunocompromised patients, newborns of mothers who develop chickenpox a few days before or after delivery, premature infants exposed to chickenpox.

Tetanus immunoglobulin (Tlg)

- Pooled human donors.
- Find out how many tetanus immunizations the patient has had.
- For a clean minor wound, no Tlg is necessary. If the patient is only partially immunized or if it is 10 years since the last shot, then give a tetanus booster vaccine.
- Table XI is a guide to treatment for a major dirty wound

Table XI: Tetanus immunization guide following a major open wound

Tetanus immunizations	Tlg	Tetanus vaccine
Uncertain or none	Yes	Yes
First immunization	Yes	Yes
Second immunization	No	Yes
Third immunization	No	No
10 yr since last shot	No	Yes

TREATMENT OF HIV INFECTED CHILDREN

Supportive care

- Psychosocial support of child and family.
- Nutrition.
- Developmental interventions.
- Pain management.

Prophylactic therapy of opportunistic infections

Early diagnosis, prophylaxis and treatment of opportunistic infections have improved the prognosis and quality of life of infected children. Common opportunistic infections in children include candidiasis, *Pneumocystis carinii* pneumonia, cytomegalovirus (nonretinal), herpes simplex and herpes zoster infections.

Less common opportunistic infections in children include: retinal CMV, toxoplasmosis and cryptococcosis.

Prophylactic therapies used for *Pneumocystis carinii* pneumonia, bacterial infections and TB are shown in Table XII.

Table XII: Prophylactic therapy of opportunistic infections

Infection	Indication	Drug	Comment
Pneumocystis carinii pneumonia (PCP)	Previous episode PCP; or all HIV infected infants age 4 wk to 12 mo; or low age related CD4 count: 1–5 yr with CD4 < 500; ≥ 6 yr with CD4 < 200; or rapid decline in CD4 counts or symptomatic disease	TMP–SMX oral: 150 mg TMP/m^2 per d with 750 mg SMX/m^2 per d in 2 doses given daily or 3 d/wk	Alternatives to TMP–SMX: aerosolized pentamidine 300 mg monthly with Respirgard inhaler (children > 5 yr); or dapsone 2 mg/kg p.o. once daily (maximum 100 mg)
Serious bacterial infections	Recurrent serious bacterial infections	i.v. immunoglobulin 400 mg/kg per mo	
Tuberculosis	PPD ≥ 5 mm induration; or exposure to high risk tuberculosis case; or anergy and exposure	Isoniazid 10–15 mg/kg per d (maximum 300 mg) for 12 mo	

Antiretroviral therapy in reducing maternofetal transmission (Table XIII)

Multicenter placebo controlled study released data in 1994 showed significantly lower rate of perinatal transmission when zidovudine was given during pregnancy, delivery and to the newborn. Transmission rate was 8.3% in zidovudine group and 25.5% in placebo group. Currently, zidovudine is offered to all pregnant HIV infected women. Therapy with zidovudine begins after 14 weeks of gestation at 500 mg/d. During delivery, a continuous intravenous infusion of zidovudine is given with a bolus of 2 mg/kg followed by 1 mg/kg per h throughout deliver. The infant receives 2 mg zidovudine syrup every 6 h, beginning 8–12 h after birth and continuing until 6 weeks of age. Careful monitoring is required and should be administered through an HIV treatment center.

Table XIII: Antiretroviral therapy

Drug	Indication	Dose	Adverse reactions
Zidovudine (ZDV)	Low age adjusted CD4 count: <1 yr with CD4 < 1,750 1–2 yr with CD4 < 1,000 2–6 yr with CD4 < 750 > 6 yr with CD4 < 500; or clinical conditions regardless of CD4: opportunistic infection, failure to thrive or wasting syndrome, encephalopathy, malignancy, recurrent invasive infection, thrombocytopenia, hypoglobulinemia	180 mg/m^2 q6h p.o. in children 1 mo to 13 yr; lower doses to 90 mg/m^2 q6h may be used in the absence of encephalopathy	Bone marrow suppression, especially anemia and neutropenia; elevated hepatic transaminases; skeletal muscle myopathy (rare); nausea, insomnia and headaches (early, usually temporary)
Didanosine (DDI)	Disease progression despite ZDV therapy: growth failure, neurodevelopmental deterioration, organ dysfunction, new or recurrent opportunistic infection, rapid decrease in CD4 count; or ZDV intolerance: severe or persistent drug related adverse reactions (especially anemia and neutropenia)	100 mg/m^2 q12h p.o.	Pancreatitis; elevated hepatic transaminases; peripheral neuropathy, peripheral retinal depigmentation; diarrhea
Zalcitabine (DDC)	Alternative to DDI in combination therapy with ZDV; not used in monotherapy; limited data in children.	0.01 mg/kg q8h p.o.	Pancreatitis; peripheral neuropathy; mouth ulcers; rash
Combination therapy: ZDV + DDI or ZDV + DDC	Disease progression despite ZDV monotherapy; ZDV intolerance at higher doses	ZDV range from 90–180 mg/m^2 q6h (120 mg/m^2 q6h studied); DDI range from 90–180 mg/m^2 q12h (90 mg/m^2 q12h studied)	See component drugs

Peter Skippen and John McCready

INTRODUCTION

Intensive medical care for critically ill children is a relatively recent development that can only be afforded by rich countries. Even the large units take less than 1,500 patients a year with an average mortality of about 5%. Most of the survivors have a very good quality of life. In global terms, this does not even scratch the surface; UNICEF's last estimate for 1994 was 12.5 million avoidable deaths of children < 5 years of age. Most of these children simply required food, clean water and immunization. Community medicine cannot match the Intensive Care Unit (ICU) for drama and fascinating gadgets that go beep, but the principles of primary health care have saved millions more lives than all the ICU's together will ever achieve.

Pediatric intensive care is still a new discipline. It borrows from the slightly older literature of adult and neonatal intensive care, and there is a growing body of relevant research. However, many clinical decisions are still made on the basis of little more than common sense. Consequently, a detailed knowledge of pathophysiology is vital for any physician working with critically ill children.

Care of critically ill children is frequently very rewarding; many of the children recover well because they are usually free of underlying chronic illness. It must be stressed, however, that changes in clinical condition happen very quickly and require an appropriately prompt response from the attending physician to avert a disaster.

The following chapter will focus on the four areas that keep the ICU full: cardiac disease, respiratory disease, central nervous system disease and major trauma. Other diseases such as renal failure, although common in the ICU, will be dealt with in another chapter. Similarly, care of the child with acute liver failure is covered in chapter 6 (Gastroenterology).

CARDIOVASCULAR SYSTEM

Basic cardiovascular physiology

The final purpose of the respiratory system is to saturate hemoglobin with oxygen on the arterial side of the circulation. The final aim of the cardiovascular system is to move the saturated hemoglobin around the body, delivering the oxygen to vital organs such as the brain and kidney. The interaction between blood flow and vascular tone generates a perfusion pressure. The relationship is complex and constantly changing. Consequently, blood pressure is a very poor second order approximation of cardiac output. Cardiac output is determined by the product of heart rate and stroke volume. In turn, stroke volume depends on the contractile state of the heart, the end diastolic volume (preload) and the myocardial load during systole (afterload). Although there is a complex interdependence between these factors, from a therapeutic point of view, these can be looked at individually.

1. Preload

Normally, the heart will pump whatever is returned to it from the tissues so the venous return not only determines cardiac output but also is cardiac output (Figure I). Venous return depends on a number of variables: intrathoracic pressure, vascular compliance, total blood volume, resistance to venous return and distribution of flow to the different vascular beds. As venous return increases, the cardiac muscle fiber length at end diastole also increases. There is a tenuous relationship between ventricular muscle fiber length and atrial pressure. A plot of atrial pressure and cardiac output gives the well known s–shaped Frank–Starling curve. There are several assumptions and a pair of lungs between the right atrium and left ventricle. Despite this problem, central venous pressure is often used as a guide to left ventricular filling pressure. Even when known, the filling pressure is still only a rough approximation because the patient's position on the Starling curve is not known. A slightly more informed opinion on the filling pressures can be obtained from a pulmonary artery occlusion wedge pressure, but this requires insertion of a Swan–Ganz catheter. In some children, following cardiac surgery, a left atrial indwelling line may be available. In any event, absolute pressure should only be used as a guide. The most important point is trend and the response and degree of change in pressure to a therapeutic intervention such as fluid challenge.

2. Contractility

The central factor in muscle contraction appears to be the presence of free cytoplasmic calcium. This changes the conformation of troponin so allowing actin and myosin filaments to bind. As calcium is pumped back into the cytoplasmic reticulum, troponin changes shape and inhibits this binding so the muscle relaxes. The function of all inotropes appears to depend ultimately on the ability to increase cytoplasmic calcium levels. It is very important to remember that the primary cause of poor cardiac output in many sick children is a physiological disturbance. It is a waste of time reaching for dopamine and adrenalin if underlying physiological problems (e.g. hypokalemia, hypoglycemia and hypoxemia) have not been addressed adequately.

3. Afterload

Afterload describes the resistance to ejection by either the right or left heart. It is mostly determined by left ventricular wall tension.

$$\text{wall tension} = \frac{\text{transmural chamber pressure} \times \text{chamber radius}}{\text{wall thickness}}$$

Other factors contributing to increased afterload include: outflow obstruction (e.g. aortic stenosis), polycythemia, a raise in intra–abdominal pressure, a raise in intrathoracic pressure and vascular bed impedance.

Infant cardiovascular differences

Small children differ from adults in many ways; the cardiovascular system is no exception:
- Cardiac output is heart rate and intravascular volume dependent.
- There are structural differences in sarcomeres of neonates or small infants, making them less able to increase contractility.
- Greater dependence on extracellular ionized calcium concentration for contractility.
- They are very sensitive to increases in afterload.
- There is parasympathetic predominance (bradycardia with hypoxemia, hypovolemia).
- Immature sympathetic innervation of heart (less response to dopamine).

The normal values for heart rate and blood pressure vary with age. It is important to have at least a rough idea of what is normal for a neonate, infant and older child. A normal right atrial pressure in children is about 5 mm Hg and a left atrial pressure is about 8 mm Hg. A newborn has a systolic pressure of 55–65 mm Hg and a pulse rate ranging from 120–160 mm Hg. Blood pressure rises to 70–80 mm Hg by 1 year of age and remains at that level until about 5 years of age. Thereafter, pressure gradually rises as pulse rate falls. An approximation of the age related pressures can be obtained by the following simple formula:

$$\text{Systolic BP} = 80 + (2 \times \text{age in years})$$
$$\text{Diastolic BP} \approx \tfrac{2}{3} \text{ of systolic BP}$$

Transitional circulation

Newborns differ so much from adults that they are almost another species: umbilical cord clamping results in increased systemic vascular resistance, hence, left atrial pressure (LAP) rises. With the first breaths and increased oxygenation, pulmonary vascular resistance decreases by 75% and pulmonary blood flow increases by 450%, consequently, right atrial pressure (RAP) falls. When LAP > RAP, the foramen ovale closes.

The pulmonary arterial pressure equals the systemic blood pressure immediately after birth but falls over the first 72 hours to less than half systemic pressures. Physiological closure of the ductus arteriosus occurs by 48 hours. Transient right to left shunting can occur through these channels for 48–72 hours.

The pulmonary circulation remains very sensitive to physiological disturbances during this time. Many children with congenital heart disease are dependent upon a persistent duct or other shunt for survival. Events such as hypoxemia, acidosis or sepsis may result in acute elevations in pulmonary artery pressure to systemic levels or greater and precipitate persistent fetal circulation (PFC). This condition has a high morbidity and mortality. Alkalosis may be life saving in children with pulmonary hypertension. Nitric oxide is useful in some of these children and has reduced the need for ECMO.

Pulmonary hypertension in children is caused or aggravated by hypoxemia, respiratory or metabolic acidosis, hypothermia or polycythemia.

ICU CARDIAC DISEASES

Cardiac arrest

Cardiac arrest in children is very different to the pattern seen in adults. Primary cardiac causes such as infarction or arrhythmias are extremely uncommon. Full cardiac arrest is usually due to hypoxia following a respiratory arrest. Children will stop breathing in response to a wide range of underlying diseases; the younger they are, the sooner they develop respiratory arrest. If caught early and treated efficiently, a respiratory arrest has a good prognosis. Once hypoxic cardiac arrest occurs, the chance of successful resuscitation is small. The list of potential causes is too large to be of use but major causes include: sepsis, trauma, asphyxia and severe respiratory disease.

The diagnosis is made in the usual way: unconscious, apneic, flaccid, pulseless child. The carotid, brachial or femoral pulses are the easiest to palpate and feel in infants. Once the diagnosis has been established, call for help. Learn local practices as a first priority when joining a new ward or hospital.

The management involves initiating basic life support (BLS):
• Position patient supine. Protect cervical spine if suspected trauma.
• Open the airway: chin lift, jaw thrust (bottom teeth override upper teeth).
• Clear airway using back blows, if foreign body suspected (care with chest thrusts).
• Provide assisted manual breathing, either mouth to mouth or using a reinflatable manual ventilation device with 100% oxygen if available.
• Assess circulation and commence external artificial circulation if pulseless:
  One person CPR: child < 6 years = 5 compression/breath.
  One person CPR: child > 6 years = 15 compression/breath.
  Two persons CPR: all ages = 5 compression/breath.
  Rates of compression for infants $\geq$ 100/min; for older children 80–100/min.

Once the basic life support has been commenced and assistance has arrived, begin advanced life support (ALS):
• Continue external chest compressions.
• Establish intravenous access or intraosseous access.
• Give isotonic fluids rapidly in volume appropriate to situation (20 mL/kg initially).
• Intubate orally using cricoid pressure, confirm position, 100% oxygen.
• Decompress stomach with nasogastric tube.
• ECG monitor to assess rhythm.
• Medications to be given by endotracheal tube if vascular access has not been established.

1. Pharmacology of cardiac arrest
• 100% oxygen.
• Adrenalin: as much as needed (actual dose is controversial; AMA recommends initially 10 µg/kg i.v., repeated every 5 min or less; much larger doses may be used).
• Bicarbonate: indicated for severe metabolic acidosis, pulmonary hypertensive crisis and hyperkalemia in a dose of 1 mmol/kg i.v. or intraosseous, repeated according to blood gas measurement of pH (not down endotracheal tube). The use of bicarbonate has not been shown to affect outcome in cardiac arrest, but correcting a severe metabolic acidosis may improve the ability of the heart to respond to adrenalin.
• Calcium: indicated for documented hypocalcemia, calcium antagonist overdose, hyperkalemia and hypermagnesemia in a dose of 0.2 mL/kg 10% $CaCl_2$, slow i.v. push.
• Atropine: indicated for bradyarrhythmias but unlikely to be of benefit if adrenalin use is unsuccessful.
• Glucose: only if documented hypoglycemia.
• Lignocaine: indicated with ventricular fibrillation or ventricular tachycardia in a dose of 1 mg/kg i.v.
• Bretylium: agent of choice for hypothermic arrhythmias; also for ventricular fibrillation (VF) or ventricular tachycardia (VT) failing to respond to usual doses of lignocaine in a dose of 5 mg/kg i.v. (up to 30 mg/kg total dose).
• Drugs safe for administration via endotracheal tube during resuscitation are: naloxone, adrenalin (0.1 mL/kg, 1:1000), atropine (40 µg/kg, minimum dose 0.2 mg), lignocaine.

2. Defibrillation
- For documented cardiac arrest associated with VF or VT, electric DC countershock is the treatment of choice after establishing basic life support.
- Correct paddle size is essential (adults, 13 cm diameter; older child, 8 cm; infants, 4–5 cm).
- Correct position for external paddles is one placed below the left nipple and the other positioned below the right clavicle.
- The first dose of DC countershock is 2 J/kg, followed by 4–5 J/kg with subsequent shocks. Attention should be paid at all times to ventilation with 100% oxygen, circulating intravascular volume and correction of metabolic acidosis.
- Consider giving lignocaine after the second shock if ventricular arrhythmia persists. Give bretylium if lignocaine use has been unsuccessful.
- Frequent reassessment for return of pulses or rhythm on the monitor is essential.

Shock

Several classifications of shock exist (e.g. cardiogenic, septic, neurogenic, etc.). In practice, these terms add little except confusion. Shock is simply the state where available oxygen delivery is insufficient to meet tissue oxygen requirements.

The causes are best viewed in terms of oxygen delivery:
- Decreased cardiac output: cardiac failure of any cause, sepsis.
- Decreased circulating volume: hemorrhage, dehydration.
- Decreased vascular tone: anaphylaxis, severe CNS injury, Addison's disease.

The clinical picture depends on the underlying cause but the common feature is insufficient oxygen delivery with areas of anaerobic metabolism:

$$\text{Oxygen delivery } (DO_2) = \text{cardiac output (CO)} \times \text{oxygen carrying capacity } (CaO_2)$$
$$DO_2 = CO \times (Hb \times SaO_2 \times 1.34 + 0.003 \times PaO_2)$$

At rest, an adult's CO is about 5 L/min and arterial oxygen contains 200 mL/L O_2. Consequently, O_2 delivery is roughly 1 L/min. Adult oxygen consumption at rest is 200–250 mL/min, giving an extraction ratio of 20–25%. If oxygen requirements increase, the system can only respond by increasing CO (oxygen carrying capacity is on a plateau and will not increase). The body's only other option is to increase the extraction ratio (so reducing S_vO_2).

In severely ill patients, particularly during sepsis, oxygen delivery is often adequate but peripheral tissues are unable to extract the oxygen. Extraction ratios may be well below 20% in the face of elevated lactic acid. The fashion for driving cardiac output to supranormal levels in an attempt to "force" the tissue to accept oxygen is falling from favor.

Compensated shock refers to a condition where blood flow to the tissues is redistributed to the vital organs while oxygen consumption is maintained by an increased extraction of oxygen. Blood pressure may be normal. Mixed venous oxygen saturation will fall. Mixed venous oxygen saturation can be a useful monitor of the balance between supply and demand but an invasive mixed venous line is necessary.

Hypovolemic shock from loss of volume of any cause results in a reduction in venous return because of a decrease in mean systemic filling pressure. Compensation occurs by altering the ratio of pre– and postcapillary resistances to allow movement of fluid from the interstitial space to the intravascular space, increasing oxygen extraction, reducing venous compliance or reducing resistance to venous return.

Cardiac failure of any cause results in a decrease in the cardiac function curve and a shift to the right for any given filling pressure. As can be seen from the combined cardiac function and venous return curves (Figure I), since the venous return curve intersects on the ascending slope of the cardiac function curve, no matter what the degree of ventricular dysfunction, cardiac output may still be improved with a judicious volume challenge.

Figure I: Guyton (venous return) and Starling (cardiac output) curves superimposed

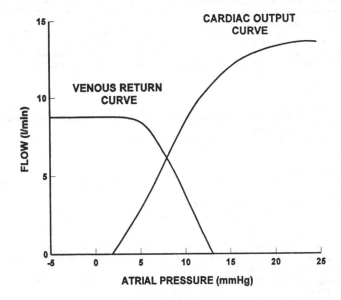

Septic shock is an extreme form of the systemic inflammatory response. In neonates, always remember congenital heart disease (particularly coarctation) and metabolic diseases in the differential diagnosis. The systemic injury in septic shock results from mediator induced circulatory and cellular metabolic abnormalities. The hemodynamic consequences are complex and change with the duration of the illness and response to therapy. Cardiac function, intravascular volume and vascular tone may simultaneously be affected. Cardiac output may be increased or decreased and a given response may be influenced by the patient's underlying cardiac reserve. Peripheral resistance and afterload may also be either increased or decreased. Capillary permeability abnormalities or bleeding diatheses and blood loss associated with sepsis contribute to the loss of intravascular volume.

The consequences of prolonged or untreated shock are often irreversible. A secondary dysoxic and reperfusion injury may result, which is largely untreatable. Secondary mediator induced cellular and circulatory disturbances can result in further organ damage. The mediator cascades result in a dysfunctional immune system. Myocardial depressant factors are probably released and contribute to the inadequacy of oxygen delivery. Coagulation and fibrinolysis are activated in a disordered and uncontrolled fashion, resulting in bleeding diatheses. The subsequent progression to failure of multiple organ systems (MSOF) is probably not as common in children as adults but, once developed, the prognosis is poor.

1. Presentation of shock
• General clinical signs:
    CVS: tachycardia, weak or impalpable pulses, cold to touch, mottled extremities, sluggish or absent capillary refill, pallor.
    Respiratory: tachypnea, irregular respirations or apnea, peripheral or central cyanosis.
    CNS: lethargy, floppy, coma.
    Renal: oliguria.
• Specific conditions:
    Hypovolemia: dehydration, poor skin turgor, sunken eyeballs, dry mucosae, distended tense abdomen, signs of multiple trauma.
    Sepsis: may be wide pulse pressure initially, flushed appearance, fever, hypothermia.
    Cardiogenic: absent femoral pulses, hepatomegaly, cardiomegaly, gallop rhythm, chest crepitations.
• Laboratory features:
    Complete blood count with differential and platelet count: white blood count may be increased, normal or decreased in sepsis, often with a left shift of immature leukocytes, thrombocytopenia, anemia.
    Coagulation screen: PT, PTT increased in sepsis; fibrinogen may be low in sepsis or shock of any cause; D–dimers elevated typically in sepsis.
    Electrolytes and renal function: exclude hypoglycemia; hyperglycemia is a common feature of the stress response; differentiate prerenal and renal causes of oliguria.
    Arterial blood gases: acidosis secondary to inadequate tissue perfusion.
    Cultures and urinary bacterial antigens.
    Metabolic screen (neonates and infants): urinary amino acids and organic acids if suspect metabolic disease, serum ammonia.
    Chest X–ray: cardiomegaly suggests a cardiac cause (do not forget endocarditis); lung infiltrates may be infective, cardiogenic or noncardiogenic.

2. Treatment of shock
- General principles:
  Priority one: pay attention to the adequacy of the airway and breathing. Avoiding hypoxemia is essential. Administer oxygen. An unconscious and moribund patient requires intubation and assisted ventilation with 100% oxygen. Position the patient in supine position and elevate the legs. If a central venous line is to be inserted, the Trendelenburg position should be used. Bloodwork should be taken at the time of insertion of the peripheral venous or central line but should not interfere with the resuscitation.
  Priority two: rapid restoration of perfusion to the critical vascular beds and hence oxygen delivery is the next priority. This is aimed at preventing the activation of the secondary and as yet largely untreatable mediator cascades.
  Priority three: treating the underlying cause occurs simultaneously. Ongoing support is essential. This involves close and careful monitoring and measuring responses to any therapeutic interventions. Constant attention to the patient's metabolic state (correction of acid–base abnormalities, correcting electrolyte abnormalities, avoiding hypoglycemia) is an essential component of ongoing care. Much of the ICU care of these patients involves patient and organ support until the homeostatic mechanisms normalize and the patient recovers. Insertion of an indwelling urinary catheter is required after the resuscitation has begun.
- Cardiovascular support:
  The principles are to normalize cardiac output and perfusion pressure rapidly and hence restore vital organ perfusion. Blood pressure and pulse rate should be normalized for age.
  Preload: large bore intravenous access is a necessary prerequisite for rapid infusion of fluids during volume resuscitation. Isotonic fluids (normal saline, Ringer's lactate, 5% albumin) should be infused rapidly over 5–10 min in a dose of 20 mL/kg normal saline or 10 mL/kg of 5% albumin, repeated as necessary if the response to the fluid challenge has been assessed to be inadequate. Monitoring adequacy of a volume challenge involves assessing the postchallenge heart rate, blood pressure, the CVP if a central line has been placed, peripheral pulse volume, base deficit, production of urine and liver size.
  Contractility: in cardiogenic shock and often in septic shock, the addition of an inotrope is required to optimize cardiac output and perfusion pressures. A neonate has immature noradrenalin stores and often has an inadequate response to dopamine. The most reliable inotrope in children, after a trial of dopamine up to 10–15 µg/kg per min, is adrenalin in a dose of 0.1–2 µg/kg per min. Amrinone is a useful inotropic agent in the postoperative cardiac surgical patient because of its effect as a peripheral vasodilator. The dose ranges from 5–10 µg/kg per min after an intravenous load of 2–3 mg/kg, given slowly over 30 min. Different inotropes can be used alone or in combination. Neonates may respond to a calcium infusion; monitor with ionized calcium levels. Be very careful with a calcium bolus as it may precipitate hypertension, bradycardia and cardiac standstill if an excessive dose is inadvertently administered. Avoid hypoglycemia. Follow glucometer levels frequently. If hypoglycemia develops, correct immediately with a bolus of 1–2 mL/kg D25W solution, followed by a dextrose infusion of 5–8 mg/kg per min, using either D5W or D10W solution.
  Afterload: neonates and infants are particularly sensitive to increased afterload. Children with a primary cardiac disorder will respond to peripheral vasodilators, e.g. nitroprusside. Inhaled nitric oxide acts specifically as a pulmonary vasodilator and hence can unload the right ventricle in states associated with acute pulmonary hypertension. Coronary blood

supply requires an adequate diastolic pressure. Children in septic shock and vasodilated will respond well to a titrated infusion of noradrenalin (same dose range as adrenalin). Children with extensive burns not only have large volume losses but also develop a systemic inflammatory response which responds well to noradrenalin.

Rate and rhythm: a child's cardiac output is rate dependent. A rate of 100 might be a critical bradycardia in a shocked baby. Bradyarrhythmias should be taken seriously (atropine, isuprel, pacing). Specific arrhythmias are initially treated by correcting the metabolic disorders commonly precipitating them (hypoxemia, systemic acidosis, electrolytes).

- Respiratory support:

   Shock results in hypoxemia because of an inadequate perfusion pressure in the lungs, with a resultant increase in dead space ventilation and increased ventilation or perfusion mismatching. Some children may have alveolar infiltrates of either cardiac or noncardiac origin which contribute to the hypoxemia.

   The patient with severe respiratory dysfunction will benefit from intubation and assisted mechanical ventilation. The application of positive pressure reverses atelectasis and improves V/Q matching.

   The patient with severe cardiac dysfunction will also benefit from assisted mechanical ventilation. Raised intrathoracic pressure decreases venous return and also reduces transmural pressure and hence afterload.

   Care must be taken to ensure that preload is optimized so a reduction in venous return does not complicate the institution of positive pressure ventilation.

- Supportive measures:

   Gastric stress ulcer prophylaxis using either H_2–antagonists or sulcrafate (both equally effective).

   Metabolic support: dialysis for renal failure, nutrition (preferably enteral), general support for liver failure, clotting factor replacement for symptomatic coagulopathy, fluid/electrolytes. Surveillance for secondary complications and nosocomial infections is critical.

   Steroids: use of large dose steroids is not of benefit in septic shock. Many patients with septic shock probably have a blunted pituitary and adrenal response and may benefit from stress replacement of hydrocortisone.

   Immunotherapy to date has been disappointing.

Myocardial ischemia

Myocardial ischemia in children is uncommon and results from an imbalance of myocardial oxygen supply versus demand. Patients present with diaphoresis after exertion (e.g. feeding), crying spells, arrhythmias or cardiac arrest. Diagnosis is made with typical ECG changes and cardiac enzyme elevation.

1. Etiologies of myocardial ischemia in children
- Congenital heart disease: anomalous coronary artery, cyanosis, hyperviscosity, pulmonary hypertension, patent ductus arteriosus (diastolic hypotension), ventricular hypertrophy.
- Noncongenital heart disease: asphyxia or severe hypoxemia, hypotension, ventricular overload, pulmonary hypertension secondary to respiratory disease, systemic hypertension, coronary artery disease, Kawasaki's disease, connective tissue diseases, metabolic disease, atherosclerosis, familial hyperlipidemias.

- Others: drugs, coagulopathy.

2. Management principles (similar to adult)
- Oxygen.
- Rest.
- Decrease cardiac work.
- Decrease oxygen consumption.
- Investigate or treat specific cause.
- May require intubation and ventilation, inotropic support or arrhythmia management.

Congestive heart failure (CHF)

The term describes a patient with a syndrome of borderline cardiac output. The most common cause of CHF in children is left to right shunt (e.g. VSD).

A simple method of discussing heart failure is:
- Forward failure: poor contractility.
- Backward failure: poor cardiac filling.
- Volume overload: L–R shunts.
- Pressure overload: aortic stenosis.

The great majority of cases will present under 1 year of age with failure due to structural cardiac abnormalities. However, there are many other causes, including cardiomyopathies, arrhythmias, chemotherapy and Kawasaki's disease.

Some guide to the cause can be obtained from the age of presentation:
- Neonate < 2 weeks:
    Volume overload: valvular regurgitations, AV fistulae, PDA in premature infant.
    Left heart obstruction: coarctation, aortic stenosis, hypoplastic left heart.
    Right heart obstruction: anomalous pulmonary venous return, double outlet right ventricle.
    Other: myocarditis (coxsackievirus, rubella), arrhythmias (heart block, SVT).
- Infant < 1 year:
    Volume overload: PDA, truncus, VSD, TGA with VSD, AV canal (presents after pulmonary pressure has fallen).
    Pressure overload: pulmonary hypertension, PS (not with tetralogy since VSD provides pressure release).
    Myocarditis: endocardial fibroelastosis, Pompe's disease, anomalous coronary arteries, postviral.
    Arrhythmias.
- Children:
    Bacterial endocarditis ± underlying structural defects.
    Hypertension: systemic or pulmonary.
    Cor pulmonale: cystic fibrosis, bronchopulmonary dysplasia.
    Myocarditis: postviral, rarely rheumatic fever, very rarely diphtheria.
    Cardiomyopathies.
    Late structural: PDA, coarctation.

The heart responds initially by hypertrophy, followed by dilatation. The sympathetic nervous system is activated and contributes to the pathophysiology of CHF. The endocrine system is activated (e.g. increased ADH, aldosterone, ANF) and contributes to the fluid retention and volume overload.

1. Clinical presentation (signs and symptoms)
- Tachypnea, tachycardia, pallor, diaphoresis with exertion, lethargy, irritability.
- Indrawing, increased work of breathing, displaced heart apex.
- Cool peripheries, feeble peripheral pulses, peripheral cyanosis.
- Jugular venous distension (difficult to identify in infancy), hepatomegaly (may be pulsatile).
- Abdominal distension if ascites, peripheral edema.
- Failure to thrive with decreased appetite and poor feeding.
- Recurrent chest infections.
- Auscultation: gallop, murmurs, abnormal heart sounds.
- Crackles and wheezes throughout the chest or predominantly basally (wheezing is a sign of bronchiolar cuffing due to interstitial edema).
- Chest X–ray: cardiomegaly, increased pulmonary vasculature, pulmonary edema, effusions.

2. General treatment
- 100% oxygen, position wherever the child is most comfortable (supine or head elevated).
- Control the fever.
- Restrict fluids unless hypotensive.
- Examine and take a detailed history to identify the cause (CHF is not a diagnosis).
- Initiate laboratory investigations, including arterial blood gases.
- Order chest X–ray.

3. Cardiac support
- Diuresis (frusemide 1 mg/kg initially).
- Inotropes (digoxin, dopamine).
- Cautious afterload reduction.
- May still require some preload support even though the patient is relatively overloaded (judicious use of 5 mL/kg aliquots of 5% albumin in an intubated patient can be helpful).
- Correct hypoglycemia.
- Calcium infusion may be considered in neonate.
- Pulmonary hypertension: priorities are avoiding hypoxemia, clearing the airway and avoiding hypercarbia and treating the metabolic acidosis. Once the basics are controlled, pulmonary blood pressure will often respond to alkalosis (either respiratory or i.v. bicarbonate 1 mmol/kg bolus) or nitric oxide.

4. Respiratory support
- 100% oxygen initially.
- Intubation: upper airway obstruction, fatigue, apnea, cyanosis, severe respiratory distress.
- Positive end expiratory pressure may be required to control the frothy pulmonary edema.
- Beware of the use of any agents that depress contractility.

5. Miscellaneous support
- Packed red cells for severe anemia.
- Phlebotomy for severe polycythemia.
- Morphine for venodilation and patient comfort.

Cyanosis

Cyanosis is usually clinically obvious when there is more than 5 g/100 mL arterial blood. The sign is not so obvious in anemic children. Peripheral cyanosis is due to sluggish capillary flow (polycythemia, heart failure, hypothermia) and can be difficult to differentiate from central cyanosis by simple inspection. The color of the tongue can distinguish between the two but, fortunately, pulse oximeters are now available to make the diagnosis easier. It should be understood that not all patients with tissue hypoxia are cyanotic. A child with severe anemia or septic shock may have tissue hypoxia and lactic acidosis, yet have quite normal blood gas values.

The list of causes is too long to remember so an orderly approach to diagnosis is essential:
- Alveolar hypoventilation: CNS depression (drugs, asphyxia), neuromuscular disease, airway obstruction (croup).
- Oxygenation failure: respiratory disease (pneumonia), congenital heart disease (tetralogy, TGA).
- Decreased oxygen transport: cardiac failure, severe anemia, carbon monoxide poisoning.
- Oxygen uptake failure: septic shock, cyanide poisoning.

In older children, the cause will usually be respiratory but the differential for neonates is large and includes cardiac, respiratory and central nervous diseases.
- A hyperoxic test is usually used as a first step in determining the cause. If the child's saturation does not improve after breathing high flow oxygen by mask, congenital heart disease is more likely.
- Transient fetal circulation patterns are confusing: a trial of prostaglandin (0.01–0.1 µg/kg per min) is relatively safe and can be tried if the diagnosis of a duct dependent lesion is in doubt (e.g. prior to transport to a referral center). The main side effect is apnea in 20% of cases. It is sensible to treat the child for sepsis while the workup takes place.
- Tet spells: place child in knee to chest position and give morphine 0.1 mg/kg i.m. If unsuccessful, give propranolol slowly by i.v. push (0.05 mg/kg); this may be repeated once.
- Methemoglobinemia: chocolate colored arterial blood following exposure to some dyes and drugs. Give methylene blue 0.1–0.2 mL/kg of a 1% solution.

Pulmonary hypertensive crisis

Pulmonary hypertensive crises typically occur following repair of congenital heart disease in a child with pre–existing pulmonary hypertension. They can be acutely life threatening with sudden right heart failure. Cardiac arrest can occur rapidly.

Management:
- Anticipate problems early.
- Control ventilation to keep alkalosis pH > 7.45. Maintain adequate saturation with high inspired

oxygen. Use nitric oxide prophylactically. Load with phenoxybenzamine while still on cardiac bypass.
• Acute crisis:
   Hand ventilate with 100% oxygen. Hyperventilate.
   Intravenous bicarbonate bolus (1 mmol/kg).
   May benefit from 10 mL/kg bolus of isotonic fluid; repeat as necessary.
   Adrenalin bolus if hypotensive 5–10 µg/kg i.v.
   Chest compressions if bradycardia–asystolic.
• Nitric oxide if available. Toxic dose not yet determined. Many start at 80 ppm, then reduce to < 20 ppm if a response is obtained.
• Several drugs are tried (PA infusions of prostaglandin or salbutamol plus systemic alpha blockade) but are usually ineffective.

Dysrhythmias

Arrhythmias in children are not uncommon. Many are associated with congenital heart disease and follow repair of a congenital cardiac defect. Other causes include: Wolff–Parkinson–White syndrome, cardiomyopathy, cardiac contusion, metabolic disorders (hypoxemia, hypokalemia, etc.) and drug overdose (digitalis, tricyclics, etc.).

Supraventricular tachycardia (SVT) is the most common form of tachyarrhythmia in children with an otherwise normal heart. The most common form of SVT is atrioventricular re–entry tachycardia due to the presence of an accessory atrioventricular bypass tract (e.g. WPW). These pathways may or may not be revealed on a resting 12 lead ECG. The next most common type of SVT is AV node re–entry tachycardia. Bradyarrhythmias are most commonly associated with hypoxemia.

Diagnosis is made following a complete history and examination and adjunctive 12 lead ECG. Esophageal leads, if available, can be very useful. In the postoperative cardiac patient, connecting the pacing wires to a standard ECG monitor allows easy and rapid diagnosis of tachyarrhythmias. Carotid sinus massage, application of ice to the face or administration of adenosine are useful adjuncts for SVT diagnosis while recording the ECG. A narrow QRS tachycardia complex excludes ventricular tachycardia in the older child, but an infant with a QRS complex < 80 ms may be in ventricular tachycardia.

Differentiating VT from SVT with aberrant conduction can be difficult. Atrioventricular dissociation, absence of an RS complex in any precordial lead or fusion beats are highly suggestive of VT.

1. Management of asymptomatic patients
Monitor, look for the cause, correct predisposing factors such as hypoxemia or electrolyte abnormalities; all require secure intravenous access.
• Supraventricular tachycardia:
   If sinus tachycardia, look for the cause (e.g. hypovolemia, sepsis, fever).
   Increase vagal tone: carotid massage; never eyeball pressure.
   Ice to face (diving reflex) but infants may develop reflex apnea for up to 10 seconds.
   Adenosine 50 µg/kg rapid i.v. push, flushed immediately with 2 mL of normal saline (repeat 100 µg/kg rapid i.v. push if no response).
   β–blockers (avoid in neonates or infants): propranolol (0.05–0.1 mg/kg i.v. slow push) or

esmolol (0.5 mg/kg i.v. slow push, 50–200 µg/kg per min for up to 48 h).
- Rapid atrial fibrillation/flutter:
  As for SVT (may be presentation of aberrant pathway).
  May use adenosine as above.
  β–blocker if aberrancy a possibility.
  Digoxin after hypokalemia has been corrected.
  Elective synchronized DC countershock under anesthesia or sedation.
- Ventricular tachycardia:
  Correct predisposing factors.
  Lignocaine bolus 1 mg/kg, followed by infusion (20–50 µg/kg per min).
  Adenosine can be used in a stable patient to help differentiate SVT from VT.
- Heart block:
  Atropine (20–40 µg/kg i.v.).
  Isoprenaline infusion (0.1–2 µg/kg per min i.v. infusion).
  Pacing.

2. Management of symptomatic patients
Patients will have varying degrees of reduction in their cardiac output, depending on the underlying rhythm. Consequently, they will be diaphoretic with weak or impalpable pulses, hypotensive and unresponsive.
- 100% oxygen, monitor, establish intravenous access, commence BLS and ALS if necessary.
- Correct cause of hypoxemia, correct airway obstruction, restore circulating blood volume, correct electrolyte disturbances.
- Bradyarrhythmia:
  Pharmacotherapy: atropine, isoprenaline bolus and infusion.
  Pacing: external, transvenous, transoesophageal.
  CPR if heart rate < 60 in infants with poor perfusion.
  Adrenalin i.v. or i.o. 0.1 mL/kg 1:10,000; repeat as necessary.
- SVT/rapid AF/flutter:
  Synchronized DC countershock: 0.5–1 J/kg.
  Adenosine (if i.v. but do not delay DC shock).
- Junctional ectopic tachycardia (JET) is usually a complication of heart surgery:
  Correct hypoxemia, hypercarbia, acidosis.
  Correct hypovolemia.
  Treat fever, cool, induce hypothermia (if intubated).
  Correct electrolyte abnormalities.
  Adequate analgesia.
  Minimize catecholamines (paralyze, sedate and wean inotropes if possible).
  Intravenous magnesium.
  Amiodarone or propafenone are both useful but should only be used after consultation.
- Torsade de pointes (prolonged QT syndrome): congenital or acquired (carditis, electrolyte disorder, medication such as quinidine or tricyclics):
  BLS/ALS.
  Correct hypocalcemia, hypomagnesemia, hypokalemia.
  Adenosine if unsure, SVT versus VT, and blood pressure stable.
  Intravenous pacing.

Intravenous magnesium 0.2 mmol/kg bolus.
DC countershock.
Isoprenaline infusion.
As for cardiac arrest.
- Ventricular tachycardia, ventricular fibrillation: as for cardiac arrest (CPR/DC shock 2 J/kg).
- The use of digoxin in the management of undiagnosed tachyarrhythmias in older patients is controversial because it may increase conduction through an aberrant pathway. However, digoxin has proven both safe and effective in children with WPW and remains the drug of choice of many pediatric cardiologists treating this condition.
- Avoid verapamil in neonates and infants; care with β–blockers in infants.

Anaphylaxis

1. Presentation
The attack may vary from mild to catastrophic:
- Cardiovascular collapse, cardiac arrest, arrhythmias.
- Cough, wheeze, stridor, cyanosis.
- Cutaneous flushing and urticaria.
- Facial, perioral or periorbital edema.
- Diarrhea.

2. Emergent therapy
If symptoms or signs already exist, treat urgently; do not wait "to see what happens".
- Discontinue infusion of the suspected offender.
- 100% oxygen. Secure airway. Intubate early if stridor or loss of consciousness.
- Ensure good intravenous access, give volume challenge 20–40 mL/kg isotonic solution rapidly.
- Adrenalin 0.1 mL/kg i.v. (1:10,000 solution), repeat as necessary.
- Hydrocortisone 5 mg/kg i.v.
- Antihistamine, diphenhydramine 1–2 mg/kg i.v.
- Transfer to ICU for ongoing support and monitoring.
- Prior to extubation, careful assessment of the airway is required to exclude significant residual laryngeal edema.

RESPIRATORY SYSTEM

Respiratory anatomy

Small children have very little respiratory reserve. Even a normal infant can go dusky while doing nothing more energetic than crying. In addition to a variety of anatomical disadvantages, children have a high oxygen demand. The combination is not ideal so that minor problems (even as innocuous as a blocked nose) can produce rapid deterioration. The main anatomical differences compared to adults are: small nasal airway, small mouth or large tongue, short neck, small anterior larynx, small immature lungs, compliant chest wall, large abdomen prone to gastric distension, high airway resistance and rapid respiratory rate.
Two primitive reflexes tend to make matters worse: neonates are obligate nose breathers except when screaming, so that simple nasal obstruction may produce apnea. In addition, the

response to airway occlusion or greatly increased work of breathing is thoracic muscle relaxation and apnea (Hering–Breuer reflex). The survival value of this reflex is difficult to imagine.

The narrow airways and high airway resistance make them prone to severe upper and lower airway obstruction. The compliant chest wall predisposes children to alveolar collapse.

Surfactant is produced by the type II pneumatocytes. It is usually present by 32 weeks gestation. It minimizes the tendency of the alveoli to collapse. Surfactant may become deficient or altered in function with many acute pulmonary processes, including pulmonary edema, acute lung injury and pulmonary infections.

Normal lung volumes are determined by the balance of the tendency of the lungs to collapse and the rib cage to expand. The equilibrium volume is called the functional residual capacity (FRC). In children > 7 years of age, the FRC is above the closing volume (CV), which is the lung volume at which the alveoli begin to passively collapse. In newborns and children, resting tidal ventilation encroaches upon the CV, predisposing to hypoxemia.

Developmental defects of the lungs, airways, pulmonary vasculature and heart may all contribute to or cause acute respiratory failure.

Basic respiratory physiology

Normal minute ventilation is determined by the product of tidal volume and respiratory rate. Alveolar ventilation is influenced by the airway's resistance, lung compliance, respiratory muscle function and chest wall elasticity. Dead space ventilation is influenced by the size of the airways, airway obstruction, alveolar volume and pulmonary blood flow.

Alveolar ventilation determines arterial PCO_2:

$$P_aCO_2 \sim \frac{VCO_2}{V_A}$$

Normally, the pulmonary blood flow is matched to the ventilating lung units. This is termed ventilation perfusion matching. Pulmonary blood flow is gravity dependent in the supine and erect position. Ventilation in a spontaneously breathing patient is preferentially distributed to the dependent regions of the lung. In a supine patient, who is on a mechanical ventilator and is receiving positive pressure ventilation, ventilation is preferentially directed to the nondependent lung units, hence V/Q matching is worsened.

Hypoxic pulmonary vasoconstriction (HPV) is the pulmonary arteriolar response to the inspiration of a hypoxic gas mixture or mismatching of ventilation with pulmonary blood flow. HPV minimizes the V/Q mismatch in acute lung disease by shifting blood away from underventilated lung units. A number of factors affect the hypoxic pulmonary vascular reflex: intravenous vasodilators, alkalosis and nitric oxide.

1. Gas exchange
Gas exchange involves the movement of oxygen from the alveolus into the pulmonary capillary and movement of carbon dioxide in the reverse direction across the alveolar membrane. It occurs because of a concentration gradient favorable to the movement of each of the respective gases. For oxygen, this is determined by the atmospheric pressure, the inspired concentration of oxygen and the vapor pressure of water (P_{swv}). Alveolar PO_2 can be determined by the alveolar gas

equation:

$$P_AO_2 = FiO_2 (P_B - P_{swv}) - \frac{P_aCO_2}{R}$$

For a patient breathing room air at sea level at 30 °C, this equates to:

$$P_AO_2 = 0.21(760 - 47) - 40/0.8 = 118 \text{ mm Hg}$$

For a patient breathing 100% oxygen at sea level at 30 °C, this equates to:

$$P_AO_2 = 1.0(760 - 47) - 40/0.8 = 681 \text{ mm Hg}$$

The difference between the alveolar and an arterial blood gas sample is called the A–a gradient (alveolar–arterial gradient) and is usually less than 10 mm Hg. An increasing A–a gradient is reflected clinically by worsening P_aO_2 and hypoxemia. Factors affecting the A–a gradient are: V/Q mismatch, R–L pulmonary or intracardiac shunt, diffusion defect such as thickened alveolar membrane from edema or fibrosis. The oxygen stores in the body are minimal and consist of the oxygen in the lungs at FRC and that carried in the blood stream.

2. Oxygen carriage
Oxygen is carried to the tissues, bound to hemoglobin. The arterial oxygen saturation reflects the amount of oxygen carried by the hemoglobin. The arterial content of blood is calculated as follows:

$$CaO_2 = 1.34 \times Hb \times \text{arterial saturation } (\%/100) + 0.003 \times P_aO_2$$

For an average healthy adult, the arterial oxygen content is about 20 mL/100 mL blood:

$$CaO_2 \sim (1.34 \times 15 \times 1) + (0.003 \times 100)$$

The unique structure of hemoglobin (mL/100 mL) causes a nonlinear binding of oxygen to the Hgb molecule, the relationship of which is expressed by the oxyhemoglobin dissociation curve (OHDC). The position of the curve on the axis is determined by the type of Hgb, body temperature, blood pH and 2,3 DPG. The P_{50} (the P_aO_2 at a saturation of 50%) of fetal Hgb is 19 mm Hg and of adult Hgb is 27 mm Hg at normothermia and pH 7.4. This means that a newborn can be 100% saturated at a much lower P_aO_2 than an older child or adult. A shift of the OHDC curve to the left means that oxygen is picked up easily from the lungs but is not released at the tissue level quite as freely.

3. Assessing oxygenation defects
A variety of formulae are used to describe the severity of an oxygenation defect in neonates and children:
- A–a gradient on 100% oxygen ($P_AO_2 - P_aO_2$).
- Oxygen index (OI) = mean airway pressure × FiO_2 × 100/postductal P_aO_2 (normal $\leq$ 10; consideration for ECMO > 40).
- P_aO_2/FiO_2 ratio (consider ECMO when < 100).

4. Carbon dioxide transport
Carbon dioxide is transported from the tissues to the lungs by three methods:
- Dissolved.
- Bicarbonate (reaction of $CO_2 + H_2O$ produces $H^+ + HCO_3^-$).
- Chemical combination with amino groups of proteins (particularly the histidine residue of Hgb), forming carbamino Hgb). Arterial blood carries roughly 50 mL CO_2/100 mL of blood.

5. Pulmonary blood flow
Pulmonary blood flow is determined by the cardiac and pulmonary vasculature, cardiac output, blood volume, alveolar and extra–alveolar vascular resistance. The pulmonary vascular resistance (PVR) is lowest at FRC. PVR is effectively the afterload of the right ventricle. Overdistension of the lungs, with excessive lung volumes or lung collapse, causes increases in the PVR.

6. Lung mechanics
- Static lung compliance is a function of the elastic properties of the lungs and describes the change in lung volume for a change in transpulmonary pressure (alveolar pressure–pleural pressure). Specific lung compliance increases slightly with age from 0.5 mL/kg per cm H_2O during infancy to approximately 1.5 mL/kg per cm H_2O at puberty.
- The pressure volume characteristics of the lung are also nonlinear. At high lung volumes, the alveoli are overstretched, resulting in a smaller increase in lung volume for a given increase in pressure. The same occurs at lung volumes below closing volume. Hysteresis describes the difference between the inspiratory and expiratory pressure volume curves (similar to inflating a new balloon). The degree of hysteresis is increased by surfactant deficiency and acute lung injury.

Respiratory failure

Respiratory failure is usually classified into two groups:
- Type 1 (oxygenation failure): usually due to V/Q mismatch from underlying parenchymal disease (pneumonia, ARDS, pulmonary edema). P_aCO_2 is usually normal in the early stages. V/Q mismatch responds to oxygen therapy. Pure shunt (V/Q = 0) is usually due to alveolar collapse and will require positive pressure ventilation.
- Type 2 (ventilatory failure): several diseases reduce the minute ventilation so inducing respiratory failure, even though the lung parenchyma might be normal (narcotic overdose, head injury, croup, foreign body and neuromuscular diseases). Mechanical ventilation provides a good temporary therapy because high pressures and high oxygen concentrations are not required.

Always remember that tissue hypoxia can occur despite adequate oxygenation (cardiac failure, anemia, septicemia), so a normal saturation is not a guarantee of normal oxygen delivery. If a patient is still acidotic after resuscitation, check the heart and hemoglobin.

Clinical features are as variable as the list of causes. Cyanosis due to some cardiac shunts is well tolerated if there is no cardiac failure.

1. Typical features of respiratory failure
- Tachypnea, irregular respirations, apnea or dyspnea.

- Intercostal recession, supraclavicular indrawing.
- Tachycardia, bounding pulses.
- Anxious, agitated, confused, lethargic, obtunded.
- Diaphoretic, increased work of breathing.
- Cyanosis.

2. Initial general supportive management
- 100% oxygen by face mask.
- Assess airway patency: degree of respiratory distress, suction oropharyngeal–nasal secretions.
- Support the airway, intubate if impending respiratory arrest, bradycardic or obtunded.
- Establish intravenous access, restore circulation as necessary.
- Initial investigations: chest X–ray, arterial or capillary blood gas, complete blood count, electrolytes, blood culture.
- Monitor closely and intubate if necessary (q.v.)

Acute lung injury (adult respiratory distress syndrome)

Acute lung injury (ALI) is a clinical syndrome that can result from either pulmonary or nonpulmonary insults to the alveolar–capillary lung unit. It may primarily involve the lung or progress to multisystem organ failure (MSOF). The most common causes in the pediatric patient are shock, sepsis and near drowning. The response of the lungs is nonspecific. The severity of injury varies somewhat unpredictably in a given patient.

1. Diagnosis
- Catastrophic events: identifiable cause (pulmonary or nonpulmonary).
- Respiratory distress, hypoxemia, reduced lung compliance, pulmonary shunt (Q_S/Q_T).
- Diffuse pulmonary infiltrates on chest X–ray.
- Previously normal lungs and the absence of left heart disease.

2. Pathology
The response of the lungs follows an exudative, proliferative and fibrotic phase. Survival is related to the extent of the fibrotic phase and the associated MSOF.
- The initial result is severe hypoxemia due to a combination of noncardiogenic pulmonary edema, dysfunctional surfactant and the consequent small airway and alveolar collapse.
- FRC is reduced, closing volume exceeds FRC, consequently shunt and V/Q mismatch are severe. Lung compliance decreases because of the low lung volumes and pulmonary edema.
- Dead space ventilation is increased but P_aCO_2 generally does not rise because of hyperventilation, unless patient fatigue occurs.
- Pulmonary artery pressure and pulmonary vascular resistance are elevated and may result in right heart failure. Left ventricular output may also be reduced because of bulging of the interventricular septum from right to left.

3. Management
The basic principles of care involve oxygen therapy or ventilatory support, general organ system supportive care and treatment of the underlying disease process.

Management of respiratory failure

1. Oxygen therapy
Oxygen is expensive and has some hazards so it should be used carefully.
- Potential side effects include:
    Suppression of hypoxic drive (vanishingly rare in children).
    Absorption atelectasis (washout of N_2 predisposes to alveolar collapse).
    Oxygen toxicity (FiO_2 < 0.5 is traditionally assumed to be safe).
    Fire hazard—not sigificant in children since they do not usually smoke in bed with their O_2 nasal prongs in place—not unknown in the adult world.
- Routes of administration include:
    Nasal prongs (well tolerated up to about 3 L/min; some mucosal drying occurs).
    Venturi masks (O_2 flow is diluted by room air through graduated Venturi valves; delivers up to FiO_2 0.6 fairly accurately).
    High FiO_2 masks (various designs of mask with reservoirs attached to achieve FiO_2 close to 1.0; they are worth trying if it avoids intubation).

2. Ventilatory support
Many of these patients require intubation and mechanical ventilation to allow adequate oxygenation. The intubation may be difficult in a hypoxemic, restless and uncooperative patient. The patient may require muscle relaxation, at least initially, until ventilation and oxygenation have improved. All ventilated patients require some sedation, e.g. judicious infusions of morphine (20–50 µg/kg per h) and midazolam (0.1–0.5 µg/kg per h), depending on patient stability and response.
- The basic modes of positive pressure ventilation include: CMV, AMV, assist control (controlled or assisted mechanical ventilation), SIMV (synchronized intermittent mechanical ventilation), VC (volume cycled), PC or PS (pressure control or pressure support). Most ventilators today allow either VC or PC in both spontaneous or controlled modes.
- Advantages of VC are:
    Desired preset volume delivered with every breath.
    Consistent minute ventilation.
    Can detect changes in lung compliance or resistance by checking the pressure manometer on the ventilator.
- Disadvantages of VC include: can get large increases in airway pressure with changing compliance or resistance.
- Advantages of PC include: the pressure delivered is preset, thereby limiting the risk of barotrauma (if set appropriately); overcomes leak around ETT; simpler machinery than VC.
- Disadvantages of PC include:
    May get inconsistent ventilation with changes in compliance or resistance.
    May miss airway obstruction unless monitoring expired volumes.
    Clinical assessment of adequacy and symmetry of chest movement is essential.
- Consider the respiratory support of these patients as two distinct problems: oxygenation (uptake of oxygen) and ventilation (clearance of carbon dioxide).
    Oxygenation:
    The main determinants of oxygenation in an intubated patient are inspired oxygen concentration (FiO_2) and mean airway pressure (MAP).

PEEP is the most useful variable to manipulate early in the illness. Correctly applied, it restores the FRC back towards normal, improves lung compliance, reduces pulmonary shunt and improves oxygenation.

"Optimal PEEP" can be most easily thought of as the lowest PEEP that will allow a reduction in the FiO_2 to < 0.6 (60%) without compromising cardiac output.

Incorrect application has complications: decreased venous return, alveolar overdistension, reduced lung compliance, increased dead space ventilation, increased pulmonary vascular resistance, reduced cardiac output, reduced renal or hepatic blood flow, increased free water retention.

Ventilation (i.e. clearance of CO_2):

The main concern is to avoid further lung injury. It has been well demonstrated that high ventilating pressures and high lung volumes induce acute lung injury and cause barotrauma. The determinants of ventilation are respiratory rate and tidal volume. The settings of each are determined by the desired blood gases for a particular patient.

It has been appreciated, surprisingly recently, that patients do not need perfect blood gases to survive and that excessive ventilation may actually make matters worse.

Permissive hypercapnia has become popular in an effort to reduce the complications of ventilation while maintaining the ability to oxygenate. The clinical effects of hypercapnia on the patient are minimal. Contraindications are few: severe head injury, severe pulmonary hypertension or pulmonary hypertensive crises, acute renal failure and severe uncorrected metabolic disturbances.

- Some initial guidelines in a patient with acute lung injury would be:

  Mode = pressure control.

  FiO_2 initially 1.0.

  PEEP 5–10 cm H_2O initially, depending on the severity of pulmonary infiltrates and hypoxemia.

  I:E ratio 1:2 initially; may need to increase inspiratory time (approach 1:1) depending on the severity of pulmonary infiltrates and hypoxemia.

  SaO_2 > 90%: wean inspired oxygen as rapidly as possible (FiO_2 < 0.6).

  Tidal volume = 8–10 mL/kg.

  Arterial pH > 7.2: this will gradually correct over the subsequent couple of days as the kidneys compensate.

  Frequent changes in patient position, including the prone position, should be included in the respiratory care if the hemodynamics are stable. This improves secretion clearance, V/Q matching and oxygenation.

3. General support

Use volume infusions to support preload but avoid volume overload as it will aggravate the low pressure permeability pulmonary edema. Inotropes should be used if necessary.

- Reduce VO_2 (paralysis and sedation, e.g. morphine, midazolam).
- Treat fever aggressively.
- Restrict unnecessary fluids.
- Maintain normovolemia.
- Stress ulcer prophylaxis (consider sucralfate).
- Support renal function (dopamine may support urine output in some patients but has not been shown to prevent renal failure).

- Nutritional support, preferably by the enteral route.
- DVT prophylaxis (e.g. after multiple trauma).

4. Monitoring
- Chest movements (adequacy, symmetry); position of endotracheal tube; color, perfusion, pulses; pulse oximetry; arterial line (arterial blood gases, pressure monitoring); central venous pressure (guide to intravascular volume, inotrope infusions); oximetry; chest X–ray (routine or urgent with acute deteriorations).
- The debate over the value of invasive hemodynamic monitoring will probably never finish. Certainly, measuring cardiac output and deriving a dozen other variables brighten up a boring ward round but does it help? Sober assessment of measurement errors (significant and usually ignored), clinical value (not proven in children) and side effects (potentially severe) make the PA catheter less fashionable in pediatric units.

Alternative therapies

Modern ventilators are very good at keeping patients alive if used properly; death from primary oxygenation failure is unusual in a referral PICU. Despite this, an enormous investment is made into therapies designed to improve oxygenation in ARDS without side effects. Apart from ECMO and nitric oxide, there are: partial liquid ventilation, various synthetic surfactants, intravenous oxygenation, extracorporeal CO_2 removal, various forms of high frequency ventilation and intravenous oxygenation. The interested reader will find plenty of literature; do not embrace new techniques until you know how to use a conventional ventilator.

1. Role of nitric oxide (NO) in ALI
- It is an endogenous endothelial relaxing factor, i.e. pulmonary vasodilator.
- Dose range is not yet fully determined but 0–40 ppm is commonly used.
- Useful in some patients with ALI: reduces pulmonary arterial pressure, improves oxygenation by reducing V/Q mismatch (in some patients).
- Mild bronchodilator.

2. ECMO and ALI
- Rescue therapy or survival depends upon indication.
- Should only be considered if the condition is potentially reversible.
- Entry criteria (Michigan):
    Fast entry criteria P_aO_2 < 50 mm Hg for > 2 hours, FiO_2 1.0 and PEEP $\geq$ 5 cm H_2O.
    Slow entry criteria P_aO_2 < 50 mm Hg for > 12 hours, FiO_2 0.6 and PEEP $\geq$ 5 cm H_2O and ventilated for < 7 days.
- Respiratory indications include: ALI (many causes), viral pneumonia (e.g. bronchiolitis), bacterial pneumonia, lung trauma.
- Advances in respiratory support mean that very few children, outside the neonatal age range, fulfill ECMO criteria.

Safe intubation techniques

Only regular practice can make you comfortable with intubation, but the following section lays out the main points that should be covered for a safe intubation.

1. Preparation for emergency intubation
- Optimal patient position: supine, cervical spine flexed, atlanto–occipital joint extended (neutral head position in infants and small children).
- Help available.
- Working, free running intravenous line.
- Oxygen source.
- Means to ventilate: self–inflating bag, Jackson–Rees circuit.
- Appropriate sized, close fitting face mask.
- Suction with Yankeur attachment (not flexible suction catheter).
- Working laryngoscope, appropriate type and size laryngoscope blade with bright light (a Miller, Macintosh or Oxford blade, depending on the patient's size).
- Have a selection of appropriate sized endotracheal tubes: (age/4) + 4 internal diameter, with a smaller tube on standby (always use an oral approach until the airway is secure).
- Ancillary pieces: stylet or Magill forceps, oral airways, patient monitors.

2. Drugs
- Sedation: noncardiodepressant, e.g. ketamine 1–2 mg/kg (care if raised intracranial pressure), midazolam 0.1 mg/kg (care if hypovolemic or cardiac dysfunction), morphine 0.1–0.2 mg/kg i.v.
- Atropine 20–40 μg/kg i.v. (minimum dose 0.15 mg): give before other medication.
- Succinylcholine 2 mg/kg: only give if no upper airway obstruction and able to assist ventilation (pretreatment with a nonfasciculating dose of a nondepolarizing muscle relaxant has become popular; it offers no advantage over regular dosing of succinylcholine and complicates the process).

3. Procedure for emergency intubation
- Preoxygenate with 100% oxygen using a tight fitting face mask, assist ventilation as necessary.
- Drugs, laryngoscope, endotracheal tube at the ready, suction turned on "maximum suction" and by the right hand of operator.
- Give atropine intravenously always.
- Assistant gently applies cricoid pressure (reduces risk of regurgitation or aspiration).
- Sedation given first, followed by suxamethonium, followed by saline flush (give drugs rapidly).
- Gently introduce laryngoscope into the right side of mouth and displace tongue to the left side of mouth. Assistant should gently pull on corner of mouth with left index finger while maintaining cricoid pressure with left hand; insert oral endotracheal tube only when cords are visualized.
- Watch the endotracheal tube pass between the cords. Stop when the black line on the endotracheal tube is at the cords (an endobronchial intubation is very easy in small children and is a common cause of hypoxemia postintubation).
- Note position at the lips, secure, check position with eyes, stethoscope and chest X–ray.
- Assist ventilation.
- Check patient color, blood pressure and pulses.
- Suction endotracheal tube if obvious secretions; collect specimen for culture and Gram stain.
- Insert orogastric or nasogastric tube (if any possibility of a bleeding disorder, use oral tube).

4. Failed intubation (two scenarios)
- Can maintain airway:
    Virtually everyone can be hand ventilated, including patients with epiglottitis and other forms of upper airway obstruction. Call for help.
    Resume assisted ventilation with 100% oxygen; oral airways may be useful if patient is unconscious and paralyzed.
    Reassess patient position.
    Stabilize as best as you can; try and assess why you have failed.
    Retry after improving patient position? Different laryngoscope blade?
    Different size endotracheal tube? Introducer angle?
- Cannot maintain airway:
    This is a disastrous situation to be in. Almost all patients can be hand ventilated by mask as long as the operator has the necessary experience.
    Insertion of a laryngeal mask airway is the best of several bad alternatives.
    Cricothyroidotomy or tracheotomy are last ditch maneuvers with little chance of success.
    The best approach is to maintain airway skills by occasional days spent in the Operating Room.

UPPER AIRWAY OBSTRUCTION

The small size of a child's airway predisposes him or her to upper airway obstruction. Superimposed swelling on an already small airway causes severe symptoms acutely. A 1 mm circumferential rim of edema in a newborn airway decreases the subglottic cross–sectional area by 60%. Reducing the endotracheal internal diameter from 3.5–3 mm increases resistance to airflow by 50%. Symptoms and signs vary with the degree of narrowing, the site of obstruction and the age of the child.

Extrathoracic obstruction produces worse inspiratory than expiratory stridor because of the natural tendency of extrathoracic structures to collapse during inspiration. Intrathoracic obstruction typically produces worse expiratory stridor and wheeze because of airflow obstruction as pleural and intrathoracic pressure rises. Acute pulmonary edema occasionally results from severe sustained airway obstruction because of the transmission of large negative intrapleural pressures to the lung interstitium. Chronic obstruction can result in chronic hypoxemia, right heart failure and pulmonary hypertension.

Clinical management

1. Presentation
- Stridor may be soft or noisy, may be more easily heard with stethoscope over the larynx (pharyngeal obstruction is lower pitched and coarser).
- Posture: may prefer to sit up, e.g. anterior mediastinal mass compressing trachea, epiglottitis.
- The voice may be altered in pitch or absent. Chest wall, sternal, supraclavicular indrawing or nasal flaring.
- Apnea: neonates and infants fatigue early and may stop breathing without warning.
- Wheeze: may be localized if foreign body.
- Chronic signs: failure to thrive, pectus excavatum, cor pulmonale, recurrent chest infections.
- Late signs: cyanosis, bradycardia, bradypnea.

2. Diagnosis and evaluation
- Clinical: history and physical examination.
- Radiology: depends on history, physical examination and, most likely, diagnoses. Reliability of a lateral neck X–ray in making a diagnosis has been shown to be poor; never of benefit with severe symptomatic airway obstruction.
- If obstruction is severe, the best investigation and management is an examination under anesthetia, followed by intubation if necessary.

3. Airway management of acute upper airway obstruction
- Inhalational induction:
    Halothane plus 100% oxygen is the preferred inhalation technique, performed by a clinician experienced in its use. Efficient suctioning apparatus. Allow the child to remain positioned where they prefer. No peeking in the airway, no radiology.
    Call for help: depends on the personnel available (anesthetist, ENT surgeon, pediatric intensivist). Arrange for an Operating Room if time allows.
    Prepare equipment for intubation: endotracheal tubes 0.5–1.5 mm smaller than predicted for age, range of laryngoscope handles and blades, stylet.
    Intravenous access: opinions vary as to the best time of establishing; if there is an obvious juicy vein, insert an i.v. prior to inducing anesthesia.
    Drugs: atropine intravenously. Halothane, anesthesia machine, tight fitting oxygen masks, Jackson–Rees circuit preferred but a pediatric circle system is suitable on the modern anesthetic machines.
- Awake intubation:
    Should only be attempted if there is an acute and complete loss of airway.
    Inhalational induction with halothane in the face of airway obstruction may take up to 20–30 min; patience is required.
    The patient must be deeply anesthetized before laryngoscopy (to avoid laryngospasm and loss of the airway).
    Monitors can be applied after the child becomes sleepy so as not to agitate further.
    Application of PEEP and gentle assistance of inspiration help to overcome obstruction.
    Laryngoscopy should only be performed when anesthesia is deep (4% halothane for at least 10 minutes; check saturations and blood pressure throughout).
    Oral intubation initially is always best; convert to nasal only after airway is secured orally and one is sure of the airway anatomy; suction endotracheal tube.
    Nasal endotracheal tube is the easiest to secure; immobilize arms.

4. Differential diagnosis
Common causes of upper airway obstruction are covered fully in chapter 21 (Respirology).

LOWER AIRWAY OBSTRUCTION

Diseases due to lower airway obstruction are the commonest single cause of admission to a Children's Hospital. The management of bronchiolitis and asthma should be second nature for any physician interested in pediatrics.

Bronchiolitis

- Usually in children during first year of life, usually caused by RSV (also by parainfluenza, adenovirus).
- Contagious.
- Those requiring intubation usually < 6 months of age.

1. Presentation
- Apnea, before onset of other respiratory symptoms.
- Cough, sneeze, rhinorrhea, wheeze, severe respiratory distress.
- Marked hyperinflation.
- Cyanosis; often have CO_2 retention on capillary blood gas.

2. Differential diagnosis in small babies
Pertussis, *Chlamydia*, other causes of apnea.

3. Pathophysiology
Mucous plugging, bronchial epithelial necrosis, sloughing and plugging of small airways.

4. Management
- Oxygen.
- Ventilatory support: decision to intubate is clinical (e.g. recurrent apnea, severe respiratory distress, patient fatigue); may require ventilatory support for over a week.
- Some patients may benefit from a trial of nebulized bronchodilator (e.g. salbutamol).
- Antiviral therapy (ribavirin) is controversial: its use is usually confined to intubated patients with associated congenital heart disease or prematurity. Recent large prospective trials have shown no clinical benefit from the drug.
- Bronchodilators (particularly adrenalin) have been shown to help in some children.
- Steroids are not of value.

5. Fluid management
- Restrict free water as there is a tendency to retain water with hyponatremia.
- Enteral feeding can be commenced early.
- Judicious use of diuretics may be beneficial if water logged and/or hyponatremic.

6. Monitoring
Clinical, oximetry, transcutaneous O_2/CO_2 transducers.

7. Ventilatory management
- Enough inspired oxygen to maintain arterial saturation > 90%.
- Tidal volume ~ 8–10 mL/kg initially.
- PEEP 5 cm H_2O initially: lungs are often already hyperinflated, with patchy areas of atelectasis. Limit peak pressure to 30–35 cm H_2O.
- pH > 7.3 initially (the P_aCO_2 may be in the 70's with this pH but is compensated and will cause no harm; overventilation to a normal P_aCO_2 will increase the risk of barotrauma).
- Allow a long expiratory time for expiration; monitor breath sounds and audible wheeze.

Status asthmaticus

Asthma is so common that it is easy to forget there is a large differential diagnosis for a wheezing child (e.g. foreign bodies, vascular compression, laryngotracheomalacia, tracheal stenosis, lung cysts, lobar emphysema, bronchiolitis).

1. Presentation
- Usually gradual progression of respiratory difficulty following URTI.
- Severe respiratory distress with marked hyperinflation, use of accessory respiratory muscles, nasal flaring, intercostal indrawing, pulsus paradoxus, diaphoresis.
- Wheeze, absent breath sounds.
- Fatigue, cannot speak in sentences, decreasing level of consciousness where severe.
- May have air leak (subcutaneous emphysema, pneumothorax).
- Hypoxemia, initially respiratory alkalosis.

2. Pathophysiology
- Increased airway resistance, air trapping, hyperinflation, decreased lung compliance.
- V/Q mismatch with hypoxemia, increased dead space ventilation.
- Increased work of breathing.
- Pulmonary hypertension, occasionally pulmonary edema.

3. General management
- Close observation, oxygen.
- Continuous nebulized bronchodilator therapy.
- Adequate i.v. hydration.
- Intravenous steroids.
- Subcutaneous adrenalin 0.01 mL/kg may buy time if the patient's poor air entry limits delivery of nebulized drugs.

4. Intubation
- Clinical decision is based on the patient's response to therapy, fatigue, neurological status; there are no absolute blood gas criteria. Treat as emergency. Most experienced operator should intubate.
- 100% oxygen, atropine 0.15 mg/kg i.v. Ketamine 1–2 mg/kg i.v. is safest (bronchodilator), followed by succinylcholine 2 mg/kg i.v.
- Always use oral approach until airway secured and patient oxygenated; confirm position with chest X–ray.
- May not be able to bag after intubation because of severe airway obstruction: suction, 100% oxygen, repeat dose of ketamine, nondepolarizing muscle relaxant, may require halothane or isofluorane inhalation 1–3%.
  Consider a bolus of magnesium sulfate 0.2 mmol/kg slow intravenous push.
- Intravenous ventolin infusions can be used (5 µg/kg over 10 min, then 1–5 µg/kg per min continuous infusion).
- Aminophylline 5 mg/kg slow i.v. bolus, followed by an infusion 0.5–1 mg/kg per h if not already started.

5. Ventilatory management
- Do no harm; similar to bronchiolitis. Do not overventilate simply to achieve normal blood gases.
- Give enough inspired oxygen to maintain arterial saturation > 90%.
- Tidal volume ~ 8 mL/kg initially. PEEP 0 cm H_2O initially; lungs are often already hyperinflated with patchy areas of atelectasis.
- Limit peak pressure to 30–35 cm H_2O.
- pH > 7.2 initially (the P_aCO_2 may be in the 70's with this pH but is compensated and will cause no harm; overventilation to a normal P_aCO_2 will increase the risk of barotrauma).
- Allow a long expiratory time for expiration; use a slow rate initially; monitor breath sounds and audible wheeze. Patients die of hypoxemia, not hypercarbia.
- Require long–acting muscle relaxants and sedation: midazolam, morphine or fentanyl.
- Monitoring: arterial line, ECG monitor, peak ventilatory pressures, chest movement, breath sounds, arterial blood gases, electrolytes (especially K^+ because of the effects of steroids and β–agonists).

CENTRAL NERVOUS SYSTEM

Basic physiology

Consider intracranial cavity and vertebral column as a single unit:
- Two fontanelles at birth: posterior closes at 3 months, anterior closes at 10–16 months.
- Low compliance system even with open fontanelles (smaller axis volume, nonstretchable dural cover).
- Components of intracranial cavity: brain parenchyma, 80%; CSF, 10%; cerebral blood volume, 10%.
- Brain at birth = 10–15% of birth weight, 335 g.
    The brain doubles its weight by 6 months; weighs 900 g by 12 months; 1,000 g at 2 years; 1,200–1,400 g by 12 years = adult weight (2% of body weight).
- Cerebral blood flow at:
    Birth: ~ 15–25 mL/100 g per min.
    12 months–12 years: ~ 80–100 mL/100 g per min.
    Adults: ~ 50 mL/100g per min.
- Global $CMRO_2$ (oxygen consumption): children ~ 5 mL O_2/100 g per min (lower in both infants and adults).
- Normal ICP infant < 5 mm Hg; adult ~ 10–15 mm Hg.
- CSF production: 0.35 mL/min.

Control of cerebral blood flow (CBF)

Cerebral blood flow is under a complex set of controls that are not fully understood, especially in children.

- Small scale regional flow probably responds to local metabolic demand.
- Global cerebral blood flow regulation occurs over a wide range of cerebral perfusion pressure (CPP = mean arterial pressure – intracranial pressure). Cerebral flow remains constant over a range from 50–150 mm Hg in adults. The range in small children is not known.

- Carbon dioxide tension controls CBF through its effect on cerebrovascular reactivity. There is a linear response between 20–80 mm Hg. CBF increases 3% for each mm Hg increase in P_aCO_2.

Pathophysiology of the craniospinal axis

The intracranial contents are encased in a fixed volume enclosure. Any increase in volume of one of the three components results in a rise in pressure within that enclosure, unless one of the other components is reduced in volume (Monro–Kelly). The compliance of the craniospinal cavity describes the relationship of small increases in volume until the compensatory mechanisms are exhausted, followed consequently by rises in intracranial pressure (ICP).

The adverse effects of elevated ICP include:
- Reduction in CPP.
- Local pressure effects (upon brain, blood supply, nerves).
- Global pressure effects, resulting in herniation syndromes.

Pathophysiology of cerebral blood flow

Following a brain insult, the response of the cerebrovasculature may be either increased CBF, reduced CBF or altered responsiveness to the usual regulators of flow.

1. CBF may be increased by
- Hypercarbia.
- Hypoxemia.
- Anemia.
- Following head trauma (less common than originally described).
- Loss of metabolic or flow coupling.
- Steal phenomena.

2. CBF may be reduced by
- Hypotension.
- Hyperventilation.
- Following head trauma (more common than originally described).
- Vasospasm.
- Reperfusion injury.
- Mechanical distortion.
- Steal phenomena.

Following an acute cerebral insult, tolerance to further insults (particularly hypoxemia and hypotension) is probably reduced. Compensatory blood flow changes may not occur normally, with a variable and time dependent response to CPP/CO_2. CBF changes occur both globally and regionally.

3. Etiology of intracranial hypertension
- Vascular: vasodilation, passive distension (loss of autoregulation), venous engorgement, hypotension with intact autoregulation.

- Nonvascular: cytotoxic, vasogenic, hydrostatic edema, mass effect, obstructed CSF flow, drainage.

4. Signs of elevated ICP
- General: vomiting, headache, full fontanelle in infants (when not crying).
- Level of consciousness: irritability, progressing through drowsiness to coma, seizures.
- Respiratory status: irregular respiratory pattern, shallow respiration, apnea in infants and neonates.
- Pupil size and reactivity: sluggish reaction, increasing size, irregular shape.
- Gaze: conjugate and roving, changing to dysconjugate, conjugate deviation.
- Posture and tone: extensor or flexor posturing.
- Circulatory status: hypertension, bradycardia.

Etiology of acute cerebral injury

1. Primary insult (beyond medical control)
- Trauma.
- Hypoxemia, ischemia, low flow states.
- Hypoglycemia.
- Hyponatremia, hypernatremia.
- Prolonged seizures.
- Hyperthermia.
- Infection (meningitis, encephalitis).

2. Delayed primary insult (possibly minimized by efficient resuscitation)
- Reperfusion injury.
- Mediator induced cascade injury (e.g. oxygen free radicals, leukotrienes, nitric oxide, excitatory amino acids).

3. Secondary insult (should be avoidable with careful management)
- Hypotension.
- Hypoxemia.
- Hypoglycemia, hyperglycemia.
- Hyponatremia, hypernatremia.
- Prolonged seizures.
- Hyperthermia.
- Elevated ICP.
- Infection (meningitis, encephalitis).

Monitoring

1. Clinical
- Glasgow Coma Scale score.
- Brain stem reflexes, especially pupillary response to light.
- Symmetrical motor movements, other focal signs.

2. Cardiovascular
Ensure normovolemia, normotension (may require invasive arterial catheter and central venous catheter for monitoring pressures).

3. Respiratory
Pulse oximetry, blood gases (ensure adequate oxygenation, avoid hypercarbia, hypocarbia).

4. ICP
- Pressure monitoring (preferably external ventricular drain) allows pressure transduction as well as an option to treat the pressure elevations with drainage of cerebrospinal fluid.
- Maintain adequate CPP for age.
- Maintain ICP < 20 mm Hg if possible.

5. Jugular venous bulb catheters to measure jugular venous (global brain) oxygenation.
- Calculate cerebral oxygen extraction ratio:

$$CEO_2 = \frac{(SaO_2 - SjO_2)}{SaO_2} \cdot 100$$

- Adjust ventilation accordingly to maintain CEO_2 within acceptable range (i.e. normal for adults < 45%; for children < 35%). High extraction ratios imply global reduction in CBF; commonly due to excessive hyperventilation.

6. Other
- Sensory evoked potentials, EEG.
- Follow–up CT scans.
- MRI (uncommon).

Brain resuscitation (therapeutic options)

- Avoid secondary injury.
- Optimize cerebral oxygen delivery.
- Minimize cerebral oxygen consumption.
- Reduce intracranial pressure or avoid elevations in ICP.

1. Avoid secondary injury
- There should be urgent attention to airway, ventilation and oxygen administration.
- Early aggressive intravascular volume resuscitation with isotonic fluids.
- Avoid glucose containing solutions unless documented hypoglycemia (hyperglycemia may potentiate lactic acid production).

2. Optimize cerebral oxygen delivery
- Aggressive ongoing support of circulating blood volume and oxygen administration.
- Support a normal cerebral perfusion pressure for patient age.
- Maintain arterial saturations above 90%.
- Maintain hematocrit above 30%.

- Avoid routine hyperventilation unless there is acute neurological deterioration.
- Minimize unnecessary increases in intrathoracic pressure but maintain enough positive end expiratory pressure to ensure adequate arterial saturation and minimize lung collapse.

3. Minimize cerebral oxygen consumption
- Avoid any elevation in body core temperature.
- Consider phenytoin loading to reduce the risk of hidden seizures if the patient is intubated and paralyzed or has a history of recent seizures.
- Sedate with morphine and/or midazolam infusions if intubated.

4. Management of elevated ICP
(ICP persistently elevated over 20 cm H_2O for over 5 minutes or alteration in pupillary responses)
- Routine use of hyperventilation is unwarranted because of potentially significant reductions in CBF. It should be reserved for acute elevations in ICP unresponsive to other interventions.
- ICP is normally elevated in healthy patients by such maneuvers as coughing and turning and is usually coincident with an elevation in blood pressure. This is normal. An elevated ICP becomes abnormal when it remains elevated and becomes a plateau rather than a spike, becomes elevated without a coincident rise in arterial blood pressure or it remains elevated for over 5 minutes with a falling arterial blood pressure.
- Open external ventricular drain (EVD); allow to drain for 5 minutes.
- Failing this, mannitol 0.25–1 g/kg for ICP > 20 mm Hg; may be used repeatedly if clinical effect persists. Maintain normovolemia at all times by replacing a proportion of the increased urine flow.
- Hypocarbia: lower CO_2 gently, preferably with the guidance of cerebral extraction ratios. Hyperventilation can obviously be used as a rescue maneuver if there is a sudden acute deterioration, e.g. a dilated pupil.
- Cool the patient (35 °C).
- Barbiturate coma: when the above maneuvers fail (but only after a repeat CT scan and after a discussion between the ICU physician and neurosurgeon), consider high dose barbiturates. Patient should always have a central line if barbiturate infusion is commenced.

5. Complications of brain injury
- Electrolyte disorders:
  Hyponatremia: excessive water retention, excessive salt wasting or inappropriate fluid management.
  Hypernatremia: excessive fluid restriction, excessive osmotic diuresis, diabetes insipidus.
- Cardiovascular: hypertension, hypotension.
- Respiratory: hypoxemia, aspiration, pneumonia, upper airway obstruction upon extubation, neurogenic pulmonary edema.
- Hypermetabolism: early nutritional support.
- Gastric stress ulceration.
- Skin: pressure sores.
- Coagulation:
  Early DIC (brain tissue thromboplastin); later, deep vein thrombosis and thromboembolism (immobilization).
- Other infections: meningitis, line sepsis, urinary tract infections.

Coma and encephalopathy

There are many causes of coma in a child, some of which are rapidly progressive if untreated, e.g. meningitis and hypoglycemia. After initial resuscitation, a comprehensive search for the underlying cause must be started immediately.

- CNS infection: meningitis, encephalitis.
- Hypoxic–ischemic insult: head trauma, suffocation, carbon monoxide, seizures, postictal state.
- Intoxication or poisoning: ASA, alcohol, recreational drugs.
- Metabolic: hyperglycemia, hypoglycemia, hyperammonemia, Reye's syndrome.

1. Early evaluation and management of coma
The basic principles remain:
- Airway: clear airway, administer oxygen, care with cervical spine if trauma suspected.
- Breathing:
    If inadequate, support with bag, mask and oxygen; prepare to intubate.
    Always preoxygenate with 100% oxygen using a well sealed face mask.
    Sedate with agents which have cardiovascular stability (e.g. opiates, ketamine, small doses of midazolam).
    Paralyze for intubation with suxamethonium (1.5 mg/kg i.v.).
    Always intubate via oral route; assume the child has a full stomach and protect against aspiration or regurgitation using cricoid pressure.
- Circulation:
    Always attempt to have intravenous access prior to intubation; secure i.v.
    Withdraw venous bloodwork at the time of insertion of i.v. if possible.
    Assess vital signs.
    Restore normovolemia and normotension aggressively.
- Immediate therapy of reversible causes of metabolic coma:
    Oxygen or ventilation.
    Glucose administration for hypoglycemia: 1–2 mL/kg D50W.
    Consider sepsis and early administration of antibiotics after blood cultures.
- Central nervous system:
    Early assessment of CNS function during preparation.
    Assess Glasgow Coma Scale score, symmetry of movement, other localizing signs.
    Pupillary, corneal, doll's eye reflexes.
- Ongoing assessment of ABC's and vital signs, ongoing support of ABC.
- Complete physical examination and detailed history.

2. History and physical examination
After stabilization, initial assessment, initiation of essential laboratory investigations, and a thorough history and complete physical examination are required:
- General appearance: unkempt, alcohol, body odor, sores, old injuries.
- Head: bruising, swelling, ear canals and drums, fontanelle, eyes (conjunctival injection or hemorrhage, light reflex, movements, fundi for hemorrhage), nose for CSF or purulent drainage, breath odor.
- Neck: if in collar, remove only after sand bag stabilization, bruising, swelling, laceration,

subcutaneous air, thyroid enlargement.
- Chest: respiratory pattern, Kussmaul respirations, adequacy of chest movements, symmetry of chest movements, heart sounds, vital signs (RR, BP, PR).
- Abdomen: organomegaly, abdominal distension or tenderness.
- Skin and extremities: color (cyanosis, jaundice, erythema), bruising or swelling, petechiae, wheals, injection marks, skin abscesses, lymphadenopathy, temperature, peripheral pulses.
- Body secretions:
    Urine color, odor, culture and urinalysis, toxicology.
    Stool consistency, culture.
    Sputum volume, color, culture and Gram stain.
    Nasopharyngeal secretions, color, culture, immunofluorescence.
    CSF color, culture, Gram stain, protein and sugar, special studies.
    Blood culture, routine and special laboratory investigations, toxicology.

3. Laboratory investigations
The investigations depend on the history, child's age and most likely etiology. Some or all of the following may be warranted:
- Bloodwork: blood culture, CBC, platelet count and differential, serum electrolytes, blood sugar, ionized calcium, magnesium, phosphate, urea, creatinine, serum osmolality, arterial blood gas, coagulation screen (PT, PTT, fibrinogen), liver function tests, ammonia.
- Urine: toxicology screen, reducing substances (e.g. glucose, fructose, galactose).
- Lumbar puncture or cerebrospinal fluid:
    If you want a quiet life, do not perform a lumbar puncture as an acute procedure on comatose patients. Leave it until the child is more stable. Obviously treat for meningitis, after taking blood cultures and while waiting for the result.
    Opening pressure, color, cell count and differential, glucose, protein, Gram stain and bacterial culture (viral, TB and fungal if suspected).
    Rapid diagnostic tests (e.g. ELISA for bacterial antigens, polymerase chain reaction for herpes simplex).
- Secondary investigations that may be necessary following the stabilization and initial workup of the comatose patient and following consultation with metabolic specialists:
    Blood: organic acids, amino acids, ketones, pyruvate/lactate, fructose, carnitine, porphyrins.
    Urine: organic acids, amino acids, ketones, carnitine, orotic acid.
    Liver or muscle biopsy.
    Freeze urine or blood specimens for further analysis at a later date.

Meningitis

Meningitis is a relatively common childhood infection and remains a cause of significant morbidity and mortality.

1. Clinical presentation
- Neonates: nonspecific signs of lethargy, fever, hypothermia, apnea, coma, seizures, bulging fontanelle, irregular respirations, systemic sepsis with poor peripheral perfusion or pulses, petechiae.
- Infant: headache, lethargy, vomiting, fever, decreased level of consciousness, seizures.

- Older child: lethargy, irritability, headache, neck stiffness, fever, vomiting, photophobia, decreased level of consciousness, petechiae.
- It is essential to respond urgently to any signs of raised intracranial pressure such as decreased level of consciousness, sluggish pupils or abnormal motor responses.

2. Meningitis management
- ABC, establish intravenous access, take bloodwork including blood culture.
- Give intravenous antibiotics early after blood cultures; do not wait to perform a lumbar puncture if the patient is unstable.
- Volume resuscitate aggressively to normalize intravascular volume and blood pressure.
- Check glucose early; give i.v. glucose bolus if low or patient obtunded, before laboratory results return.
- Restrict free water intake, not intravascular volume.
- Steroids remain controversial. CT scan taken during acute meningitis often reveal a pattern of vasculitis, consequently some centers give a short course of dexamethasone. The evidence for benefit is small and it is certainly much less important than efficient resuscitation and appropriate antibiotic treatment.
- 0–3 months: commonest organisms are group B *Streptococcus*, group D *Streptococcus*, Gram negatives, rarely *Listeria*. Empiric treatment: ampicillin and gentamicin or ampicillin and cefotaxime.
- 3 months–10 years: commonest organisms are *H. influenzae*, *S. pneumoniae*, *N. meningitidis*. Empiric treatment: ceftriaxone or cefotaxime or ampicillin and chloramphenicol.
- > 10 years: commonest organisms are *S. pneumoniae*, *N. meningitidis*. Empiric treatment: penicillin.
- Immunocompromised/shunt infection: empiric treatment includes vancomycin and cefotaxime.
- Tuberculous meningitis is often forgotten; it is probably more common than *Listeria*. It can present acutely. Drug resistant pneumococci are developing. If incidence is high in local area, use vancomycin until the cultures are back.

Status epilepticus

Management principles are based upon:
- Stabilization: ABC, oxygen. Establish intravenous access. Draw necessary bloodwork. Correct acute metabolic derangements, e.g. glucose.
- Stop the seizures.
- Prevent seizure recurrence.
- Prevent or treat systemic complications.
- Look for the cause of the seizures.
- Protect the brain.
- Antiseizure therapy requires knowing a few drugs very well. All the medications currently used have significant complications. Initially, the seizure should be stopped using an agent with rapid onset and maintained with a longer–acting agent. Always be prepared to support the child's ventilation and intubate if poor respiratory efforts, apnea or cyanosis develop. Prolonged seizures will often require airway protection, ventilation, cardiovascular support and neurological monitoring in the ICU.

Brain death

The diagnosis of brain death requires clinicians experienced in pediatric neurological ICU. Guidelines for neonatal brain death are less clear because of immaturity of the brain stem reflexes, but follow the same principles as for the older child and adult. If in doubt, request advice from the referral pediatric center. The issue of organ transplantation has made brain death both an emotional and ethical dilemma.

1. Pre–assessment requirements
- Cause of brain death determined.
- Normal blood pressure.
- Normal metabolic environment (electrolytes, pH, temperature > 35 °C).
- No sedative agents.
- Muscle relaxants discontinued and reversed. Confirm with neuromuscular monitor.

2. Clinical examination criteria
- Unresponsive to noxious stimuli (trigeminal distribution).
- Fixed dilated pupils.
- Absent corneal reflex.
- Absent spontaneous eye movements.
- Absent oculovestibular (caloric) reflex.
- Absent oculocephalic (doll's eye) reflex.
- Absent cough to deep tracheal stimulation.
- Absent suck, gag and rooting reflexes.
- Absent spontaneous respiratory effort with P_aCO_2 > 50 mm Hg (with normal arterial saturation).
- Clinical examination repeated at least once more by an independent specialist. The time to repeat examination depends on the etiology of the brain death. Uncertainty of cause would require a longer period between examinations.

3. Auxiliary tests
- EEG.
- Cerebral blood flow study.
- Indications for auxiliary tests to confirm the diagnosis of brain death include:
    Cause unknown.
    Residual effects of drugs, e.g. barbiturate coma.
    Unstable cardiorespiratory system so unable to perform the apnea test.

PEDIATRIC TRAUMA

Priorities in management

The "golden hour" describes the initial assessment and management of any patient who has suffered from trauma during which the priorities of care are established. The medical management of the patient during this crucial time determines subsequent survival. This short period allows the best opportunity for the physician to prevent the development of the mediator induced cascade injury which can ultimately result in multi–organ failure and is the most common cause of death following trauma.

• Exclude life threatening injuries during the primary survey: airway obstruction, hypovolemia, tension pneumothorax, cardiac tamponade.
• Prevent brain stem compression; avoid aggravating spinal cord injury.
• Assess the need for urgent or immediate surgery.
• Assess the need for referral to a dedicated pediatric center.
• A thorough secondary survey.

Primary survey (initial assessment)

Vital signs should be taken automatically, immediately upon arrival in the Emergency Room. Simultaneously, apply essential monitoring but beware; noninvasive blood pressure and pulse oximetry may be unreliable and give false reassurance in a cold shocked patient with poor peripheral pulses.

1. Assess airway
• Administer 100% oxygen by face mask.
• Lift chin, pull mandible forward (pulls tongue with it): avoid hyperextension of the neck, avoid fingers directly on the soft tissues under the chin.
• Suction secretions, blood, vomitus, foreign bodies.
• Maintain cervical spine precautions and institute C–spine precautions if not already done; rigid board with rigid collar or sand bags on either side of head or manual stabilization.
• Indications to intubate:
    Airway inadequate or not tolerating oral airway (caution: an oral airway in an awake patient may promote retching or regurgitation and aspiration of gastric contents).
    Head injury with Glasgow Coma Scale score < 8.
    Associated facial burns: prepare to intubate early.
• Contraindications to rapid sequence induction:
    Maxillofacial injury, facial burns, upper airway obstruction, suspected difficult airway. These injuries should be managed either by an anesthetist or with consideration of tracheostomy under controlled conditions.
    Beware: prolonged bag/mask ventilation may distend the stomach with air, resulting in aspiration of gastric contents and increasing difficulty with ventilation because of the elevation of diaphragm and raised intra–abdominal pressure.
    Orotracheal intubation is the preferred approach.
    Blind approach contraindicated with any head, facial or neck injuries: use cricoid pressure until the airway is secured, insert nasogastric tube (preferable to insert orogastric tube if there are head or facial injuries).
    Chest X–ray; confirm ETT position.

2. Breathing inadequate and/or signs of respiratory distress
• Search for correctable causes (e.g. pneumothorax). Check position of ETT and patency if already intubated.
• Support ventilation manually with bag/mask and oxygen.
• Chest X–ray. Insert intercostal catheter to drain pneumothorax.

3. Circulation
- Assess pulses or perfusion: tachycardia is the earliest sign of hypovolemia; bradycardia is a terminal sign of hypovolemia.
- Control active bleeding sites with pressure.
- Establish i.v. access, preferably in the upper limbs if intra–abdominal trauma suspected (as large a cannula as possible). More than one i.v. often required; collect blood for urgent group and cross–match, electrolytes, liver function tests, amylase and blood sugar.
- Options for i.v. access (only by persons experienced in the techniques) include: peripheral veins (anywhere), intraosseous needle, saphenous cutdown, femoral vein (difficult in a shocked or hypovolemic infant), central access (internal jugular or subclavian).
- Aggressive fluid resuscitation with isotonic crystalloid or colloid:
   20–30 mL/kg of normal saline or Ringer's lactate, or 15–20 mL/kg of 5% albumin given as fast as possible (often require to syringe the volume in to overcome resistance of small bore i.v.).
   Repeat as necessary to restore normovolemia and normotension; frequent reassessment of vital signs (3 mL crystalloid ~ 1 mL colloid or blood as replacement).
   Replace with packed cells for ongoing blood loss (reconstitute with normal saline prior to administration).
   Correct hemostatic problems (platelets, factor replacement) as they arise.
   Signs of mechanical obstruction to cardiac output (persisting tachycardia and/or low blood pressure despite "adequate" volume replacement, distended neck veins (suspect pneumothorax or cardiac tamponade). If the situation is too grave to wait for a chest X–ray, blind needle aspiration is acceptable if performed by a knowledgeable operator.

4. Disability
- Assess Glasgow Coma Scale score after resuscitation; correction of hypoxemia and hypotension.
- Assess pupillary reflexes, symmetry of motor movements, presence of lower limb movements.

5. Exposure
- Essential for complete examination (head to toe, front and back).
- Large surface area, rapidly cool on exposure.
- Use overhead radiant heaters.
- Warm inspired gases.
- Cover as soon as examination is completed.

6. "Missed or hidden" sites of blood loss
Scalp, pleural space, pericardial space, abdominal cavity, retroperitoneal space, pelvic fractures, femoral fractures, blood loss at the scene of the accident.

7. Investigations
- Blood withdrawn at the time of establishing vascular access: CBC, electrolytes, group and cross–match, PT, PTT, liver function tests, amylase, blood sugar.
- Arterial blood gas.
- Urine for urinalysis.
- Radiology.

8. Emergency radiology
The extent of radiology will depend upon the history and suspected injuries.
- Routine radiology:
     Skull: rarely of value.
     Cervical spine: anterior and lateral films down to T1.
     Chest: always.
     Abdomen: supine or lateral decubitus if suspect free air.
     Pelvis.
     Long bones: easy to miss a small fracture.
     Vertebral column: AP/lateral X–ray for high velocity trauma, lap belt injuries, falls from heights.
- Special radiology: abdominal ultrasound, head CT scan, abdominal CT scan, thoracic CT scan, angiography (suspected aortic arch injury, other vascular injury).
- Special investigations: transesophageal echocardiogram for suspected aortic arch injury, cardiac tamponade.

9. Monitoring
- Vital signs, clinical, ECG.
- Urinary catheter (caution if pelvic fractures, blood in meatus), urine volume and color.
- Pulse oximetry (unreliable with poor peripheral perfusion), central venous pressure.

Secondary survey

During this period, ongoing resuscitation and monitoring continues.

Detection of other possible life threatening injuries now begins. Consider the following:
- Immediate: hypoxemia or airway obstruction, hypovolemia, cardiac tamponade, tension pneumothorax, large flail chest.
- Potential: hemothorax, pulmonary contusion, aortic disruption, tracheobronchial tear, traumatic diaphragmatic hernia, esophageal tear, myocardial contusion.
- Head: lacerations, bruising, swelling, ear canals, tympanic membranes, mobility of midface (be careful), teeth (firm or missing).
- Neck (take off the collar, maintain midline position with sand bags): tenderness, lacerations, swelling, tracheal position.
- Chest: tracheal position, respiratory rate, chest movements (symmetry, flail), bruising, tenderness, crepitations, breath sounds, check all distal pulses for equality (aortic disruption).
- Abdomen: check for distension, tenderness, bowel sounds. Pass a gastric tube if not already done; log roll to inspect the back (tenderness, linear bone contour, lacerations, abrasions, unsuspected penetrating injury).
- Pelvis: springing of pelvic bones, perineum for hematoma or laceration, rectal examination.
- Extremities: deformity, hematomas, tenderness, abrasions, lacerations.
- Perform careful neurovascular examination if conscious, compartment pressure or firmness: immobilize fractures if not already done.
- CNS: if not intubated, response to verbal commands and painful stimuli, symmetry of motor movement, full cranial nerve assessment.
- Review history in detail: of injury (high velocity, acceleration or deceleration, witnessed or

unwitnessed, distance thrown, level of consciousness at the scene, movements at the scene), past history (illnesses, hospitalizations, immunizations, medications, allergies, family history, anesthetics and complications).

CHILD ABUSE

Most commonly inflicted upon children < 2 years of age, particularly < 1 year of age. A high index of suspicion is required. Accidental bruising before 9 months of age is very uncommon and occurs primarily on the knees, shins, forehead and elbows in crawling or ambulatory children.

Common circumstances

- Single parent.
- Parent was abused as a child.
- Single mother with male partner acting as babysitter while mother is working.
- Premature infant.
- Strong association with poor socioeconomic situation.
- Parental substance abuse.
- Previous history of suspected child abuse.

Diagnostic clues

1. Warning signs
- Multiple injuries.
- Injuries do not match history (e.g. child in coma with a history of a fall from a sofa onto the carpet).
- Multiple injuries at various stages of healing.
- Different forms of injury present concurrently.
- Delays in seeking medical help.
- Spontaneous or unexplained injury.
- Repetitive patterns of injury.
- Conflicting stories.
- Absent, unavailable, uninterested, overreacting parent.
- History incompatible with child's neurodevelopmental capability.
- History incompatible with force required to cause the injury.

2. Suspicious fractures
- Metaphyseal "chip" or "bucket handle" fracture.
- Posterior rib fracture.
- Avulsion fracture of distal clavicle.
- Diaphyseal spiral or transverse fracture before 9 months of age.
- Anterior compression fracture of vertebral body.
- Middle or proximal humeral fracture.

3. Suspicious other injuries
- Retinal hemorrhages.

- Cigarette burns.
- Scald injuries (stocking, buttock with doughnut pattern).
- Bite marks.
- Ligature or gag marks.
- Multiple bruises of different ages.

A common presentation to ICU is an infant in coma, with surface bruising of multiple ages and an inconsistent history. These children require aggressive critical care and neurosurgical support but the prognosis is often poor.

Management

Priorities of management are the same as for any case of trauma. Any child suspected of a nonaccidental injury must be admitted to hospital pending investigation. A child presenting in coma following a nonaccidental injury may require drainage of intracranial hematomas and the insertion of an ICP monitor.

Investigations

- Brain CT scan for any child in coma, seizures of unexplained etiology or other features of nonaccidental injury.
- Full skeletal survey is essential after stabilization.
- Photographic documentation of surface injuries may be required.
- Further investigations depend on the suspicion of sexual abuse.
- Collection and documentation of evidence must be done carefully by people experienced in this area. Complete documentation and early referral to a child protection team is essential.

BURNS

A severe burn is regarded as:
- Involving > 15% BSA.
- Full thickness burn > 5% BSA.
- High voltage electrical burn.
- Inhalational burn.

Burns are systemic injuries, producing a "systemic inflammatory response" (SIRS). Complications may arise either directly from the burn, from the SIRS or as a consequence of the severe immunocompromise that occurs with loss of the integument.

Complications of a burn

- Cardiovascular: volume loss (edema or permeability defects, insensible losses, blood loss, hemolysis), hypotension (volume loss, low systemic vascular resistance), SIRS or sepsis, myocardial depression, occasionally hypertension (volume overload, pain, sympathetic overdrive).
- Respiratory: inhalation injury, upper airway obstruction, hypoxemia (hypoxia, CO inhalation,

aspiration, atelectasis, pneumonia, acute lung injury, pulmonary edema, severe bronchospasm).
- Integument: edema, infection, heat or fluid loss.
- Hematological: thrombocytopenia (consumption or sepsis), coagulopathy, hemolysis, DVT's.
- GI tract: jaundice, stress ulceration, gastric stasis, acalculous cholecystitis, paralytic ileus.
- Metabolic: catabolic, many electrolyte abnormalities, hyperosmolar state (hyperglycemia), elevated basal body temperature (38–38.5 °C).
- Immunity: sepsis (skin, respiratory, renal, invasive lines).
- CNS: encephalopathy, hypoxic injury on presentation.
- Renal: ATN (hypovolemia, myoglobinuria, hemoglobinuria, sepsis).

Estimating burn size/depth

See chapter 24 (Appendix) for a chart used to calculate burn area. Rule of 9's for children > 15 years of age (infants require different criteria): head 10% BSA, chest or abdomen 18% each front and back, arms 9% each, legs 18% each, perineum 1%, one hand 1%.

Full thickness burns involve the epidermis, dermis and hypodermic fat and may involve deep injury to the muscle and deep fascia. Partial thickness burns involve the epidermis and may involve the dermis but with sparing of the deepest portion of the dermal papillae and epidermal appendages. The capillary leak resolves by 24 hours in the uncomplicated burn. (Partial thickness burns can be converted to full thickness burns by delayed resuscitation, inadequate resuscitation, hypotension, inadequate oxygen delivery or infection.)

Management

There are three priorities:
- Assess degree of airway compromise.
- Stop the burning process: remove all burnt clothing, wash off chemicals.
- Establish intravenous access, commence fluid resuscitation; restore/optimize oxygen delivery to the burn wound and vital organ systems.

1. Airway
- If a child presents in coma or with facial burns or signs of respiratory distress, prepare to intubate. Intubate early if airway injury suspected, before airway edema makes visualization of the airway difficult or impossible.
- Fiberoptic intubation or inhalational induction should be used if signs of airway obstruction are already present.
- Succinylcholine remains the drug of choice in the acute phase of a burn injury. However, beginning 48 hours after the burn, the patient's response changes; a major risk of succinylcholine induced hyperkalemia exists and persists for as long as the burn wound is healing.
- Inhalational injury associated with a decreased level of consciousness requires consideration of active therapy of carbon monoxide poisoning (hyperbaric oxygen). A carboxyhemoglobin level drawn after transfer to the Emergency Room may be normal but the patient may still have suffered a significant poisoning.

2. Breathing
Increased requirements for O_2 exist because of increased oxygen consumption, V/Q mismatch and pulmonary shunting:
- Liberal use of appropriate PEEP important.
- Severe bronchospasm can occur (airway injury, smoke inhalation resulting in reactive airways, mediator release similar to asthma). In this situation, in addition to bronchodilator therapy, ventilation should be managed to limit barotrauma.

3. Circulation
The priority is simple: restore adequate oxygen delivery to the burn wound and other vital organs.
- May require a central line for assessment of volume status; occasionally may require a pulmonary artery catheter.
- Fluid therapy begins and requirements are calculated from the time of the injury.
- Numerous formulae are available: best is based on BSA because of the larger BSA of children compared with adults.

General principles of fluid therapy

- Replace deficits (from time of burn). Assess deficits by clinical examination (time from injury) and vital signs.
- Replace ongoing losses.
- Replace maintenance requirements.
- Restore oxygen delivery to normal.
- An initial easy to remember formula is the Parkland formula: 4 mL/kg per %BSA + daily maintenance requirements using an isotonic solution, half given in the initial 8 hours postburn. Once the weight and length of the patient have been more accurately measured, the following formula should be substituted for greater accuracy (see chapter 24, Appendix, for BSA chart).

    Day 1:   2,000 mL/m^2 BSA per 24 h (maintenance requirements)
                                    plus
              5,000 mL/m^2 BSA burn per 24 h (burn injury replacement)

- Half of 24 hour requirement administered over first 8 hours (including catch–up time), with remaining half over the remaining 16 hours.
- For children < 12 months: use 5% dextrose in Ringer's lactate in combination with 5% albumin (volume ratio of 4:1, crystalloid:colloid).
- For children > 12 months: use 5% dextrose in Ringer's lactate alternating with half normal saline, in combination with 5% albumin (volume ratio of 4:1, crystalloid:colloid).
- Monitoring fluid replacement: general appearance, sensorium, mucous membranes (if not burnt), peripheral pulse volume or pulse pressure, urine output (fluctuates widely: 15–45 mL/m^2 per h during initial 48 h after the burn, depending on intravascular volume changes, release of aldosterone ADH and atrial natriuretic factor); urine output can be a poor indicator of adequacy of resuscitation.
- Laboratory: hematocrit, blood sugar, electrolytes, urea, arterial blood gases.
- Invasive monitoring (essential for the intubated patient with a major inhalational injury): invasive arterial catheter, CVP monitor, pulmonary artery catheter (occasionally).

Day 2:   1,500 mL/m² BSA per 24 h (maintenance requirements)
                                plus
          3,750 mL/m² BSA burn per 24 h (burn injury replacement)

- Most losses now secondary to evaporation, hence less sodium requirements.
- Most of the fluids by 48 hours should be given by the enteral route.
- Potassium requirements may become large.
- Follow electrolytes closely.
- Enteral feeds can be commenced by 24 hours in all patients including those intubated. Those patients with gastric stasis can be fed with the positioning of a duodenal/jejunal feeding tube.

Burn wound assessment and management

- Depth and size as described above.
- Need for escharotomy: essential to assess the pulses of a circumferential wound. Consider escharotomies for decreasing pulse volume and poor peripheral perfusion for limb burns or increasing ventilatory pressures with chest wall burns. Blood loss can be extensive following escharotomy.
- Topical antimicrobial therapy (silver sulfadiazine in 1% soluble cream base commonly used because of its broad antimicrobial spectrum and minimal systemic absorption).

Pain control or sedation

- Require large doses of morphine (10–100 µg/kg per h) and midazolam (1–5 µg/kg per min) as a constant infusion.
- Burn showers and dressing changes require extra:
    Ketamine 1–2 mg/kg i.v.
    Morphine 0.1–0.2 mg/kg i.v.
    Fentanyl bolus 1–2 µg/kg i.v.

CONTINUOUS INFUSION GUIDELINES FOR INFANTS AND CHILDREN
John McCready

The continous infusion tables are intended to be used only as a guideline to provide the minimum amount of information necessary to start the most common intravenous infusions. Ultimately, the requirements of the dose and administration of these medications are dictated by each individual clinical situation.

The information is presented in a six column format, which relates the dilution of the drug given by continuous infusion to the dose delivered.

Definitions

- Patient group: these guidelines normally apply to infants and children. Where information is available for neonates, it has been included.
- Dilution: this column gives the number of mg or mL of each drug to be added to the diluent up to a total volume of 50 mL.
    The dilutions represented here are applicable for use in children of 5–20 kg body weight. Younger children (< 5 kg), or those who are fluid restricted, may require more concentrated solutions (double–quadruple strength), especially for drugs noted by **. Older children may tolerate more dilute solutions of these drugs. (For children > 20 kg, calcium chloride, dopamine and norepinephrine are to be diluted to half strength.)
    The dilution and dose recommendations in this chart do not apply to neonates for drugs noted by *. Consult special neonatal references and use extra care when treating this age group.
    It should be noted that:
    The dilution may be indicated as either mg/kg of drug product per 50 mL (e.g. dopamine) or mg or mL of drug product per 50 mL (e.g. aminophylline, sodium bicarbonate). It is the responsibility of the prescriber and the nurse to verify that the dilution used will deliver the correct dose.
    Some drugs (e.g. alcohol, diazepam, paraldehyde) are recommended to be given at the fixed concentrations indicated in the dilution column.
    The maximum recommended infusion concentration of each drug is stated in the comments section.
- Infusion rate: the standard initial infusion rate is given for an average child.
- Dose delivered: the dose delivered at the standard infusion rate.
- Dose range: the recommended infusion dose range is given in column five but unusual clinical situations may dictate higher doses.
- Comments: other pertinent information pertaining to the infusion of each drug is presented, including:
    Loading dose, where applicable.
    Central or peripheral line recommendations.
    Protect from light, where noted.
    Maximum recommended concentration for infusion.
    Solution expiry noted; change tubing at specified time.

Drug	Dilution (#mg or mL to total of 50 mL i.v. fluid)	Infusion rate	Dose delivered	Dose range	Comments
* Alcohol, Ethyl 99%	5 mL (to make 10% dilution) normal saline or SWI	*No dialysis:* 1.4 mL/kg per h *Dialysis:* 3.0 mL/kg per h	109 mg/kg per h (s.g. = 0.79) 237 mg/kg per h	Titrate i.v. rate to keep blood ethanol level in range that will block alcohol dehydrogenase (> 22 mmol/L)	Loading dose is 7.6 mL/kg i.v. (of 10% solution) over 30 min; to make 10% dilution, mix 5 mL ethanol 99% with 45 mL i.v. fluid; peripheral or central line; maximum concentration is 10% solution; consider early hemoperfusion, peritoneal dialysis if methanol levels are > 15 mmol/L if acidosis is refractory to NaHCO₃; 24 h
* Aminophylline 25 mg/mL pH: 8.6–9.0	50 mg D5W, normal saline	1 mL/kg per h	1 mg/kg per h	Reduce dose for children < 1 yr or > 9 yr; titrate to keep theophylline blood level in therapeutic range (55–110 µmol/L)	Loading dose is 6 mg/kg i.v. over 20 min; peripheral or central line; maximum concentration is 10 mg/mL; 72 h
Amiodarone 150 mg/3 mL	15 mg/kg D5W only; infuse at concentrations 0.6–4.8 mg/mL	1 mL/hr	5 µg/kg per min	5–15 µg/kg per min	Loading dose is 5 mg/kg slow i.v. over 20 min–1 h; the duratin of injection should never be < 3 min; avoid the use of direct undiluted injections; central line preferred; adsorbs to PVC bags and tubing; change buretrol and tubing at 24 h

Drug	Dilution (#mg or mL to total of 50 mL i.v. fluid)	Infusion rate	Dose delivered	Dose range	Comments
Aminone 5 mg/mL pH: 3–4 $33.00/amp	15 mg/kg; 0.45, 0.9% saline only	1 mL/h	5 µg/kg per min	5–10 µg/kg per min *Neonates:* 3–5 µg/kg per min	Infuse at concentration of approximately 1–5 mg/mL; incompatible with dextrose, however, may be run through a Y–site connector into a line containing dextrose; peripheral or central lines; 72 h
** Calcium chloride 10% 100 mg/mL pH: 5.5–7.5	150 mg (1.5 mL)/ kg (CaCl₂) D5W, normal saline (for children > 20 kg, dilute to ½ strength)	1 mL/h	0.5 mmol/kg per d or 1 mEq/kg per d (Ca²⁺)	0.5–1.5 mmol/kg per d or 1–3 mEq/kg per d (Ca²⁺)	Central venous (RA) line only; avoid extravasation; maximum concentration is 10%, 100 mg/mL; 1 mEq = 20 mg Ca²⁺; 27 mg Ca²⁺ = 1.36 mEq = 0.68 mmol/mL
Calcium gluconate 10% 100 mg/mL pH: 6–8.2	Dilute to 20 mg/mL or less and mix in maintenance fluids			*Neonates:* 200–400 mg (2–4 mL of 10% solution)/kg per d *Infants and children:* 200–1,000 mg (2–10 mL of 10% solution)/kg per d	Central line where Ca > 400 mg/100 mL or peripheral line; do not give by scalp, vein; maximum concentration is 20 mg/mL peripherally; 9 mg Ca²⁺ = 0.47 mEq = 0.24 mmol/mL
* Diazepam emulsion 5 mg/mL (Diazemuls)	10 mg D5W only (0.2 mg/mL) or undiluted	0.5 mL/kg per h	0.1 mg/kg per h	Titrate dose to clinical response	Peripheral or central line; maximum concentration is 0.2 mg/mL diluted in D5W; 24 h; diazemuls may also be infused undiluted via syringe pump; antidote is flumazenil 0.01–0.025 mg/kg i.v. p.r.n.

Drug	Dilution (#mg or mL to total of 50 mL i.v. fluid)	Infusion rate	Dose delivered	Dose range	Comments
** Dobutamine 12.5 mg/mL pH: 2.5–5	15 mg/kg D5W, normal saline	1 mL/h	5 µg/kg per min	2–20 µg/kg per min	Central venous line preferred; pink discoloration okay; maximum concentration is 10 mg/mL; 72 h
** Dopamine 40 mg/mL pH: 2.5–4.5	15 mg/kg D5W, normal saline (for children > 20 kg, dilute to ½ strength)	1 mL/h	5 µg/kg per min	2–20 µg/kg per min	Central venous line only; avoid extravasation; for infiltration, notify doctor immediately regarding phentolamine protocol; do not use discolored solutions; maximum concentration is 5 mg/mL; 72 h
* Epinephrine 1:1,000 1 mg/mL pH: 2.5–5	0.3 mg/kg D5W, normal saline	1 mL/h	0.1 µg/kg per min	0.05–1 µg/kg per min	Central venous line preferred; avoid extravasation; do not use discolored solutions; maximum concentration is 500 µg/mL; 72 h
Esmolol 100 mg/10 mL pH: 4.5–5.5 $10.00/vial	100 mg/10 mL vial is ready for use	0.6 mL/kg per h	100 µg/kg per min	50–200 µg/kg per min	Infusion control device; loading dose 500 µg/kg per min over 1 min; maximum concentration is 10 mg/mL (i.e. undiluted); 72 h; not compatible with sodium bicarbonate

Drug	Dilution (#mg or mL to total of 50 mL i.v. fluid)	Infusion rate	Dose delivered	Dose range	Comments
** Fentanyl 0.05 mg/mL pH: 4–7.5	0.05 mg/kg D5W, normal saline	1 mL/h	1 μg/kg per h	1–4 μg/kg per h	Loading dose is 1–2 μg/kg i.v. over 1–3 min; peripheral or central line; maximum concentration is 50 μg/mL; monitor for respiratory depression in nonventilated patients; antidote is naloxone 0.01–0.1 mg/kg i.v. p.r.n.; 72 h
* Furosemide 10 mg/mL pH: 8.5–9.3	25 mg/kg D5W, normal saline	1 mL/h	0.5 mg/kg per h	0.1–1 mg/kg per h	Peripheral or central line; do not use discolored solutions; maximum concentration is 10 mg/mL; furosemide is an alkaline drug and does not mix well with catecholamines such as dopamine, epinephrine, etc.; 72 h
Heparin 1,000 unit/mL pH: 5–7.5	1,000 unit/kg D5W, normal saline	1 mL/h	20 unit/kg per h	15–25 unit/kg per h individualized based on PPT results	Loading dose is 50 unit/kg i.v. once; peripheral or central line; maximum concentration is 400 unit/mL; 72 h
Insulin (Toronto, regular) 100 unit/mL pH: 7–7.8	5 units normal saline, 0.45 saline, D5W	1 mL/kg per h	0.1 unit/kg per h	0.05–0.1 unit/kg per h based on serum glucose concentrations	Loading dose is 0.1 unit/kg i.v. over 1–2 min; only regular insulin is given i.v.; preflush tubing with 25–50 mL insulin solution; peripheral or central line; maximum concentration is 5 unit/mL

Drug	Dilution (#mg or mL to total of 50 mL i.v. fluid)	Infusion rate	Dose delivered	Dose range	Comments
** Isoproterenol 0.2 mg/mL pH: 3.5–4.5	Chronotrope or inotrope: 0.075 mg/kg	1 mL/h	0.025 µg/kg per min	0.025–0.1 µg/kg per min	Peripheral or central line; discard solution if darkens or a precipitate is present
	Bronchodilator: 0.3 mg/kg D5W	1 mL/h	0.1 µg/kg per min	0.1–1.0 µg/kg per min	Maximum concentration is 0.2 mg/mL; 72 h
* Ketamine 50 mg/mL	30 mg/kg D5W, normal saline	2 mL/h	20 µg/kg per min	20–40 µg/kg per min	Watch airway closely; peripheral line; maximum concentration is 50 mg/mL
Labetalol 5 mg/mL pH: 3–4 $16.00/amp	50 mg D5W or normal saline (mix 100 mg to total 100 mL i.v. fluid)	1 mL/kg per h	1 mg/kg per h	1–3 mg/kg per h	Peripheral or central line; incompatible with NaHCO₃; maximum concentration is 5 mg/mL (undiluted); 72 h
Lidocaine 200 mg/mL pH: 5–7 (200 mg/mL strength only for dilution)	30 mg/kg D5W	1 mL/h	10 µg/kg per min	20–50 µg/kg per min; therapeutic range of lidocaine is 4.5–21 µmol/L	Loading dose is 1 mg/kg q10 min p.r.n. up to 5 mg/kd; peripheral or central line; maximum concentration is 20 mg/mL; incompatible with phenytoin and NaHCO₃; 72 h

Drug	Dilution (#mg or mL to total of 50 mL i.v. fluid)	Infusion rate	Dose delivered	Dose range	Comments
** Midazolam 5 mg/mL pH: 3–3.6 $3.00/5 mg vial $19.00/50 mg vial	3 mg/kg D5W, normal saline	1 mL/h	1 µg/kg per min	0.5–6 µg/kg per min *Neonates:* 0.5 µg/kg per min	Use midazolam cautiously and avoid load dose in postoperative open heart patients, septic shock or meningococcemia; loading dose for neonates is 0.05 mg/kg i.v. over 15 min; for other patients, loading dose is 0.05–0.1 mg/kg i.v. over 3 min; peripheral or central line; maximum concentration is 5 mg/mL; 72 h; antidote is flumazenil 0.01–0.025 mg/kg i.v. p.r.n.
** Morphine 10 mg/mL pH: 2.5–6	0.5 mg/kg D5W, normal saline	1 mL/h	10 µg/kg per h	Postoperative analgesia or sedation 10–40 µg/kg per h (dose for neonates < 1 mo is 5–20 µg/kg per h) *Burn patients:* have received doses as high as 0.5–2.5 mg/kg per h	Peripheral or central line; maximum concentration 10 mg/mL; monitor for respiratory depression in nonventilated patients; antidote is naloxone 0.01–0.1 mg/kg i.v. p.r.n.; incompatible with lasix and NaHCO₃; 72 h
**Nitroglycerine 5 mg/mL pH: 3–6.5	3 mg/kg D5W, normal saline	1 mL/h	1 µg/kg per min	0.5–10 µg/kg per min	Peripheral or central line; administer via syringe pump with non-PVC tubing; maximum concentration is 1 mg/mL; 72 h

Drug	Dilution (#mg or mL to total of 50 mL i.v. fluid)	Infusion rate	Dose delivered	Dose range	Comments
** Nitroprusside 50 mg/vial pH: 3.5–6 $15.00/vial	3 mg/kg D5W only	1 mL/h	1 µg/kg per min	0.5–8 µg/kg per min; keep thiocyanate < 0.8 mmol/L *Neonates:* begin at 0.025–0.5 to maximum 6 µg/kg per min	Check thiocyanate levels in high dose prolonged (> 48 h) use or renal failure; do not admix; peripheral or central line; protect infusion solution and tubing from light with aluminum foil; maximum concentration is 5 mg/mL; 24 h
Norepinephrine 1 mg (base)/mL pH: 3–4.5	0.3 mg/kg D5W only; do not mix in normal saline (for children > 20 kg, dilute to ½ strength)	1 mL/h	0.1 µg/kg per min	0.02–0.1 µg/kg per min; titrate to bp	Do not mix in normal saline or use if solution turns brown; central venous line only, avoid extravasation; for infiltration, notify doctor immediately regarding phentolamine protocol; incompatible with alkalis; maximum concentration is 0.5 mg/mL; dose and calculations in terms of norepinephrine base, i.e. 1 mg base = 2 mg bitartrate; 24 h
Paraldehyde (100%) 1 g/mL	2.5 mL (to make 5% dilution) normal saline, ⅔ and ⅓ D5W, ⅔ and ⅓	0.4 mL/kg per h	20 mg/kg per h	20 mg/kg per h	Do not admix; protect infusion from light; change i.v. administration set and solution q8h; discard solution if it has a brown color or a sharp odor of acetic acid; maximum concentration is 5% solution; 8 h; peripheral or central line

Drug	Dilution (#mg or mL to total of 50 mL i.v. fluid)	Infusion rate	Dose delivered	Dose range	Comments
Procainamide 100 mg/mL pH: 4–6 $10.00/100 mg vial	60 mg/kg normal saline only	1 mL/h	20 µg/kg per min	*Children:* 20–80 µg/kg per min; monitoring levels of procainamide and NAPA recommended; *Range:* procainamide 15–37 µmol/L; sum of procainamide and NAPA < 110 µmol/L	Peripheral or central line; must be diluted prior to use; load dose for children is 2–5 mg/kg per dose (maximum 100 mg), dilute i.v. over 5 min, q5–10 min to maximum 15 mg/kg (hypotension); 72 h
Propafenone 70 mg/20 mL	12 mg/kg D5W only	1 mL/h	4 µg/kg per min	4–8 µg/kg per min	Central or peripheral line; incompatible with normal saline, KCl; loading dose is 0.2 mg/kg i.v. q10 min until heart rate decreases to 150 beat/min; 72 h
Prostaglandin E$_1$ 500 µg/mL pH: 4.3/D5W $130.00/amp	Ductal dilatation: *Newborns:* 0.05 mg (50 µg) D10W (this also delivers maintenance fluids); *Ductal dilatation or pulmonary vasodilation:* 0.15 mg/kg (150 µg/kg) D5W, normal saline (no maintenance fluid delivered)	3 mL/kg per h 1 mL/hr	0.05 µg/kg per min 0.05 µg/kg per min	0.01–0.1 µg/kg per min 0.01–0.1 µg/kg per min	For ductal dilatation make initial dilution (50 µg/mL) by adding 1 mL prostin VR (500 µg/mL) to 9.0 mL normal saline in 10 mL vial; label, refrigerate, discard vial in 7 d; incompatible with NaHCO$_3$; peripheral or central line (central line preferred for concentration ≥ 10 µg/mL); maximum concentration is 20 µg/mL; compatible with NaCl, KCl (concentration of 2 mmol/100 mL); 24 h

Drug	Dilution (#mg or mL to total of 50 mL i.v. fluid)	Infusion rate	Dose delivered	Dose range	Comments
* Salbutamol 0.5 mg/mL pH: 3.5 $11.00/amp	May run full strength (25 mg/50 mL or diluted)	0.12 mL/kg per h	1 µg/kg per min	0.2–10 µg/kg per min	Peripheral or central line; may use undiluted or diluted to ½ strength or less; maximum concentration is 0.5 mg/mL; 72 h
Sodium bicarbonate 1 mEq/mL 1 mmol/mL pH: 7.4–8.5	25 mmoL (25 mL) (0.5 mmol/mL, 4.2%)	1 mL/kg per h	0.5 mmol/kg per h	Sufficient to control acidosis 0.5–2 mmol/kg per h	Do not admix; peripheral or central line (preferred); maximum concentration is 1 mmol/mL central line, 0.5 mmol/mL peripheral line; 72 h
Streptokinase 250,000 unit/vial 750,000 unit/vial (high dose systemic thrombolytic therapy) $85.00 per 250,000 units $230.00 per 750,000 units	50,000 unit/kg	1 mL/h	1,000 unit/kg per h	300–2,000 unit/kg per h	Loading dose is 3,000–5,000 unit/kg over 30 min; reconstitute vial with 5 mL normal saline by rolling and tilting; avoid shaking; further dilute in normal saline prior to infusion; discard solutions containing precipitate; 24 h
Streptokinase 250,000 IU/vial 750,000 IU/vial (low dose local thrombolytic therapy)	2,500 unit/kg D5W	1 mL/hr	50 unit/kg per h	50–100 unit/kg per h	Low dose local infusion via small plastic catheter; 24 h

Drug	Dilution (#mg or mL to total of 50 mL i.v. fluid)	Infusion rate	Dose delivered	Dose range	Comments
Thiopental 25 mg/mL, 2.5% pH: 10–11	200 mg (0.4%) D5W or normal saline	0.25 mL/kg per h	1 mg/kg per h	1–5 mg/kg per h	Central line only; avoid extravasation; maximum concentration is 25 mg/mL (2.5%); incompatible with catecholamine; 72 h
Urokinase 250,000 unit/vial (high dose systemic thrombolytic therapy)	100,000 unit/kg D5W or normal saline (mix sufficiently for 24 h D5W or normal saline only)	2 mL/h	4,000 unit/kg per h	300–5,000 unit/kg per h, increase dose if fibrinolysis is not effected; doses up to 50,000 unit/kg per h have been used	Loading dose is 4,000–6,000 unit/kg per dose i.v. over 10 min; reconstitute vial with 5.2 mL sterile water without preservative; roll & tilt; do not shake; use solution immediately after
(low dose local thrombolytic therapy) 250,000 unit/vial $250.00 per 250,000 units	10,000 unit/kg	2 mL/h	400 unit/kg per h	300–500 unit/kg per h	preparation; discard solution after 24 h after reconstitution of powder
Vasopressin 20 unit/mL pH: 2.5–4.5 $5.00/20 unit amp $45.00/100 unit amp	*Central diabetes insipidus* 1 unit/kg D5W, normal saline	1 mL/h	0.0003 unit/kg per min	0.00003–0.0003 unit/kg per min (0.1–1 mL/h) or begin at 1 mL/h (0.003 unit/kg per min) and titrate infusion downward as control is achieved;	Central line preferred, peripheral; maximum concentration is 1 unit/m; avoid extravasation; for upper GI hemorrhage, begin therapy with a loading dose of 20 unit/1.73 m², then start infusion; use only with expert consultation; hemostatic techniques may be indicated
	Gastrointestinal hemorrhage 50 units	0.12 mL/kg per h	0.002 unit/kg per min	0.002–0.01 unit/kg per min (a higher dose might be required but complications are more frequent)	

Drug	Dilution (#mg or mL to total of 50 mL i.v. fluid)	Infusion rate	Dose delivered	Dose range	Comments
Vecuronium 10 mg/vial pH: 4 $18.00/10 mg vial	3 mg/kg D5W, normal saline	1 mL/h	1 µg/kg per min	1–10 µg/kg per min	Reconstitute with SWI to 1 mg/mL; central or peripheral line; maximum concentration is 2 mg/mL; 72 h

Note:
* The dilution and dosage recommendations for these drugs do not apply to neonates.
** For children: < 5 kg, more concentrated solutions (2 ×, 4 ×) may be used.
  > 20 kg, less concentrated solutions may be used.

INTRODUCTION

Definitions

- Congenital anomalies are structural or anatomical defects of varying significance:
    Major anomalies require medical or surgical attention or are of social concern.
    Minor anomalies are those that are neither medically nor socially significant.
- Syndromes are etiologically related congenital anomalies occurring together.
- An association consists of congenital anomalies that are found together more frequently than chance alone would predict, but that are not known to be etiologically related.
- A sequence is a group of congenital anomalies that are related through a common primary event.

Prevalence of genetic anomalies

- Major congenital anomalies occur at similar rates regardless of ethnicity or place of birth. They may present at any age, consequently the prevalence increases with age:
    2–3% of newborn infants are found to have major congenital anomalies. This increases to 5% in the first year of life.
    7–10% of children > 5 years of age have identified major congenital anomalies or learning disorders.
    Congenital anomalies may also present in adulthood or at postmortem examination.
- Two–thirds of pediatric deaths in hospital in developed countries are related to an underlying congenital anomaly.

Etiologies

- Most congenital anomalies occur during the first 8 weeks of gestation (Table I).
- There are a variety of etiologies for congenital anomalies:
    Single gene defects: 7.5%.
    Chromosomal abnormality: 6%.
    Multifactorial: 20%.
    Congenital infection (herpes, cytomegalovirus, rubella, HIV, toxoplasmosis, syphilis, parvovirus) or maternal illness: 5–8%.
    Unknown: > 50%
- The most common teratogen in pregnancy is alcohol. Other drugs or chemicals that may be teratogenic include anticoagulants, anticonvulsants, vitamin A, isotretinoin and cocaine. Environmental teratogens include radiation and hyperthermia, drugs or chemicals.

Table I: Embryological timing of some congenital anomalies

Tissues	Malformation	Defect in	Prior to	Comment
CNS	Anencephaly	Closure of the anterior neural tube	26 d	Subsequent degeneration of forebrain
	Meningomyelocele	Closure in a portion of the posterior neural tube	28 d	80% lumbosacral
Face	Cleft lip	Closure of lip	36 d	42% associated with cleft palate
	Cleft maxillary palate	Fusion of maxillary palatal shelves	10 wk	
	Branchial sinus ± cyst	Resolution of branchial cleft	8 wk	Preauricular and along the line anterior to sternocleidomastoid
GI	Esophageal atresia + tracheoesophageal fistula	Lateral septation of foregut into trachea and foregut	30 d	
	Rectal atresia with fistula	Lateral septation of cloaca into rectum and urogenital sinus	6 wk	
	Duodenal atresia	Recanalization of duodenum	7–8 wk	
	Malrotation of gut	Rotation of intestinal loop so that cecum lies to right	10 wk	Associated with incomplete or aberrant mesenteric attachments
	Meckel's diverticulum	Obliteration of vitelline duct	10 wk	May contain gastric ± pancreatic tissue
GU	Diaphragmatic hernia	Closure of the pleuripotential canal	6 wk	
	Extroversion of bladder	Migration of infraumbilical mesenchyme	30 d	Associated Müllerian and wolffian duct defects
	Bicornate uterus	Fusion of the lower portion of the Müllerian ducts	10 wk	
	Hypospadias	Fusion of the urethral folds (labia minora)	12 wk	
	Cryptorchidism	Descent of testicle into scrotum	7–9 mo	

Tissues	Malformation	Defect in	Prior to	Comment
Heart	Transposition of great vessels	Directional development of bulbus cordis septum	34 d	
	Ventricular septal defect	Closure of ventricular septum	6 wk	
	Patent ductus arteriosus	Closure of ductus arteriosus	9–10 mo	
Limb	Aplasia of radius	Genesis of radial bone	38 d	Often accompanied by other defects of radial side of distal limb
	Syndactyly, severe	Separation of digital rays	6 wk	
Complex	Cyclopia, holoprosencephaly	Prechordial mesoderm development	23 d	Secondary defects of midface and forebrain
	Sirenomelia (sympodia)	Development of posterior axis	23 d	Associated defects of cloacal development

Classification of dysmorphisms

The importance of classifying dysmorphic features lies not only in the understanding and identification of etiological factors or events but also in the assessment of recurrence risk, therapeutic intervention and prognosis (Table II).

- Malformations are usually genetic in nature and result from abnormal developmental processes that begin at conception (e.g. hypoplastic radii and congenital heart defects associated with Holt–Oram's syndrome).
- A disruption is an alteration in normal development due to extrinsic interference, including maternal factors (e.g. thalidomide embryopathy).
- Deformations are usually asymmetric in nature and occur secondary to external mechanical forces (eg. twin pregnancies, oligohydramnios).
- Dysplasia is the abnormal differentiation of tissue secondary to either inherited conditions and/or extrinsic factors.

INHERITED GENETIC DEFECTS

Chromosomal imbalance

- Normally, there are 46 chromosomes in the human genome; 23 derived maternally and 23 paternally.
- Aneuploidy results from an error during cell division—the creation of too many or too few chromosomes. The best example of aneuploidy is Down's syndrome or trisomy 21, where an additional chromosome 21 is present.
- Trisomies are the most common form of aneuploidy, while the absence of a chromosome, or

monosomy, other than Turner's syndrome (monosomy X) is relatively rare.
- Polyploidy results from the addition of a complete set of chromosomes (eg. 69, XXY).

Breakage

- During cell division, breakage and rearrangement of chromosome segments may occur. This may result in an overall increase or decrease in the amount of DNA present.
- Translocation occurs when a portion of one chromosome breaks off and joins to another chromosome. These are said to be balanced if the overall content of DNA remains unchanged and unbalanced if there is either a net gain or loss of genetic material.
- A deletion results from the loss of a segment of a chromosome during cell division, whereas a duplication is the addition of a chromosome segment.

Gene defects

- Each individual normally receives a set of 23 chromosomes from each parent, resulting in each gene being present in two copies.
- The phenotype or clinical expression of a specific gene defect will depend on whether that defect present is dominant (i.e. only one of the two alleles needs to be defective to produce phenotypic anomaly) or recessive (i.e. both copies of the gene must be defective to result in the anomaly). Autosomal defects affect nonsex chromosomes and, as such, generally affect males and females equally.
- X–linked disorders result from defective genes on the X chromosome. The majority of these disorders are recessive and therefore affect males much more commonly than females .
- Multifactorial anomalies recur in families but inheritance results from a poorly understood combination of genetic and environmental factors rather than from specific single gene defect or chromosomal imbalance. While the particular pattern is not predictable, empiric recurrence risks are available based on epidemiological data.

Nontraditional

- Gonadal mosaicism occurs when a number of gametes (and thus a number of potential offspring) are affected by a new mutation (e.g. osteogenesis imperfecta type 2).
- Uniparental disomy occurs when both alleles in a pair originate from the same parent. Identification is by specific polymorphic markers (e.g. Beckwith–Wiedemann's, Prader Willi's, and Angelman's syndromes).
- Imprinting results in the expression of a gene depending on the parent of origin. Examples are that of Prader Willi's and Angelman's syndromes, both of which are the result of uniparental disomy of chromosome 15, with the former derived maternally and the latter paternally.
- Contiguous gene syndromes result from a chromosomal deletion large enough to affect a number of genes along the chromosome (e.g. DiGeorge's syndrome).
- Mitochondrial inheritance occurs when there is an abnormality in mitochondrial DNA and primarily affects the energy metabolism of the individual. As cytoplasmic mitochondria are passed on through the ovum, these disorders are inherited maternally.

Table II: General aspects of selected congenital anomalies/syndromes

Clinical condition	Incidence	Genetic defect	Clinical features	Prenatal diagnosis	Recurrence risk (%)
Trisomy 21 Down's syndrome	• 1:800 live births	• Trisomy 21 (95%) • Translocation (4%) • Mosaicism (1%)	• Hypotonia • Facies: brachycephaly, small ears, upslanting palpebral fissures, flat nasal bridge, protruding tongue, Brushfield spots • Extremities: transverse palmar creases, fifth finger clinodactyly, large space between first and second toes • Congenital heart defects (40%) • IQ 25–50; premature senility	• Amniocentesis • Chorionic villus sampling • Triple screen: amniocentesis, chorionic villus sampling • Triple screen: AFP, hCG, estriol	• Trisomy: approximately 1% overall • Age specific risk: > 35 yr old • Translocation (4/21): maternal 5%, paternal 2%
Trisomy 18	• 1:8000 • Spontaneous abortion in 95% • Mortality rate: 50% in first 48 h, 90% in by 1 mo	• Trisomy 18 (> 90%) • Translocation (< 5%) • Mosaicism (rare)	• Hypertonia • IUGR • Facies: triangular face, small mouth • Short sternum • Extremities: clenched fist with second and fifth overlapping third and fourth fingers, absent distal flexion creases, nail hypoplasia • Increased association with congenital anomalies (such as omphalocele, esophageal atresia)	• Amniocentesis • Chorionic villus sampling • Ultrasound: IUGR	• < 1%

Clinical condition	Incidence	Genetic defect	Clinical features	Prenatal diagnosis	Recurrence risk (%)
Trisomy 13	• 1:25,000 • Spontaneous abortions in most • Mortality rate: 100% by 6 mo	• Trisomy (25%) • Unbalanced translocation (20%) • Mosaicism (5%)	• Severe CNS abnormality (such as holoprosencephaly) • Facies: microphthalmia, bulbous nasal tip, cleft lip and palate • Extremities: polydactyly • Congenital heart defect	• Amniocentesis • Chorionic villus sampling • Ultrasound	• < 1%
Turner's syndrome		• 45, X (50%) • 46, X, iso (Xq) (10%) • Mosaicism or other karyotypes (40%)	• Intellect normal • Short stature • Facies: laterally protruding ears, neck webbing, low posterior hair line • Extremities: edema of hands and feet at birth • Gonadal dysgenesis (streak gonads, infertility) • Congenital heart defects (especially coarctation 20%) and renal defects	• Amniocentesis • Chorionic villus sampling • Ultrasound	• Depends on karyotype
Klinefelter's syndrome		• 47, XXY	• Long legs, thin body habitus, prepubertal microrchidism • Mild intellectual impairment • Infertility expected	• Amniocentesis • Chorionic villus sampling	

Table II: (cont.) General aspects of selected congenital anomalies/syndromes

Clinical condition	Incidence	Genetic defect	Clinical features	Prenatal diagnosis	Recurrence risk (%)
Neurofibromatosis	• 1:3–5,000	• Autosomal dominant • Many cases are new mutations	• Café au lait spots, neurofibromas • Malignancies (5%) • Mental retardation (5%) • Learning disabilities (15%)	• Linking DNA markers possible in some	• 50%
Tuberous sclerosis		• Autosomal dominant • High mutation rate • 9q, 16p	• Hypopigmented skin macules • Mental retardation, seizures • Hamartomas: CNS, kidneys, heart	• DNA techniques	• 50%
Marfan's syndrome	• 1–2:100,000	• Autosomal dominant • 15–30% new mutations	• Tall stature • Arachnodactyly • Lens dislocation • Aortic root dilatation, mitral valve prolapse		• 50% for affected patients
Cystic fibrosis	• 1:2,000 in whites	• Autosomal recessive • 7q31 with single gene mutation in 70% (ΔF508)	• Pulmonary disease • Pancreatic insufficiency	• DNA techniques	• 25%
Sickle cell anemia	1:4–600 African–Americans	• Autosomal recessive • 11p	• Severe hemolytic anemia • Splenomegaly or infarction • Recurrent infectious	• DNA diagnosis	• 25%

Clinical condition	Incidence	Genetic defect	Clinical features	Prenatal diagnosis	Recurrence risk (%)
Tay–Sachs' disease	• 1:3,600 Ashkenazi Jewish population • Death by 3 yr of age	• Autosomal recessive • 15q23–q24	• Severe mental retardation and CNS deterioration • Enzyme analysis (hexosaminidase A)	• DNA techniques	• 25%
Fragile X syndrome	• 1:2,000 • 1:1,000 female carrier freq	• X-linked • Fragile site Xq27.3 • Over-amplification of CGG repeat segments of variable lengths	• Males: general overgrowth with prominent jaws and foreheads and large ears; postpubertal macrorchidism; hyperextensibility, high arched palate, flat feet, mitral valve prolapse; IQ 30–65; 20% are clinically and intellectually normal • Females: carriers may be normal (⅓), have learning disabilities (⅓), or be mildly retarded (⅓); 30% have clinical features similar to male carriers	• Cytogenic analysis • Molecular testing	
Hemophilia A	• 1/10,000 male carriers	• X-linked • Xq28	• Prolonged bleeding, bruising, joint and muscle hemorrhages • Deficiency of factor VIII	• DNA techniques	• 50% boys affected • 50% girls affected

Table II: (cont.) General aspects of selected congenital anomalies/syndromes

Clinical condition	Incidence	Genetic defect	Clinical features	Prenatal diagnosis	Recurrence risk (%)
Duchenne's muscular dystrophy	• 1:3,000 • New mutation (⅓) • Death in teens	• X–linked • Xp21 (many mutations)	• Progressive muscle weakness • Calf pseudohypertrophy • Elevated CPK, absent protein dystrophin in muscle	• DNA techniques	• 50% boys affected
Pyloric stenosis	• (M:F) 5:1	• Multifactorial inheritance			• Males affected: 2–5% • Females affected: 7–20%
Cleft lip ± palate	• (M:F) 1.6:1	• Multifactorial inheritance	• Unilateral CL: 4% • Unilateral CL + P: 5% • Bilateral CL: 6.7% • Bilateral CL + P: 8%		

APPROACH TO THE DYSMORPHIC CHILD

Important historical information

1. Pregnancy
- Ages of both parents and ethnicity.
- Length of gestation.
- Complications (bleeding, preterm labour, premature rupture of membranes, infections, other medical illnesses, fevers, hypertension, gestation diabetes).
- Onset and consistency of fetal movement.
- Diagnostic investigations (e.g. ultrasound, amniocentesis, chorionic villus sampling).
- Umbilical cord or placental pathology.

2. Postnatal
- Appearance of congenital anomaly and age at presentation.
- Review of symptoms, specifically related to the anomaly.
- Developmental milestones or intellectual abilities.
- Previous, present and future investigations, treatment, plans.

3. Previous pregnancy history
- Number and outcome (e.g. stillbirths, miscarriages, abortions, prematurity, live born).
- Diagnostic investigations.
- Complications.
- Family history: three generation pedigree, looking for
  Other family members with congenital anomalies.
  Medical illnesses or early death.
  Stillbirths or miscarriages.
  Consanguinity.

Physical examination

When assessing congenital anomalies, an accurate description of the malformation and surrounding structures is essential.
- Noted characteristics should include the size, shape, color, consistency of the anomaly as well as any additional malformations or birthmarks.
- Accurate anthropometric measurements are important, starting with weight, height/length and head circumference, and extending to characteristic facial (e.g. hypotelorism, short palpebral fissures) or other body features (e.g. short limbs, chest circumference). These measures can be compared to standardized tables in chapter 24 (Appendix).
- All organ systems should be carefully examined for associated anomalies not apparent from external features.

Concepts in approach

1. Variability
Individuals with the same disorder may differ considerably in structural anomalies. As such, a

specific anomaly, or lack there of, should not be relied upon for diagnosis.

2. Heterogeneity
The same structural anomaly may be characteristic or present in a number of disorders which is important for diagnosis, prognosis and recurrence risk counselling. For example, the anomalies included in the VACTERL association (vertebral, anal, cardiac, tracheoesophageal, renal, limb) may also be found in Fanconi anemia, an autosomal recessive disorder with guarded prognosis.

3. Using rarest feature
While some anomalies are common to many disorders, others are rare and limited to a small number of conditions. By using rarer malformations for investigation, there is a greater chance of arriving at the correct diagnosis.

4. Dating onset
In any case where diagnosis of a specific disorder is not possible, an attempt should be made to date the onset of each anomaly (prenatal, intrapartum or postnatal). Malformations that are due to defects in embryogenesis can be dated and events during that part of the pregnancy can be reviewed.

Diagnosis

1. Identification of all anomalies
The presence of one congenital anomaly increases the likelihood that other anomalies are present. As such, having identified one malformation, a careful search for others should be undertaken. This will be helpful for prognostic and treatment interventions as well as aiding in the diagnosis of the underlying condition.

2. Chromosomal analysis
- Routine chromosomal analysis is useful for evaluation of numerical and large structural abnormalities. It consists of a three day culture (a two day preliminary result may be requested) of peripheral blood lymphocytes. Light and dark banding pattern is characteristic for each chromosome.
- High resolution chromosomal analysis is a time consuming process that allows the detection of smaller structural abnormalities. Cell division is stopped earlier in mitoses with the chromosomes more elongated.
- Other tissues that are commonly used for chromosomal analysis include bone marrow (which provides immediate results), amniocytes and skin.

3. Special studies
- Fragile X–analysis uses culture media deficient in thymidine or folate, enhancing the fragile site. Molecular analysis is also available.
- Chromosomal fragility uses different techniques to enhance chromosomal fragility based on the disorder suspected (e.g. Fanconi anemia, Bloom's syndrome, ataxia telangiectasia).
- Fluorescent in situ hybridization (FISH) and chromosome painting are techniques that provide increased resolution of chromosomal structure.

4. Prenatal diagnosis
Prenatal diagnosis provides information to parents and medical personnel regarding the well being of the fetus. It may provide reassurance to high risk couples including those with increased risk for specific genetic disorders. While termination may be a consideration for a severe congenital condition, even when termination is not an option, the information obtained may help physicians plan for the labor and birth and may help parents prepare for the child's birth and postnatal care.
- Indications: advanced maternal age, other affected children or strong family history of genetic disorder, known structural chromosomal abnormality in parent.
- Techniques:
  Ultrasound is important for the assessment of morphological abnormality. Fetal age, growth and viability, as well as multiple pregnancy and the associated complications, can be accurately identified.
  Amniocentesis allows the analysis of chromosome number and structure. Amniotic fluid may be assessed for alpha$_1$–fetoprotein (AFP) levels, which may be elevated in twin pregnancies, fetal demise and fetal structural anomalies such as neural tube defects and abdominal wall abnormalities.
  Chorionic villus sampling (CVS) is performed earlier than amniocentesis and allows more time for decision making if abnormal results are discovered; however, amniotic fluid AFP levels cannot be assessed with this technique.
  Fetal blood sampling may be taken for chromosomal analysis and indications of fetal infection, including antibody titers.

Treatment

1. Medical/surgical
Surgery is possible for correction or palliation of many structural congenital anomalies. Multiple congenital anomaly disorders may require a multidisciplinary team.

2. Surveillance
Some congenital anomalies are associated with disorders that present outside of the neonatal period. For example, an infant born with aniridia has a greatly increased risk of developing Wilm's tumor. Regular abdominal ultrasounds would help to identify the tumor early, thus increasing survivability.

3. Gene therapy
For certain disorders resulting from the deficiency of a specific protein or gene product, replacement of that product may be possible in the future.

4. In utero fetal treatment
Therapeutic interventions are possible in utero when certain abnormalities are present. These include medical (e.g. digitalizing mothers when fetal supraventricular tachycardia is discovered) and surgical (e.g. decompressing urinary tract obstructions). Fetal bone marrow transplantation may permit engraftment of transplanted tissues prior to the development of immunocompetence.

Genetic counselling

Discussions with the family following the identification of a congenital anomaly are essential. Usually a number of sessions is required, depending on the significance of the anomaly and the individuals involved; the processing of the information provided may be limited initially. Therefore, accurate and timely information must be provided to the parents or guardians so that decisions regarding the affected child's care or treatment and/or future pregnancies may be made.

Recurrence risks

The risk of the recurrence of a particular anomaly will depend on its mode of inheritance (such as 25% for autosomal recessive conditions). While multifactorial inheritance is more difficult to predict, recurrence risks are available based on epidemiological studies (Tables II and III).

Table III: Other abnormalities

Abnormality	Normal parents affected child incidence	One affected parent risk for first child	Identical twin
Cleft lip and palate (1:1,000)	4%	3.2%	31%
Cleft palate alone (1:2,000)	2%	6%	40%
Club foot (1:2/1,000)	3%	3%	33%
Congenital heart disease: VSD PDA Tetralogy ASD	4–5% 1.4% 2–3% 3%	3–4% 2.8% 1.6% 3.5%	5:1,000 1:2,000 1:1,000 1:1,000
Neural tube defect British Columbia (1:700) Great Britain	2% 4.4%	2% 3%	21% 1:330
Congenital dislocated hip (2:1,000)	3.5%	3–5%	35%
Pyloric stenosis	3.2% brother affected 6.5% sister affected	4.2% father affected 25.4% mother affected	3:1,000
Scoliosis	7%	5%	20:1,000
Atopy (20–30:1,000)	5.8%		24%
Asthma (30–40:1,000)	10%	26%	
Idiopathic epilepsy	5%	5%	5:1,000
Down's syndrome	1%		1:1,000

NEONATOLOGY AND NEONATAL DRUG DOSAGE GUIDELINES CHAPTER 13
Susan Albersheim and Emily Ling

The following doctors contributed to the Neonatology chapter:
A. Antrim, Z. Cieslak, J. Eason, A. Kingo, K. Lannon, A. Leung, E. Ling, B. Lupton, T. Oberland, A. Solimano and A. Tang.

DELIVERY ROOM RESUSCITATION

Labor, delivery and the first minutes of life carry a high risk for asphyxia in the newborn. Anticipation and prompt skillful intervention can prevent the sequelae of asphyxia, minimizing neonatal morbidity and mortality.

The goals of resuscitation are to:
• Maintain body temperature within the normal range.
• Establish adequate respiratory function.
• Intervene early and prevent complications.

A minimum of two persons skilled in neonatal resuscitation should be immediately available for every birth. Personnel should seek periodic theoretical and practical training in this area.

The delivery room environment

• Thermoregulation is an immediate priority in managing any newborn. The delivery room area should be maintained draft free and at a temperature between 22 °C and 26 °C.
  This recommendation also applies to an Operating Room set up for a cesarean section.
• The level of lighting should be regulated. Low levels of lighting may be requested by the parents of well babies but should not affect the capacity of staff to observe the baby's color.
• The noise levels should be kept low.
• All equipment needed for neonatal resuscitation, including a wall clock with second hand, should be available, easily accessible and in good working order.
• Separate oxygen, air and suction outlets should be available for both mother and neonate.

Equipment list

• Overhead warmer: turn the warmer on prior to delivery. Ensure that a skin probe is available and the temperature control is set at 37 °C in automatic mode. Check alarm function.
• Oxygen source: verify the oxygen source. If a blender is available, set it to provide 100% O_2. Verify that oxygen tanks are full or contain no less than 1 hour of use at 10 L/min. This corresponds to 100 psi in a size E tank. Oxygen delivered to the free flow oxygen mask or tubing and to the bagging system should be set at a flow of 5 L/min. Ensure that self–inflating bags are connected to an appropriate reservoir, otherwise they will not provide close to 100% oxygen.
• Positive pressure source: check connections to oxygen source and pressure gauge. Check that the pressure relief valve in self–inflating bags "pops" at pressure between 35 and 45 cm H_2O.

Check that oxygen is flowing to the bag by confirming that the reservoir is inflated.
- Masks: face masks should cover from the chin to the bridge of the nose but not reach the eyes.
- Suction: a #10 Argyle catheter should be attached to the suction tubing and a vacuum pressure of 100 mm Hg preset.
- Intubation equipment: equipment should be assembled before delivery. Choose appropriate laryngoscope blade and test the light source. If planning to use a stylet, place it inside the endotracheal tube and ensure that its tip is 0.5 cm proximal to the tip of the tube. Always have the suction system ready before attempting intubation.
- Resuscitation drugs and intravenous equipment: drugs are seldom needed in neonatal resuscitation. They do not need to be set up routinely but ensure they, and means for administration, are accessible and current.
- Gloves: we recommend that gloves be routinely worn to handle the newborn at the time of delivery.

Anticipation of problems

Babies most likely to need resuscitation are called "high risk". The following constitute high risk conditions: gestational age < 34 weeks, multiple pregnancy < 37 weeks, severe intrauterine growth retardation (IUGR), severe oligohydramnios, severe perinatal infections, severe congenital anomalies, fetal distress, meconium, prolapsed cord, hydrops fetalis, severe hemolytic disease, twin–to–twin transfusion syndrome.

Establishment of adequate cardiorespiratory function

At every delivery, the heart rate, respiratory effort, color (oxygen requirement), muscle tone and reflex activity are determined and recorded as an Apgar score at 1 and 5 minutes.

If the infant needs resuscitation, three parameters of the Apgar score must be checked without delay and served as an ongoing guide to resuscitation requirements (Tables I and II):
- Respirations: Is the baby breathing?
- Heart rate: What is the heart rate?
- Color: Is there central cyanosis?

Table I: Initial resuscitation of the newborn

Assessment	Action
Regular breathing and central cyanosis	Free flow oxygen
Apnea after stimulation or heart rate < 100 beat/min	Positive pressure
Positive pressure ventilation for 30 s and heart rate < 60 beat/min or heart rate 60–80 beat/min and not increasing	Cardiac compressions
Heart rate is 0 or heart rate < 80 beat/min after 30 s of positive pressure and cardiac compressions	Epinephrine

1. Airway
- To achieve this, place the infant's head in a semi–extended or "sniffing" position and suction the oropharynx. Avoid hyperextension or flexion of the neck as this can obstruct the airway.
- If a patent airway cannot be established by positioning and suctioning of the baby, endotracheal intubation must be performed.

2. Breathing
- If the airway is patent but respiratory effort is insufficient, or if the heart rate is < 100 beat/min, positive pressure ventilation should be commenced with 100% oxygen and a face mask. Begin with inspiratory pressures of 20–30 cm H_2O and a rate of 40 breath/min.
- Observe the baby's chest for symmetrical chest wall movement and auscultate to ensure equal breath sounds bilaterally. The heart rate should rapidly rise over 100 beat/min and the child's color improve from blue or pale to pink.
- If the heart rate remains < 100 beat/min and/or no chest expansion, check:
    Seal: ensure that a good seal exists between mask and face.
    Airway: reposition the head to the "sniffing position". Suction the upper airway if secretions are present. Ensure the baby's mouth is slightly open (consider use of oral airway).
    Pressure: increase pressure to 30–40 cm H_2O.
    If this sequence fails, intubate and provide positive pressure ventilation and 100% oxygen until the baby is pink.

Table II: The Apgar score

Sign	0	1	2
Heart rate	Absent	< 100	> 100
Respiratory effort	Absent	Slow, irregular	Good crying
Muscle tone	Limp	Some flexion of extremities	Active motion
Reflex irritability	No response	Grimace	Cough or sneeze
Color	Blue, pale	Body pink, extremities blue	Completely pink

- Withdrawal of positive pressure support should be gradual to allow for assessment of the baby's respiratory effort and regularity.
- The stomach may become distended with air after prolonged positive pressure ventilation with face mask; a 8 Fr. feeding tube should be inserted and aspirated intermittently with a 10–20 mL syringe to prevent regurgitation.
- Indications for intubation:
    Failure to establish adequate gas exchange with a bag and mask.
    Need for prolonged positive pressure ventilation.
    In the presence of thick or particulate meconium (for efficient airway suctioning).
- When attending the delivery of premature infants, particularly those ≤ 1,000 grams, ≤ 28 weeks gestation or those with respiratory distress, it is important to anticipate that they are prone to respiratory failure. In these circumstances, early intubation may be beneficial.

3. Circulation
- Cardiac massage is seldom needed in neonatal resuscitation. The most common cause of severe persistent bradycardia in the newborn is hypoxia. Establishment of adequate airway and ventilation is mandatory to improve circulatory status. Cardiac massage should not be performed during intubation.
- There are two methods of external cardiac massage in the newborn:
    With both hands encircling the chest, the fingers support the back and the thumbs compress the sternum. Do not apply pressure to the ribs. This is the most comfortable method and the one that is likely to achieve the highest cardiac output.
    Place the infant on a firm surface and compress the chest with the first two fingertips. Use this method when the fingers cannot reach the paravertebral area to support the back or when trying to access the umbilical cord.
- Pressure is applied over the lower third of the sternum, under the nipple level. Avoid the xiphoid where abdominal organ damage may result.
- Compressions should be 1–2 cm in depth, with the compression and relaxation phases given equal time ("sinus wave pattern").
- Recommendations regarding the compression–ventilation sequence for newborns are that 3 compressions be followed by a pause to allow delivery of an effective breath. The rate of compressions combined with ventilation should be 120/min which will result in 90 compressions and 30 breaths each minute.
- Effectiveness of cardiac massage should be assessed by palpating the umbilical or femoral pulses.
- The heart rate should be checked after 30 seconds of chest compressions; discontinue compressions after the heart rate reaches 80 beat/min.

Drugs and volume expanders

Drugs and volume expanders are uncommonly needed during resuscitation of the newborn (Table III). Their usefulness is limited to situations where prolonged resuscitation has occurred.

Table III: Resuscitation drug doses in the newborn

Drugs/ETT	1 kg	2 kg	3 kg	4 kg
ETT (size)	2.5	3.0	3.0	3.5
Epinephrine (mL) (1:10,000) i.v. or ETT	0.3	0.6	0.9	1.2
Bicarbonate (mL) (4.2%) UV, i.v.	4	8	12	16
Volume expander (mL) UA, UV, i.v.	10	20	30	40
Narcan (mL) (1 mg/mL) UA, UV, i.v., ETT, i.m.,s.c.	0.1	0.2	0.3	0.4

UA/UV = umbilical artery/vein

Evaluation

Most newborns respond quickly to normal resuscitation techniques. If a child is still cyanosed after intubation, then a careful examination should be conducted to determine the cause. The main culprits will be either complications of delivery or resuscitation (pneumothorax or blood loss) or underlying developmental problems (diaphragmatic hernia, congenital heart disease).

Check:
- Is the endotracheal tube in the trachea?
    Mist should be seen in the ETT on expiration.
    Chest should expand with positive pressure.
    Air entry should be equal and symmetrical over the chest.
    Abdomen should not become distended.
    If still in doubt, confirm ETT position with laryngoscope.
- Are there any mechanical problems with ventilation?
    Check that oxygen source is on.
    If manometer is registering, check the pressure being delivered.
    If using a self–inflating bag, check that reservoir is present and inflated.
- Is there right main stem bronchus intubation?
    Black line in ETT should be at level of vocal cords.
    Centimeter mark at lips (rule of thumb: 8 cm for 1 kg baby; 9 cm for 2 kg; 10 cm for 3 kg).
    Air entry is decreased on the left side.
- Is there airway obstruction?
    Air entry usually decreased in spite of high pressures.
    Adventitious chest sounds may be present.
    Precordium usually in midline.
    Baby is more hypercarbic than hypoxic.
    If suspected cause is a plug, suction using ETT; plugs are associated with meconium at birth and severe oligohydramnios.
    If suspected cause is anatomical (vascular rings, tracheomalacia, etc.), attempt bypassing affected area, advancing ETT to near carina.
- Is there acute bleeding or volume depletion?
    History of maternal bleeding, evidence of placental abruption or previa, site of bleeding present in infant. All may be absent in feto–maternal bleed.
    Air entry and chest expansion are usually good.
    Peripheral perfusion is poor; capillary refill is slow (> 3 seconds).
    Pulse is difficult to palpate.
    Heart sounds distant.
    Marked metabolic acidosis is present.
- Is infection a possibility?
    History of prolonged rupture of membranes or maternal infection.
    Air entry and chest expansion are usually good.
    Peripheral perfusion is poor; capillary refill is slow (> 3 seconds).
    Metabolic acidosis may be present.
- Is there a pneumothorax?
    Is precordium in the midline (more likely to be shifted to the left as right–sided pneumothorax is more common during resuscitation).
    Occurs more commonly in preterm infants with respiratory distress syndrome or term infants with meconium aspiration syndrome, but spontaneous pneumothorax in nonresuscitated infants may occasionally occur.

- Is there a diaphragmatic hernia?
    Air entry is more commonly decreased in the left side.
    Is precordium in the midline (more likely to be shifted to the right as 90% of diaphragmatic hernias occur in the left side).
    Scaphoid abdomen is characteristic.
    More common in term than preterm infants; normal obstetrical history, sometimes history of polyhydramnios and borderline small for gestational age.
    Baby tends to be more hypoxic than hypercarbic.
    Avoid positive pressure with mask.
- Is there lung hypoplasia?
    Air entry usually decreased in spite of high pressures.
    Precordium is in midline.
    Baby has severe hypercarbia and hypoxia.
    It is a diagnosis of exclusion.
    Associations: severe prolonged oligohydramnios (rupture of membranes before 25 weeks, fetal renal malformation, severe fetal neuromuscular disease).
    Chest X–ray: lungs usually clear but small; in neuromuscular disease, fine tubular ribs are often seen.

After a successful resuscitation, the infant should not be assumed to be normal. Trained observers should carefully monitor the baby in a special area.

Prevention of meconium aspiration syndrome (MAS)

The main goal in prevention of MAS should be to minimize intrauterine hypoxia, which is now accepted to result not only in passage and aspiration of meconium (in utero and during birth) but also in pulmonary arteriolar muscularization that makes babies prone to pulmonary hypertension.

As secondary prevention, aggressive and effective intervention at the time of birth is thought to have greatly reduced the incidence and severity of MAS.

- In the presence of thick particulate meconium, the physician delivering the baby must suction the pharynx of the baby at the perineum as soon as the head is delivered and before the rest of the body is born. This may be the most important step in the meconium prevention sequence during birth. Suctioning is best done by inserting a finger in the baby's mouth and guiding a 10 Fr. catheter connected to 100 mm Hg wall suction to the infant's pharynx. A bulb syringe is inadequate for suctioning meconium.
- Immediately after delivery, and before drying or any other maneuver, insert a laryngoscope and suction the pharynx under direct vision. While doing this, it may be possible to pass the suction catheter between the vocal cords and suction the trachea.
- Suctioning below the vocal cords can be done more easily by intubating and applying suction on the ETT. Because of concerns about transmission of infection to the operator, an adaptor should be used such as the meconium aspirator, which allows direct connection of the suction line to the ETT adaptor.
- Suction catheters inserted through the ETT are inadequate unless the baby has been intubated with a 3.5 ETT and the catheter being used is a 10 Fr. (catheters smaller than 10 Fr. are too small to effectively suction thick meconium).

- If meconium is obtained from below the vocal cords, suctioning may be repeated if the baby tolerates it. Suctioning once is usually sufficient to clear most of the meconium in the airway when continuous wall suction is used and when thorough suctioning at the perineum has already been done.
- Following this, the infant will require positive pressure ventilation to allow prompt recovery and achieve adequate oxygenation.
- Remember, the stomach may be full of meconium and should be suctioned before the baby leaves the delivery room area.
- The presence of watery meconium stained amniotic fluid does not require endotracheal intubation.
- The procedure in a vigorously crying baby born in the presence of thick meconium is controversial. Provided there has been adequate suction "at the perineum", we currently do not recommend routine tracheal suctioning of these babies. Suction below the vocal cords only if, under direct laryngoscopic vision, meconium is seen in the pharynx.

RESPIRATORY DISEASES OF THE NEWBORN

Respiratory distress syndrome (RDS)

This presents as patchy atelectasis due to surfactant deficiency with capillary exudative leak (hyaline membranes).

1. Predisposing factors
- Prematurity.
- Perinatal asphyxia.
- Hypovolemia and hypothermia.
- Maternal diabetes.
- Incidence and severity reduced by prenatal steroids administered 1–7 days before delivery, prior to 34 weeks gestation.

2. Diagnosis
- Tachypnea starting within 4 hours of birth.
- Expiratory grunting and costal recession.
- Often cyanosed, requiring oxygen.
- Chest X–ray: reticulogranular pattern with air bronchogram.

3. Treatment (initial management)
- Respiratory:
    Check saturations are between 88 and 95% and supply humidified oxygen if they are lower. If FiO_2 is > 40% or the child is ventilated, then an arterial line should be inserted (usually in the umbilical artery). Nasal or nasopharyngeal CPAP at 4–8 mm Hg may be tried before intermittent positive pressure ventilation (IPPV) when there is only moderate respiratory distress.
    Intubation required if:
    Severe respiratory distress.
    Moderate distress with increasing respiratory acidosis with pH < 7.25 and CO_2 > 55–60.

Increasing oxygen requirements (FiO_2 > 60% in an infant < 1,500 grams and > 80% in an infant > 1,500 grams).
Suggested ventilation settings:
IPPV rate 40–60/min; inspiratory time 0.35–0.5 second; PIP 18–24 mm Hg (set to obtain moderate chest expansion); PEEP 4–6 mm Hg.
Monitor blood gases, initially every 4 hours if ventilated.
Consider surfactant if patient requires ventilation and supplemental O_2, (usually the arterial–alveolar PO_2 ratio < 0.22).
- Sedation: asynchronous infants are more difficult to ventilate. This may be caused by a high pCO_2, which should be corrected. Other strategies are to try and match the baby's respiratory rate with the ventilator or to use sedation. Rarely paralysis is indicated.
- Routine: maintain neutral thermal environment and check glucose and calcium.
- Fluids: provide intravenous fluids and keep n.p.o. until respiratory distress is settled enough to start enteral feeds.
- Cardiovascular: check hematocrit and give blood if below 0.4. Maintain normal blood pressure with volume expanders 5% albumen or normal saline 10–15 mL/kg. Consider fresh frozen plasma if sepsis suspected. Consider dopamine.
- Sepsis: difficult to differentiate RDS from early pneumonia, particularly group B, beta hemolytic *Streptococcus*, therefore, take blood cultures, WBC and differential. Start on ampicillin and gentamicin.

4. Continued management
- It is not necessary to aim for a normal pH unless there is also significant pulmonary hypertension. Do no harm—hyaline membrane disease is usually a self–limiting disease. Respiratory progress can be monitored with blood gases as well as transcutaneous CO_2 and saturation monitor.
- Maintain: pH > 7.25; pCO_2 40–60 mm Hg; PaO_2 50–80 mm Hg.
- Natural history is for improvement around day 2 or 3, however, may be quicker with surfactant.
- Falling FiO_2 requirement and increasing urine output usually indicate improvement allowing weaning.
- Initially, reduce PIP, followed by rate, aiming to extubate from a rate of 10–15 breath/min.

Pneumonia

Pneumonia may be acquired transplacentally (usually viral or *Listeria* monocytogenes) or during labor and delivery. Further discussion is limited to ascending infection which is more common and usually caused by group B *Streptococcus* or Gram negative bacteria.

1. Predisposing factors
- Prolonged rupture of membranes.
- Maternal intrapartum fever.
- Maternal group B *Streptococcus* carriage.

2. Diagnosis
- Respiratory distress.
- Associated signs of sepsis with fever, shock, apnea.

- Chest X–ray: group B *Streptococcus* may give a picture indistinguishable from RDS.

3. Management
- Respiratory support as for RDS.
- Septic screen with blood cultures and full blood count. Note low WBC seen in overwhelming infection. Lumbar puncture may need to be delayed until child is stable.
- Antibiotics: meningitic doses of ampicillin and gentamicin until cultures available.

Meconium aspiration syndrome (MAS)

Meconium stained amniotic fluid occurs in about 8–10% of all deliveries. However, only a small percentage of them develop MAS.

1. Diagnosis
- Respiratory distress.
- Presence of meconium below vocal cords at birth.
- Chest X–ray may show patchy areas of increased density or hyperinflation. There may be complications of pneumothorax or pneumomediastinum.

2. Treatment
- Mildly affected infants may just need supplemental oxygen. However, infants often develop persistent pulmonary hypertension or air leak complications which will require more aggressive support.
- Blood cultures and antibiotics should be given because of risk of underlying infection in respiratory distress.

Pulmonary air leak syndromes

Gas leaking out of an alveolus rarely ruptures subpleurally but instead may accumulate in the interstitial space, causing pulmonary interstitial emphysema. It may, however, track along the bronchovascular bundles to the mediastinum to cause a pneumomediastinum. From there, it can rupture into the pleural cavity to give a pneumothorax or into the pericardium to cause a pneumopericardium. Rarely, gas dissects through to the peritoneum.

Spontaneous pneumothorax occurs in 1–2% of "normal" babies, however, the incidence is higher in the following situations:
- After resuscitation with bag and mask or ETT.
- Meconium aspiration or severe RDS.
- Mechanical ventilation with IPPV and/or PEEP.

1. Pulmonary interstitial emphysema
- Diagnosis: made on chest X–ray usually following deterioration in infant's respiratory status with increasing hypoxia and hypercapnia. Chest X–ray shows round or linear lucencies, particularly at the periphery of the bronchovascular tree. May be generalized or focal.
- Management:
  Try to oxygenate adequately by increasing FiO_2. Try to reduce ventilatory settings (PIP,

PEEP and inspiratory time), accepting higher CO_2 if maintaining pH > 7.25.
Position infant with affected lobes down.
Consider trial of high frequency ventilation and dexamethasone.

2. Pneumothorax
- Significance of a pneumothorax depends on the degree of tension it is under and the amount of respiratory distress it is causing.
- Small nontension pneumothorax in an infant with minimal or no respiratory distress and no significant underlying lung disease may be left to resolve spontaneously. If the baby is not at risk of retinopathy of prematurity, then resolution can be speeded up with a high inspired oxygen concentration.

3. Tension pneumothorax
- Diagnosis:
  Sudden deterioration in a child's respiratory and/or cardiovascular status.
  Shift of heart sounds more noticeable with a left–sided pneumothorax.
  Abdominal distension due to diaphragm being pushed down; abdomen may look asymmetrical.
  Transillumination of chest with a bright light source.
  Chest X–ray: mediastinal shift and distortion of diaphragm are better indicators of the degree of intrapleural tension than the volume of extrapulmonary gas.
  (Note: clinical signs and symptoms may be absent in a baby receiving high frequency ventilation.)
- Management:
  Tension pneumothoraces require draining quickly. As an emergency procedure, aspiration with a syringe and butterfly needle can be done as long as it is followed by insertion of a chest tube. If the baby is more stable, a chest tube is the treatment of choice. (Use of trocar is not recommended because of risk of injury to the lung. Sufficient skin incision should be made so that curved forceps can be tunnelled over the underlying rib and into the pleural space. Positioning should be along the anterior clavicular line and the chest tube positioned anteriorly.)
  Repeat chest X–ray to assess re–expansion of lung. A lateral X–ray will show whether the chest tube is anteriorly or posteriorly placed. May need to position the patient in order for the chest tube to evacuate the collection of air.
  Check blood pressure and perfusion and correct with albumen as required
  Consider head ultrasound (significant association between tension pneumothorax and IVH).

4. Pneumomediastinum
- Diagnosis: made on chest X–ray. A lateral chest film is often helpful.
- Management: infants are usually asymptomatic. A pneumomediastinum cannot be drained.

5. Pneumopericardium
- Diagnosis: often an incidental finding in a child with a large air leak but may occasionally present with sudden and profound hypotension, distant heart sounds and arrest if left untreated. Chest X–ray characteristically shows a ring of air around the heart.
- Management: emergency treatment consists in removing the air by inserting a catheter into the

pericardial sac by subxiphoid approach, but only if clinically necessary.

6. Pneumoperitoneum
Air from a tension pneumothorax sometimes tracks retroperitoneally or may also pass directly into the peritoneum through small diaphragmatic defects. The gas usually resolves spontaneously but it should be differentiated from a ruptured bowel.

Persistent pulmonary hypertension

The pulmonary artery pressure usually falls rapidly following institution of normal respiration. In many seriously ill neonates, this fails to happen (sepsis, meconium aspiration, congenital heart disease). Subsequently, right to left shunting at atrial level and through a patent ductus arteriosus produces cyanosis and acidosis.

1. Predisposing factors
- Perinatal asphyxia, meconium aspiration, diaphragmatic hernia, pneumonia or severe RDS, polycythemia.
- More common in the term infant.
- May be transient but often is not. It is impossible to predict the severity.

2. Diagnosis
- Cyanosis unresponsive to oxygen.
- Difference between pre– and postductal PaO_2 > 10–15 mm Hg on blood gases.
- Chest X–ray may be normal or represent the predisposing cause.

3. Treatment (initial management)
- Ventilate with 100% oxygen, aiming for PaO_2 > 100 mm Hg, $PaCO_2$ 30–40 mm Hg.
- Maintain a metabolic alkalosis with infusion of sodium bicarbonate, starting with 1 mmol/kg per h.
- Sedation with fentanyl and paralysis with pancuronium.
- Cardiovascular: maintain blood pressure at upper limit of normal. Term infant: 45–55 mm Hg. Initially give 10–20 mL/kg albumen, followed by dopamine 5 kg/min, increasing to 20 µg/kg per min as required. Perform an echocardiogram to exclude congenital heart disease (also to assess pulmonary pressures and cardiac contractility). Consider epinephrine or dobutamine if contractility is poor.
- Vascular access: arterial line and double lumen umbilical venous catheter are usually required.
- Routine care: check CBC, differential, platelets, calcium and glucose. Use a urinary catheter to monitor urine output. Consider exogenous surfactant ± nitric oxide ± dexamethasone for very sick infants. Monitor oxygen index (OI):

$$OI = \frac{Paw \times FiO_2 \times 100}{PaO_2}$$

to assess treatment (Paw = mean airway pressure).
- Sepsis: give ampicillin and gentamicin after taking blood cultures.

Transient tachypnea of the newborn

Mild self–limiting respiratory distress is thought to be due to slow resorption of lung fluid which can occur in term and preterm infants.

1. Predisposing factors
- Cesarean section (particularly if mother is not in labor).
- Congenital hypothyroidism.

2. Diagnosis
- Tachypnea with minimal recession or grunting.
- Chest X–ray shows increased perihilar marking with fluid in pleural fissures and blunting of diaphragm.

3. Treatment
- Check oxygen saturations as sometimes require supplemental oxygen (occasionally require ventilation).
- Blood cultures and antibiotics should be considered for a child with marked respiratory distress or any risk factors for sepsis, i.e. maternal fever, prolonged rupture of membranes or maternal group B, beta hemolytic *Streptococcus* carriage.
- Fluids: provide intravenous fluids and keep n.p.o. until respiratory distress is settled enough to start enteral feeds.

Apnea of prematurity

Premature infants often have periodic breathing with short pauses between breaths which are normal. Longer periods of apnea over 10–15 seconds, particularly associated with bradycardias and desaturations, are a problem with decreasing gestational age.

1. Underlying causes need to be considered and excluded on an individual basis
- Infection: septicemia, meningitis, necrotizing enterocolitis.
- Respiratory: hypoxemia from lung disease or upper airway obstruction.
- Cardiovascular: heart failure, especially secondary to PDA.
- Metabolic: hypoglycemia, hypocalcemia, metabolic acidosis.
- Central nervous system: seizures.
- Thermal: incubator temperature high or low.
- Maternal drugs: opiates and magnesium sulfate.

2. Management
- The majority of apneas will correct with cutaneous stimulation of infant's back, however, sometimes mask IPPV is required.
- Prevention of further apnea needs to be addressed:
      Correction of any underlying causes.
      Consider stopping feeds.
      Theophylline i.v. or p.o. Aim for a trough level of 55–70 µmol/L.
      Apnea mattress.

Oxygen may help apneas.
Nasal CPAP around 6 mm Hg.
IPPV may be required.

Bronchopulmonary dysplasia (BPD)

There is no single satisfactory definition of BPD and neonatal chronic lung disease is probably a better description. The majority of these infants have had mechanical ventilation, required prolonged supplemental oxygen for 28 days and have an abnormal chest X–ray. Occasionally, chronic progressive lung disease develops in a premature infant without a preceding history of mechanical ventilation. The ultimate radiological appearances are identical to BPD. Slow resolution after the age of 6–12 months is the usual course. Several terms are used, including Mikity–Wilson's syndrome and chronic pulmonary insufficiency of prematurity.

The chest X–ray findings include cardiomegaly, emphysema, hyperexpansion, fibrosis or interstitial abnormalities. These findings may be categorized as mild, moderate or severe.

1. Predisposing factors
- Prematurity particularly < 28 weeks.
- Mechanical ventilation and barotrauma.
- PDA and fluid overload have been associated with BPD.
- Oxygen toxicity.
- Inflammation and infection.

2. Management
- Therapy is aimed at maintaining adequate oxygenation while trying to minimize barotrauma and oxygen toxicity. This means accepting higher pCO_2 if pH is compensated.
- Prompt treatment of PDA.
- Pulmonary edema is often a complication requiring diuretics, either furosemide (short–term) or spironolactone and hydrochlorthiazide (long–term).
- Steroids:
    Dexamethasone improves pulmonary mechanics and facilitates weaning from mechanical ventilation. However, potential serious side effects mean that its use should be limited to the more severe cases.
    Use of inhaled steroids (budesonide) may be beneficial with fewer side effects.
- Bronchodilation with specific beta–2 agonists (salbutamol) is helpful in patients with evidence of air trapping.
- Deterioration in respiratory status may reflect infection.
    Investigate with blood count and blood cultures followed by broad spectrum antibiotics.
    Search for *Ureaplasma urealyticum* and consider treating if present. Respiratory viruses should be considered in older infants.
- Nutrition:
    Infants with BPD require increased calories to grow and therefore need high calorie intake (120–150 Cal/kg per d).
    As fluid overload may be a problem, enteral feedings with higher caloric content should be considered.

NEUROLOGICAL DISEASES OF THE NEWBORN

Perinatal asphyxia

An asphyxial insult occurs when there is lack of oxygen (hypoxia) and/or lack of blood flow (ischemia). In practice, such insults comprise, in varying degrees, components of both hypoxia and ischemia (hypoxic–ischemic insult). When of sufficient magnitude, a hypoxic–ischemic insult will lead to injury which may be transient or permanent. Although brain injury is usually the paramount concern, all organs may sustain injury.

The type, extent and clinical presentation of injury from a given insult are potentially altered by a number of factors:

- Gestational age (term or preterm): different regions of the brain are most vulnerable to HIE insult at different gestational ages due to differences in brain blood flow patterns, metabolic rate and tissue composition. Clinical signs of encephalopathy are less apparent at lower gestational ages.
- Acuity of insult: different patterns of brain injury are predicted by variation in the insult such as total acute, partial prolonged, etc.
- Temporal relationship of insult to delivery: an interval between insult and delivery may affect need for resuscitation at birth and clinical features and temporal pattern of encephalopathy.
- Nature of the insult: predominantly hypoxic or predominantly ischemic.

The constellation of abnormal neurological signs resulting from an HIE insult is called hypoxic–ischemic encephalopathy. Although HIE brain injury can occur in the absence of encephalopathy (e.g. the preterm), the vast majority of term newborns sustaining permanent HIE brain injury close to the time of delivery have obvious encephalopathy. In clinical practice, the diagnosis of perinatal asphyxia is not based on the presence of any single finding but rather on the summation of historical, clinical and investigational findings which support this diagnosis and exclude other potential differential diagnoses. Indeed, it may be useful to consider HIE as a diagnosis of exclusion. This clinical approach prevents unwarranted assumptions that the cause of a neonatal encephalopathy is perinatal asphyxia. Commonly considered differential diagnoses include sepsis (meningitis, encephalitis), hypoglycemia, electrolyte disorders, inborn errors of metabolism, intracranial hemorrhage (including traumatic), congenital infection and congenital structural brain abnormalities.

1. Management of asphyxia

Preventive measures are a key component of an effective management strategy. Easy access to good antenatal care and a population highly receptive to this care, along with optimal management of labor and delivery, reduces the risks for perinatal asphyxia. Preventive measures include ensuring that resuscitation equipment and personnel trained in its use are available for each delivery. Where additional neonatal care is required, it should be accessible and safely practiced.

2. Identification of asphyxia

Early recognition of the occurrence of a hypoxic–ischemic insult assists management. Consequently, antenatal risk factors should be noted (e.g. late deceleration of fetal heart rate) and the condition of the newborn assessed at delivery (e.g. cord gas, need for and response to resuscitation, etc.). Although low cord pH and low Apgar scores at 1 and 5 minutes do not accurately define infants with HIE injury (most such infants are normal), these assessment tools identify a subgroup at higher risk of sequelae. This is particularly so when profound metabolic acidosis or protracted low Apgar scores are noted. Following resuscitation, newborns at risk should be observed for potential multi–organ injuries. Serial clinical examination will identify signs of encephalopathy.

3. Management of hypoxic–ischemic encephalopathy
• Correct hypoxic–ischemic insult:
   Correct blood gas (ventilation, volume, bicarbonate).
   Correct intravascular volume (5% albumin, packed cells, plasma, normal saline).
   Ensure adequate blood pressure (volume, inotropes such as dopamine 5–20 mg/kg per min).
   Correct significant anemia.
• Prevent additional insults:
   Ensure thermoregulation.
   Continuously monitor vital signs.
   Monitor renal, cardiac, pulmonary lung and other organ function.
   Monitor and maintain electrolytes (Na^+, K^+, Ca^{2+}, Mg^{2+}) in normal range.
   Monitor and maintain blood sugar in normal range (serum glucose levels may be increased or decreased following asphyxia due to varying effects on glyconeogenesis and utilization).
   Observe and monitor for coagulopathy (platelet count, PT, PTT).
   Increased risk for intestinal ischemia (ileus, NEC). Consider delay in oral feeding. (Although therapies which may decrease brain edema have been identified, it is currently unclear whether resultant reduction in edema confers any benefit for outcome. A more fruitful avenue for potential intervention involves blocking the biochemical cascade, which occurs some hours after asphyxia and leads to later cell death. Animal studies are in progress using glutamate antagonists, calcium channel blockade and free radical scavengers, and inhibitors in an attempt to modify this injurious biochemical cascade.)
• Respiratory intensive care:
   May be required because asphyxia destroys surfactant and leads to atelectasis; there are risks for associated aspiration of meconium. Asphyxia may also cause myocardial injury, leading to heart failure and consequent respiratory embarrassment.
   Hypoxic–ischemic insult may contribute to pulmonary arteriolar constriction and persistent pulmonary hypertension of the newborn (PPHN).
   Blood gas targets for ventilation PCO_2 35–45 mm Hg, oxygen saturation 88–95%, PO_2 50–80 mm Hg (except PPHN).
   Monitor for cardiac dysfunction and support poor myocardial contractility.
• Restrict fluids (50 mL/kg per d):
   Risk of inappropriate antidiuretic hormone (ADH) or acute renal failure.
   Follow weight, input/output, serum Na^+, K^+, BUN. Avoid added Na^+, K^+ or accumulation of drugs eliminated in urine. May slowly increase fluids if urine output and electrolytes are stable.
• Treat seizures:
   Load with phenobarbital 20 mg/kg i.v.
   If seizures persist, either give additional phenobarbital intravenously in 5 mg/kg aliquots to

maximum total dose of 40 mg/kg or phenytoin 20 mg/kg i.v.
Monitor anticonvulsant levels.
- Assess etiology:
  HIE is a diagnosis of exclusion. Differential diagnosis includes congenital abnormality of
  the brain, intracranial hemorrhage, sepsis, metabolic disease.
  Complete history.
  Serial neurological examination.
  Examination for dysfunction of other organs and structural abnormalities.
  Consider imaging studies (head ultrasound scan on day 1 is usually appropriate).
  Consider lumbar puncture or metabolic studies (e.g. ammonia, lactate).
  Neurology consultation.
- Assess prognosis:
  Because the severity of hypoxic–ischemic encephalopathy has prognostic significance,
  careful and serial clinical examinations (including fontanelle tension) are of importance.
  Clinical features of mild, moderate and severe HIE and associated outcomes are listed
  below (Table IV).
  The use of adjunct investigations has a role in the assessment of the extent of brain injury.
  Such investigations include CT or MR scanning, intracranial pressure monitoring, imaging
  of brain with ultrasound, assessment of electrophysiological function using EEG or evoked
  potentials, and assessment of brain blood flow using Doppler ultrasound, nuclear medicine
  studies or near infrared spectroscopy.
  Consider paired day 1 and day 3 head ultrasound scans imaged using identical equipment
  settings. EEG. CT scan 72 ± 12 hours after the insult. (In the asphyxiated term newborn,
  significant brain swelling indicates irreversible injury, consequently, investigations which
  can identify the presence of brain swelling have prognostic utility. A CT scan at 72 ± 12
  hours, demonstrating generalized decreased attenuation (greatly increased brain water
  content), has been shown to correlate with a poor long–term outcome.

Table IV: Prognostic clinical signs following hypoxic–ischemic encephalopathy

Severity	Features	Outcome
Mild	Hyperalert, brisk reflexes, sympathetic stimulation, < 24 h duration	Good prognosis
Moderate	Lethargy or stupor, hypotonia, suppressed primitive reflexes, seizures	20–30% die or have permanent neurological abnormalities
Severe	Coma, flaccid, suppressed brain stem function, seizures, increased intracranial pressure	Vast majority die or have permanent neurological abnormalities

- Follow–up:
  Undertake serial assessments of growth (including head circumference) and development
  (motor, intellectual and behavioral function, vision and hearing).
  Provide feedback to parents about assessment findings and prognosis.
  Arrange for appropriate developmental interventions (e.g. developmental physiotherapy).
  Review risks for seizures, decisions regarding anticonvulsants.

Consider follow–up EEG or brain imaging studies.

Neonatal seizures

Seizures are a common sign of serious neurological disease in both the term and preterm newborn. It is important to begin diagnosis and treatment early since delays can have adverse implications. Studies suggest ongoing seizure activity can potentiate further neuronal injury.

Clinical presentation in the newborn varies somewhat from that in older age groups. A summary of the principle seizure types are listed in Table V.

1. Jitteriness
- Jitteriness should be differentiated from seizures.
- Jitteriness has a tremor–like appearance, is stimulus sensitive and can be stopped by flexing the affected limb.
- EEG recordings assist in the diagnosis of a neonatal seizure disorder.

2. Etiology
- Studies of etiology of neonatal seizures have defined a long differential diagnosis. Sometimes more than one factor is involved in the genesis of the seizure. The most common association which has been identified is hypoxic–ischemic brain injury, accounting for almost half of all cases.
- Some important etiologies are: hypoxic–ischemic encephalopathy, infection, intracerebral hemorrhage, infarction, hypoglycemia, congenital structural abnormality of CNS, inborn errors of metabolism, subarachnoid hemorrhage, hypocalcemia, drug withdrawal.
- The diagnosis of seizures requires a careful history, physical examination and some investigations which are guided by history and examination findings. Treatable causes such as hypoglycemia, hypocalcemia, hypomagnesemia and infection should be sought. Lumbar puncture or treatment with antibiotics for meningitis and acyclovir should be considered. EEG and brain imaging studies may assist diagnosis.

Table V: Clinical presentation of neonatal seizures

Type	Clinical features
Subtle	Repetitive blinking, mouth or tongue movements, staring, apnea
Tonic	Focal or generalized tonic extension of limb(s); sometimes upper limb flexion and lower limb extension
Clonic	Focal or multifocal repetitive, jerky limb movements; sometimes localized with preserved consciousness
Myoclonic	Generalized or focal, single or several flexion jerks of limbs; differentiate myoclonic seizures (serious) from benign neonatal sleep myoclonus

3. Treatment
- Treat underlying disease such as hypoglycemia, hypocalcemia, etc.
- Anticonvulsant therapy: phenobarbital (first line), phenytoin (second line); refractory seizures

may respond to other anticonvulsants.
- Supportive measures.
- Prognosis depends on the underlying disease process. Hypocalcemia and subarachnoid hemorrhage have a relatively good prognosis; structural CNS abnormalities have a poor prognosis.

Intraventricular hemorrhage (IVH)

Intraventricular hemorrhage (IVH) is a common occurrence in the premature infant born prior to 32 weeks gestation; the incidence is inversely related to birth weight with the highest incidence observed in those of birth weight < 1,000 grams. The incidence in infants of < 1,500 grams has fallen slightly in recent years to around 25–30%.

1. Site and timing
- The site of origin of IVH is the subependymal germinal matrix (GM), which lines the ventricles of the preterm brain and involutes just prior to term. The most common location is in the GM of the thalamostriate groove at the head of the caudate nucleus and close to the foramen of Monro.
- In 80% of subependymal hemorrhages, blood also enters the neighboring ventricular system. More extensive bleeding may affect CSF dynamics, obstructing flow and leading to ventricular dilatation.
- Between 10 and 15% of subependymal hemorrhages are associated with periventricular cerebral infarction.
- About 50% of subependymal hemorrhages have occurred by day 1 of life and 90% by day 4. These hemorrhages may later extend during the first week of life.

2. Clinical features and pathogenesis
- Although most IVH's are clinically silent, larger hemorrhages are occasionally associated with clinical features such as bulging fontanelle, abnormalities of perfusion, activity and tone, and even seizures. Consequently, the diagnosis is usually made by routine head ultrasound scan examination.
- The pathogenesis of IVH is multifactorial. Intravascular factors principally relate to defects in hemostasis and to perturbations of perfusion of the subependymal germinal matrix, including local changes in flow and pressure in arterial and venous systems. Vascular factors relate to fragility of the GM blood vessels and their susceptibility to hypoxic–ischemic insult. Extravascular factors relate to the integrity of supporting tissues, including potential effects from fibrinolysis or postnatal decreases in extracellular brain water content.
- The most important mechanisms of brain injury associated with IVH are posthemorrhagic hydrocephalus and periventricular hemorrhagic infarction. Additional potential mechanisms of injury include the presence of concomitant periventricular leukomalacia, local hemorrhagic injury to the subependyma (directly or via pressure effects), focal ischemia and injury mediated by vasoactive metabolites from blood clot.

3. Complications of IVH
- Posthemorrhagic hydrocephalus: significant hemorrhage into the ventricular system may affect CSF drainage either by obstruction of flow within the ventricular system from blood clot or,

more commonly, by affecting CSF resorption by the arachnoid villi. This results in ventricular dilatation which sometimes resolves spontaneously or, following temporary drainage procedures (e.g. serial lumbar puncture), sometimes persists. In the latter circumstance, a ventricular shunt is required for management. Fortunately, such intervention is required in only 1–2% of very low birth weight infants.

- Periventricular hemorrhagic infarct: this serious lesion often occurs unilaterally or at least asymmetrically and most frequently involves periventricular frontal or parietal white matter lateral to the angle of the lateral ventricles. This lesion often affects an extensive area of the brain and, mostly, is associated with a large IVH.
- It is proposed, based on pathological studies, that asymmetrical periventricular hemorrhagic infarction complicating IVH is due to obstruction of the venous drainage of medullary and terminal veins, leading to venous stasis, venous infarction and hemorrhage. The stimulus may be the mass effect of a subependymal hemorrhage or intraventricular clot. This may result in a wedge–shaped (fan–shaped) region of hemorrhagic infarction.

4. Prognosis
- Subependymal hemorrhage with or without intraventricular hemorrhage and without ventricular dilatation is associated with risks for major neurological injury of a similar order of magnitude as infants of similar birth weight without hemorrhage.
- Posthemorrhagic hydrocephalus is often, but not invariably, associated with significant neurological sequelae.
- Periventricular hemorrhagic infarcts have a relatively poor prognosis, the nature and extent of sequelae depending on many factors including size and location of lesions.

5. Prevention
- Because the genesis of IVH is multifactorial, prevention involves addressing a matrix of risk factors. In the absence of prevention of prematurity, neonatal management includes avoiding stress to the subependymal GM via vascular, intravascular and extravascular factors. Consequently, avoiding asphyxia, decreasing respiratory distress (a condition which in turn predisposes to unstable GM perfusion) and using synchronized ventilation or sedation, etc., are considered to decrease risks for IVH.
- Pharmacological interventions have been proposed and tested with mixed success. Claims have been made for drugs such as ethamsylate (not available in Canada) and indomethacin. The latter has the theoretical advantage of inhibiting prostaglandin activity, blunting vasodilation and inhibiting free–radical production. However, it must be noted that the goal of effective management is good long–term outcome. Few managements are entirely free of side effects, and treatments which decrease risks of IVH also require assessment for safety.

Periventricular leukomalacia (PVL)

Periventricular leukomalacia is a common pattern of hypoxic–ischemic cerebral injury which occurs in the premature newborn. It involves principally the watershed zones of arterial supply in the periventricular white matter, most predominantly posteriorly in the region of the trigone of the lateral ventricles. In addition to hypoxic–ischemic insults, other possible pathogenic factors include endotoxin exposure associated with infection or disturbed glucose metabolism.

The diagnosis of PVL during the neonatal period cannot be based reliably on clinical criteria and is established by detection of abnormalities on cranial ultrasonography, that is increased echogenicity in periventricular white matter during the first days of life, followed by later development of cysts in these regions in severe cases. The lesion is usually bilateral and often symmetrical.

The importance of PVL as a cause of significant brain injury is becoming increasingly recognized. Sequelae include injury to motor function (particularly spastic diplegia), corticovisual impairment (due to injury to the optic radiation) and variable cognitive dysfunction.

Head ultrasound in preterms

Because of portability and safety, head ultrasound examination has become the standard routine imaging modality for assessment of neonatal brain injury in the preterm.

Cranial ultrasonography can identify with a high degree of accuracy the presence of subependymal GM hemorrhage with or without intraventricular blood. In addition, it is an excellent imaging modality for identifying and following posthemorrhagic ventricular dilatation. Improved ultrasound technology permits better assessment of parenchymal lesions than previously. Despite such improvements, ultrasound assessment of parenchymal integrity has deficiencies. Blood, edema and calcium deposition all produce echodensities. Furthermore, assessment of parenchymal echogenicity is subjective and affected by choice of ultrasound settings.

It is important to take all these factors into account when assessing the significance of ultrasound findings. Consequently, in the preterm, cranial ultrasound assessment will report presence or absence of each of the following: subependymal hemorrhage, intraventricular blood, ventricular dilatation, intraparenchymal echogenicity (a CT scan is useful for differentiation between edema, hemorrhage and structural or other abnormalities).

FLUIDS AND ELECTROLYTES

Fluids

Body fluid compartments, renal function and fluid requirements all vary with age.

Fluid compartments

1. Total body water (TBW)
Total body water = 78% of body weight at birth and decreases to adult levels of 60% by 1 year of age. Total body water consists of several compartments whose relative size changes from conception through the first 9 months of postnatal life.

2. Extracellular water (ECW)
This fluid decreases from 35–40% at birth to constitute 20–25% of body weight by 1 year of age. It is made up of plasma water (5%), interstitial water (15%) and transcellular water (1–3%). Transcellular water is mostly made up of gastrointestinal secretions, cerebrospinal, intracellular, pleural, peritoneal and synovial fluids.

3. Intracellular water (ICW)
This constitutes about 35–40% of body weight throughout life. It consists of the total fluid in the

cells of the various tissues and organs in the body (Table VI).

Regulation of water

Plasma osmolality is maintained at 285–295 mOsm/kg H_2O, balancing water intake and production from oxidation against losses from kidneys, lungs, skin and gastrointestinal tract.

1. Intake
- Regulated by thirst in term babies.
- Volume restoration has a priority.
- Disorders can occur with CNS diseases, hypokalemia and malnutrition.

Table VI: Variations in body fluid compartments with age

Age	TBW (% body weight)	ECW (% body weight)	ICW (% body weight)
24–26 wk	84–88	58–62	24–28
Newborn	75–80	35–45	35–40
1 wk	70–75	30–40	35–40
1 yr	60–65	20–25	35–40

2. Absorption
- This occurs primarily with the active transport of solutes.
- Interference with active transport will affect water absorption.

3. Excretion
- This involves evaporation from the lungs and skin as well as renal losses from solute excretion and the mechanisms controlling the rate and dilution of urine. Evaporation will be affected by surface area, temperature, respiratory rate, humidity and sweating.
- Renal losses are affected by ADH, diet, glomerular filtration rate (GFR), renal tubular function and steroids (Table VII).
- ADH is regulated by osmotic pressure of the ECW (Na^+, Cl^-) and acts by increasing the permeability of the renal collecting ducts to water, conserving water and concentrating urine. Decreased responsiveness by the collecting duct to ADH leads to diabetes insipidus. Release of ADH may be stimulated by pain, trauma, surgery, burns and opioids. It may be inhibited by emotional factors, alcohol and certain drugs.

Renal function

Renal function is relatively poor in infancy and does not reach adult values until 1.5–2 years of age. Table VII shows the relative increase in GFR as age increases. Urine flow in the newborn infant is 1–4 mL/kg per h after the first day of life.

The blood pressure of an infant is normally much less than that of an older child (Table VIII). The difficulty is to know when to treat or what you are treating. The figures quoted are guidelines only. It is very difficult to find information on what the blood pressure should be at a particular gestation. Most physicians would try to maintain even a 24 week gestation baby with a mean blood pressure near to 30 mm Hg. At the other end of the scale, a term baby with a mean blood pressure > 70 mm Hg would be regarded as hypertensive.

Table VII: Change in renal function with age

Age	GFR (ml/min per m²)
< 37 wk	< 15
Newborn	10–20
1–2 wk	20–35
2–4 mo	35–45
6–12 mo	45–60

Table VIII: Normal blood pressure in the newborn

Age	Systolic (mm Hg)	Diastolic (mm Hg)	Mean (mm Hg)
Newborn: 1–2 kg	50	25	30
Newborn: 2–3 kg	60	30	40
Newborn: > 3 kg	65	40	50
1 yr	75	50	60

- Hypotension is caused by: poor cardiac function, acute blood loss, sodium depletion, low oncotic pressure.
- Treatment of hypotension: replacement of sodium, replacement of fluid or colloid loss (blood, 5% albumin), treatment with dopamine as an inotrope (0–20 µg/kg per min); possible use of dexamethasone.
- Hypertension is caused by:
    Cardiac: coarctation of the aorta, hypoplastic aortic arch, umbilical catheterization, renal artery stenosis.
    Renal: polycystic kidneys, dysplastic kidneys.
    Endocrine: adrenal hyperplasia, pheochromocytoma.
    Drugs: steroids.
    Others: hypervolemia, raised intracranial pressure.
- Treatment of hypertension:
    Significant: hydralazine ± captopril ± diuretic ± β–blocker.
    Mild: captopril ± diuretic.

Serum proteins

The capillary endothelial wall is a barrier between plasma and interstitial fluid. While water and small molecules can move through it freely, its pores are too small for plasma proteins to pass through in significant amounts in a healthy person. Plasma proteins are colloids and the pressure they create is the oncotic pressure.

Hydrostatic pressure in the vascular system encourages filtration but oncotic pressure keeps fluid in the blood vessels. Oncotic pressure and total body sodium determine the size of the circulating volume.

Albumin is the most important serum protein affecting oncotic pressure. When serum albumin is low, the oncotic pressure is low and the perfusion to the kidneys decrease. The kidneys compensate by conserving salt and water, and a sodium and water excess is achieved. This results in edema and a low serum sodium. A low serum albumin is found in sick and immature infants, infants with necrotizing enterocolitis and infants with an abdominal wall defect. Treatment: 25% albumin 1 g/kg over 1 h.

Fluid requirements

Modification of fluid requirements is often necessary with general anesthesia, renal disease, central nervous system disease and particularly in the neonatal period.

During the neonatal period, maintenance requirements in the first 2 days are approximately 70% of requirements, increasing gradually to 100% by day 5. Low birth weight infants require relatively more water due to the greater surface area and increased water losses. Table IX shows some fluid guidelines for the neonate.

Table IX: Fluid requirements for newborn children

Birth weight (g)	Days 1–2	Day 3	Day 7*
Term infant	70	80	120–150
1,751–2,000	80	110	120–160
1,501–1,750	80	110	130–160
1,251–1,500	90	120	130–160
1,001–1,250	100	130	140–180
751–1,000	105	140	140–200
501–750	105	140	140–200

*Many factors in the management of neonates may require modification of fluid intake. These include phototherapy, radiant heaters, gestational age, humidity, fever and high metabolic rates. Modifications are also made in conditions where high fluid loads are thought to have an adverse effect, e.g. patent ductus arteriosus, hyaline membrane disease, bronchopulmonary dysplasia and necrotizing enterocolitis.

Increased requirements

Maintenance fluids often need to be increased in the following cases:
- Fever: in neonates, the normal thermal environment can be lowered on the incubator. In larger infants, increase fluids 10% per °C rise above 38.
- Renal losses: diabetes insipidus or recovery phase of tubular necrosis.
- GI losses: nasogastric tube, gastrostomy, ileostomy, pancreatic fistula, diarrhea. These should be replaced volume for volume with the appropriate electrolyte solutions (Table X).

In practical terms, saline is used to replace most losses with or without the addition of potassium. Replacement should be considered when losses exceed 5–10 mL in a 24 hour period.

Table X: Electrolyte composition of GI fluids

GI source	H⁺ (mmol/L)	Na⁺ (mmol/L)	K⁺ (mmol/L)	Cl⁻ (mmol/L)	HCO₃⁻ (mmol/L)
Gastric	40–80	20–80	10–20	120–150	0
Small bowel	0	100–140	10–15	90–130	20–40
Biliary	0	120–140	10–15	80–120	30–50
Pancreatic	0	120–140	10–15	80–120	30–50
Diarrhea	0	40	40	40	40

Decreased requirements

Some situations will require strict fluid restrictions:
- Renal failure: severely restrict to insensible losses (40–60 mL/kg in a neonate or 25 mL/kg in an infant) if undialyzed.
- SIADH: caused by head injury, meningitis, surgery, etc. Give two-thirds maintenance and closely follow the serum sodium and clinical condition. This is a water restriction only, not an electrolyte restriction.

Electrolytes

Sodium is the main positive ion in the ECW and there is little in the ICW. It is actively kept out of normally functioning cells by the cell membrane sodium pump. Potassium is the main cation in the ICW.

The amount of sodium in the body determines the size of the extracellular space. Assessing the sodium balance involves assessing the ECW. Since the ECW is a large part of an infant's total body weight, an increase in the ECW will cause an increase in weight.

Enlargement of the ICW causes edema, while enlargement of the circulating volume causes hypertension, congestive cardiac failure and pulmonary edema.

Requirements are met by the following standard solutions (Table XI). Treatment of electrolyte disorders is covered in chapter 5 (Fluids and Electrolytes).

Table XI: Standard neonatal maintenance solution

Fluid	D10W	Range
Sodium	2.5 mmol/100 mL	0–12 mmol/100 mL
Potassium	2.0 mmol/100 mL	0–6 mmol/100 mL
Calcium gluconate	200 mg/100 mL	0–600 mg/100 mL

Calcium can cause severe chemical burns if it extravasates. High concentrations of glucose or calcium should only be given via a central line.

NUTRITION

Breast feeding

More and more families appreciate the nutritional superiority of breast feeding with its immunological, psychological and developmental benefits. Given that breast feeding is becoming a more common choice of infant feeding, these families may desire to breast feed but need further support and teaching in the skill.

1. Factors in successful breast feeding
* Supportive environment:
    In 1992, the World Health Organization and UNICEF introduced the concept of "baby friendly hospital initiatives". These are: have a written breast feeding policy, train all health staff to implement this policy, inform all pregnant women about the benefits of breast feeding, help mothers initiate breast feeding within 30 minutes of birth, show mothers the best way to breast feed, give newborn infants no food or drink other than breast milk (unless medically indicated), practice "rooming in" by allowing mothers and babies to remain together 24 hours a day, encourage breast feeding on demand, give no artificial pacifiers or soothers, help start breast feeding support groups and refer mothers to them. A supportive environment also includes family members and friends with realistic expectations for the nursing pair (e.g. maternal rest and nutrition, low priority of housework versus infant nutrition).
* In most cases, a woman can successfully breast feed, given teaching and support.
    Maternal factors that may inhibit (I) or contraindicate (C) breast feeding include:
    Severe maternal illness (postpartum hemorrhage, pregnancy induced hypertension) (I).
    Inverted or flat nipples (I). Breast surgery, particularly reduction (I).
    Maternal substance use of alcohol (C), heroin(C), cocaine(C).
    HIV infection in Western society (C).
    Hepatitis C infection (C).
    Certain prescribed drugs (C or I); very few in fact are absolute contraindications.
    Separation from the infant.
    New diagnosis of breast cancer.
    Some infant factors can make breast feeding difficult to establish (D) or contraindicated (C):
    Galactosemia (C).
    Phenylketonuria (amount of breast feeding may be prescribed).

Prematurity (immature suck, swallow, breath reflex and weak suck) (D).
Significant illness (e.g. sepsis, respiratory distress) (D).
Hypotonia (e.g. asphyxia, congenital disorders or syndromes) (D).
Cleft palate (D).

2. Getting started...the act of breast feeding
• Maternal posture: there are a number of feeding positions. The positions should be comfortable to the mother as she will spend a lot of time feeding her child.
• Infant position: the baby should be close to the mother in a way that the body and head are well supported:
     With body and head facing the mother.
     With the mouth just below the nipple as the infant prepares to feed.
     With the head, neck and back in a straight line.
•   How the infant takes the breast:
     Position the infant's nose at the level of the nipple. Wait till the baby's mouth is open wide before bringing him/her onto the breast. The mother may need to stimulate the upper lip or cheek to encourage the infant to open his/her mouth wide. Bring the infant quickly onto the breast.
     When the infant is well latched on, one will notice that the chin is against the breast; the mouth is wide open with the lips flared out and the lower lip is pressed down and back onto the chin; the nose lies against the breast; the nipple (at least half an inch of the areola) is taken into the infant's mouth. There may be some initial tenderness with the feed but it should resolve as the feeding progresses. If the infant is just on the nipple, there will be discomfort throughout the feed (and lead to cracked nipples), insufficient drainage of the milk sinuses (leading to malnutrition of the infant and engorgement for the mother) and insufficient stimulation of the breast to support adequate milk production (engorgement also leads to lower prolactin levels which decreases milk supply).
• How the infant feeds:
     Sucks strongly and rhythmically, perhaps with occasional rests.
     Remains latched on and comes off when ready. Once nursing is established, a feeding usually takes a minimum 10–15 minutes for the infant to obtain the hindmilk in the breast (the high fat, high calorie milk).
     Feeds eagerly at least 8 times per day in the first 3 weeks.
• Assessing baby's health: given early hospital discharge prior to establishment of lactation, the mother and infant should be assessed within 1 week of birth if solely breast feeding. At that time:
     The infant should be gaining steadily (15–45 g/d) after the initial nadir in weight after birth. The infant should be back at birth weight (on average) by 10–14 days of age. The infant significantly wets 6 disposable or 8 cloth diapers per day and the urine is odorless and pale yellow or clear. Once meconium has all been passed, there should be at least one mustard yellow, soft stool per day, that is, more than a smear on the diaper. The infant should have alert periods, is not excessively sleepy or irritable and seems satisfied after a feeding of 10 or more minutes.
     Problems with inadequate nutrition of the infant can lead to poor growth, dehydration, severe hypernatremia and the sequelae of these complications. It is important to develop basic knowledge in assessing breast feeding or to refer to someone with expertise. While

you do not want to cause undue anxiety in a mother–baby pair that is learning a new skill, it is essential to be able to evaluate adequacy of breast feeding in a friendly and supportive manner.

3. Specific Issues
- Prematurity:
  Expressed breast milk is an excellent source of nutrition for the preterm infant. Compared to formula, it is associated with a lower incidence of necrotizing enterocolitis, less infections and a small but significant advantage in developmental scores of preterm infants solely given breast milk. If a mother of a sick or preterm infant wishes to breast feed, she should start pumping the breasts as soon as is feasible after birth. She should pump at least 6 times per day using an efficient, large electric pump. The milk can be refrigerated or frozen and given to the baby at a later date when the child is ready. For preterm infants < 35 weeks gestation and < 2 kilograms, mature expressed breast milk (EBM) has inadequate minerals and calories to sustain good bone deposition and growth. A milk fortifier (powder or liquid forms available) can be added to the milk that supplies extra protein, calcium, phosphorus, sodium, glucose polymers and multivitamins. A fortifier is added when an infant demonstrates clinical tolerance to human milk feedings at a volume of 100 mL/kg per d.
- Supplements:
  The Canadian Pediatric Society recommends that infants solely breast fed should receive a vitamin D supplement of 400 IU orally once daily.
  In premature infants, start iron supplements 2 weeks after complete enteral feeding achieved. In healthy term infants, iron supplementation is not necessary. A source of iron, other than breast milk, is needed by 6 months or so and is usually supplied by fortified cereals and infant foods.
  Fluoride: there is no data about the fluoride needs of the preterm infant. Prematurity is, however, associated with an increase incidence of dental caries. Therefore, fluoride is likely to be important for the preterm infant.

ACUTE ABDOMEN

Necrotizing enterocolitis (NEC)

NEC is the most common life threatening acquired GI disease that affects premature infants in ICU. It occurs in about 5% of the infants admitted into ICU. Mortality rate is not high but long–term morbidity from sepsis, strictures and feed intolerance is significant. NEC is characterized by partial or full thickness bowel wall necrosis, usually involving the terminal ileum and the colon.

1. Pathogenesis and risk factors
The pathogenesis of NEC is not fully known. It is a multifactorial disorder and represents the end response of the immature GI tract to multiple risk factors causing gut ischemia and mucosal injury. Subsequent colonization and invasion by microorganisms causes bowel wall necrosis. Predisposing factors identified include cyanotic congenital heart disease, polycythemia, umbilical catheterization, exchange transfusion, perinatal asphyxia and rapid advancement of hypertonic

feeds, etc. Coagulase negative staphylococci, which are delta toxin producing, have been identified in very high colony counts in the stools of infants developing NEC. However, after multiple case control studies, the most consistently identifiable epidemiological precursors for NEC are prematurity and GI feeding.

2. Clinical features
NEC is characterized by a combination of systemic and GI symptoms, signs and typical radiological features.
• Systemic: the infant is ill with temperature instability, lethargy, recurrent apneas, circulatory collapse and bleeding tendency.
• Gastrointestinal: increasing gastric residuals and abdominal distension are usually one of the earliest clinical signs. Other symptoms include bloody stool, absent bowel sounds and abdominal tenderness. In advanced cases, there is erythema and induration of the abdominal wall with signs of peritoneal irritation due to bowel perforation.
• Radiological:
    Early diagnosis: dilated bowel loops (localized or generalized), uneven bowel wall thickening.
    Late diagnosis: *Pneumatosis intestinalis*, portal venous gas, pneumoperitoneum and ascites.
    Ultrasound findings: sonographic detection of portal venous gas, intramural gas and bowel wall thickening may precede the plain film findings of these pathological hallmarks of NEC and is therefore a good adjunct to diagnosis. The modified Bell's staging criteria for NEC (Table XII) are useful and widely used clinically. Because of the high morbidity and mortality associated with NEC, it is important to diagnose NEC as early in the illness as possible. A high index of suspicion is justified even though this will lead to the treatment of some infants with suspicion of NEC but no pathognomonic signs.

3. Management
• Withhold oral feeding and institute nasogastric decompression.
• Perform sepsis workup and provide broad spectrum antibiotic coverage, e.g. vancomycin and cefotaxime pending further culture results.
• Follow–up progress clinically and use clinical judgment with abdominal films to monitor for signs of perforation and pneumoperitoneum.
• Consultation with pediatric surgeon because of the possibility of surgical intervention.
• Indications for operation:
    Absolute indications include: pneumoperitoneum, intestinal gangrene (positive results of paracentesis).
    Relative indications include: clinical deterioration such as persistent metabolic acidosis, oliguria and shock, thrombocytopenia, leucopenia or leucocytosis, portal venous gas, erythema of abdominal wall, fixed abdominal mass, persistent dilated loops.
• Supportive treatment for shock, DIC, electrolyte disturbance and oliguria. Mechanical ventilation for apnea and shock.
• On recovery, enteric feed should be introduced gradually. Maternal expressed breast milk is used when available. Depending on injury, a lactose free formula or elemental formula (such as pregestamil) may be required. Check the stool for reducing substance and occult blood. In case of epidemic, institute infectious disease control measures.

4. Complications of NEC
- Short gut syndrome after extensive bowel resections.
- Metabolic complications of prolonged TPN.
- Recurrent NEC occurs up to 10%.
- Intestinal obstruction due to stricture of the involved bowel. A small number of infants will develop stricture disease following NEC. This may present as ongoing GI symptoms, including ongoing blood loss in the stools or with GI obstruction. Beware of infants with significant blood loss in stool following NEC. Infants with stricture disease can rapidly become seriously ill.

Table XII: Modified Bell's staging criteria for neonatal necrotizing enterocolitis

Stage	Systemic signs	Intestinal signs	Radiological signs
IA–suspected NEC	Temperature instability, apnea, bradycardia, lethargy	Elevated pregavage residuals, mild abdominal distension, emesis, stool positive for occult blood	Normal or intestinal dilation, mild ileus
IB–suspected NEC	Same as above	Bright red blood from rectum	Same as above
IIA–definite NEC: mildly ill	Same as above	Same as above, plus diminished or absent bowel sounds with or without abdominal tenderness	Intestinal dilation, ileus, *Pneumatosis intestinalis*
IIB–definite NEC: moderately ill	Above plus mild metabolic acidosis and mild thrombocytopenia	Above plus definite abdominal tenderness, with or without abdominal cellulitis or right lower quadrant mass, absent bowel sounds	Same as stage IIA with or without portal vein gas, with or without ascites
IIIA–advanced NEC: severely ill, bowel intact	Same as IIB plus hypotension, bradycardia, severe apneas, combined respiratory and metabolic acidosis, disseminated intravascular coagulation (DIC), neutropenia, anuria	Above plus signs of generalized peritonitis, marked tenderness, distension of abdomen, and abdominal wall erythema	Same as stage IIB, definite ascites
IIIB–advanced NEC: severely ill, bowel perforation	Same as stage IIIA	Same as stage IIIA	Same as stage IIB plus pneumoperitonuem

CONGENITAL INFECTION

General features

The newborn infant's host defense mechanisms, particularly those of the sick preterm infant, may be immature and easily overcome by invading organisms. Infections may become fulminant and cause death within a few hours or days. The fetus may be infected in utero (congenital), at the time of birth (natal) or after birth and during the neonatal period (postnatal).

Transplacental route is the most common means of transmission in utero. As well as stillbirth, abortion, malformation, IUGR and premature birth, infection may lead to acute disease in the newborn or asymptomatic but persistent infection in the infant. The most common organisms are rubella, CMV, *Toxoplasma gondii*, *T. pallidum*, HIV, parvovirus and EBV. Others include herpes and hepatitis virus.

Congenital infection may be suspected if there is a history of maternal intravenous drug use, unexplained illness, immunosuppression, active herpes lesions, ingestion of raw meats, exposure to cats, exposure to CMV, exposure to rubella and findings such as poor fetal growth or microcephaly on the antenatal visits.

1. Clinical presentation
In the majority of congenital infections, there are no symptoms evident at birth. General findings such as SGA, jaundice, prematurity, congenital defects of heart, malformations of the CNS, hepatosplenomegaly, purpura, petechiae, lesions of the bones, cataracts, chorioretinitis, microcephaly, and intracerebral calcification may be present. There are specific manifestations for each infectious agent.

2. Diagnosis
- Mother:
     Vaginal culture; serology (IgM, IgG for specific organisms, acute and convalescent titers).
     Placenta: culture; histological examination.
     Cord blood: IgM (if elevated, suggests an infection has occurred).
- Infant:
     CBC; differential (hemolytic anemia, thrombocytopenia).
     Serology (IgM, IgG for specific organisms, acute and convalescent titers, IgG for rubella, toxoplasmosis, VDRL, RPR for syphilis, surface Ag for hepatitis B, PCR, ELISA, Western Blot for HIV).
     Culture of oropharynx, urine, rectum, blood, CSF, eye.
     Smears of skin lesions for FA stain, Darkfield exam, Tzank.
     Liver functions (include PT, PTT), hyperbilirubinemia, hepatitis.
     Lumbar puncture (pleocytosis).
     Radiographical (chest X–ray, head ultrasound, CT scan, X–rays of long bones).
     Ophthalmology examination; audiological examination.

3. Management and treatment
- Mother: antenatal, intrapartum, postpartum monitoring for next pregnancy.
- Infant: specific therapy, supportive care and feeding, isolation, prevention and follow–up depend on the causative organism.

Cytomegalovirus (CMV)

- Highest risk is with maternal primary infection, risk of transmission 50%, highest in first trimester.
- Majority of infected newborns are asymptomatic; 5–10% present with microcephaly, periventricular calcifications, mental retardation, hepatosplenomegaly, dermal erythropoiesis, hearing loss, chorioretinitis; 90% develop late sequelae such as sensorineural hearing loss; mortality rate in the symptomatic is 20–30%.
- Virus identified in urine and blood, specific IgM.
- No specific therapy, possibly CMV hyperimmunoglobulin.
- Breast feeding is acceptable.
- May excrete virus for months or years.
- Avoid contact with pregnant women and careful handwashing for nonimmune pregnant women in high risk environments (daycares, nurseries).

Hepatitis A

- Severe disease has not been reported in neonates.
- Asymptomatic at birth.
- If mother jaundiced 2 weeks before delivery or up to 1 week after, treat with immunoglobulin.
- Breast feeding acceptable.
- Contact isolation.

Hepatitis B

- May be transplacental, most occur during delivery, highest risk (80%) for fetus is active maternal infection in last trimester and chronic carrier state (70%) in mother.
- Most newborns are asymptomatic; 90% of untreated develop chronic infection, hepatitis, cirrhosis; primary hepatocellular carcinoma with a 25% mortality from liver disease.
- To reduce infection rate and chronic carrier state in 85–95% of cases, give HBIg and HBV concurrently but at different sites within first 12 hours after birth (85–95% effective); repeat HBV in 1 and 6 months; check antibody response at 9 months.
- Mother HB_sAg^+: give both HBIg and HBV.
- Mother HB_sAg?: give HBV and if mother becomes positive, give HBIg not later than 1 week after birth.
- Mother HB_sAg^-: give HBV.
- Center for disease control recommends hepatitis B vaccination for all infants regardless of mother's status.
- Screen all pregnant women; vaccinate those that are negative but high risk during pregnancy.
- Infant requires blood and body fluid precautions.
- Breast feeding acceptable.

Hepatitis C

- Infection probably occurs but risk and consequence to the infant are yet to be defined.
- No treatment; routine universal precautions apply.

Herpes

- Most frequently transmitted during passage through infected vaginal canal but ascending infection through intact membranes has been reported. Postnatal transmission from mouth, hands and nipples. Fifty percent risk of transmission if maternal primary vaginal infection at time of delivery; only 0–8% risk in recurrent maternal disease; most infected newborns occur without maternal lesion or history of infection.
- Infant may have localized infection of skin, eyes, mouth or CNS. There may be multi–organ disseminated disease with mucocutaneous vesicular rash, conjunctivitis, keratitis, severe meningoencephalitis, chorioretinitis, sepsis or DIC, hepatitis. Symptoms are usually evident in first 3 weeks of life but may take up to 6 weeks. High mortality with disseminated disease, significant neurological and/or ocular impairment.
- Tzanck smear of any vesicles from infant or mother and culture of nasopharynx, mouth and conjunctiva, direct fluorescent antibody staining and enzyme immunoassay of HSV antigens can be done. PCR of cerebrospinal fluid for HSV; DNA may be helpful. Look for a rise in the convalescent HSV antibody titer.
- If infant is infected or cultures obtained 24–48 hours after birth suggests infection, or mother has had primary infection, treatment is indicated. Treat with acyclovir.
- Contact isolation if infection is suspected or clinical disease is present, infants at low risk (cesarean section or asymptomatic mother without lesion at delivery) do not require isolation.
- Cesarean section may be recommended if mother has genital lesion present at time of delivery.

Rubella

- Clinical severity worsened by first trimester infection.
- Microcephaly, mental retardation, chorioretinitis, cataracts, glaucoma, microphthalmia, hearing loss, congenital heart defects, dermal erythropoiesis (blueberry muffin baby), IUGR, bone radiolucencies, thrombocytopenia.
- Culture of throat, urine and CSF.
- IgM and IgG serology.
- No specific therapy.
- May excrete virus for months, contact isolation.
- Avoid contact with nonimmune pregnant women.
- Women of childbearing years, if nonimmune, should be vaccinated at least 3 months prior to conception.

Toxoplasmosis

- Only occurs with primary maternal infection with highest incidence of fetal infection in third trimester. Severity of infection is inversely related to gestational age at time of primary maternal infection.
- Most are asymptomatic but 15% have chorioretinitis; 10% have intracranial calcifications, hydrocephalus, microcephaly, hepatosplenomegaly, thrombocytopenia, jaundice, elevated CSF protein and pleocytosis.
- Fundoscopic exam, CT scan, IgM in blood and CSF.
- Treat with spiramycin, pyrimethamine, sulfadiazine, folinic acid, ID consult.

- Breast feeding acceptable.
- No isolation necessary.
- Pregnant women should avoid cat feces, litter box, raw meats.

Syphilis

- Infection may occur at any time in pregnancy with any maternal stage of infection. Primary maternal infection risk to fetus is 70–90%, secondary syphilis risk is 90% and latent is 30%.
- Twenty-five percent of infections result in fetal death. Live born infants with syphilis have a rash on soles and palms, rhinitis, hepatosplenomegaly, osteochondritis, periostitis, low birth weight, jaundice. Some may be asymptomatic.
- Serological diagnosis in both infant and mother are either nontreponemal (VDRL, RPR, RST, EIA) or treponemal (MHA–TP, FTA–ABS). Blood and CSF should be examined. Direct visualization of the organism from skin lesions, nasal discharge, placental tissue or amniotic fluid is diagnostic.
- Treat with penicillin if symptomatic, highly probable disease or mother has syphilis. Asymptomatic infants in appropriately treated mothers need careful follow–up. Asymptomatic infants in inadequately treated mothers may receive a single dose of penicillin or a full course. ID consult is advised.
- Contact isolation until 24 hours after antibiotics started.
- Prenatal screening and treatment for all serologically confirmed cases is the ideal approval.

Varicella

- The risk of embryopathy is about 2% after maternal varicella infection during the first 20 weeks of pregnancy. Infections occurring within 4–5 days of delivery may result in fulminant infection as maternal antibody transfer has yet to occur.
- Physical findings of embryopathy include limb hypoplasia, chorioretinitis, neurological abnormalities. Otherwise cicatricial skin lesions may be present.
- Diagnosis confirmed by persistence of anti–VZ IgG.
- Newborn infants whose mothers had onset of chickenpox within 5 days before delivery or 48 hours after delivery should be given VZIg as soon as possible after delivery.
- Infants of early pregnancy infection do not need isolation. Neonates born to mothers with active varicella should be placed in isolation at birth and, if still hospitalized. until 21–28 days of age (depending on whether they received VZIg). Premature babies ($\geq$ 28 weeks gestation) whose mothers do not have a history of chickenpox or any premature babies (< 28 weeks or $\leq$ 1,000 grams), regardless of maternal history who cannot be discharged home, should be placed in strict isolation from day 8–21 after onset of rash in mother (day 28 for those who received VZIg).

Parvovirus

- Maternal infection may occasionally lead to fetal infection, overall risk 1%.
- First half of pregnancy highest risk for fetal death and abortion.
- Congenital infection leads to anemia and hydrops.
- Culture of bone marrow, IgG and IgM.

- No specific treatment.
- High prevalence of virus in the community with low risk of infection, therefore, maternal precautions are not recommended.

Enterovirus (polio, coxsackievirus, echo)

- May be acquired in third trimester but most are acquired perinatally.
- Infant is often well at birth and most disease is mild but may develop severe septicemic–like disease, myocarditis, aseptic meningitis, DIC, hepatitis, high mortality.
- Diagnosis established by isolating virus from the CSF, feces, nasopharynx.
- Supportive therapy, immunoglobulin therapy.

HIV

- Risk of infection, without use of AZT, is about 25%.
- Generally no clinical evidence of infection in the first weeks after birth; earliest signs may be persistence of oral and diaper *Candida* infection.
- HIV antibody will be present in infants born to a seropositive mother; if the infant is not infected the titer should decline during the first year; infection is suggested when the titer is persistent or rising.
- Universal precautions recommended.
- Breast feeding in the seropositive mother is not recommended in developed nations due to the risk of transmission in breast milk secondary to cracked nipples.

IMMUNIZATION FOR PREMATURE INFANTS

Routine immunizations

Infants born preterm, whose clinical condition is satisfactory and who have attained a weight of 1.5 kilograms or more, should be immunized with full doses of vaccines starting at 2 months (8 weeks) chronological age. Prematurity is not a reason to defer immunization; the reduced levels of maternal antibody afford premature infants little protection, necessitating the earliest possible inducement of active immunity against infections.

DTP–P/Hib conjugate combination vaccine (PENTA)

1. Dose and administration
- Dose: 0.5 mL i.m. in the anterolateral thigh.
- Give the first dose at 2 months chronological age (minimum 6 weeks), then second and third doses at approximately 2 month (8 weeks) intervals.

2. Precautions/contraindications
- Pertussis vaccine is contraindicated in infants with progressive developmental delay or changing neurological findings, recent convulsions, or known or suspected neurological deterioration. It is prudent to defer pertussis in infants with recent or changing neurological findings until a progressive disorder is excluded. Prematurity, developmental delay and

cerebral palsy pose no increased risk of seizures following pertussis immunization in the absence of other evidence of predisposition to seizures. Infants with well controlled seizures, or in whom a seizure is not likely to recur, may be vaccinated.
- Give acetaminophen (Tylenol) 15 mg/kg per dose starting at the time of the vaccine injection and again at 4 and 8 hours later. Continue treatment if fever is present.

Vaccination in special circumstances

1. Hepatitis B
- Infant born to hepatitis B surface antigen positive mother:
  Give hepatitis B vaccine; Engerix–B, 0.5 mL (10 µg) or Recombivax HB, 0.25 mL (2.5 µg), i.m. in the anterolateral thigh, at birth or before 12 hours of age.
  Administer using a separate syringe: hepatitis B immunoglobulin (HBIg) 0.5 mL in the opposite anterolateral thigh (preferably within 12 hours of age). Give second dose of vaccine at 1 month and third dose at 6 months of age, regardless of gestational age or birth weight. For infants < 2,000 grams, add postvaccination testing because some may not respond.
- Infant of a mother at high risk for hepatitis B (e.g. drug using), whose HB_sAg status is unknown at delivery should be immunized at birth with the vaccine dose recommended for infants of HB_sAg positive mothers. Additional administration of HBIg should depend on serological screening of the mother, which should be done as soon as possible (maximum 72 hours).
  Note: For infants < 2,000 grams who are vaccinated routinely, delay until 2 months when other vaccines are given or weight > 2,000 grams.

Neonatal varicella exposure

Varicella zoster immunoglobulin (VZIg) is recommended for the following infants, providing significant exposure has occurred:
- Newborn infants whose mother had onset of chickenpox within 5 days before delivery or within 48 hours after delivery.
- Hospitalized premature infants exposed during the first weeks of life.
  Exposed premature infants < 28 weeks gestation or < 1,000 grams regardless of maternal immune status.
  Exposed premature infants > 28 weeks gestation whose mother was not immune.

Dose and administration:
- 125 units i.m. in the anterolateral thigh.
- For maximal effectiveness, VZIg should be given within 48 hours of and not more than 96 hours after exposure.

INFECTION CONTROL IN THE NURSERY

There are a few issues which are important when considering infection control in neonates. Most importantly, good handwashing technique cannot be overemphasized to all personnel coming into the nursery. Anyone coming into direct contact with an infant should keep any clothing on the arms pushed up above the elbow, remove all jewelry and ensure that hands (including under the nails, wrists and forearms) have been washed with a microbial soap, before and after each contact with an infant.

When a question arises about infection control, most hospitals have infection control nurses or officers on call as well as infectious diseases subspecialists.

Who needs to be isolated?

- A very common question relates to varicella exposure: treatment of infants born to mothers with chickenpox or exposure. Premature infants (28 weeks or older) exposed to varicella when mother has no history of chickenpox and all premature infants (< 28 weeks) should receive VZIg. All exposed susceptible patients who cannot be discharged should be placed on strict isolation from days 8–21 after onset of rash in index case. For babies who received VZIg, strict isolation should continue for 28 days.
- Contact isolation is recommended for the following infections: rubella, hepatitis A, HSV, respiratory viruses, multiply resistant bacterial infection (especially staphylococci or *E. coli*).
- Isolation is not necessary for the following infections: CMV*, toxoplasmosis*, hepatitis B+, hepatitis C+, HIV+ (* pregnant women should not handle these infants; + universal precautions should be strongly reinforced).

SEPSIS NEONATORUM

Most infants with septicemia present with nonspecific signs and symptoms such as temperature instability, feeding intolerance, apnea, increased oxygen or ventilatory requirements. A complete history and physical examination will aid in decision making. If there is clinical suspicion of sepsis, order a CBC, differential and platelets as well as a blood culture; start antibiotics pending culture results. If there is respiratory or GI mischief, also do appropriate X-rays, which may aid in the diagnosis. A lumbar puncture is often recommended for an infant > 7 days old, particularly with nonspecific, nonlocalizing signs of sepsis. Suprapubic urine culture may be helpful in the diagnosis of renal tract infection.

Group B, beta hemolytic *Streptococcus* (GBS)

This is the most common Gram positive bacterium found on blood culture from infants with sepsis in North America. GBS is found on vaginal or anorectal cultures in 35% of asymptomatic pregnant women. One difficulty which arises is that vertical transmission occurs in 50–70% of maternal–infant pairs, and colonization is relatively common, with a rate of 8–25%. Most infected women have normal babies but 1–2% result in stillbirth or neonatal disease. The mortality rate from early onset GBS sepsis is quite high, at about 20%. Late onset disease may occur at 2–4 weeks of age, with meningitis occurring in 60% of infants and a 10–15% mortality rate.

The present thrust is to identify high risk mothers and to treat them intrapartum. Treatment is recommended if a woman is found to be culture positive for GBS during pregnancy or in labor and has one or more of the following risk factors: preterm labor at < 37 weeks gestation, premature rupture of membranes at < 37 weeks gestation, fever during labor, multiple births, rupture of membranes > 18 hours at any gestation. If the mother has had a previous child with invasive GBS disease, she should be treated intrapartum in all subsequent pregnancies.

Ampicillin or penicillin plus an aminoglycoside (such as gentamicin) is the initial treatment of choice for a neonate with presumed invasive GBS disease. Treatment of the neonate depends on the gestational age, the condition at birth and the maternal history. If the mother has received intrapartum antibiotics and the infant has evidence of sepsis or is premature (< 37 weeks gestation), the baby should be cultured and treated. If one of a set of twins is found to be positive for GBS disease, treatment of the other twin is indicated because of the high frequency of coinfection.

Other bacterial infections

Neonates, particularly prematurely born neonates, are immunocompromised hosts. They are at risk for acquiring any infection.

Other common Gram positive neonatal infections are:
*   Coagulase positive staphylococcal disease: this is particularly important due to the severity of the illness and the concern of epidemics in nurseries. Meticulous handwashing technique is essential.
*   Coagulase negative staphylococcal disease: though usually a contaminant in older children and adults, this is an important pathogen in neonates, particularly premature infants and/or infants with indwelling lines. These bacteria are responsible for 10% of cases of sepsis in neonatal intensive care units. Treatment with vancomycin and cephotaxime is recommended.
*   Listeria monocytogenes disease: presents similarly to GBS disease and should be treated similarly due to the severity of the illness and the response to antimicrobial therapy.
*   Gram negative infection: in North America, E. coli is the most common Gram negative organism causing septicemia during the neonatal period, followed by Klebsiella and Enterobacter.
*   Fungal Infections: occur in 5% of low birth weight infants, mostly due to Candida species.

ENTERAL FEEDING IN THE NURSERY

Particularly in premature babies the feeding–related questions are:
*   What to feed: breast milk is the feeding of choice for babies, particularly premature babies. However, when mothers do not wish to breast feed, or on the rare occasion that they cannot breast feed, there are several modified cows' milk formulas available for premature and for term infants. Premature infants may not grow well on breast milk alone. Therefore, there are two types of supplements available to add to breast milk to increase caloric content and promote growth. In the past, polycose (carbohydrate polymer) or MCT oil was added to breast milk or to formula in order to increase caloric intake. This is no longer recommended in the presence of more balanced supplements.
*   When to feed: there are no definite guidelines on when to start feeding neonates, aside from term healthy infants who should be put to breast within half an hour of birth. Generally speaking, decisions about timing of feeds are made depending on the degree of asphyxia in the perinatal period, the condition of the baby and the gestational age. Once the baby is stable from a respiratory and cardiovascular standpoint, enteral feeding should be considered. Healthy premature babies, at approximately 34 weeks gestational age, are able to suck and swallow in a coordinated way. At 32 weeks, babies with no respiratory problems may be stable enough to begin the learning process for the mother–infant pair, on the road to breast feeding.
*   How to feed: prior to 34 weeks gestation, babies who can be enterally fed will need to be fed by gavage tube. Stable babies on ventilators (with unprotected airways) are also candidates

for gavage feeding. The use of the cup or medicine dropper is finding more acceptability in neonatal nurseries.
- How much to feed: to begin feeds, the amount will depend on the weight or gestational age and clinical condition of the baby. Babies < 750 grams may be started at 1 mL every 12 hr as educational feeds and then slowly increased in frequency to every 2 hr, with slow increases in volume subsequently. Babies < 1,000 grams may be started at 1 mL every 2 hr and then slowly increase the volume, depending on how well tolerated the feeding is. Larger babies should be started on higher volumes (5–10 mL) of feeds, increasing more quickly, depending on the condition of the baby and how well the feed is tolerated. In a stable term infant, one might try an ad lib feed by breast or bottle rather than setting a specific amount of feed, keeping in mind that the term neonate may take 30–60 mL in a feed.

GROWTH CHARTS

Evaluation of adequacy of intake is assessed by daily measurements of growth. It is important to calculate caloric intake. This needs to be assessed in relation to caloric expenditure, such as in an ill baby with significant BPD who has a high work of breathing and will require a high caloric intake, which may need to come in a restricted volume. See chapter 24 (Appendix) for growth charts of preterm infants.

NEONATAL HEMATOLOGY

Hematological values in the newborn

- Normal hemoglobin (Hgb) at birth: term, 155–170 g/L; preterm (28 wks), 145 g/L.
- After birth, there is a steep increase in Hgb from a mean of 168 g/L in cord blood to a mean of 193 g/L by 1–2 hours of age, after which there is a gradual fall to about 95–110 g/L at 6–12 weeks of age in full–term infants.
  In preterm infants, the nadir is lower (70–80 g/L) and at an earlier age (4–8 weeks).
  At birth, up to 0.5×10^9 /L nucleated red cells may be present in the blood of the normal term neonate (up to 1.5×10^9 /L in preterm infant). These disappear within 48 hours of delivery.
  In the first few days, the reticulocyte count is $150–200 \times 10^9$ /L (4–5%) and then stays below 50×10^9 /L (1–2%) for most of the first 1–2 months in all infants.
- The white blood count varies considerably during the first month of life in term and preterm infants. The neutrophil count varies greatly in the first 4 days of life.
- The platelet count in the neonate averages $250–300 \times 10^9$ /L, but it may be $50–150 \times 10^9$ in normal preterm infants and up to 600×10^9 /L by 2–4 months.

Anemia

Causes of anemia:
- Acute perinatal blood loss via placenta or cord, including feto–maternal and feto–fetal (twin–to–twin) transfusions.
- Postnatal bleeding: subgaleal cephalhematoma, large intraventricular hemorrhage, adrenal hemorrhage, ruptured liver, arterial line accidents, etc.
- Hemolytic disease.

- Poor placental transfusion due to early cord clamping or nuchal cord.
- Iatrogenic conditions, e.g. repeated blood sampling.

Note:
- Site of sampling: Hgb is higher in capillary blood than central venous or arterial blood by 25–40 g/L; peripheral venous blood value is intermediate.
- After major acute hemorrhage, it takes time for the Hgb or hematocrit (Hct) to fall (hemodilution).
- Feto–maternal transfusion can be detected by the Kleihauer test (detecting fetal red cells in maternal blood).

Blood transfusion

In case of an emergency (the infant is pale and showing signs of shock) and a history suggestive of an acute blood loss, give an immediate transfusion of uncross–matched O negative blood 10–20 mL/kg over 5–10 min (most easily through a UVC).

In the critically ill neonate with RDS, sepsis, birth asphyxia, etc., it is important to keep the Hgb > 140 g/L (Hct > 0.40). In the stable infant with anemia and no hypotension, the need for transfusion will be determined by the clinical condition of the infant such as whether the infant is symptomatic (i.e. tachycardia, tachypnea, apnea, etc.). For hydropic infants with fetal heart failure, a single volume (80 mL/kg) exchange transfusion using packed cells is the safest way of raising the Hgb without exacerbating the heart failure.

For "anemia of prematurity", the value of maintaining a relatively high Hgb to prevent apnea of prematurity and improve weight gain is not established. Guidelines for blood transfusion should remain flexible, dependent on whether the infant has symptoms attributable to anemia and on whether the infant is oxygen–dependent. Trials of recombinant human erythropoietin are being reported.

Serious complications of transfusions are rare in the neonate. Volume overload can be minimized by slow infusion over several hours or by simultaneous administration of furosemide. There is a potential risk of infection, although screening for HIV, hepatitis B and C is now routine and only CMV seronegative blood is used in the neonatal period.

Formula for calculation of blood replacement:
- Volume packed RBC's = body weight (kg) × 85 × (desired rise in Hct/Hct of the donor unit).
- Volume is usually 10–15 mL/kg.

Neonatal polycythemia

The viscosity of blood increases linearly up to a Hct of 0.65 and exponentially above this level. Furthermore, at a given Hct and shear rate in vitro, neonatal blood is more viscous than adult blood. Polycythemia should only be diagnosed if the venous Hct is > 0.65–0.70 since capillary Hct may be 0.15 greater than the true central Hct.

1. Causes of polycythemia
- Transfusions: feto–fetal, feto–maternal, placental.
- Placental insufficiency in SGA and postmature infants.

- Associated with hyperinsulinism (e.g. infant of diabetic mother).

2. Signs and symptoms
- Respiratory: tachypnea, cyanosis, PPHN.
- Cardiac: tachycardia, heart failure.
- Neurological: lethargy, poor suck, irritability.

3. Complications
- Jaundice.
- Thromboses of renal vein, cerebral or mesenteric artery.
- Congestive heart failure.
- Seizures, possible long–term neurodeficits.
- Metabolic: hypoglycemia, hypocalcemia.

4. Partial exchange transfusion
- The Hct can be lowered by carrying out an exchange transfusion using normal saline or plasma. Long–term results of treated versus untreated patients are controversial; immediate hemodynamic consequences may benefit some infants. Some authorities recommend treatment for all infants with a venous Hct of 0.65–0.70, while others consider that partial exchange transfusion should be performed only in the presence of symptoms at Hct of 0.70–0.80 or when the central Hct exceeds 0.80.
- Calculation of volume of partial exchange transfusion (with normal saline):

$$\text{Volume} = \text{patient's blood volume (mL)} \times \frac{\text{observed} - \text{desired Hct}}{\text{observed Hct}}$$

Neonatal thrombocytopenia

1. Causes
- Isoimmune: maternal antibody against antigenically different fetal platelets.
- Autoimmune: maternal ITP or SLE with transplacental passage of her antiplatelet IgG.
- Rare inherited abnormalities or marrow abnormalities.
- Others: congenital infections (TORCH), hemangiomatosis, sepsis (bacterial, viral, fungal), DIC, exchange transfusion, placental insufficiency.

2 Treatment
- Isoimmune (alloimmune): give mother's washed platelets or platelets of known PIA_1–negative donor.
- Autoimmune: high dose intravenous immunoglobulin (IVIg) at 1 g/kg per d for 2 d and/or prednisone (4 mg/kg per d p.o.) are current first line therapies. Random donor platelet transfusions and exchange blood transfusion are of questionable value. The antenatal management is controversial.
- Other causes: treat cause; give platelets as necessary.

3. Platelet transfusion
- Platelet transfusions are rarely indicated in the immune thrombocytopenias since the

transfused platelets are destroyed as rapidly as the baby's own, except in isoimmune thrombocytopenia when transfusions of the mother's washed platelets, with which the baby will be compatible, can be given. In nonimmune thrombocytopenia (e.g. DIC or marrow abnormalities), the general indication for platelet transfusion in the absence of bleeding is a platelet count of < 20,000/μL in a stable infant or < 100,000/μL for invasive procedures.
• Dose: give 10 mL/kg of platelet concentrate. Usually 1 unit is given (1 unit is approximately 20–30 mL).

Hemorrhagic disorders

The neonate, particularly premature neonate, is deficient in all the factors involved in the intrinsic clotting mechanism, with the exception of fibrinogen, factors V and VIII. The levels rise to adult values within a few weeks.
The level of the natural anticoagulants antithrombin III and proteins C and S are low in neonatal plasma, as are levels of plasminogen.
Coagulation in the neonate is usually evaluated by a platelet count plus the prothrombin time (PT) and activated partial thromboplastin time (APTT). Other useful tests include fibrinogen concentration, fibrin degradation products (FDP) and thrombin time.

1. Hemorrhagic disease of the newborn
This is due to a deficiency of the vitamin K–dependent factors (II, VII, IX and X) and usually presents on the second to the fifth day of life. As it can be prevented by routine administration of 1 mg of vitamin K at birth, hemorrhagic disease of the newborn is now rare. Clotting factor synthesis can be further impaired by asphyxia or maternal anticonvulsant therapy and by breast feeding, which provides an inadequate vitamin K intake.

2. Congenital deficiencies of coagulation factors
These may present in the neonatal period, usually with bleeding from surgical incisions such as circumcision but rarely from other sites (e.g. with vacuum extraction). If bleeding in a neonate does not respond to vitamin K and DIC is not present, specific assays for these coagulation factors should be done. The commonest is factor VIII deficiency (hemophilia) in about 90% of cases.

3. Disseminated intravascular coagulopathy (DIC)
This is seen in neonates with severe birth asphyxia, placental abruption, septicemia, hypothermia, hypotension, hypoxia and acidemia. Thrombin formation, triggered in vivo by microbial endotoxin or by thromboplastin released from damaged tissues and endothelial cells, results in intravascular coagulation which consumes platelets, factors II, VIII, XIII and fibrinogen. The fibrinolytic system is also activated and the fibrin degradation products (FDP) further aggravate the bleeding tendency by interfering with fibrin polymerization.

4. Treatment
• Treat the underlying disease (e.g. sepsis, correct hypotension or acidosis).
• Replace clotting factors by transfusing fresh frozen plasma (FFP) at 10–15 mL/kg ≤ random donor platelets. Consider exchange transfusion in severely affected infants or those with continuing DIC despite intravenous FFP.

Neutropenia

Neutrophil counts vary greatly in well infants during the first 4 days of life. The definition of neutropenia varies from $< 1.0 \times 10^9$ /L to $< 2.0 \times 10^9$ /L.

1. Causes
• Fulminant infections, especially bacterial.
• Infants of mothers with pregnancy induced hypertension.
• SGA infants.
• Perinatal asphyxia.
• Primary neutropenias (very rare).

2. Neutrophil transfusion
Results of clinical trials on the efficacy of leukocyte transfusions in neutropenic neonates with bacterial sepsis were not conclusive. In addition to the general risks associated with transfusion, other side effects may include immunoreactions and leukoagglutination. Therefore, neutrophil transfusion therapy is not generally recommended.

JAUNDICE IN THE NEWBORN

The normal newborn is anticipated to develop hyperbilirubinemia (i.e. a total serum bilirubin above 22–26 µmol/L (the upper limit for the normal adult). Indeed 50% will develop visible jaundice (total serum bilirubin > 85 µmol/L). In the newborn, a set of normal developmental circumstances lead to hyperbilirubinemia. This is physiological jaundice.

Disease processes affecting bilirubin production, transport, metabolism or excretion may further increase serum levels. This is pathological jaundice. Thus, physiological and pathological jaundice are defined on the basis of presence or absence of pathology and not simply by determination of serum bilirubin concentration. A rise of bilirubin on the first day > 8 µmol/L per h or total serum bilirubin exceeding 350 µmol/L suggests pathology.

The degree and time course of hyperbilirubinemia noted in physiological jaundice are affected by factors such as racial characteristics, gestation, feeding practices, etc.

An understanding of bilirubin physiology is key to appreciating the concepts of neonatal jaundice. Bilirubin is present in the bloodstream in conjugated and unconjugated forms, "bound" to albumin or "free" in serum. The level of unconjugated bilirubin is loosely associated with the risk of bilirubin encephalopathy. The small fraction of unconjugated bilirubin which is "free" in serum may cross the blood brain barrier and cause neuronal injury. Currently, however, measurements of "free" bilirubin or albumin binding are not utilized clinically.

Bilirubin cycle

In the normal newborn, bilirubin concentration in serum is dependent on three factors: bilirubin synthesis, bilirubin metabolism (transport, conjugation or excretion) and bilirubin enterohepatic circulation.

• Bilirubin synthesis is increased due to: high numbers of erythrocyte precursors, short neonatal RBC lifespan and increased metabolism of cytochrome, myoglobin, etc.

- Rate limiting steps in neonatal bilirubin metabolism are: conjugation (low levels of the enzyme glucuronyl transferase) and uptake by hepatic cells.
- In the newborn, the enterohepatic circulation favors decreased excretion of bilirubin due to higher conversion of intestinally unstable bilirubin glucuronide, which is hydrolyzed to unconjugated bilirubin and reabsorbed. This is favored by high levels of beta glucuronidase in intestine, relatively alkaline pH, high monoglucuronide concentration, sterile gut unable to convert to urobilinogen and sterobilirubin, and good gut mucosal absorption of bilirubin.

Causes of unconjugated hyperbilirubinemia

- Increased bilirubin synthesis: isoimmunization (Rhesus, ABO), enzyme defects in red cell (G6PD, pyruvate kinase), red cell membrane defects (spherocytosis), extravasated blood (bruising, cephalhematoma), polycythemia, sepsis, DIC.
- Causes of abnormal bilirubin metabolism and excretion include: decreased conjugation (Crigler–Najjar's syndrome, Gilbert's syndrome), prematurity, hypothyroidism, hepatitis (viral, toxic, galactosemia, metabolic), biliary obstruction, GI obstruction, feeding related.

Investigations

Obtaining a careful history and physical examination is the single most important diagnostic procedure.

The following bloodwork should be taken:
- Bilirubin: conjugated and unconjugated.
- Full blood count, platelets, peripheral blood film, reticulocytes.
- Blood group (mother and newborn).
- Coombz' test.

The need for further tests depend on history, examination and results of above. The following is an incomplete list of investigations which may be considered in some situations: urinalysis, blood and urine culture, thyroid function, galactosemia screen, alpha$_1$–antitrypsin, TORCH studies, liver enzymes, G6PD, red cell fragility, clotting studies, abdominal ultrasound scan.

The risk of bilirubin encephalopathy from high levels of unconjugated bilirubin in the healthy term newborn may be much less than considered previously. This is still a point of considerable discussion. It is noteworthy that newly formulated recommendations from the USA increase the minimum level of unconjugated bilirubin which constitutes a risk for healthy term infants from 340–420 µmol/L and perhaps even 510 µmol/L. This should be borne in mind when weighing the risk of exchange transfusion against the risk of bilirubin encephalopathy in a healthy term newborn.

Causes of conjugated hyperbilirubinemia

Conjugated hyperbilirubinemia is due to defects in hepatocellular transport or insufficiency of bile secretion or flow and is defined as a level in serum of > 34 µmol/L or > 10% total bilirubin.

The pathology requires to be identified and the cause diagnosed as the etiology may be serious but ameliorated by early diagnosis and intervention.

A differential diagnosis includes:
- Neonatal hepatitis (idiopathic or caused by identified infectious agent).
- "Toxic" hepatitis (secondary to sepsis, ischemic, parenteral nutrition, etc.).
- Metabolic disease (alpha$_1$–antitrypsin, galactosemia, tyrosinemia, storage diseases, cystic fibrosis).
- Bile duct excretion disturbances (diseases causing intra– and extrahepatic bile duct obstruction including biliary atresia).

Hyperbilirubinemia and breast feeding

There are two types of breast feeding problems that are related to neonatal bilirubinemia.

1. Breast feeding jaundice of early onset ("too little breast milk" jaundice)
This exaggeration in physiological jaundice is related to inadequate breast milk intake and faulty breast feeding techniques which accentuate enterohepatic recirculation of bilirubin. Treatment consists of establishing proper breast feeding techniques, increasing breast milk production, ensuring breast feeding frequencies are adequate (10–12 times per day) and avoiding water or glucose–water supplements.

2. Breast milk jaundice of late onset
This is due to enhanced reabsorption of unconjugated bilirubin due to an unidentified factor which seems present in the majority of human milk and is noted in the second week of life and may persist for some weeks.

Treatment

Treatment of unconjugated hyperbilirubinemia is based on the concern that high levels are associated with bilirubin encephalopathy. Well term infants without abnormal red cell hemolysis constitute the lowest risk group.

Risk for neurotoxicity is increased by:
- Red cell hemolysis (e.g. Rhesus disease).
- Prematurity.
- Systemic illness (acidosis, hypoxia, hypoalbuminemia, drugs, etc.).

Although there is some literature concerning the use of phenobarbitone, and even tin, in the treatment of hyperbilirubinemia, treatment mainly relies on phototherapy or exchange transfusions. Underlying causes (sepsis, metabolic disease) must also be addressed.

1. Phototherapy
There will never be recommendations that are agreed upon by all neonatologists but most people would agree with the guidelines for the institution of phototherapy as noted in Table XIII. Phototherapy is most effective when started early in conjunction with oral feeds. Side effects of phototherapy are usually mild and include dehydration, hyperthermia, loose stools and damage to eyes. Treated children should have their fluids increased by 30% and wear eye patches.

Table XIII: Recommended bilirubin levels for instituting phototherapy

	Bilirubin μmol/L	
Weight	Well child	Sick child
> 2.5 kg	250	200
1.5–2.5 kg	200	150
< 1.5 kg	150	100

2. Exchange transfusion
There is not even agreement on the acceptable level of unconjugated bilirubin in a healthy term infant (340 μmol/L is commonly quoted but some authors allow 500 μmol/L). It would take a brave author to give dogmatic recommendations for sick premature infants. Often, the rate of rise is more important than absolute upper values. Consider exchange transfusion if:
• Severe hydrops fetalis, if first cord blood Hgb < 100 g/L.
• Hemolytic disease of newborn, if first cord blood bilirubin is already > 100 μmol/L.
• Bilirubin continues to rise rapidly in a premature infant despite use of double phototherapy.
Side effects of exchange transfusions are potentially significant and include the effects of the procedure (emboli, sepsis, fluid overload) and the dangers of a blood transfusion (infection, mismatch).

PATENT DUCTUS ARTERIOSUS (PDA)

During fetal life, the lungs receive only 10% of the cardiac output and blood is oxygenated in the placenta. The ductus arteriosus, which is well developed by the sixth week of gestation, forms an important communication that shunts blood from the pulmonary artery into the aorta. In the full term infant, functional closure of the ductus occurs in 90% of babies by 38 hours of age. That process is delayed or may not occur in preterm babies. Persistence of the ductus arteriosus (PDA) results in increased pulmonary blood flow and will either produce no symptoms or be symptomatic depending on PDA size and pulmonary vascular resistance. In relation to birth weight, symptomatic PDA has been found after 48 hours in 42% of 500–999 grams, in 21% of 1,000–1,499 grams and 7% of 1,500–1,750 grams babies. PDA is frequently found in premature babies with hyaline membrane disease and in sick premature newborns; it can also be found in combination with other congenital cardiac defects such as coarctation of the aorta as well as in other medical conditions such as congenital rubella (60–70% of affected infants).

1. Factors which may alter ductus closure
The constriction of the ductus arteriosus results from a complex interaction between multiple factors such as oxygen tension, levels of circulating prostaglandins and available smooth muscle of the ductus (all of them depend on the level of maturity and gestational age).

2. Complications of PDA
Even in the absence of congestive heart failure, PDA related increased pulmonary blood flow and increased lung water result in greater ventilator and oxygen requirements. This is considered an important factor in the genesis of BPD. The PDA may also lead to decreased diastolic tissue

perfusion, resulting in a higher incidence of renal dysfunction, necrotizing enterocolitis, intraventricular hemorrhage and cerebral periventricular (watershed) ischemia.

3. Diagnosis
- Diagnosis of a significant PDA is based on a combination of clinical, radiological and ECHO findings. The clinical examination usually reveals a systolic, sometimes continuous, murmur, hyperdynamic precordium, full or bounding peripheral pulses, and increased pulse pressure > 20 mm Hg.
- Signs of congestive heart failure or decompensated PDA include tachycardia > 170 beat/min, excessive weight gain > 3% per day, increasing ventilatory requirements or failure to make respiratory improvement, metabolic acidosis, hepatomegaly.
- Chest X–ray usually shows increased pulmonary vascular markings, pulmonary edema and cardiomegaly.
- The most specific and sensitive method of diagnosis of PDA at present is two–dimensional echocardiography and color Doppler.

4. Prevention and management of PDA
- Prenatal steroids lower the incidence of PDA and reduce RDS, BPD and grades III/IV IVH.
- In babies with suspected or symptomatic PDA, in anticipation of treatment with indomethacin, an early assessment of cardiac anatomy and function are recommended to rule out congenital heart disease with ductus dependent pulmonary or systemic circulation (e.g. coarctation of the aorta, critical aortic stenosis, etc).
- In a symptomatic premature newborn, the treatment options include:
    Supportive medical treatment: transient fluid restriction to 20–30% below estimated daily requirements, adequate oxygenation, hematocrit ≥ 0.4 and minimal handling of the infant. Pharmacological treatment with indomethacin (an inhibitor of prostaglandin synthesis), surgical ligation in cases when pharmacological treatment fails, or in the presence of contraindications to pharmacological treatment.

5. Indomethacin treatment
- Several different regimens have been developed to administer indomethacin but most of them use a standard of 3 doses (usually 0.1–0.2 mg/kg doses), given 12–24 hours apart intravenously (see the section on Neonatal Drug Dosage Guidelines).
- Pre–indomethacin administration assessment includes:
    Cardiac anatomy and function, ruling out congenital heart disease with ductus dependent pulmonary or systemic circulation (e.g. coarctation of the aorta, critical aortic stenosis, etc.).
    Assessment of renal function (BUN).
    Platelet count.
    Documentation of pretreatment weight and urine output.
- In anticipation of some degree of transient renal failure and decreased splanchnic circulation, a decrease in total fluid intake by 20–25% as well as holding enteral feeds around the time of indomethacin administration should be considered.
- Reported rate of ductal closure after first indomethacin dose is approximately 50%, after 2 doses 75% and after 3 doses 89%. There is, however, a significant recurrence: approximately 30–40% of previously "closed" PDA require one or two more courses of indomethacin or surgery.

- Side effects of indomethacin are mainly renal (decreased urine output, increased BUN, hematuria, proteinuria), metabolic (hyperkalemia, hyponatremia, hypoglycemia), GI (bowel ischemia, which may predispose to NEC) and hematological (decreased platelet function).
- Contraindications for indomethacin therapy include: poor urinary output < 0.5 mL/kg per h, serum BUN 10.5 mmol/L, platelet count < 50,000, signs of NEC and evidence of GI bleeding. Pulmonary hemorrhage, evidence of recent periventricular or intracranial hemorrhage, persistent fetal circulation and high bilirubin levels (> 200 g/L) may constitute additional contraindications.

6. Surgical closure of PDA
- Premature infants with persistent PDA and respiratory failure requiring continued ventilatory support beyond the first 1–2 weeks of life are prime candidates for surgical ligation of PDA. In some circumstances, the decision to treat surgically can be made earlier, e.g. an extremely premature neonate with significant clinical symptoms or a baby with a large PDA and major containdication(s) to indomethacin therapy. The decision to ligate is made jointly by the attending neonatologist, cardiology consultant and cardiac surgeon. Parental informed consent must be obtained. Neonates must have good intravascular access and be kept n.p.o. for at least 4 hours prior to surgery.
- Although most babies tolerate the procedure well, it is important to remember that acute morbidity related to PDA ligation includes hypothermia, pneumothorax, atelectasis, pulmonary edema, hyperglycemia, general instability, infection and pain. Recurrent laryngeal nerve damage is occasionally seen. Postoperative care includes close observation of general and cardiorespiratory function and adequate pain control for the first 24–48 hours.

INFANTS OF SUBSTANCE USING MOTHERS (ISUM)

The treatment of infants of substance using mothers (ISUM) is more than the symptomatic treatment of the baby. The family unit also requires assessment and may require treatment. In fact, the social situation may be of greater importance than the treatment of withdrawal in the newborn. In the development of an effective program to treat ISUM, the most important aspect is a nonjudgmental attitude and an understanding that addiction is a process with remissions and relapses to be anticipated and not perceived as failures. This complex, high risk situation is best managed by a multidisciplinary team, which includes pediatrics, obstetrics, family practice, a hospital social worker, nurse and Ministry of Social Services/Child Protective Services, all with expertise in dealing with ISUM.

In summary, the goal is to provide the best possible care for ISUM and their families. All members of the team should be consulted as early as possible in the pregnancy. Women should be given information about the concerns related to intrauterine substance exposure and counselled about what to expect once the baby is born. Involvement of the Ministry of Social Services/Child Protective Services should be initiated prior to birth in order to expedite the discharge process after delivery.

Admission

It is very important to document mother's current address and contact phone number.

1. History
- The assessment should begin as soon as the mother and infant enter the room. Unspoken words and body language can be important clues to both mental and physical health. The history and physical examination should be done in a comfortable, unhurried and empathetic atmosphere. Questions should be nonjudgmental and nonthreatening. This setting should convey a sense of interest, belief and support.
- Setting the scene:
    "I'd like to ask you some routine questions about drugs and alcohol use during your pregnancy".
    The history should be obtained with open–ended questions:
    Questions such as "did you use drugs during your pregnancy?" could lead to a dead–end. If there is a high suspicion of drug use, do not try at the outset to establish the fact but rather elicit information, as if it is a known fact, with questions such as: "When you used heroin during the pregnancy, did you use more at the beginning or towards the end?" In this way the conversation may avoid the unnecessary dead–ends caused by questions that are perceived as threatening or judgmental and will convey a sense that it is acceptable to talk about drug and alcohol use.
    The history should obtain specific details regarding:
    What was used? Ask specifically about prescription and nonprescription medications, cigarettes, alcohol and street drugs used before and during the pregnancy. Commonly used street drugs include: heroin, cocaine, marijuana, Talwin ± Ritalin (T's and R's), methadone (from a clinic or off the street) and other substances such as glue and solvents.
    How were the drugs used? Smoked, injected, inhaled or consumed orally?
    Were there periods of withdrawal? What were the symptoms? How frequent?
    When did you use it during the pregnancy? How often did you use it and how much did you use?
    When was the last time you used drugs or alcohol before delivery?
    Who do you use it with (i.e. partner, friends, relatives)? Who else uses drugs, drinks or smokes at home?

2. Physical examination
The physical examination should include a complete newborn examination with particular attention to possible clues of intrauterine drug or alcohol exposure. These include:
- Vital signs: temperature, heart rate, respiratory rate (e.g. respiratory distress may be the presentation of a metabolic acidosis, which could be the result of maternal solvent sniffing).
- Vasomotor instability: mottling, cyanosis during feeds, sweating, nasal stuffiness, sneezing, GI symptoms.
- Evidence of growth retardation: birth weight, head circumference, length.
- Behavior: resting versus handling state of arousal; how easy is it for the infant to make a state transition (i.e. awake alert to sleep state); response to light, sound and touch; evidence of specific acute narcotic withdrawal symptoms (see Neonatal Withdrawal Sheet for specific details)
- Skin: hemangioma.
- Minor physical anomalies: hair, ears, mouth, nose, eyes, etc.
- Organ malformation: GI, renal, cardiac, etc. Infants exposed to drugs in utero who later show evidence of withdrawal or fetal alcohol syndrome/fetal alcohol effect (FAS/FAE) can have an

entirely normal initial physical examination. Symptoms of withdrawal can be identical to symptoms of a concurrent illness (e.g. sepsis). Multiple conditions can coexist.

3. Neonatal and pediatric complications of maternal substance use
- Low birth weight.
- Prematurity.
- Microcephaly.
- Respiratory distress (including meconium aspiration and transient tachypnea of the newborn).
- Asphyxia.
- Infections (HIV, hepatitis, venereal diseases).
- Postnatal growth delay.
- Neonatal stroke.
- Neurobehavioral abnormalities (with long–term developmental delay).
- Increased incidence of sudden infant death syndrome (SIDS).

4. Clinical associations of fetal cocaine exposure
- Prematurity.
- Intrauterine growth restriction (IUGR).
- Neurodevelopmental abnormalities.
- Intracranial hemorrhage.
- Nonduodenal intestinal atresia or infarct.
- Limb reduction defects.
- Urinary tract anomalies.

5. Mnemonic for neonatal withdrawal
Wakefulness.
Irritability.
Tremulousness, temperature instability, tachypnea.
Hyperactivity, high pitched cry, hyperacusis, hypertonus.
Diarrhea, disorganized suck, difficult to comfort, diaphoresis.
Respiratory distress, rhinorrhea, rub marks.
Apnea.
Weight loss or failure to thrive.
Alkalosis.
Lacrimation.
Sneezing, seizures.

Infections in infants of substance using mothers

1. Hepatitis B
Mothers who have active hepatitis B infection or are chronic carriers of this infection pose a significant risk to their babies. Neonates born to mothers who are infected with hepatitis B virus (HBV) during the last trimester have approximately an 80% chance of acquiring the infection. Neonates born to mothers who are chronic carriers of hepatitis B surface antigen (HB_sAg) have approximately a 70% chance of becoming infected with hepatitis B virus. The virus carrier state develops in up to 90% of infected infants with a lifetime risk of 25% of death from chronic liver

disease or hepatocellular carcinoma. The administration of hepatitis B immunoglobulin (HBIg) soon after delivery, followed by 3 doses of hepatitis B vaccine, has proven successful in preventing perinatal HBV transmission in about 85–95% of cases. This vaccination regimen has proved to be effective because intrauterine infection is rare (about 5%) and most infants are exposed at the time of birth (an incubation period for hepatitis B is 6 weeks to 6 months). Since immunoprophylaxis is most effective if started as soon as possible after delivery, prenatal identification of pregnant women who are carrying HBV (HB$_s$Ag positive) is essential. The virus may also be transmitted to personnel who come in contact with blood or body secretions from these mothers. All mothers should be screened for HB$_s$Ag.

- HB$_s$Ag status: although there are particularly high risk groups (e.g. immigrants from countries with a high incidence of hepatitis B such as Asian countries, multiple transfusions of blood or blood products, or a history of injection drug use), there are many women with no identifiable risk factors who acquire HBV and therefore universal screening antenatally is recommended. The HB$_s$Ag status, by recent testing, of all mothers engaged in high risk activity should be known at the time of delivery or very soon thereafter.

- Labor and delivery: if the HB$_s$Ag status during the pregnancy (recent testing for women engaged in high risk activity) is not known on entry to the labor and delivery rooms, maternal blood sampling should be done as soon as possible. If the hepatitis B status is unknown and will not become available within 12 hours, immunoprophylaxis should be given.
  Immunoprophylaxis consists of HBIg and hepatitis vaccine which should be given at separate sites as soon as possible after delivery, preferably within 12 hours of delivery.
  If the mother is HB$_s$Ag negative on a recent test, but is still engaged in high risk activity or other members of the household are engaged in high risk activity, the baby should receive a course of hepatitis B vaccine, beginning within 12 hours of birth.

- Personnel protection: personnel attending the delivery or coming in contact with blood or body secretions of an infected mother should wear gloves, protective gown, mask and protective eyewear. All personnel should be immunized against HBV.

- Baby: practice universal precautions. These babies should be washed free of all blood in the delivery room. (Temperature control is important in neonates). If the infant's condition necessitates immediate transfer to the nursery, then the baby should be washed on admission to the nursery. Once the infant has been washed free of blood, (s)he poses no further hazard for several weeks. However, precautions for blood and body secretions should be exercised until the infant's blood (not cord blood) is shown to be free of Hb$_s$Ag, ruling out prenatal infection (5% risk).

- Laboratory investigations: the presence of HB$_s$Ag is indication of an acute infection. The presence of HB$_e$Ag, HB$_c$Ab, HB$_s$Ag is evidence of chronic infection. There may, however, be a "window period" where the mother is HB$_e$Ag negative and this is a time when HB$_s$Ab is being developed but IgM HB$_c$Ab is present. This is also evidence of an acute infection. The presence of IgG may mean an old infection.

- Prevention (Table XIV):
  If the infant is preterm or very ill, we recommend giving HBIg 0.5 mL i.m. at birth and every 6 weeks if the infant is not stable and has not received the hepatitis vaccine.
  Seroconversion rates in very low birth weight infants in whom vaccination was initiated shortly after birth have been reported in some studies to be lower than in those preterm infants vaccinated later or in term infants vaccinated shortly after birth. Therefore, delay vaccination in premature infants (< 2 kg) whose mothers are HB$_s$Ag negative until just

before hospital discharge. Infants of HB$_s$Ag positive mothers should be tested at 9 months (or at least 1 month after the third dose of hepatitis vaccine) for HB$_s$Ag and antibodies to HBV (to determine the outcome of the immunoprophylaxis).

2. Hepatitis C

- Hepatitis C virus (HCV) is the cause of parenterally transmitted non A, non B hepatitis. High risk groups include parenteral drug users, persons transfused with blood or blood products, health care workers with frequent blood exposure, persons with sexual or household contact with an infected person and persons with multiple sexual partners.
  HCV is vertically transmitted from mother to infant in 6–13% of cases according to recent studies.
- The consequences in the pediatric population have not been well defined. In approximately 50% of adult cases, HCV may result in chronic liver disease, which may include cirrhosis and hepatocellular carcinoma. There is a serological test available for anti–HCV. However, anti–HCV may be absent during acute illness and there are no confirmatory tests. Of note, screening in low risk populations has demonstrated a 50% false positive rate. Since plasma donors are screened for anti–HCV, immunoglobulin does not contain antibodies to HCV and is therefore not recommended in the treatment of infants born to HCV positive women.

Table XIV: Hepatitis B prevention for ISUM

Infants of	Dose	Age
HB$_s$Ag–positive mothers	HB vaccine 1 HBIg (0.5 mL i.m.) HB vaccine 2 HB vaccine 3	Birth within 12 h Birth within 12 h 1 mo 6 mo
HB$_s$Ag–unknown mothers	HB vaccine 1 HBIg (0.5 mL i.m.) HB vaccine 2 HB vaccine 3	Birth within 12 h Birth within 12 h 1 mo after vaccine 1 5 mo after vaccine 2
Mothers who are documented HB$_s$Ag–negative at the time of delivery	HB vaccine 1 HB vaccine 2 HB vaccine 3	 1 mo after vaccine 1 5 mo after vaccine 2

It is recommended to give the HB vaccine and the HBIg within 12 h of birth. However, if this is missed, in high risk cases such as ISUM, it is recommended to give the HB vaccine and the HBIg as soon as possible, up until 7 d of age. The efficacy of the HBIg after 48 h is unknown. After 7 d, give HB vaccine alone.

3. HIV

- Infants born to mothers engaging in high risk behavior (multiple sexual partners and intravenous drug users) are at risk of developing human immunodeficiency virus (HIV–1) infection. It appears that in approximately 80% of cases, the spread of the virus to the baby occurs just prior to or at the time of the delivery; in 20% of cases, the virus may infect the fetus during intrauterine life. Infants born before 34 weeks gestation have a higher rate of vertical transmission of HIV–1.
- The mother's infection is diagnosed by the presence of antibody to HIV. As it takes some time

to develop the antibody (usually within 6–12 weeks) there is a small chance of a negative antibody response even though the individual has the virus (window of recent seroconversion). Because the mothers have antibody present in essentially all instances and because mothers pass immunoglobulin to their baby, the baby will have maternally acquired antibody to the HIV. Therefore, all mothers who are seropositive (antibody positive) for HIV will have babies who are antibody positive for HIV. Approximately 20–30% of the babies born to seropositive mothers will actually be infected by the virus, that is two–thirds of the infants will not be infected and will not develop AIDS. The problem occurs in trying to diagnose which babies are truly infected by the virus as assays to detect the viral antigens or to culture the virus are only available through units which treat children with HIV. Long–term follow–up of the clinical and immunological well–being of all infants born to seropositive mothers is critical in specialized HIV units. Babies who are HIV positive are usually normal at birth, seldom symptomatic within the first 6 months of life and rarely require treatment at this stage. However, they should not receive oral polio vaccine nor BCG vaccine.

- See chapter 10 (Infectious Diseases) for treatment of HIV positive pregnant mothers.
- In order to handle the families in whom the mother is a member of a high risk group, there must be a balance between the rights of the mother, the rights of the baby, the safety of the staff and the need to maintain confidentiality.

Monitoring of children born to mothers with HIV infection

Babies born to mothers who are infected with the human immunodeficiency virus (HIV) are at risk for developing the infection themselves. Global studies show that transmission risk varies 10–50% and may be correlated to the degree of symptomatology suffered by the mother. Studies in developed countries show a lower risk of transmission, generally from 20–30%. There are multiple factors that may determine whether a child will become infected (maternal factors, viral factors and infant factors).

Diagnosing HIV infection in the baby can be difficult as the maternal antibody passes via the placenta to the baby and all babies will have the same HIV seropositivity as the mother at birth. Hence, all of the babies will be antibody positive whereas only approximately 20–30% of them may have the virus. In uninfected infants, the maternally acquired antibody will gradually decrease and only disappear in 12–18 months. Though the risk of transfer of HIV in breast milk is small, it is recommended that the baby be bottle fed.

For those babies who are infected with the HIV virus, approximately 20% of them will develop symptoms by 1 year of age and up to 80% will have later onset of AIDS defining conditions. Clinical features that should prompt diagnostic assessment for HIV infection in babies: infections (opportunistic or recurrent bacterial infections), lymphadenopathy and/or hepatosplenomegaly, lymphocytic interstitial pneumonitis, developmental delay (particularly language), failure to thrive, chronic parotitis, persistent oral thrush.

There are currently three ways of determining whether or not the child is infected with HIV: HIV culture, HIV p24 antigen detection and polymerase chain reaction (PCR). Antibody serology is not useful since it is contaminated with maternal antibody. HIV culture has a sensitivity of 60–100%. Antigen detection by commercially available kits is provided by the provincial laboratories. Polymerase chain reaction (PCR) has a low sensitivity in neonates but improves after 1–2 months to > 90%. One must take caution regarding testing of cord blood as a minute amount of maternal cells can contaminate the specimen. Therefore, testing cord blood with these assays is not recommended.

The following clinical assessment and laboratory investigations are recommended to follow the child born of an HIV infected mother, so as to determine as early as is feasible whether or not an HIV infection is present.

1. Clinical follow–up
- Growth and development (HIV infected babies grow more slowly).
- Milestones (HIV infected babies may be slow to achieve or lose milestones).
- Infections.
- Hepatosplenomegaly or lymphadenopathy.

2. Laboratory follow–up
- The infant should be studied at birth or at 1 month, then every 8 weeks until age 6 months, then every 12 weeks for the first 15–18 months. Using antigen detection test, most infants who are HIV infected (i.e. carry the virus) can be diagnosed by age 3 months.
- Every 3 months:
  CBC, differential, ESR (watch for neutropenia, lymphopenia, thrombocytopenia, or elevated ESR).
  T–cell markers (T_3, T_4, T_8, T_4/T_8) (watch for falling T_4 or T_4/T_8 ratio < 1.0).
  HIV serology (consistently decreasing titer may suggest maternal antibody only).
  HIV culture and p24 antigen and PCR testing (a positive culture and PCR would indicate HIV infection).
- Every 6 months:
  Liver and renal function tests (watch for liver abnormalities or elevated LDH, indicating lung disease).
  T–cell mitogens (PHA, PWM) (watch for falling proliferative response but one–third of babies with AIDS may have normal proliferation).
  IgG, IgA, IgM (watch for hyper– or hypogammaglobulinemia).
- As indicated: chest X–ray, ECG, cultures of various sources.
- Monitoring should be continued until HIV infection is proven (e.g. positive HIV culture, PCR or antigen test) or highly probable (e.g. opportunistic infection, severe drop in T_4 cells or T–cell mitogen responses), or when the serology is negative and the child is progressing well. It is unusual to have seroreversions (i.e. become seronegative) without some clinical or immunological abnormality if the infant is indeed infected.

Recommended immunization schedule for proven or suspected HIV positive babies

Routine immunizations are recommended with the following exceptions:
- BCG should not be given.
- Live attenuated oral polio should not be given due to the risk of acquiring polio. The killed, Salk polio vaccine is recommended.

The following immunizations are recommended:
- Hepatitis vaccine, as indicated.
- Diphtheria, pertussis, tetanus (DPT) and injectable polio vaccine (IPV).
- *Haemophilus influenzae* B vaccine.

- Flu shots for the entire household and for babies 6 months of age and older to be given in October or November.
- Measles, mumps, rubella vaccine (MMR).

Urine drug screening

The mainstay of laboratory testing for maternal substance use has been urine toxicology. There are several problems inherent in urine drug screening. The test is dependent on the concentration of the drug in the specimen tested, therefore, its accuracy in assessing drug use depends on the timing of the drug exposure prior to testing and the metabolism of the drug by the individual. A minimum of 10 mL of urine is required in order to run the drug screen, but 20 mL is the recommended volume of urine for testing the neonate and should be collected as soon as possible after birth. Samples can be pooled daily but subsequent day collections should be sent in separate containers so that the first day's sample is not diluted.

For storage and shipping, refrigerate (4 °C). If possible, send urine specimen to the laboratory within 24 hours of collection. If the laboratory is a distance from the nursery, the specimen (in cold packs) should be sent by courier to prevent the sample from warming up during shipment. If the sample will require more than 4 days for storage and shipping, it should be frozen at −20 °C.

Meconium testing and hair analysis are being used in some centers. Check with your toxicology laboratory to determine the screening tests used, the drugs routinely screened for and the confirmatory assays employed.

Social work consultation

Parents will be seen automatically and should be given high priority by the hospital social worker as these cases are identified as being high risk child protection situations.

The hospital social worker should interview the parent(s) with a view to collecting the following kinds of information concerning the mother's circumstances and attitude:

- Address: length of time at this address and previous address.
- Phone number: if no phone number, obtain one or more contact phone numbers where messages may be left.
- Drug and alcohol history in detail.
- Current living situation.
- Partner's name, status of relationship with the mother, baby's paternity, the partner's drug history.
- Support system.
- Attitude toward drug dependency and her interest and willingness to seek help.
- Plans for baby.
- Insight into their situation, that is, are they realistic about coping abilities, etc.?
- Willingness to become involved with community agencies, including the Ministry of Social Services/Child Protective Services and drug rehabilitation programs.
- Understanding of baby's medical condition and staff's treatment plans.
- Willingness to cooperate with medical recommendations, including the recommended transfer plans for baby.

Universal blood precautions

Universal blood precautions (UBP) are intended to prevent transmission of blood borne pathogens, primarily hepatitis B (HBV) and human immunodeficiency virus (HIV). This requires handling all blood and visibly bloody body fluids as though they are potentially infectious because infected infants may not always be recognized.

Environmental recommendations

Neonatal intervention is largely supportive and dependent on the type of substance the mother has used. Infants born to women who have used various substances can be irritable and easily excited by sensory stimuli. Therefore, the environment of these infants should be regulated by the caregiver to reduce the quantity and variety of sensory input. Methods of accomplishing this are dimming the lights in the nursery and reducing noise. If the nursery lights cannot be dimmed, a blanket can be placed over the incubator or bassinet. Many noises can be eliminated by not talking loudly at the bedside, keeping radios and intercom volumes low, silencing alarms quickly and quietly closing incubator doors. ISUM benefit from a private, isolation room or a quieter area of the nursery. Nursing care of the infant should be grouped and unnecessary handling should be avoided. Swaddling the infant, combined with gentle up and down rocking, has been shown to console them.

Recommendations for the feeding of infants of substance using mothers

While breast feeding is considered the best initial feeding for infants, at this time it is not recommended for infants of mothers who currently or had been using substances of addiction (such as opioids, cocaine and benzodiazepines). There are, as yet, no data indicating how long freedom from drug use prior to delivery will allow for drug free breast milk.

There are concerns of transmission of HIV in breast milk. Therefore, at this time, breast feeding is not recommended for mothers who are HIV positive.

Babies with evidence of withdrawal do not grow well on routine infant formula (20 Cal/30 mL). Therefore, a higher caloric formula (i.e. 24 Cal/30 mL) is recommended. Table XV gives a suggested observation sheet for use during drug withdrawal.

Pharmacological treatment of neonatal withdrawal

1. Indications
Treatment of neonatal withdrawal should be considered, having ruled out other medical conditions, when there is a constellation of the following signs and symptoms unresponsive to environmental control:
- Convulsions.
- Inconsolable or crying continuously for 3 hours.
- Persistent tremors or jitteriness when undisturbed.
- Continuous central nervous system irritability including hyperactive moro reflex, tremors or jitteriness, increased muscle tone and unprovoked muscle jerks.
- Persistent vomiting or projectile vomiting over a 12 hour period.
- Explosive diarrhea of 2–3 consecutive episodes.

Neonatal withdrawal is a constellation of signs and symptoms found in term infants showing evidence of withdrawal. Premature infants may not show the same signs and symptoms but may still be experiencing withdrawal.

2. Medications for narcotic withdrawal
*   Pediatric (neonatal) opium solution (0.04% = 0.4 mg/mL morphine equivalent); solution is prepared by Pharmacy to provide a 25 fold dilution of tincture of opium.
    Initial dose: 0.07 mL/kg* q3h p.o. If signs and symptoms persist, give half of this dose p.r.n. in between the maintenance doses (* pediatric opium is ordered in mL/kg; morphine is ordered in mg/kg). After the initial dose, treatment should be titrated according to clinical effect, recognizing the short half–life of morphine.
    Maintenance dose: continue initial dose. If p.r.n. doses are still necessary after 36 hours of treatment, increase maintenance dose by 20–50%, depending on the severity of symptomatology. (There has been no established upper limit of pediatric opium dosage for this purpose.) Maintain at optimal dosage for 72 hours before attempting to wean.
    To wean: decrease by 10% of effective dose (above) every other day. If withdrawal symptoms increase during weaning, give p.r.n. doses of half the last dose, no more frequently than q3h. This will allow for more rapid weaning. If medication is still required once the baby is weaned off the regular dose, give p.r.n. doses for symptomatic withdrawal.
*   Oral or intravenous morphine solution (1 mg/mL morphine):
    Initial dose: 0.028 mg/kg* q3h (* pediatric opium is ordered in mL/kg; morphine is ordered in mg/kg).
    Maintenance dose: same protocol as above.
    To wean: same protocol as above.
*   Medications for non–narcotic withdrawal: phenobarbital
    Initial dose: 10 mg/kg p.o. or i.v., followed by a second 10 mg/kg p.o. or i.v. 15 min later.
    Maintenance dose: 3–5 mg/kg q24h; first dose given 24 hours after loading. Phenobarbital levels should be followed.

Table XV: Neonatal withdrawal observation sheet

Gestational age at birth: _____   Birth weight: _____

	Signs and Symptoms √ = present 0 = not present	Interval of Observation									Comments (Date & time)
		Age										
		Date										
		Time										
METABOLIC/VASOMOT	Temperature											
	Heart rate											
	Respiratory rate											
	Sweating											
	Frequent yawning > 3–4 times/interval											
	Mottling											
	Nasal stuffiness											
	Sneezing > 3–4 times/interval											
	Nasal flaring											
CENTRAL NERVOUS SYSTEM	Cry: high pitched											
	Cry: inconsolable											
	Sleeps < 1 h after feeding											
	Sleeps < 2 h after feeding											
	Sleeps < 3 h after feeding											
	Hyperactive moro reflex											
	Tremors or jitteriness when disturbed											
	Tremors or jitteriness undisturbed											
	Abnormal muscle tone (↑ or ↓)											
	Unprovoked muscle jerks											
	Convulsions											
	Incoordinate sucking or swallowing											
GI	Regurgitation or vomiting (amount)											
	Projectile vomiting (amount)											
	Loose, watery or explosive stools (L/W/E)											
	Seedy, pasty or formed (S/P/F)											
OTHERS	Feeding: weak or absent suck (W/A)											
	Feeding: duration (min)											
	Excoriation/abrasions (specify area)											
	Weight											
	Pediatric opium solution: p.r.n. dosage											
	Observer's initials											

Developmental follow-up

It is important to recognize that no specific developmental dysfunction has been linked to a particular drug. Typical measures of a child's development may not provide specific information that can be related to the altered neurotransmitter activity in the developing nervous system caused by cocaine. Nor is it clear how altered autonomic function, state regulation and abnormal response to sensory stimuli are potentially related to impulsivity and altered mood in older children with prenatal cocaine exposure. Some recent work has shown that in early childhood, cocaine exposure has been associated with an increased incidence of individual children with subnormal developmental scores and difficulty with unstructured tasks that require initiation and goal setting. Drug exposed children have been shown to have a preference for easy tasks, attentional difficulties and may be more disruptive in a classroom setting. These behavioral problems may continue on into the school age and adversely influence IQ scores. Higher levels of depression, thought problems and aggressive behavior have also been reported among drug exposed children. These type of behavioral problems may not be easily identified in a typical structured assessment setting.

Prenatal exposure to illicit drugs is part of a larger set of social, economical and biological variables that put infants and children at risk for adverse growth and development. The environment that accompanies drug use often occurs in the midst of multiple risk factors which include poverty, inadequate nutrition, limited prenatal care, poor maternal mental health, HIV/AIDS, violence and family chaos that interfere with effective parenting. The presence of this combination of risk factors and the frequent use of multiple drugs make it extremely difficult to isolate the precise effects of one drug from other risk variables. Similarly, the long–term developmental and behavioral effects are also hard to determine because of the difficulty of controlling for all the variables that coexist in the postnatal environment.

Given this situation, child development in this setting can be best understood by considering an inter–relationship between pre– and postnatal factors. In such a multifactoral model, prenatal drug exposure creates a biological vulnerability that renders the child more susceptible to the effects of a poor environment. This may be either expressed as a developmental dysfunction or may be partly or completely compensated for by postnatal brain growth and development and/or competent caregiving. Therefore, our job as clinicians is to carefully identify these variables, determine their contribution to the child's and family's growth and development and develop, with the families and a multidisciplinary team of professionals, strategies to support the child and family to reduce the impact of these factors.

Family and social functioning should be an integral component of the comprehensive program developed for the high risk child. Therefore, care for the child should occur concurrently with an intervention program that promotes parenting skills, drug treatment and harm reduction as well as promoting child development. Ideally, this should occur in one clinical program where pediatric care, child development services and drug treatment occur in one location. Parents should be involved in all aspects of the assessment and treatment program. In this way, developmentally appropriate activities can be modelled and can engage parents in supporting their child's development. Recent experience suggests that mothers are more likely to comply with drug treatment if they see it as a part of their child's care. Child development services needed to address the effects of prenatal drug exposure should occur in a family context.

NEONATAL DRUG DOSAGE GUIDELINES
Emily Ling

These guidelines are intended to be used in an intensive care nursery with appropriate cardiorespiratory monitoring and therapeutic drug monitoring. Special note should be made of the comments column, which indicates special precautions regarding drug dosage or administration.

Table of contents

Reprinted with permission from the Department of Pharmacy, British Columbia's Children's Hospital, Vancouver, B.C., Canada

I. Antibacterial agents (mg/kg per dose)

Antibiotics	Routes of Admin.	Weight < 1,200 g Age 0–4 wk	Weight 1,200–2,000 g Age 0–7 d	Weight 1,200–2,000 g Age > 7 d	Weight ≥ 2,000 g Age 0–7 d	Weight ≥ 2,000 g Age > 7 d	Comments
Amikacin	i.m., i.v.	0–7 d (use GA*) < 28 wk 7.5 q24h 28–34 wk 7.5 q18h ≥ 35 wk 7.5 q12h		> 7 d (use PCA**) < 28 wk 7.5 q24h 28–34 wk 7.5 q18h ≥ 35 wk 7.5 q8h			1,3,5
Ampicillin *Meningitis*	i.v., i.m.	50 q12h	50 q12h	50 q8h	50 q8h	50 q6h	1
Other diseases		25 q12h	25 q12h	25 q8h	25 q8h	25 q6h	
Cefazolin	i.v., i.m.	20 q12h	20 q12h	20 q12h	20 q12h	20 q8h	1
Cefotaxime	i.v., i.m.	50 q12h	50 q12h	50 q8h	50 q12h	50 q8h	1
Ceftazidime	i.v., i.m.	50 q12h	50 q12h	50 q8h	50 q12h	50 q8h	1
Chloramphenicol	i.v., p.o.	25 q24h	25 q24h	25 q24h	25 q24h	25 q12h	1,2,3,5
Clindamycin	i.v., i.m., p.o.	5 q12h	5 q12h	5 q8h	5 q8h	5 q6h	2,5,6
Cloxacillin	i.v., i.m.	25 q12h	25 q12h	25 q8h	25 q8h	25 q6h	1; double dose for meningitis
Cotrimoxazole (Septra, Bactrim)	p.o., i.v.	Minor infections: p.o.: 4 mg TMP + 20 mg SMX/kg per dose q12h (= 0.5 mL/kg per dose q12h) Prophylaxis (urinary tract infection): p.o.: 4 mg TMP + 20 mg SMX/kg once daily (= 0.5 mL/kg q24h) Serious infections: i.v.: 5 mg TMP + 25 mg SMX/kg per dose q6–8h					2,5,6; not for use in infants < 1 mo; contains trimethoprim (TMP)/sulfamethoxazole (SMX) in a ratio of 1 to 5
Erythromycin	i.v., p.o.	10 q12h	10 q12h	10 q8h	10 q12h	10 q8h	1,2; hypertrophic pyloric stenosis noted in 5 infants
Gentamicin	i.v., i.m.	0–7 d (use GA*) < 28 wk 2.5 q24h 28–34 wk 2.5 q18h ≥ 35 wk 2.5 q12h			> 7 d (PCA**) < 28 wk 2.5 q24h 28–34 wk 2.5 q18h ≥ 35 wk 2.5 q8h		1,3,5

I. Antibacterial agents (mg/kg per dose)

Antibiotics	Routes of Admin.	Weight < 1,200 g — Age 0–4 wk	Weight 1,200–2,000 g — Age 0–7 d	Weight 1,200–2,000 g — Age > 7 d	Weight ≥ 2,000 g — Age 0–7 d	Weight ≥ 2,000 g — Age > 7 d	Comments
Metronidazole	i.v., p.o.	Loading: 15; then 7.5 q48h	Loading: 15; then 7.5 q24h	Loading: 15; then 7.5 q12h	Loading: 15; then 7.5 q12h	15 q12h	1,6; neutropenia
Penicillin G — Meningitis	i.v.	50,000 units q12h	50,000 units q12h	50,000 units q8h	50,000 units q8h	50,000 units q6h	1
Penicillin G — Other diseases		25,000 units q12h	25,000 units q12h	25,000 units q8h	25,000 units q8h	25,000 units q6h	
Penicillin G benzathine	i.m.		50,000 units (one dose only)	50,000 units (one dose only)	50,000 units (one dose only)	50,000 units (one dose only)	
Penicillin G procaine	i.m.		50,000 units q24h	50,000 units q24h	50,000 units q24h	50,000 units q24h	
Piperacillin	i.v., i.m.	75 q12h	75 q12h	75 q12h	75 q8h	75 q6h	1
Rifampin	p.o.	10 q12h	10 q12h	10 q12h	10 q12h	10 q12h	2,5,6
Ticarcillin	i.v., i.m.	75 q12h	75 q12h	75 q12h	75 q8h	75 q6h	1
Tobramycin	i.v., i.m.	Same as gentamicin					1,3,5
Vancomycin	i.v.	*(see table below)*					1,3,4; infuse over 60 min to avoid red-man syndrome

Vancomycin:

PCA**	Dose (mg/kg per dose)	Dosing interval
< 27 wk	18	q36h
27–30 wk	16	q24h
31–36 wk	18	q18h
≥ 37 wk	15	q12h

1. Increase dosing interval in renal impairment.
2. Reduce dose in liver impairment.
3. Monitoring of serum drug concentration recommended.
4. Check special protocol for administration.
5. Close clinical monitoring for dose related and idiosyncratic toxicity recommended.
6. Inadequate pharmacokinetic studies in neonates; only indicated in very unusual situations.

GA* = gestational age; PCA** = postconceptional age

Clearance of amikacin, gentamicin, and vancomycin is influenced both by the gestational age and the postnatal age. Therefore, in infants > 7 days old, it might be useful to consider the postconceptional age in the dosing schedule. The dosage is in mg/kg per dose.

II. Other drugs

Drug	Route	Dosage	Comments
Acetaminophen (Tylenol) 80 mg/mL oral solution; 120 mg suppository	p.o., p.r.	*Preterm:* 5 mg/kg per dose q6–8h p.r.n. *Term:* 10–15 mg/kg per dose q6–8h p.r.n.	• Contraindicated in infants with G6PD deficiency • Overdose results in delayed hepatotoxicity
Acyclovir 500 mg vial for injection	i.v.	<u>Herpes simplex:</u> 10 mg/kg per dose q8h for 10–14 d <u>Varicella:</u> 15 mg/kg per dose q8h for 10–14 d	• Adverse reactions noted: transient renal dysfunction associated with rapid infusion or large doses • Increase in dosing interval required in patients with significant renal impairment
Adenosine (Adenocard) 3 mg/mL injection	i.v.	Supraventricular tachycardia (SVT): *Initial dose:* 0.05 mg/kg; if not effective within 2 min, may repeat p.r.n. every 2 min in the following doses: 0.1 mg/kg, 0.15 mg/kg, 0.2 mg/kg, 0.25 mg/kg (i.e. dose is increased in 0.05 mg/kg increments to a maximum of 0.25 mg/kg) *Median dose:* 0.15 mg/kg	• Clinical effects occur rapidly and are brief • Must be given by rapid i.v. push as quickly as possible (half–life < 10 s); administer at i.v. site closest to infant; follow dose with normal saline flush; monitor ECG, heart rate, and blood pressure • Contraindicated in second or third degree AV block or Sick–sinus syndrome unless pacemaker placed • Adverse effects (transient): dyspnea, flushing, irritability, dysrhythmias, nausea; minimal hemodynamic effects • Theophylline antagonizes effects • Do not refrigerate; precipitation may occur
Aminophylline 5 mg/mL injection; 3 mg/mL, 25 mg/mL oral solution	i.v., p.o.	<u>Apnea of prematurity:</u> *Loading:* 6 mg/kg per dose *Maintenance:* Initiate with 2.5–3.75 mg/kg per dose q12h Bronchodilation for infants > 6 wk <u>postnatal age:</u> *Loading:* 6 mg/kg per dose *Maintenance:* 3 mg/kg per dose q6h	• Ethylenediamine salt of theophylline • Contains 80% theophylline

II. Other drugs

Drug	Route	Dosage	Comments
Amphotericin B 50 mg vial for injection	i.v.	Initiate with 0.5 mg/kg per 24 h and increase by 0.25 mg/kg per 24 h up to 1 mg/kg per 24 h (Note: dilute in D5W or D10W only; minimum dilution recommended is 0.1 mg/mL; in fluid restricted patients or central line patients 0.2 mg/mL; infuse over 4–6 h)	• Adverse reactions: hypotension, thrombophlebitis, renal dysfunction (hypokalemia, azotemia, distal renal tubular acidosis, hyposthenuria), hematologic (anemia, thrombocytopenia, granulocytopenia) • Monitor closely hematological and renal status (CBC, platelet count, serum creatinine, BUN, electrolytes) • Interrupt therapy for 2–5 d when renal function falls to < 25% normal; adverse effects appear to be less common in neonates
Atropine 0.4 mg/mL injection	i.v. over 1 min; endotracheal	0.01 mg/kg per dose; to be repeated q10–15 min with the total maximum dose of 0.04 mg/kg	• Indicated for bradycardia; presumed to be vagal in origin
Budesonide (Pulmicort) suspension for inhalation: 0.5 mg/mL; 0.25 mg/mL	via nebulizer	Bronchopulmonary dysplasia: 1 mg via nebulizer b.i.d. (given together with ventolin 0.25 mL and diluted to total volume of 3 mL with normal saline)	• Adverse effects: oral thrush; routine prophylaxis with nystatin suspension used by some; for other potential steroid effects, see dexamethasone • Ampoules must be shaken prior to withdrawing dose • Unused contents must be discarded after 12 h • Rinse patient's mouth after every dose and wash face if using mask to prevent oral thrush
Calcium gluconate 10% injection	i.v.	Cardiac resuscitation: 1–2 mL/kg per dose (over 10 min) Symptomatic hypocalcemia: 1–2 mL/kg by slow infusion over 30 min Maintenance: 2–4 mL/kg per 24 h (200–400 mg/kg per 24 h) mixed in compatible i.v. fluids	• Contains elemental Ca^{2+} 0.23 mmol/mL or 9 mg/mL • Monitor closely for bradycardia, dysrhythmias and extravasation • Infusion rate not to exceed 20 mg Ca^{2+}/kg per min

II. Other drugs

Drug	Route	Dosage	Comments
	p.o.	400–800 mg/kg per 24 h (36–72 mg/kg per 24 h elemental Ca^{2+}) div. equally among feedings; start with 400 mg/kg per 24 h (36 mg/kg per 24 h elemental Ca^{2+}) and increase gradually as tolerated	• i.v. preparation can be given orally to supplement nutritional intake in preterm infants to a total intake of 150 mg/kg per 24 h of elemental calcium including content of feedings • Less irritating to GI tract than calcium chloride
Calcium polystyrene sulfonate (Resonium calcium)	p.o., p.r.	Acute hyperkalemia: 1 g/kg per dose q6h as needed	• 1 g/kg decreases serum K^+ by 0.5–2.0 mmol/L; exchanges approximately 1.6 mmol K^+/g of resin
Captopril 1 mg/mL oral solution	p.o.	Initial dose: 0.01 mg/kg per dose q6–8h; increase dose by 50–100% to titrate BP to desired range (usual dosage range 0.03–1.5 mg/kg per 24 h)	• Adverse effects: rash, hypotension, oliguria, hyperkalemia, proteinuria, agranulocytosis • Contraindicated in neonates with bilateral renal artery stenosis or unilateral renal artery stenosis with single kidney • Dosage reduction required in patients with renal impairment (decreased clearance with decreased GFR)
Chloral hydrate 100 mg/mL syrup	p.o., p.r.	10–30 mg/kg per dose q6–8h p.r.n. Maximum dose: 120 mg/kg per 24 h	• Can cause gastric irritation; laryngospasm if aspirated • Caution in preterm infants: reported cases of coma 24–48 h following doses; postulated to be due to delayed gastric emptying and/or immature liver function • Avoid large doses in severe cardiac disease • Contraindicated in severe hepatic/renal impairment
Cimetidine 150 mg/mL injection; 60 mg/mL oral syrup	p.o., i.v.	Preterm: 2–4 mg/kg per dose q12h Term neonates: 2–4 mg/kg per dose q8h Infants: 2–4 mg/kg per dose q6h	• Use in neonates still experimental • Eliminated, mostly unchanged by kidney • Reduction of dosage required in renal dysfunction • Can cause CNS side effects

II. Other drugs

Drug	Route	Dosage	Comments
Cisapride oral suspension 1 mg/mL	p.o.	Gastric stasis and GE reflux: 0.15 mg/kg per dose t.i.d. or q.i.d. (generally given 20–30 min prior to feeds)	• Prokinetic agent similar in efficacy to metoclopramide and domperidone but with no dopamine antagonist properties • No extrapyramidal effects • Limited data on dosage or efficacy in neonates
Defibrillation		Approximately 1 watt sec/kg Maximum: 10 watt sec/infant	
Dexamethasone sodium phosphate (Decadron) 4 mg/mL injection; 0.5 mg/mL oral solution	i.v., p.o.	Bronchopulmonary dysplasia: 0.25 mg/kg per dose q12h i.v. or p.o. for first 3 d then 0.15 mg/kg per dose q12h for next 3 d; this dose is reduced by 10% q3 d until a dose of 0.1 mg/kg per 24 h is reached; following 3 d at this dose, the drug is given on alternate days for 7 d and then discontinued Speculative use for edema of trachea postextubation: 0.5 mg/kg per dose q8h; therapy generally not continued beyond 1 d	• Short–term adverse effects: hyperglycemia, glucosuria, and hypertension (these effects often observed early in course of treatment), hypokalemia, hypocalcemia, edema, hypertrophic cardiomyopathy • Long–term adverse effects: increased risk of sepsis, nephrocalcinosis (in infants on furosemide), osteopenia, growth suppression • Acute adrenal insufficiency may develop if abruptly discontinued after treatment for > 1 wk • Contraindicated in patients with active untreated infections • Dilute i.v. preparation to 0.2 mg/mL with D5W; administer by slow i.v. over 5 min
Diazepam (Valium) 5 mg/mL injection	i.v.	0.1–0.2 mg/kg slow i.v. push over 2 min; repeat q5–10 min as needed up to a total dose of 1 mg/kg	• Indication: not used as a first line anticonvulsant; short–term adjunctive therapy in status epilepticus • Risk of CNS and respiratory depression, hypotension, and phlebitis • Contraindicated in hyperbilirubinemia due to sodium benzoate preservative in injectable vehicle
	p.r.	0.5–1 mg/kg; parenteral preparation to be used in conjunction with a syringe and catheter inserted in the rectum	

II. Other drugs

Drug	Route	Dosage		Comments
		Loading[a] (μg/kg) i.v.[c]	Maintenance[b] (μg/kg per dose) i.v.[c]	
Digoxin 0.05 mg/mL injection; 0.05 mg/mL oral solution	i.v., p.o.	Preterm[d] 20 μg Full-term 30 μg Infant > 2 mo 40 μg Above dosages are for CHF, producing levels of 1.3–2.7 nmol/mL; higher doses may be needed for treatment of arrhythmias	2–3 μg q12h 3–4 μg q12h 5 μg q12h	a. Loading dose is given in 3 div. doses (½, ¼, ¼) q6h; start maintenance 24 h after last digitalizing dose in preterm and 12 h after in full-term neonates b. Maintenance dose is generally 25% of the total loading dose c. The p.o. dose is 25% more than the i.v. dose d. At 1 mo of age, increase maintenance dose to that of full-term neonates
Dobutamine 12.5 mg/mL injection	i.v.	2.5–15 μg/kg per min *Maximum:* 20 μg/kg per min		• Acts directly on β_1–receptors to increase myocardial contractility • No dopaminergic effect to selectively increase renal and mesenteric blood flow • Adverse effects: dysrhythmias, systemic hypertension or increase in pulmonary capillary wedge pressure • May be preferred over dopamine as an inotrope in the neonate with cardiogenic shock

II. Other drugs

Drug	Route	Dosage	Comments
Dopamine (Inotropin) 200 mg/5 mL injection	i.v.	Continuous i.v. infusion: *Initial*: 2–5 µg/kg per min increasing gradually up to 20 µg/kg per min for desired cardiac or vascular effects; minimum dilution = 0.8 mg/mL in D5W or D10W Suggested method for calculation of dopamine and isoproterenol solutions: Dilute with D5W or D10W Select: desired drug dose and desired i.v. fluid rate Calculation: mg/100 mL = wt(kg) × 6 × desired dose (µg/kg per min) / desired i.v. fluid rate (mL/h)	• Dose dependent pharmacological actions: Renal: 2–4 µg/kg per min i.v. Inotropic (β_1): 5–10 µg/kg per min i.v. Vasoconstrictive (α): > 10 µg/kg per min i.v. • Care must be exercised to prevent local infiltration since vasoconstrictive activity will lead to vasospasm and tissue necrosis • The manufacturer recommends reinfiltrating the area with an α–blocker, phentolamine 5–10 mg (1 mg/mL in normal saline) in adults as soon as possible after extravasation; but there is no clinical experience in neonates as to dosage or efficacy • Experimentally, only a few drops of the 1 mg/mL solution are needed to reverse the vasoconstriction; benefits should be weighed against potential risks (local effect of infiltration in tiny baby; systemic effect of hypotension)
Epinephrine 1:10,000 (0.1 mg/mL) injection; 1:1,000 (1 mg/mL) injection	i.v., ETT, rarely intracardiac	Cardiac arrest: 0.1–0.3 mL/kg per dose of 1:10,000 concentration i.v. push, ETT or rarely intracardiac Refractory hypotension (refractory to dopamine/dobutamine): *Continuous infusion*: 0.1–1 µg/kg per min; use 1:1,000 (1 mg/mL) concentration to make up infusion solutions	• Never use 1:1,000 (1 mg/mL) concentration to prepare i.v. push doses; use 1:10,000 (0.1 mg/mL) • Adverse effects: cardiac arrhythmias (PVC's and ventricular tachycardia); decreased renal and splanchnic blood flow
Exosurf neonatal		See surfactant	

II. Other drugs

Drug	Route	Dosage	Comments
Fentanyl citrate (Sublimaze) 0.05 mg/mL injection	i.v.	Pain or sedation: Intermittent: 2.5–5 µg/kg per dose over 10 min q2–4h p.r.n. Continuous infusion: 5–10 µg/kg loading dose over 10 min followed by 5–10 µg/kg per h (in some neonates, doses as high as 60 µg/kg per h may be required during prolonged therapy due to development of tolerance)	• Preferred agent for use in infants with PFC or cardiovascular instability • Adverse effects: respiratory depression and apnea, bradycardia, chest wall rigidity (with large doses), functional ileus, urinary retention, neonatal abstinence syndrome • Tolerance develops rapidly to sedative effects, necessitating increases in dosage • It is recommended to gradually taper fentanyl when patient has received therapy for > 1 wk • Assess analgesic and/or sedative effects frequently; if dosage increase required, give loading dose of 5 µg/kg over 10 min; increase infusion rate in 20–25% increments
Flucytosine 20 mg/mL oral suspension; 10 mg/mL injection	p.o.	25–37.5 mg/kg per dose q6h (Note: i.v. preparation is investigational; infuse over 30 min and monitor serum concentrations)	• Adverse reactions noted: enterocolitis, nausea or vomiting, diarrhea, hepatotoxicity, bone marrow suppression • Monitor closely hematological, renal, and liver function status • Increase dosing interval to q12h when renal function is 50% normal and to q24h when renal function is < 10% normal
Fludrocortisone (Florinef) 0.1 mg tablet	p.o.	Congenital adrenal hyperplasia: 0.1–0.2 mg once a day	• Excessive therapy can cause hypertension
Furosemide (Lasix) 10 mg/mL injection; 10 mg/mL oral solution	i.v., i.m., p.o.	Initial: 1 mg/kg per dose q24h in preterm; q12h in full-term; up to q6h > 1 mo; maximum single i.v. dose is 2 mg/kg (i.v. push over 2–3 min)	• Adverse effects: hypovolemia, hyponatremia, hypokalemia, hypocalcemia, hypomagnesemia, hypochloremic alkalosis, nephrocalcinosis, ototoxicity

II. Other drugs

Drug	Route	Dosage	Comments
Glucagon 1 mg vial for injection	i.m., i.v.	30 µg/kg i.m.; may repeat p.r.n.; 0.5–2 mg/24 h as continuous infusion (dilute in D5W or D10W)	• Limited use in neonates; indicated in persistent hypoglycemia despite aggressive glucose infusion (> 14 mg/kg per min) or problem of fluid overload
Heparin 1,000 unit/mL injection (10 unit/mL injection reserved for central venous line or peripheral line heparin locks)	i.v.	To keep indwelling lines open: 1 unit/mL in flushing and parenteral solutions For heparinization: Initial: 50 unit/kg Maintenance: 20–25 unit/kg per h	• Monitor baseline and subsequent coagulation studies: clotting time, PT, activated PTT, INR, platelet count, and fibrinogen
Hepatitis B immunoglobulin (HBIg)	i.m.	0.5 mL as soon after birth as possible (within 12 h)	• For prophylaxis in newborns whose mothers are hepatitis B antigen (HB$_s$Ag) positive
Hepatitis B recombinant vaccine (Engerix–B)	i.m.	0.5 (10 µg) administered within 7 d of birth and again at 1 and 6 mo of age	• Hepatitis B vaccine may be given at the same time as HBIg but should be given in a separate site
Hydralazine (Apresoline) 20 mg/mL injection 1 mg/mL oral suspension	i.v. p.o.	Initial dose: 0.2 mg/kg per dose q4–6h as required for BP control; dose may be gradually increased by 0.1 mg/kg per dose as needed; usual dose range: 1–4 mg/kg per 24 h p.o. dose generally twice the effective i.v. dose	• Causes direct relaxation of smooth muscle in peripheral vascular bed • Give by slow i.v. push at rate not exceeding 0.2 mg/min • May cause tachycardia, SVT, diarrhea, emesis, agranulocytosis • Decrease dosage in renal failure • Oral bioavailability generally 50% that of i.v. route
Hydrochlorothiazide (Hydrodiuril) 2 mg/mL oral suspension	p.o.	1–2 mg/kg per dose q12h	• Common adverse effects: hypovolemia, hyponatremia, hypokalemia, hypomagnesemia, hypochloremic alkalosis • Rare adverse effects: hypercalcemia, hyperglycemia

II. Other drugs

Drug	Route	Dosage	Comments
Hydrocortisone 100 mg vial for injection	i.v.	For adrenal crisis: 25 mg i.v. bolus, followed by continuous infusion 50–100 mg/m² per 24 h until improvement occurs	• Wide variation in glucocorticoid requirements • Dose must be individualized according to growth and hormone data • Can cause adrenal suppression, growth retardation, fluid and electrolyte disturbances, hyperglycemia, increased susceptibility to infections
	p.o.	Maintenance dose for congenital adrenal hyperplasia: 6–8 mg/m² per dose t.i.d.	
	i.v.	Neonatal hypoglycemia: 1–2 mg/kg per dose q8h	• Indicated in persistent hypoglycemia despite aggressive glucose infusion (> 14 mg/kg per min) or problem of fluid overload
Immune serum globulin (Human)	i.m.	Prophylaxis for hepatitis A: 0.02 mL/kg Replacement therapy for hypogamma-globulinemia: 100 mg/kg per mo (= 0.6 mL/kg per mo)	
Immunoglobulin IV (Gamimune 5%) (Sandoglobulin 3%)	i.v.	Replacement therapy for congenital or acquired antibody deficiency: 100–200 mg/kg q2–4 wk Treatment of severe systemic viral or bacterial infections: Preterm: 0.5 g/24 h over 3 h for 6 d Term: 1 g/24 h over 3 h for 6 d Neonates with passive autoimmune thrombocytopenia: 1 g/kg per 24 h for 2 d (reconstitute in 0.9% saline solution as a 5% solution, and infuse over 12 h on each of 2 consecutive days)	• Can cause anaphylactoid and hypersensitivity reactions • Start infusion at very slow rate and increase slowly • Adjunctive therapy in severe infections with theoretical benefits

II. Other drugs

Drug	Route	Dosage	Comments
Indomethacin (Indocin) 1 mg vial for injection	i.v.	*0–7 d:* 0.2 mg/kg per dose at hour 0 0.1 mg/kg per dose at hour 12 0.1 mg/kg per dose at hour 36 *> 7 d:* 0.2 mg/kg per dose at hour 0 0.2 mg/kg per dose at hour 12 0.2 mg/kg per dose at hour 36 Infuse over 30 min	• Adverse effects: transient renal dysfunction (oliguria, hyponatremia, hyperkalemia, elevated BUN, creatinine), platelet dysfunction, hypoglycemia • May reduce renal clearance of aminoglycosides, digoxin, theophylline, vancomycin; close monitoring of serum concentrations of these drugs is required
Insulin human (regular) (Humulin R) 100 unit/mL	i.v.	Hyperglycemia: Start with 0.05 unit/kg per h as a continuous infusion (add 10 units of insulin to 100 mL of fluid; 1 mL/kg per h = 0.1 unit/kg per h); titrate infusion to maintain blood glucose concentration between 5.6 and 8.3 mmol/L Hyperkalemia: Start with 0.3 unit insulin/g glucose; increase glucose and insulin proportionately according to serum glucose and potassium levels	• Use syringe pump and microbore tubing if possible to reduce adsorption and improve delivery; flush with 5 mL of solution prior to infusion • If standard tubings used, flush with solution, double the volume of the dead space of the tubing
Ipratropium bromide (Atrovent) 0.25 mg/mL solution	inhalation	Inhalation solution: 0.125 mg (0.5 mL) diluted to 3 mL with normal saline q6h	• Not generally approved for use in children < 5 yr old • Use only after consultation with neonatologists • Little systemic absorption from respiratory or GI tract
Iron (Ferrous sulfate) 25 mg Fe²⁺/mL oral drops	p.o.	Treatment of iron deficiency: 6 mg/kg per 24 h elemental iron Prevention of iron deficiency: 2 mg/kg per 24 h elemental iron	

II. Other drugs

Drug	Route	Dosage	Comments
Isoproterenol (Isuprel) 0.2 mg/mL injection	i.v. infusion	*Initial:* 0.05 µg/kg per min; may increase q4 min by 0.05 µg/kg per min as required	• β₁ and β₂ adrenergic agonist; dose dependent inotropic and vasodilator effect • May decrease coronary and renal blood flow; adjust rate of infusions to keep heart rate < 200/min
Ketoconazole (Nizoral) 2% topical cream; 20 mg/mL oral suspension	p.o.	<u>Oral candidiasis (thrush):</u> 5 mg/kg per 24 h div. q12–24h; continue treatment for 2 d after lesions clear (usual course of therapy is 2–3 wk); discontinue therapy if no improvement after 1 wk <u>Cutaneous candidiasis (unresponsive to nystatin):</u> Apply 2% cream topically b.i.d.–t.i.d.	• Limited data on efficacy and toxicity in neonates • Adverse reactions: hepatotoxicity, nausea and vomiting, adrenal cortical insufficiency (reported with high doses in adults) • Drug interactions: increases serum concentrations of phenytoin, theophylline, cyclosporine, warfarin; decreases serum concentrations of rifampin and isoniazid; decreased GI absorption when given concomitantly with H₂-blocker or antacid • Perform periodic liver function tests; monitor for signs of adrenal insufficiency
Lidocaine (Xylocaine) 20 mg/mL injection	i.v., ETT	<u>Ventricular arrhythmias:</u> *Initial:* 0.5–1 mg/kg i.v. over 5 min; may repeat once after 5 min *Subsequent infusion:* 10–50 µg/kg per min	• For short-term control of ventricular arrhythmias; may cause hypotension • Should be used in critical care areas only • Monitor serum concentrations: therapeutic range: 6–21 µmol/L; toxic: > 21 µmol/L
Lorazepam 4 mg/mL injection	i.v.	*Initial:* 0.05–0.1 mg/kg per dose, may repeat dose in 15 min *Maintenance:* dose not determined, but suggest 0.05–0.1 mg/kg per dose q6–8h p.r.n.	• May be useful in seizures refractory to phenobarbital and phenytoin • Lorazepam has a distinct advantage over diazepam as a result of its significantly longer duration of action and equally effective onset of action • Same dosage can be used for sedation (limited information)

II. Other drugs

Drug	Route	Dosage	Comments
Magnesium sulfate 50% (500 mg MgSO$_4$/mL) injection (4 mEq Mg^{2+}/mL or 2 mmol/mL)	i.v., i.m., p.o.	For hypomagnesemia: 25–50 mg MgSO$_4$/kg (0.1–0.2 mmol Mg^{2+}/kg), may repeat q6h for 3–4 doses Maintenance: 31.2–62.5 mg MgSO$_4$/kg per 24 h (0.125–0.25 mmol Mg^{2+}/kg per 24 h) to be added to total i.v. fluid	• For i.v. use, the solution should be diluted to 1% (add 1 mL 50% injection to 49 mL normal saline or sterile water) and the required dose infused over a minimum of 60 min • For i.m. use, dilute to a concentration of 200 mg/mL MgSO$_4$ • For oral administration, use injection and dilute 1:10 with sterile water or formula • Monitor blood pressure, serum magnesium, calcium, and phosphate levels
Midazolam HCl 5 mg/mL injection	i.v.	Sedation: Continuous infusion: 0.05 mg/kg loading dose over 15 min followed by continuous infusion of 0.5 μg/kg per min	• Major adverse effect: hypotension (neonates with compromised intravascular volume or receiving opioids appear to be at greatest risk) • Monitor blood pressure closely during administration of loading dose • Use a dilution of 1 mg/mL for administration of loading dose • Assess sedative effects frequently; if dosage increase required, give loading dose of 0.025 mg/kg over 15 min and increase infusion rate (0.1 μg/kg per min increments) • Limited data on use in neonates

II. Other drugs

Drug	Route	Dosage	Comments
Morphine sulfate 2 mg/mL injection; 10 mg/mL injection; 1 mg/mL oral solution	i.v., i.m., p.o.	Neonatal withdrawal: *Initial:* 0.028 mg/kg per dose p.o. or i.v. q3h; gor maintenance dose and p.r.n. doses, see guidelines under pediatric opium solution Postoperative pain: *Bolus:* 0.05 mg/kg over 5 min followed by initial infusion of 0.03 mg/kg per h Sedation: *Bolus:* 0.05 mg/kg over 5 min followed by initial infusion of 0.02 mg/kg per h	• Can cause respiratory depression and apnea, hypotension, bronchospasm, functional ileus, and possibly physical dependence • Tolerance to sedative and analgesic effects may develop, necessitating dosage increases • Specific antidote for narcotic overdose: naloxone 0.1 mg/kg i.v. • Monitor for pain and sedative effects frequently; if more medication is required, give bolus dose (0.05 mg/kg) and increase infusion rate (generally by 0.01 mg/kg per h)
Nitroglycerin 5 mg/mL injection	i.v.	Start with 0.1 µg/kg per min and titrate infusion rate to desired response	• The role of nitroglycerin therapy in the neonate is at present unclear and its use is considered experimental • It may be preferred over nitroprusside in the treatment of severe cardiac failure to reduce afterload
Nitroprusside 50 mg vial for injection	i.v.	*Initial:* 0.25 µg/kg per min; titrate infusion rate by doubling rate of infusion until desired or adverse effects are observed; maximum rate of infusion is 6 µg/kg per min; for infusion, dilute to a concentration of 100 µg/mL; protect solution and line from light	• Indicated in refractory hypertension • Toxicity manifested by hypotension, reflex tachycardia, methemoglobinemia, cyanide toxicity with metabolic acidosis • Wean dose slowly as acute withdrawal may precipitate hypertensive crisis
Nystatin 100,000 unit/mL suspension	p.o.	100,000–200,000 unit/dose q6h	
	topical	Applied as ointment or cream 3–4 × daily (100,000 unit/g)	

II. Other drugs

Drug	Route	Dosage	Comments
Pancuronium 2 mg/mL injection	i.v.	*0–1 wk:* 0.03 mg/kg *1–2 wk:* 0.06 mg/kg *2–4 wk:* 0.09 mg/kg *4 wk:* 0.10 mg/kg Infuse slowly over 3–5 min; repeat as required q2–4h	• Indicated in infants requiring mechanical ventilation who continue to have inadequate oxygenation despite optimal supportive care • Can cause tachycardia • Effects potentiated in hypothermia, acidosis, renal dysfunction, hypokalemia, hypermagnesemia, and with concomitant use of aminoglycosides
Paraldehyde 1 g/mL injection	i.v.	Seizures refractory to standard anticonvulsants: *Loading:* 3 mL/kg per h (150 mg/kg per h) of a 5% solution × 3 h *Maintenance:* 0.4 mL/kg per h (20 mg/kg per h) of 5% solution	• For i.v. administration, add 5 mL (5 g) to 100 mL normal saline or D5W to make a 5% solution • Administer via syringe pump with a glass syringe; i.v. tubing and syringe must be protected from light by wrapping • i.v. tubing (and syringe if plastic) should be replaced every 4 h • Adverse effects: pulmonary edema and hemorrhage, hypotension, local irritation, displacement of bilirubin from albumin • Routine use discouraged except for treatment of status epilepticus, resistant to initial therapy with phenobarbital, phenytoin, diazepam, or lorazepam • Contraindicated in pulmonary or hepatic disease
	p.r.	0.3 mL/kg per dose (300 mg/kg) q4–6h p.r.n.; dissolve dose in equal volume of olive oil prior to administration; irregularly absorbed by rectal route	

II. Other drugs

Drug	Route	Dosage	Comments
Pediatric opium solution (0.04% = 0.4 mg/mL morphine equivalent)	p.o.	**Neonatal withdrawal:** *Initial:* 0.07 mL/kg per dose p.o. q3h; if signs and symptoms persist, give 50% of this dose p.r.n. in between maintenance doses *Maintenance:* same as initial dosage schedule: increase dosage by 20–50% as necessary based on the severity of symptoms; maintain at the effective dosage for 72 h before attempting to wean *Weaning:* decrease effective dosage by 10% every other day; if withdrawal symptoms occur, give p.r.n. doses (50% of last dose) no more frequently than q3h	• For neonatal withdrawal • Can cause constipation and CNS depression • May use oral or i.v. morphine instead
Phenobarbital 30 mg/mL injection	i.v., i.m, p.o.	**Neonatal seizures:** *Loading:* 15–30 mg/kg i.v. slowly (maximum rate of infusion 2 mg/kg per min) *Maintenance:* 3–5 mg/kg q24h (first dose given 24–48 h after loading) **Asphyxiated infants:** 1–3 mg/kg q24h	• Indication: neonatal seizures • If seizures continue after the initial i.v. loading dose, additional doses of 5 mg/kg (spaced at 20–30 min intervals) can be given, up to a total loading dose of 40 mg/kg to achieve a plasma level of 170 μmol/L (must ensure adequate respiratory control if using high dose) • Adverse effects: lethargy, sedation, and hypersensitivity reactions • Long half-life in neonates • Drug levels increased with alkalosis • Drug interactions: reduces serum levels of chloramphenicol; plasma phenobarbital levels increased by phenytoin and valproate

II. Other drugs

Drug	Route	Dosage	Comments
Phenytoin (Dilantin) 50 mg/mL injection; 6 mg/mL oral suspension; 50 mg chewable tablet	i.v., p.o.	*Neonatal seizures:* *Loading:* 20 mg/kg i.v. slowly (maximum rate of infusion 0.5 mg/kg per min *Maintenance:* 2–3 mg/kg per dose q12h; if > 1 wk old, may require increases in dosage or increases in frequency of administration (frequent drug monitoring essential in the first 3 wk of age due to rapid changes in elimination rate)	• Infuse in normal saline only • Rapid i.v. administration may cause hypotension and bradycardia • Indication: neonatal seizures refractory to phenobarbital alone • Adverse effects: drowsiness and behavioral changes, hypersensitivity reactions • Drug interactions: increases serum levels of chloramphenicol; diazepam or phenobarbital may increase or decrease phenytoin levels
Phosphate supplements		i.v. injection preparations can be given orally to supplement nutritional intake in preterm infants to a total intake of 75 mg/kg per 24 h of phosphorus, including content of feeds; begin with 20–25 mg/kg per 24 h and gradually increase dose to full supplement to prevent diarrhea	• Monitor serum Ca^{2+}, PO_4, and alkaline phosphatase
Potassium phosphate injection	i.v., p.o.	1 mL = 93 mg (3 mmol) phosphorus (as mono– and dibasic phosphate) = 4.4 mmol K^+	• Dilute in compatible solutions for i.v. administration • Note high K^+ content
Sodium phosphate (Lyphomed) injection	i.v., p.o.	1 mL = 93 mg (3 mmol) phosphorus = 4 mmol Na^+	• Dilute in compatible solutions for i.v. administration
Prednisone 5 mg/mL oral suspension	p.o.	1 mg/kg per dose q12h	• Rare indications, e.g. hemangiomatosis • All side effects of steroids

II. Other drugs

Drug	Route	Dosage	Comments
Propranolol (Inderal) 1 mg/mL injection; 1 mg/mL oral suspension	i.v., p.o.	Tachyarrhythmia: i.v.: Acute: 0.01–0.02 mg/kg per dose over 10 min; may repeat q10 min to total of 4 doses Maintenance: Initiate with 0.01–0.02 mg/kg per dose q6h; increase as needed to maximum of 0.15 mg/kg per dose q6h p.o.: 0.5–1 mg/kg per dose q6h Hypertension: i.v.: Initiate with 0.01–0.02 mg/kg per dose q6h; increase as needed to 0.15 mg/kg per dose q6h p.o.: 0.5–1 mg/kg per dose q6h Neonatal thyrotoxicosis: p.o.: 2 mg/kg per 24 h div. q6h	• Drug dosages are increased in a stepwise fashion until desired therapeutic effect is achieved or side effects develop • May cause hypotension, bradycardia, bronchospasm • EKG and blood pressure should be monitored during i.v. administration
Prostaglandin E₁ (Prostin VR) 500 μg/mL injection	i.v.	Initial: 0.05–0.1 μg/kg per min i.v. (or IA) Maintenance: once stable improvement, decrease dosage to ½ or less Suggested protocol: Dissolve 500 μg of PGE₁ in 100 mL of D5W (5 μg/mL) Initial: 0.05 μg/kg per min i.v. (0.6 mL/kg per h of 5 μg/mL concentration); solution stable for 24 h	• For maintaining blood flow through patent ductus in certain congenital heart diseases • Maximal effect: cyanotic lesions < 30 min, acyanotic average < 3 h • Major adverse effects: hypotension and apnea
Pyridoxine 100 mg/mL injection	i.v., p.o.	Initial: 50–100 mg i.v. over 1–2 min Maintenance: 50–100 mg p.o. daily	• Indication: for diagnosis and treatment of pyridoxine dependent seizures • Initial dosing should be accompanied by EEG monitoring • No toxicity reported with therapeutic doses

II. Other drugs

Drug	Route	Dosage	Comments
Ranitidine 15 mg/mL oral suspension; 25 mg/mL injection	i.v., p.o.	For the prevention and treatment of stress ulcers and GI hemorrhage: *p.o.:* *Preterm, term:* 1–1.5 mg/kg per dose q12h *i.v.:* *Preterm:* 0.5–0.75 mg/kg per dose q12h *Term:* 0.5–0.75 mg/kg per dose q8h *Continuous infusion:* 0.06–0.1 mg/kg per h	• Limited data on use in neonates; no adverse effects have been reported in infants and children • Reduce dose in renal dysfunction • Lack of adverse effects on endocrine system strongly supports use over cimetidine • For i.v. administration, dilute to final concentration of 2.5 mg/mL in D5W or D10W and infuse over 15 min; concentration of 5 mg/mL can be used for central line administration • Monitor AST, ALT during therapy
Ribavirin (Virazole) 6 g vial	aerosol	Administer using a SPAG–2 aerosol generator provided by the company; the drug is delivered via an oxygen hood or through the inhalation tubing of a ventilator; concentration of drug in reservoir (20 mg/mL) is not varied with patient weight; treatment is carried out for 12–18 h/d for 3–7 d	• Rash and conjunctivitis have been observed • Special precautionary measures need to be taken when drug is being given through a ventilator to avoid drug deposition and consequent malfunctioning of expiratory valve
Salbutamol (Ventolin) 5 mg/mL solution	via nebulizer	0.25–0.5 mL/dose of inhalation solution diluted to 2–3 mL with normal saline q2–6h p.r.n.	• Monitor heart rate • Major adverse effect is tachycardia
Sodium polystyrene Sulfonate resin (Kayexalate)	p.r., p.o.	1 g/kg per dose q6h	• For treatment of hyperkalemia associated with oliguria or anuria • Exchanges: 1 mmol of K⁺/g resin • Monitor for hypocalcemia, hypomagnesemia, hypokalemia, and hypernatremia
Spironolactone (Aldactone) 2 mg/mL oral suspension	p.o.	1–3 mg/kg q24h	• Used in conjunction with other diuretics for potassium sparing effects • Monitor serum potassium levels to avoid hyperkalemia

II. Other drugs

Drug	Route	Dosage	Comments
Surfactant beractant (Survanta)	endotracheal	Treatment of hyaline membrane disease: 4 mL/kg per dose up to 4 doses at least 6 h apart in infants requiring assisted ventilation and an $FiO_2 \geq 0.3$; administer in 4 aliquots through a catheter inserted into the endotracheal tube (see manufacturer's administration guidelines)	• Modified natural surfactant extract from bovine lung • Close monitoring of transcutaneous O_2 saturation, arterial blood gases, tidal volumes, and ECG is essential to follow rapid changes in lung compliance and to prevent postdosing hyperoxia and hypocarbia • Adverse effects: pulmonary hemorrhage, ETT blockage, apnea
Colfosceril palmitate (Exosurf neonatal) 108 mg/8 mL suspension	endotracheal	Treatment of hyaline membrane disease: Initiate with a 5 mL/kg dose, administered in two 2.5 mL/kg half-doses via a sideport endotracheal tube adapter (see manufacturer's administration guidelines); give second dose 12 h later in infants who remain on the ventilator	• A protein free synthetic surfactant (dipalmitoyl phosphatidylcholine, hexadecanol, and tyloxapol) • Close monitoring of transcutaneous O_2 saturation, arterial blood gases, NVM (tidal volumes), and ECG is essential to follow rapid changes in lung compliance and to prevent postdosing hyperoxia and hypocarbia • Reconstitute vials with 8 mL of preservative-free sterile water for injection; resulting suspension is stable for 12 h at 2–30 ºC • Adverse effects: pulmonary hemorrhage, ETT blockage, apnea
Survanta		See surfactant	

II. Other drugs

Drug	Route	Dosage	Comments
Theophylline	i.v., p.o.	*Apnea of prematurity:* *Loading:* 5 mg/kg *Maintenance:* 2–3 mg/kg per dose q12h *Bronchodilation for infants > 6 wk postnatal age:* *Loading:* 5 mg/kg *Maintenance:* 2.5 mg/kg per dose q6h	• With advancing postnatal age, the clearance of the drug increases; may need to give q8h to maintain therapeutic levels • May cause tachycardia, hyperglycemia, jitteriness, diuresis, and seizures • Increase dose by 20% to convert to aminophylline • Monitor serum levels to avoid toxicity • Monitor peak and trough levels when used for bronchodilation in older infants > 6 wk postnatal age
L–Thyroxine (Synthroid) 0.025 mg (25 µg) tablet	p.o.	Initial dose is 10 µg/kg once per d; increase dose by 12 µg/24 h q2 wk until TSH < 20 mU/L and T₄ 130–190 nmol/L; generally 25–50 µg is given daily	• Make a 5 µg/mL suspension in oral syringe following supplied instructions
Tolazoline (Priscoline) 25 mg/mL injection	i.v.	*Load:* 0.5–1 mg/kg *Maintenance:* 0.5–1 mg/kg per h	• Pulmonary vasodilator • Major side effects: hypotension, oliguria, and GI bleeding
Vitamin D (D–Vi–Sol) 400 IU/0.6 mL oral solution	p.o.	*Preterm, term:* 400 IU/24 h	
Vitamin K₁ 1 mg/0.5 mL injection	i.m., s.c., i.v.	*Prevention of hemorrhagic disease of newborn:* *i.m. or s.c.: Term:* 1 mg at birth; if body weight < 1,500 g, 0.5 mg at birth *p.o.:* 2 mg with first clear feed *Treatment: i.v.:* 1 mg/kg; give slowly, not exceeding 1 mg/min	• When given i.v., monitor blood pressure
Vitamins (Poly–Vi–Sol)	p.o.	0.6 mL/d	• Contains (in 0.6 mL): vitamin A 1500 IU, vitamin D 400 IU, ascorbic acid 30 mg, thiamine 500 µg, riboflavin 600 µg, niacinamide 4 mg

III. Drugs used in neonatal resuscitation

Drug	Indication	Dose	Route	Response	Complications
Albumin 5% Fresh frozen plasma	Hypovolemic shock	10–20 mL/kg	i.v.	Increased perfusion	Circulatory overload in cardiogenic shock
Calcium gluconate (10%)	Low cardiac output	1–2 mL/kg per dose	i.v. over 2–5 min	Improved cardiac output	Bradycardia dysrhythmias
Dopamine	Low cardiac output, shock	5–15 µg/kg per min to maintain blood pressure	i.v.	Increased cardiac output, increased peripheral vascular resistance	Dysrhythmia?; decreased renal perfusion if dose > 12–15 µg/kg per min
Epinephrine 1:10,000 (0.1 mg/mL)	Asystole or severe bradycardia	0.1–0.3 mL/kg	i.v. or ETT, rarely intracardiac	Increased heart rate, blood pressure, and cardiac output	Hypertension, ventricular fibrillation
Glucose (10%)	Hypoglycemia	0.5 g/kg (5 mL/kg) followed by infusion 5 mL/kg per h (approximately 8 mg/kg per min)	i.v.	Increased blood glucose	
Glucose (25%)	Hypoglycemia	0.5 g/kg (2 mL/kg)	i.v.	Increased blood glucose	Rebound hypoglycemia, hyperosmolar
Group O–Rh negative blood	Acute blood loss	10–20 mL/kg	i.v.	Increased perfusion and oxygen carrying capacity	Cross-match against mother's serum
Naloxone (Narcan) 1 mg/mL	Narcotic depression (rare)	0.1 mg/kg per dose repeated p.r.n.; give rapidly; may repeat p.r.n.	i.v., i.m., s.c., or ETT	Improved respiratory effort	Acute withdrawal syndrome in infants of narcotic addicted mothers
Sodium bicarbonate (4.2%)	Metabolic acidosis	2–3 mmol/kg per dose	i.v. over 2–5 min	Increased pH if adequate ventilation	Hypernatremia, hyperosmolarity, IVH?

IV. Guidelines for therapeutic drug monitoring a. Antibacterial agents			
Drug	Optimal sample time	Optimal serum concentration range	Time to steady state after dose change
Amikacin	Peak: 30 min after 30 min infusion	25–30 mg/L	24–48 h
	Trough	3–5 mg/L	
Gentamicin	Peak: 30 min after 30 min infusion	6–10 mg/L	24–48 h
	Trough	0.5–2 mg/L	
Tobramycin	Peak: same as gentamicin	6–10 mg/L	24–48 h
	Trough	0.5–2 mg/L	
Vancomycin	Peak: 1 h after 1 h infusion	25–35 mg/L	24–72 h
	Trough	5–10 mg/L	

Trough serum drug concentration: sample taken within 30 min prior to the next dose.
Serum measurements are routinely obtained at a steady state, which is usually around the third dose after start or change of dosage and then once weekly. Earlier measurements may be necessary in very sick infants with fluctuating renal conditions.
Not necessary to draw serum levels of drugs unless patient will be maintained on therapy > 3 days.

IV. Guidelines for therapeutic drug monitoring b. Other drugs			
Drug	Optimal sample time	Optimal serum concentration time	Time to steady state after dose change
Digoxin	Trough	1.3–2.7 nmol/L	4–7 d with total digitalization and 1–2 wk without digitalization
Flucytosine	Peak (30 min after 30 min infusion)	50–100 mg/L	
Phenobarbital	Trough	65–170 µmol/L	14 d
Phenytoin	Trough	40–80 µmol/L	4 d after i.v. doses (rapid increase in elimination rate over the first weeks of life necessitates frequent monitoring of drug levels)
Theophylline	Trough Peak Trough	For apnea: 55–70 µmol/L For bronchodilation (for infants > 6 wk postnatal age: 80–110 µmol/L 55 µmol/L	3–4 d

Trough serum drug concentration: sample taken within 30 min prior to the next dose.
Peak serum drug concentration: sample taken 1 h postdose.

V. Recommended concentrations and infusion times for intravenous medications		
Medication	Final concentration for i.v. administration	Infusion rate
Acyclovir	7 mg/mL	60 min
Adenosine	3 mg/mL	Rapid i.v. push
Amikacin	5 mg/mL	30 min
Aminophylline	5 mg/mL	20 min
Amphotericin B	0.1 mg/mL: peripheral lines 0.2 mg/mL: central lines	4–6 h
Ampicillin	50 mg/mL	5 min
Atropine	0.4 mg/mL	1 min
Cefazolin	100 mg/mL	20 min
Cefotaxime	100 mg/mL	20 min
Ceftazidime	100 mg/mL	20 min
Chloramphenicol	50 mg/mL	30 min
Cimetidine	15 mg/mL	15 min
Clindamycin	6 mg/mL	15 min
Cloxacillin	100 mg/mL	20 min
Dexamethasone	0.2 mg/mL	5 min
Diazepam	5 mg/mL	5 min
Digoxin	0.05 mg/mL	5 min
Erythromycin	2.5 mg/mL	60 min
Fentanyl	0.05 mg/mL	10 min
Furosemide	10 mg/mL	5 min
Gentamicin	10 mg/mL	30 min
Heparin (loading doses)	1,000 unit/mL	5 min
Hydralazine	0.2 mg/mL	5 min
Hydrocortisone	1 mg/mL	5 min
Indomethacin	0.5 mg/mL	30 min
Lidocaine (loading doses)	20 mg/mL	5 min

V. Recommended concentrations and infusion times for intravenous medications		
Medication	Final concentration for i.v. administration	Infusion rate
Lorazepam	0.1 mg/mL	5 min
Metoclopramide	0.5 mg/mL	15 min
Metronidazole	5 mg/mL	60 min
Midazolam	1 mg/mL	15 min
Morphine	2–10 mg/mL	5 min
Pancuronium	0.2 mg/mL	5 min
Penicillin G	100,000 unit/mL	20 min
Phenobarbital	30 mg/mL	not > 2 mg/kg per min
Phenytoin	50 mg/mL	not > 0.5 mg/kg per min
Phytonadione (Vitamin K1)	1 mg/0.5 mL	not > 1 mg/min
Piperacillin	90 mg/mL	20 min
Propranolol	1 mg/mL	10 min
Pyridoxine	100 mg/mL	1–2 min
Ranitidine	2.5 mg/mL	15 min
Ticarcillin	50 mg/mL	20 min
Tobramycin	10 mg/mL	30 min
Trimethoprim/sulfamethoxazole (Bactrim)	1.6 mg/mL trimethoprim in D5W	60 min
Vancomycin	5 mg/mL	60 min

SEIZURES AND EPILEPSY

An epileptic seizure is a clinical event related to a paroxysmal electrical discharge in the cerebral cortex. Many paroxysmal events in children are not epileptic seizures. It is important to distinguish these events from epileptic seizures because of differences in treatment and natural history. An accurate description of an episode from an eyewitness is important. Particular attention should be paid to the description of the setting, stimulus, prodrome or aura, onset, course, and termination of the event. Laboratory investigations are usually not helpful. An EEG is of limited value unless an episode is captured during the recording.

Paroxysmal nonepileptic events which mimic seizures:
- Behavioral: daydreaming, aggressive outbursts, self–stimulation, psychogenic seizures.
- Involuntary movements: jitteriness, rigors, tics, dystonias.
- Anoxic ischemic events: reflex anoxic seizures, cyanotic and pallid breath holding attacks, syncope, migraine.
- Sleep related: night terrors, sleep walking, enuresis, sleep myoclonus, narcolepsy–cataplexy, suffocation (Münchausen's syndrome), cardiac arrhythmias.
- Vertigo.

Classification of epileptic seizures and epilepsies

An epileptic seizure is a symptom of underlying brain dysfunction. Optimal management of the patient requires an understanding of the underlying brain disorder. Determination of the seizure type (seizure classification) and the biological setting in which the seizure occurs (epilepsy classification) may suggest the nature of the underlying cause of the seizures. Seizure classification is based on the clinical features of the seizure and the EEG pattern both during and between seizures. In most patients, an ictal EEG recording is not obtained.

1. Partial
Consciousness and/or memory are not affected in a simple partial seizure but are in a complex partial seizure. The clinical features are related to the localization of the epileptic focus. Simple partial seizures may become complex partial. Partial seizures may secondarily generalize.
- Simple partial: motor (focal, Jacksonian), sensory (tingling, visual phenomena, smells), autonomic (pallor, flushing), psychic (déja vu, music, fear).
- Complex partial: simple partial onset, impairment of consciousness at onset.
- Partial becoming generalized.

2. Generalized
Absence, tonic–clonic, clonic, tonic, myoclonic, atonic.

3. Other
Epileptic spasms.

Etiology of seizures

Management of seizures is made easier by determining if the seizures are: symptomatic of an acute brain insult, due to a genetic form of epilepsy or symptomatic of an underlying chronic brain abnormality.

1. Acute symptomatic seizures

Some seizures in children occur as a symptom of an acute brain insult. Prompt diagnosis of the underlying cause may be extremely important, e.g. hypoglycemia, bacterial meningitis.

*   Common causes of acute symptomatic seizures are:
    Infection: meningitis, encephalitis, brain abscess.
    Metabolic: glucose, sodium, calcium, magnesium or acid–base disturbances.
    Hypoxic–ischemia. Trauma.
    Vascular: hemorrhage, thrombosis, emboli.
    Toxic: endogenous (renal or hepatic failure), exogenous (drugs, lead).

2. Genetic causes of seizures without underlying brain abnormality

Many seizures in children occur in the absence of an underlying brain abnormality and are related to a genetic predisposition. The past medical history and neurological examination are usually normal and there is often a family history of seizures. Four common syndromes occur in children:

*   Febrile convulsions:
    A seizure occurring in a child between 6 months and 5 years of age, in association with fever but without evidence of central nervous system infection or defined cause, is a febrile seizure. Approximately 98% of children who have a febrile seizure have a self–limiting form of recurrent seizures, which occur only with a febrile illness and which stop by 5 years of age. These children do well at school and antiepileptic drug treatment does not influence the outcome.
    Approximately 2% of children who present with a febrile seizure develop recurrent afebrile seizures.
    Risk factors for the development of epilepsy include: complex seizures (i.e. focal, prolonged more than 15 minutes, or multiple seizures in same illness), family history of epilepsy in parent or sibling, and/or neurological abnormality.
    The risk of recurrent afebrile seizures is approximately 7% with one risk factor, 20% with two risk factors, and 50% with three risk factors. EEG and CT head scan are not helpful in the prediction of later epilepsy and are rarely indicated in the management of febrile seizures.
    It is appropriate to use diazepam and phenytoin to stop a prolonged febrile seizure but prophylactic antiepileptic treatment is rarely indicated.
*   Benign rolandic epilepsy:
    This is the single most common cause of partial seizures in children. The seizures start between 4 and 10 years of age. The seizure involves focal clonic movements or somatosensory symptoms of the hand or face. Drooling is often a prominent feature. These seizures usually occur during sleep and only 10% become generalized. The EEG demonstrates a characteristic epileptiform abnormality. These children outgrow their seizures by 14 years of age. Antiepileptic drug treatment does not influence the outcome but may be useful if the seizures are occurring during the day and resulting in social stress.

- Childhood absence epilepsy:
    This common form of epilepsy starts between 3 and 10 years of age and is characterized by brief staring episodes accompanied by characteristic 3 cycles/second spike–wave discharges on EEG. A routine EEG with hyperventilation almost always demonstrates the classical abnormalities in the untreated patient. Ethosuximide and valproic acid are the most effective drugs. Thirty to 50% of patients with absence epilepsy will develop tonic–clonic seizures during their teenage years.
- Juvenile myoclonic epilepsy:
    This syndrome is characterized by myoclonic seizures and tonic–clonic seizures occurring in an otherwise normal person. The myoclonic seizures usually occur shortly after wakening and are often not reported unless questioned directly. The tonic–clonic seizures occur during sleep and may be precipitated by sleep deprivation, alcohol consumption and menstruation. This type of epilepsy starts between 8 and 20 years of age and the predisposition to seizures is lifelong. Valproic acid is the treatment of choice.

3. Seizures due to underlying brain abnormality

An underlying brain disorder can be demonstrated in only 30% of children with epilepsy. Cerebral dysgenesis is the commonest etiology but is often not demonstrated on CT or MRI head scans. The presence of dysmorphic features may suggest such a diagnosis. Neurocutaneous disorders such as tuberous sclerosis, neurofibromatosis and Sturge–Weber's syndrome may be recognized by careful examination of the skin. Hypoxic–ischemic brain injury, trauma and previous CNS infection are usually suggested by the history. Brain tumors and vascular malformations are a rare cause of epilepsy in children. Brain tumors causing seizures are usually benign and slow growing. Genetic metabolic disorders and progressive neurodegenerative disorders are a rare cause of epilepsy but early diagnosis may have important genetic implications.

Investigation of a patient with epilepsy

The purpose of the investigation of the child with seizures is to determine the nature of the underlying brain disorder. In many patients, such as the child with febrile seizures, the clinical history and examination suggest the diagnosis, so further laboratory investigations are not indicated. In other patients with characteristic clinical syndromes, which suggest a genetic epilepsy, an EEG is the only investigation needed. The chance of missing an underlying treatable cause, such as a brain tumor, is small but it is not zero. Most physicians are cautious and would order a CT scan if any doubt existed after the inital examination.

An interictal EEG may be extremely helpful in the identification of the type of epilepsy in the patient with definite seizures. The interictal EEG is often of limited value, however, in determining the nature of episodes, particularly in the child under 3 years of age. The occurrence of an episode during an EEG can usually establish if there is an epileptic basis for the episode.

Treatment of seizures in children

1. Drug treatment

Many children with seizures have an age related self–limiting disorder and do not require therapy. Furthermore, approximately 50% of children who present with an afebrile seizure will have no further seizures. The risk of recurrence in these children is increased when there is a family history of seizures in a close family member, a history of previous neurological insult or previous febrile seizure, and an epileptiform abnormality on the EEG. Most children are not treated after their first seizure unless the risk of recurrence is high. Table I describes first and second line drug choices for the different seizure types.

Table I: Antiepileptic drug selection

Seizure type	First line drug	Second line drug
Partial seizures	Carbamazepine, clobazam	Phenytoin, vigabatrin, lamotrigine, gabapentin
Generalized seizures:		
Tonic clonic	Valproic acid, carbamazepine[1]	Clobazam, phenytoin
Absence	Ethosuximide, valproic acid	Lamotrigine, clonazepam
Myoclonic	Valproic acid, clobazam	Clonazepam, nitrazepam, lamotrigine
Infantile spasms	ACTH, vigabatrin[2]	Nitrazepam, valproic acid

[1] *May precipitate seizures in patients with generalized spike–wave discharges on EEG.*
[2] *First line choice for children with tuberous sclerosis.*

Drug doses and therapeutic monitoring are covered in other parts of the manual. Phenobarbitone is often used in the treatment of partial and generalized seizures in children under 1 year of age but there are concerns regarding the effect of phenobarbital on the developing brain.

Most children outgrow their seizures. Withdrawal of medication is usually considered if the child has been seizure free for more than 2 years, has a normal EEG and has no clinical evidence of neurological abnormality.

2. Patient and parent education
The diagnosis and prevention of seizures during antiepileptic medication are only part of the overall management of the child with epilepsy. Education of the child and parents is a critical part of the modern management of epilepsy. The family needs to know the anticipated natural history of the child's epilepsy (if this is known) and what to do if another seizure occurs. Oral and written instructions on the use and adverse effects of medication improve compliance and effectiveness of medical therapy. Many children have associated difficulties, such as educational and social difficulties, which may be a greater handicap than the seizures.

ACUTE HEMIPLEGIA

The sudden onset of an acute focal neurological deficit suggests either a vascular or an epileptic mechanism. Transient hemiparesis may be due to a Todd's paresis, migraine or hypoglycemia.

Evaluation

A careful clinical assessment is important. The neurological examination should demonstrate the localization of the lesion and may provide clues to the etiology. A neurological consultation should be obtained. An underlying diagnosis is made in about one–third of children with ischemic stroke.

Etiology of stroke in childhood:
- Idiopathic.
- Traumatic.
- Cardiac: congenital or rheumatic heart disease, endocarditis, atrial myxoma, arrhythmias, mitral valve prolapse.
- Hypertension.
- Hematological: sickle cell disease, leukemia, bleeding diathesis, polycythemia, severe dehydration.
- Vascular: arteriovenous malformation, cerebral aneurysm, Moya–Moya, carotid artery injury or fibromuscular dysplasia.
- Vasculitis: hemolytic uremic syndrome, Henoch-Schönlein purpura, Kawasaki's disease, systemic lupus erythematosus, polyarteritis nodosa, Takayasu's arteriopathy, carotid arteritis.
- Metabolic: mitochondrial, homocystinuria.
- Embolic: fat, air, blood clot, tumor.
- Infection: bacterial meningitis, encephalitis.
- Drug induced: L. asparaginase, high dose methotrexate.

Investigations

The initial investigation should be a CT head scan to determine if there is a hemorrhagic or ischemic stroke.

Other investigations may include:
- CBC, ESR, PT, PTT, protein C, protein S, antithrombin III, lipoprotein A, lupus anticoagulant, anticardiolipin antibodies, antiphospholipid antibodies, antidouble stranded DNA.
- Serum lactate, urinalysis, urine homocysteine.
- Echocardiography and electrocardiogram.
- MRI, angiography.

ATAXIA

Ataxia is an abnormality of coordination and balance. Ataxia may be due to dysfunction of the vestibular apparatus, cerebellum, central white matter, posterior columns, peripheral nerve, or muscle. A careful neurological examination is essential to the localization of the abnormality.

Etiology

Ataxia may present as an acute, chronic, or progressive disorder.

Causes of ataxia:
- Acute:
     Peri–infectious: acute cerebellitis (especially chickenpox), Guillain–Barré's syndrome, tick paralysis.

Drugs: phenytoin, most psychoactive drugs, antihistamines.
Toxins: alcohol, lead, glue sniffing.
Increased ICP: hydrocephalus, brain tumor.
Trauma: postconcussion, brain hemorrhage.
Vascular: migraine, benign paroxysmal vertigo.
Epilepsy: myoclonic seizures, nonconvulsive status.
Metabolic: aminoacidurias, mitochondrial disorders.
Infectious: acute labyrinthitis, bacterial meningitis.
Others: acute intermittent ataxia may be a manifestation of basilar migraine, benign
paroxysmal vertigo, myoclonic epilepsy, autosomal dominant acute intermittent ataxia and
certain genetic metabolic disorders.
- Chronic: ataxic cerebral palsy and congenital malformations of the cerebellum and posterior
fossa may manifest with chronic ataxia.
- Progressive:
Tumors: posterior fossa tumors.
Degenerative: Friedreich's ataxia, ataxia telangiectasia, genetic metabolic disorders.
Demyelination: multiple sclerosis.

Investigations

The investigations depend on the clinical localization of the lesion and the differential
diagnosis. In the absence of an obvious case, a CT head scan should be performed and
neurology consultation obtained in a patient with acute ataxia.

ALTERED CONSCIOUSNESS

A child with altered consciousness must be assessed rapidly because of the potential for
sudden deterioration.

Evaluation

A careful history should include events leading up to the change in consciousness, exposure
to drugs or toxins, previous seizures or migraine, recent fever, infectious disease or systemic
illness, and a family history of seizures, migraine or encephalopathy.

Clinical examination should include a specific search for evidence of occult trauma (retinal
hemorrhages, unexplained bruises), meningismus, papilloedema, brain stem abnormalities and
focal neurological signs. The presence of focal neurological signs and asymmetric cranial nerve
abnormalities suggests a structural cause of coma. A CT head scan should be performed urgently
in these children and neurosurgical consultation obtained. Absence of focal neurological signs
and normal cranial nerve function suggests a nonstructural cause of coma.

Etiology of coma

1. Structural
- Trauma: intracranial hemorrhage, diffuse brain injury.
- Vascular malformation.

- Acute hydrocephalus.
- Brain tumor: rarely manifests with coma unless hemorrhage into tumor.

2. Nonstructural
- Infection: bacterial, viral, or rickettsial meningoencephalitis.
- Vascular: stroke, vasculitis, or hypertensive encephalopathy.
- Epilepsy: postictal, nonconvulsive status epilepticus.
- Hypoxic–ischemia.
- Metabolic: glucose, electrolyte, or acid–base disturbance; hyperammonemia, inborn errors of metabolism.
- Toxic: endogenous (hepatic, renal failure), exogenous (drugs, substance abuse, lead).
- Endocrine: hypothyroidism, adrenal failure.

Investigations

The investigations should be based on the presumed cause and type of coma. A lumbar puncture should never be performed in a comatose child without a neurological or neurosurgical consultaton. The absence of papilloedema does not preclude the presence of raised intracranial pressure.

1. Structural
- CT head scan.
- Neurosurgical consultation.

2. Nonstructural
- Blood culture, CBC, blood film, platelets, PT, PTT and ESR.
- Drug toxicology screen.
- Glucose, electrolytes, calcium, phosphorus, urea, liver function tests, blood gases, ammonia, lactate, plasma amino acids, urine organic acids.
- CT brain scan, EEG.

HEADACHE

Migraine and stress headaches are responsible for most chronic headaches. Headaches lasting longer than 6 months and not associated with abnormal neurological signs are rarely associated with intracranial pathology. Headaches of recent onset or those that cause the child to waken during the night should be assessed particularly carefully.

Evaluation

Children old enough to give a reliable history of their headache should be asked about precipitating and relieving factors, frequency and duration, location and quality, timing and severity, and associated features (nausea, vomiting, and visual symptoms). Stress is a major provocation in childhood headache.

Examination should include a search for evidence of focal neurological signs, increased intracranial pressure and meningismus. Assessment should include blood pressure, examination of teeth and a search for focal scalp or sinus tenderness. Investigations should be individualized.

Etiology of headache

- Vascular: migraine, hypertension, vasculitis.
- Trauma: post–traumatic headache.
- Muscular: tension headache.
- Ocular: eye strain, glaucoma.
- Infection: meningitis, sinusitis, dental infection.
- Increased ICP: pseudotumor cerebri, hydrocephalus, brain tumor, subdural collections.
- Seizures: ictal or postictal.
- Skeletal: neck injury, temporomandibular syndrome.

PROGRESSIVE NEUROLOGICAL DETERIORIATION

Progressive neurological diseases are often inherited. Consequently, early diagnosis is important. The most important point is to establish whether the child is losing skills. Early onset of seizures, dementia and macular changes suggest grey matter involvement. Spasticity, accelerated reflexes and optic atrophy imply white matter involvement. Dystonia suggests basal ganglia involvement, and cranial nerve dysfunction indicates involvement of the brain stem.

Evaluation

The history should focus on family history, consanguinity, age at onset, rate of progression, previous medical history, presence of seizures and degree of intellectual deterioration. Further history from a teacher, play school worker, etc., may be useful. A careful physical examination is important.

The following abnormalities can be important diagnostic clues:
- Fundoscopy: cherry red spot, optic atrophy, corneal clouding, cataracts.
- Head size: macrocephaly (storage disorders).
- Abdomen: hepatosplenomegaly (storage disorders).
- Craniofacial or skeletal dysmorphism.

Etiology of progressive neurologic deterioration

- Grey matter: mucopolysaccharidoses, ceroid lipofuscinosis, GM2 gangliosidoses (Tay–Sachs, Sandhoff), GM1 gangliosidosis, Gauchers and Niemann–Pick, mitochondrial disorders.
- White matter: leukodystrophies (metachromatic, adrenoleukodystrophy, Krabbes), multiple sclerosis, Canavan's and Alexander's diseases.
- Mixed: Wilsons, SSPE, hypothyroidism, chronic lead poisoning.

Investigations

A neurology consultation should be obtained and investigations will be individualized.

HYPOTONIA

Hypotonia may be caused by diseases of the central nervous system (cerebrum, cerebellum, and spinal cord) and the lower motor unit (anterior horn cell, peripheral nerve, neuromuscular junction and muscle). Central causes of hypotonia account for 90% of cases in infancy and early childhood. Weakness is a pathognomonic feature of a lower motor unit cause of hypotonia.

Evaluation

The history should include a detailed enquiry into the pregnancy and perinatal period, family history of neuromuscular disease, past and present medical history and the child's general neurological development. Neurological examination is performed to localize the lesion.

Clinical localization of cause of hypotonia

- Cerebrum: dysmorphic features, fisting of the hands, brisk deep tendon reflexes.
- Anterior horn cell: muscle wasting common, marked weakness, fasciculations, markedly reduced or absent deep tendon reflexes, sensation never affected.
- Neuropathy: distal wasting and weakness, decreased reflexes, possibly decreased sensation distally.
- Neuromuscular junction: fatiguability, normal reflexes, sensation never affected.
- Muscle: proximal wasting and weakness, decreased reflexes proximally, normal sensation.

Etiology of hypotonia

1. Central hypotonia
- Cerebral: cerebral dysgenesis, idiopathic mental retardation, chromosomal abnormalities (trisomies, Prader Willi's syndrome), peroxisomal disorders (cerebrohepatorenal syndrome, neonatal adrenoleukodystrophy), other neurogenetic disorders (familial dysautonomia, oculocerebrorenal).

2. Lower motor unit
- Anterior horn cell: spinal muscular atrophy (Werdnig–Hoffman).
- Peripheral nerve: hereditary, inflammatory (Guillain–Barré's syndrome), other (vasculitis, toxic, diabetic, vitamin deficiency, renal failure).
- Neuromuscular junction: myasthenia, botulism.
- Muscle:
    Congenital myopathy (e.g. myotubular, nemaline rod, central core, etc.).
    Dystrophy (Duchenne's muscular dystrophy, limb–girdle, facioscapulohumeral).
    Metabolic (glycogen and lipid storage diseases, periodic paralysis, steroid myopathy).
    Inflammatory (viral, parasitic, dermatomyositis).
    Myotonia (myotonia congenita, dystrophica myotonica).
- Connective tissue: Marfan's syndrome, Ehlers-Danlos' syndrome.

Investigations

Investigations are tailored to the differential diagnosis in each case. The following may be indicated.

1. Central
Cerebral imaging.

2. Lower motor
- Serum CPK performed before any muscle trauma if myopathy is suspected.
- Thyroid function, electrolytes (Ca, Mg, K).
- Tensilon test; i.v. edrophonium chloride (0.2 mg/kg) with intravenous atropine (0.01 mg/kg) to prevent cholinergic side effects.
- Stool for *Clostridium* culture if indicated.
- Lumbar puncture if Guillain-Barré's syndrome is suspected.
- Electromyography and nerve conduction studies are important in the investigation of lower motor unit dysfunction but are painful and not good screening tests.
- Muscle or nerve biopsy may be indicated in selected cases.
- Specific molecular studies are indicated in certain disorders.

PARENTERAL NUTRITION

Development of malnutrition in hospital is a frequent occurrence. The consequences of malnutrition include delayed healing, a higher incidence and severity of infection, prolonged hospitalization and death. The onset of malnutrition may be insidious or acute; nutritional repletion is usually a longer process than the development of malnutrition.

Indications for nutritional support

1. Gastrointestinal
- Inflammatory bowel diseases.
- Postoperative complications, e.g. prolonged ileus, fistulae.
- Short bowel syndrome.
- Protracted diarrhea of infancy.
- Radiation or chemotherapy enterocolitis.
- Delayed gastric emptying.
- Gut motility disorders.
- Esophageal disease.
- Rare enteropathies.
- Chronic liver disease or hepatic failure.
- Pancreatitis or pancreatic insufficiency.

2. General
- Anorexia 2° to tumor or systemic disease or 1° anorexia nervosa.
- Malnutrition prior to major surgery.
- Prematurity.
- Major trauma.
- Severe burns.
- Oropharyngeal disease.
- Coma or CNS disease.
- Congenital heart disease.

Evaluation of nutritional state

The following parameters are used to define the degree of malnutrition.

1. Ideal body weight for height
See chapter 24 (Appendix) for standard growth charts.

2. Mid–arm muscle circumference (MAMC)
Skeletal muscle mass is assessed by measuring the circumference of the nondependent upper arm between elbow and shoulder. Mid–arm muscle circumference (MAMC) is corrected from

mid–arm circumference (MAC) by the equation:

$$\text{MAMC} = \text{MAC (cm)} - (0.314 \times \text{TSF mm})$$

where TSF is triceps skin–fold thickness. See chapter 24 (Appendix) for standard values of MAMC. Values below fifth percentile are abnormally low for hospitalized patients.

3. Skin–fold thickness
A measure of fat stores. See chapter 24 (Appendix) for standard charts of skin–fold thickness.

4. Serum proteins
The long half–life of albumin makes it a less sensitive indicator of current nitrogen balance; even in the presence of acute malnutrition, the serum albumin may remain normal for 10–14 days. Transferrin, ceruloplasmin and retinal binding protein indicate more recent changes because of shorter half–lives. Nevertheless, in daily clinical practice, serum albumin is the most commonly used parameter. A low serum albumin may result from protein loss through kidneys or gut, malabsorption or decreased hepatic synthesis (liver disease). Other than the circumstance of renal albumin losses, a low serum albumin indicates the presence of chronic protein malnutrition. A normal serum albumin excludes chronic malnutrition of less than 10–14 days but not acute malnutrition.

5. Cellular immune status
Total lymphocyte count is decreased in malnutrition. Counts of 1,200–1,600 are found in mild malnutrition. Levels may be below 800 in severe cases. In malnutrition, response to skin test antigens (e.g. mumps, *Candida*) and PPD is also depressed.

Rates of administration

1. Peripheral TPN
- Peripheral TPN is provided through peripheral veins. Its advantages are readiness and simplicity of use. Because only a maximum concentration of 10% or 12.5% dextrose can be used through peripheral veins, full calories can be provided only by very high fluid volumes. In the majority of cases, full caloric requirements cannot be met by peripheral TPN (see examples below).
- Peripheral TPN has a lower incidence of infection, but it is not risk free. Phlebitis, local skin infections, sepsis and extravasation of solutions into subcutaneous tissues may all occur.

2. Central venous TPN
- Central venous TPN is provided through a silicon catheter placed into the SVC under fluoroscopic guidance. Anesthesia is necessary since the surgeon tunnels part of the catheter subcutaneously.
- Advantages of a central venous catheter (CVC) are:
    The ability to provide full calories in the least fluid volume using concentrated solutions (e.g. 25% dextrose).
    No need for peripheral i.v.'s.
    All blood tests can be drawn through the catheter, saving a chronically ill patient frequent

needlesticks.
Blood products can be infused through all but the smallest CVC.
• Risk of infection is greater with CVC's than peripheral veins, however, central venous catheters placed using aseptic technique and maintained according to strict protocols may be used for months or years without becoming infected.

Guidelines

In general, TPN is given if it is anticipated that enteral nutrition will not be possible for 7 days. Peripheral TPN is used if the anticipated duration of parenteral nutrition is 14 days or less. Central venous TPN is used for patients expected to require more than 14 days of parenteral nutritional support. Central TPN is necessary in cases of moderate to severe malnutrition and for patients with catabolic states, e.g. fever, burns, active colitis. Patients with renal, cardiac or chronic lung disease requiring TPN require a central catheter to provide nutrition in limited volumes.

There are two infusion regimens used for parental nutrition (PN): continuous or cyclic. Using a continuous administration, the patient is receiving an infusion throughout 24 hours each day.

Cyclic PN is given over only a portion of the day (e.g. the line may be capped for up to 16 h/d). This, when possible, allows patients to attend school, be ambulant in the hospital, go out on passes, etc. The decision to discontinue parenteral nutrition intermittently rests with the physician supervising PN. Newborns are not placed on cyclic PN as they have a greater tendency to hypoglycemia.

Documentation

Most hospitals recommend that a TPN physician must be consulted whenever a patient is to be started on central venous TPN. This applies to patients outside the Intensive Care Unit and Special Care Nursery.

Before starting a patient on TPN, document the following in the chart:
• Patient identification.
• Indication for TPN.
• Nutritional assessment as above, to include:
    Growth chart in patient's chart.
    Present body weight.
    Ideal body weight for height.
    Visceral (biochemical, hematological) parameters of nutrition.
• Fluid, calorie and protein requirements.
• Expected duration of TPN.
• End–point.

TPN Solutions

1. Amino acid–dextrose solutions
These contain standard amino acid mixtures with varying concentrations of dextrose. Each solution can usually be ordered with dextrose concentrations of 10%, 12.5%, 15%, 20%, 25%.

Peripheral veins cannot tolerate more than D12.5W.

2. Fat emulsions

10% and 20% are available. When denser calories are required (more calories in less volume), 20% fat is used. The brand of fat solution used is usually either Intralipid or Travamulsion. These are soy derived, oil–water emulsions, stabilized with egg phospholipid and glycerin. (Safflower oil derived solutions also exist.) Fat emulsions supply high density calories (i.e. maximum calories in minimal fluid volume) and essential fatty acids.

3. Minerals

NaCl, KCl, phosphate, calcium gluconate, magnesium sulfate.

4. Trace elements

Trace mineral solutions provide zinc, copper, manganese, chromium, selenium and iodide.

5. Vitamins

Standard vitamin preparations are available.

Calculations

1. Standard TPN solutions

Most hospitals have developed standard premixed TPN solutions for premature infants and older children in the ICU. The need for customized solutions is rare outside the nursery. Each component of the amino acid–dextrose solution does not have to be ordered separately. For example, when Travasol/D25W is ordered, the solution contains 25% dextrose and standard appropriate quantities of amino acids, minerals, trace metal solution and vitamins.

All the physician has to decide is:

- Concentration of dextrose (10%, 12.5%, 15%, 20%, 25%).
- Volumes and rates of administration.

2. Individualized TPN solutions

- Customized solutions are usually only required for patients with marked fluid restrictions. In defining a parenteral nutrition regimen, calculate fluid requirements for patient's present weight and calorie requirements for patient's ideal body weight, i.e. if you want the patient to gain weight, as is usually the case, provide calories in excess of basal calories for present weight.

Table I: Energy and fluid requirements for children

Weight	Calories (Cal/kg)	Fluids (mL/kg)
Neonate	100–120	150–180
First 10 kg	100	100
Next 10 kg	50	50
Above 20 kg	20	20

- These are basal requirements. They are modified upwards by arbitrary "fudge factors" for burns, surgery, fever, etc. Calories are available from three sources in parenteral nutrition solutions: dextrose, fat emulsion and amino acids. Amino acids provide 0.4 Cal/mL, however, do not include those calories provided by amino acids as these are not calories to be used for energy production. The aim is to provide nonprotein calories for protein sparing.
- Usually no more than 40% of total daily calories should come from fat emulsion. A maximum of 3 g/kg per d of fat is used. However, 3 g/kg per d of fat may comprise more than 40% of daily calories in a patient receiving limited dextrose (carbohydrate) calories via peripheral vein. It is permissible to give up to 60% of total daily calories as fat only for short–term TPN, i.e. less than 14 days.
- Extra care with :
    - Patients on respirators: they are unable to "blow off" CO_2 generated by carbohydrate catabolism if they are on fixed tidal volumes.
    - Patients in renal or hepatic failure.
    - Patients with cardiac or pulmonary insufficiency who may be unable to tolerate even usual maintenance volumes.
- Now juggle different dextrose concentrations and lipid flow rates to provide the calculated calories in an acceptable fluid volume.

Example: a 9 year old girl with an acute relapse of inflammatory bowel disease weighs 22 kg on admission and is to be n.p.o. Her ideal body weight for height is 28 kg. She is febrile and is started on i.v. methyl prednisone. Serum albumin is 22 g/L.

Question: Calculate her fluid and calorie requirements.
Her maintenance fluid requirement per 24 hours for her current weight is 1,540 mL. She has extra insensible water loss, as she is febrile, and normal renal function so you decide to give slightly more than 1–1½ maintenance, i.e. 2,400 mL/24 h. Her basal caloric requirement for ideal body weight is 1,660 Cal/24 h. Adding extra for fever and the negative nitrogen balance due to active disease and need for catch–up growth brings her requirement to about 2,500 Cal/24 h.

Question: Can you provide this with peripheral venous TPN?
Suppose we give 3 g/kg 20% fat = 66 g = 330 mL/h = 660 Cal. To provide the other 1,840 Cal would require about 5.5 L of D10W. Not only that, she is predicted to require a minimum of 3–4 weeks before she will be in full remission and on full calories p.o. You don't want her to get too few calories to exacerbate malnutrition; you want to turn the situation around. Moreover, you don't want her stuck daily for blood drawing. She needs central venous TPN.

Question: Calculate her central venous TPN.
Give 3 g/kg 20% fat = 66 g = 330 mL/h = 660 Cal.
Give Travasol/D25W 2,100 mL/24 h = 1,785 Cal.
Total Cal/24 h = 2,445 in 2,430 mL.
Travasol contains 2% protein, therefore, 2,100 mL contains 42 g of protein ~ 2 g/kg for present weight.

Question: What else do you watch for closely in this patient with diarrhea and ongoing fluid losses?

Hypokalemia and metabolic acidosis due to losses, e.g. potassium and bicarbonate in stools.

3. Ward management
• Calculate the total intake daily using Table II.
• Follow the patient's metabolic status with regular bloodwork.

Table II: Energy, fat and protein contents of typical TPN solutions

Solution	Energy (Cal/L)	Fat (g/L)	Protein (g/L)
D10W	340	–	–
D15W	510	–	–
D20W	680	–	–
10% lipid	1,100	100	–
20% lipid	2,000	200	–
Travasol 2%	*	–	20
Travasol 3%	*	–	30

* Energy calculations should not include the caloric value of amino acid solutions.

Changing from continuous to cyclic nutrition:
• Day 1: reduce the duration of the infusion by 4 hours, i.e. order the same volume of parenteral nutrition to run in over 20 hours by increasing the rate accordingly.
• Thereafter: reduce the duration of parenteral nutrition by 2 h/d until the patient is receiving parenteral nutrition over 10–14 hours, or whatever length of time is desired. Maintain the same nutritional intake by correspondingly increasing the rate of the infusion.

Discontinuing parenteral nutrition:
• Parenteral nutrition must never be stopped abruptly especially if using dextrose concentrations above 10% when treating infants.
• When discontinuing the infusion or placing a patient on cyclic parenteral nutrition:
    Halve the rate for 15 minutes, then halve again for 15 minutes.
    Stop the infusion, flush CVC line with heparinized saline and cap the catheter.
    When TPN is stopped for the administration of antibiotics or other drugs, check with Pharmacy to see if the drug can be given in D10W to prevent hypoglycemia.

ENTERAL NUTRITION

Levels of nutrition intervention

• Oral supplements.
• Tube feeding via nasogastric, gastrostomy or jejunostomy tube.

The enteral route for nutritional support is preferred over the parenteral route because it is safer, more economical, more nutritionally complete, has fewer side effects and maintains the structural and functional integrity of the small intestine. Even inpatients with diarrhea or those unable to tolerate full volume and strength of enteral formula should be provided with at least some enteral intake. Enterocytes and colonocytes derive significant benefits from minimal exposure to direct or preferred gut fuels such as glutamine and short chain fatty acids. In addition, enteral intake stimulates secretion of bile, pancreatic juice and gut hormones such as CCK and enteroglucagon which are trophic for the GI mucosa. This speeds repair and regeneration of enterocytes and colonocytes and decreases cholestasis and the likelihood of gallstone formation.

Indications for enteral nutrition

Generally, patients with functioning gastrointestinal tracts and who are unable to ingest adequate nutrients to meet their metabolic demands can benefit from supplemental or tube feedings.

Indications for tube feedings include:
- Gastrointestinal disease: Crohn's disease or ulcerative colitis, short bowel syndrome, esophageal disorders, delayed gastric emptying, malabsorption, partial obstruction or distal small bowel fistula, hepatic or pancreatic insufficiency.
- CNS disorders: neurological impairment.
- Hypermetabolic states: burns, trauma, surgery.
- Neoplasms.
- Oropharyngeal disease:
    Obstructive lesion of pharynx or esophagus.
    Fractured jaw, surgery or neoplasm.
- Psychiatric disease: anorexia nervosa or severe depression.

Tube feedings are contraindicated in patients with adynamic ileus, complete intestinal obstruction, intractable vomiting, proximal high output enterocutaneous fistulas and upper GI bleeding. Diarrhea with or without malabsorption may or may not be a contraindication and often can be managed by an adjustment in flow rate or type of formula.

Nasogastric tube selection

If a patient is to be fed by nasogastric tube, select a small bore silastic tube which is weighted at the tip, e.g. Keofeed 7.3 Fr. These soft silastic tubes are well accepted and tolerated. Patients should not receive feedings for more than a week through tubes not designed for feeding such as Salem sump tubes, red Robinson tubes, etc. These are associated with patient discomfort, nasal and pharyngeal ulcers, gastric irritation and chronic GE reflux occasionally leading to esophageal stricture.

Gastrostomy

For most patients requiring long–term intragastric feeds, a gastrostomy is indicated. For most patients, percutaneous gastrostomy tube (PEG) is preferred; placement by the endoscopic route, i.e. "incisionless" gastrostomy, avoids laparotomy and its risks and allows same day G–tube use. In addition, diagnostic upper GI endoscopy with biopsies is performed at the same procedure, if indicated. Contraindications to PEG placement include previous abdominal surgery and ascites, in which case surgical gastrostomy may be indicated.

Nasojejunal tube

Enteral feeding is limited in many severely ill children because of gastric stasis, although small bowel function is usually preserved. If a tube can be passed through the pylorus, jejunal feeds offer a more attractive option than short–term TPN.

- Use a nonweighted feeding tube with stylet: if patient < 5 kg, use 6 Fr., 36"; if patient > 5 kg, use 8 Fr., 43".
- Mark the tube for guidance.
    Gastric mark: ear–nares–xiphoid process.
    Pylorus mark: add distance from xiphoid to mid–axillary line.
    Jejunal mark: add 5–10 cm.
- Pass a nasogastric tube and keep it on continuous suction. Pass the jejunal tube through the other nostril and into the stomach.
- Administer metoclopramide 0.1–0.2 mg/kg i.v.; after 1 min, advance jejunal tube while simultaneously injecting air.
- Check position by injecting dyed pedialyte into the nasogastric tube; it should not return through the nasojejunal tube. Confirm by X–ray.

Formula selection

The choice of enteral feeding formula should be made only with an understanding of the patient's physical condition, including any abnormalities in the nutritional metabolic profile and should be preceded by a history of the previous diet. Dietary consultation is very helpful in the initiation and maintenance of specific enteral feedings.

Consider the following in selecting the appropriate enteral feeding formula.

1. Feeding route
Oral supplementation versus tube feeding. Palatability is a major concern if the formula is to be given orally. Preparations containing intact proteins, carbohydrates and fat are more palatable than those containing digested or simpler forms. Some formulas are designed to supplement oral intake while others (e.g. Isocal) are designed for tube feeding.

2. Digestive and absorptive ability of patient
If the GI tract is fully functional, nutritionally complete formulas which require digestion are indicated. However, patients with impaired digestive capacity (pancreatic or hepatic insufficiency, bile duct obstruction) or reduced absorptive ability (small bowel mucosal damage, short bowel syndrome, Crohn's disease, enterocutaneous fistulas) may require feeding in a simple, readily available form, i.e. free amino acids plus oligosaccharides with a low fat content. These chemically defined formulas are costly, high in osmolality and may precipitate gastrointestinal symptoms if

not administered properly.

3. Formula osmolality
The osmolality of a formula has a direct effect on GI side effects and thereby on tolerance to enteral therapy. Enteral formula osmolality ranges from 300–800 mOsm/kg. Hyperosmolar solutions (i.e. more than 300 mOsm/kg water) can cause water secretion into the intestinal lumen, producing nausea, vomiting, cramps and diarrhea.

4. Lactose intolerance
A number of children are lactase deficient and will have GI symptoms if given lactose containing formulas. In addition, lactase deficiency can develop in hospitalized patients who have had nothing by mouth for prolonged periods.

5. Cost
Many enteral nutrition formulas are relatively inexpensive. However, specialty formulas such as Pregestemil, Alimentum, Vivonex Plus, Vivonex Pediatric, Pediasure, Peptamen, Hepatic–Aid, etc., are expensive and have specific circumstances in which they are indicated, therefore, careful consideration must be made before use.

Types of formulas

Several types of enteral feeding formulas are available. Enteral nutrition formulas can be classified into four broad categories.

1. Nutritionally complete formulas
These formulas are composed of protein, carbohydrate and fat in high molecular weight form and thus are lower in osmolality, require normal digestive proteolytic and lipolytic capacity and are less expensive.
- Standard infant formulas: these have intact cow's milk protein (Similac, SMA, Enfalac) or soy milk protein (Isomil, Prosobee), triglycerides and lactose, sucrose or glucose. They contain 0.67 Cal/mL. Alactamil is cow milk–based and lactose–free.
- Supplementary formulas: formulas such as Ensure and Ensure Plus are palatable and taken p.o. Isocal is given by tube. Most of these formulas are lactose free and provide 1–1.5 Cal/mL. Higher caloric density formulas are also available for use in patients where fluid and sodium intake must be limited. Nutritionally complete formulas should be used in any patient with an intact GI tract.

2. Chemically defined formulas
- These formulas are low in residue and provide amino acids or oligopeptides as their protein source, oligosaccharides or monosaccharides as their carbohydrate source and contain little or no tryglyceride or starch. They may contain some medium chain triglycerides (MCT) and therefore bypass some of the complex mechanisms required for fat absorption. They are hyperosmolar, do not require proteolytic or lipolytic capacity and are moderately expensive. Thus, these formulas should be restricted to use in patients with impaired digestive capacity (pancreatic or hepatic insufficiency) or impaired absorptive capacity (severe mucosal damage, short bowel syndrome, Crohn's disease, enterocutaneous fistulas).

- This category includes: Pregestemil, Alimentum, Vivonex Plus, Vivonex Pediatric, Pediasure, Peptamen.

3. Modular formulas
These are not nutritionally complete and contain single nutrients such as fat, carbohydrate and protein and can be added to currently available standard enteral products to modify their nutrient content in patients with increased nutritional needs, e.g. Polycose (glucose polymer), MCT.

4. Specialty formulas
Specialty formulas for use in patients with renal or hepatic failure are available. There is some controversy over their use as detailed below:
- Hepatic disease: nutritional products high in branched chain amino acids and low in methionine and aromatic amino acids such as the enteral formula Hepatic–Aid (and the parenteral formula Hepat–Amine) are useful in patients with altered serum amino acid profiles and who develop hepatic encephalopathy. Although the data evaluating these formulations is encouraging, it must be recognized that hepatic encephalopathy is a multifactorial disorder. If the hepatic encephalopathy is due to volume depletion, hypocalcemia, alkalosis, sepsis, GI bleeding or other factors, it will not respond to these special formulas alone. No data to date has shown a change in mortality with these formulas.
- Renal failure: nutritional support of patients with renal disease is aimed at minimizing nitrogenous wastes and solutes presented to the failing or impaired kidney. Nutritional products containing amino acids as their sole source of protein, such as the enteral formula Amin–Aid or parenteral formula Nephramine, have been shown to be beneficial in patients with renal failure and who are not being dialyzed. Their use is controversial since no benefit can be shown when these formulations are compared with standard amino acid formulations containing both essential and nonessential amino acids.
- Hypermetabolic states: hypermetabolic states such as multiple trauma, sepsis, burns and major surgery with complications are associated with severe derangements in the metabolism of carbohydrate (insulin resistance and hyperglycemia), fat (hypertriglyceridemia) and protein (increased protein catabolism, negative nitrogen balance and immunoincompetence). Recent studies in hypermetabolic patients indicate that during stress there is an increased use of amino acids as a caloric source, particularly the branched chain amino acids (leucine, isoleucine and valine). Clinical trials have shown that during stress, nutritional support with branched chain enriched amino acid solutions, such as Fre–Amine HBC and BranchAmin, decreases the patient's skeletal muscle catabolism.

Writing orders

Any tube feeding prescription should contain the following:
- Name of formula and strength of formula.
- Total volume of formula and number of calories required per 24 hours.
- Special nutritional needs: the commercially available nutritionally complete formulas, when administered in calorically adequate amounts, will meet the protein, electrolyte, vitamin and trace element needs of most patients. If any restrictions or additions of these components are required in a given patient, these must be specified in the diet order.
- Rate of administration: The volume and concentration of formula should be individually

tailored to the patient's needs based on prior intake, feeding site, formula selected and current medical status. Isotonic formulas do not require the dilution necessary when using highly hypertonic solutions. Generally, when initiating therapy, continuous drip is preferred over intermittent feedings. Too rapid a rate of administration may produce cramping or diarrhea and improved absorption results from continuous infusion. If there is any question about the patient's digestive and absorptive ability, 24 hour infusion is preferred. To avoid uncontrolled changes in flow rate, an infusion pump is recommended. Intermittent feedings can be used if there is no history of diarrhea or malabsorption and if the GI tract is intact. For adolescents and adults, intermittent feedings should be administered at a rate not exceeding 240 mL/30 min. Obviously, considerably smaller volumes and slower rates are required in younger children. Orders should be written to give the volume and number of feedings desired per day over a specified time. If nausea, vomiting, cramping or diarrhea occurs, the rate of administration or concentration should be decreased. Avoid altering both rate and strength at the same time. For most patients, adaptation to an adequate volume of full strength formula should take no more than 3–4 days. Formulas should be given at room temperature to facilitate GI tolerance.

Monitoring

Proper monitoring of patients receiving enteral nutrition is necessary to prevent and detect complications. The following are guidelines. Infants and patients in unstable fluid balance may require more frequent checking.

- Confirm placement of feeding tube before initiating therapy.
- Check gastric residuals every shift. If the volume is greater than the volume infused in one hour, the physician is to be contacted.
- Maintain accurate intake/output records.
- If patient is on a formula containing glucose or lactose, check all liquid stools or ileostomy output for reducing substances on the ward.
- Record patient's weight daily.
- Check the following:
    Every 8 hours: vital signs, urine for glucose.
    Twice weekly: electrolytes including Mg, Ca, P, blood glucose, BUN or creatinine.
    Once weekly: total protein, albumin, CBC, differential, liver function tests.

Complications

Complications with the use of the small diameter tubes are relatively rare and are largely preventable with proper formula selection, administration technique and careful monitoring.

Complications with enteral feedings are generally divided into three types: mechanical complications, gastrointestinal complications and metabolic complications.

1. Mechanical complications
- The commonest mechanical complications of tube feeding include: obstruction of the tube lumen, pharyngeal irritation, esophageal erosion and aspiration of gastric contents. They are all rare if a small bore feeding tube is used. Complications of G–tubes include perforation of

large or small bowel at the time of placement, infusion of formula into the peritoneal cavity and infection of the gastrostomy site. Aspiration can be minimized by elevating the head of the bed 30° or more while the patient is being fed. Nasogastric tube feeding should be avoided in patients at high risk for aspiration. In these patients, jejunostomy feedings or TPN may be preferred.
• If a feeding tube becomes clogged, an attempt should be made to unplug it by flushing it with water or cranberry juice, which is slightly acidic. When administering drugs through a feeding tube, the tube should be flushed with water both before and after to prevent any clogging of the feeding tube.

2. Gastrointestinal complications
• Sudden nausea, vomiting or diarrhea which develops after initiation of tube feeding may be caused by:
  Irregular or too rapid administration of the formula or disaccharide intolerance.
  Hyperosmolar reactions from a formula with high osmolality.
  Concurrent drug therapy.
  Improper positioning of the tube.
  Bacterial contamination of the formula.
• Generally, these problems are preventable when appropriate feeding formulas are given by slow continous drip and gradually increased as tolerated.

3. Metabolic complications
The most common electrolyte abnormalities seen in patients on the tube feedings include: hypernatremia, hyponatremia, hypercalcemia and azotemia. These complications are largely preventable with proper monitoring of fluid intake and adjustment of the electrolyte content of the formula if needed.

DIET IN DISEASE

In the following conditions, dietary management is a major factor in the treatment program.

Galactosemia

• Autosomal recessive, incidence about 1:50,000.
• Due to deficiency of galactose–1–phosphate uridyl transferase.
• Several variants exist.
• Accumulation of metabolites damages liver, renal tubules, central nervous system and lens.
• A milder disease is caused by galactokinase deficiency.
• Treatment consists of the complete exclusion of galactose from the diet.
• Galactose is essential for the production of galactolipids, but these needs are met by endogenous production so complete exclusion can be achieved without harmful effects.
• Galactose is found mainly in the form of lactose (glucose and galactose) in milk and its products. It is also widely used in processed food and drug manufactured.
• Newly diagnosed patients are followed closely by erythrocyte glucose–1–phosphate levels, which should be < 10 mg%.

The following dietary restrictions are imposed:
- Milk: cow, goat and human milk may not be used. Soy milks include short chain starches, which contain galactose such as stachyose and raffinose; however, these starches are not metabolized in humans so soy–based formulas are safe to use. Nutramigen or meat–based formulas are expensive alternatives.
- Vegetables: fruit and vegetables are safe to use. Legumes contain galactose in the form of nonmetabolized starches so are safe to use; however, green peas continue to be excluded from the diet since they appear to be a source of free galactose.
- Protein: plain meat, poultry, fish, eggs and nuts are all safe. Several organs store galactose such as liver, pancreas, brain and kidneys, so may not be used.

The diet must be continued for life. If a fetus is shown to be galactosemic by amniocentesis, some centers recommend that the mother follows a galactose restricted diet during her pregnancy.

Phenylketonuria (PKU)

- Autosomal recessive.
- Incidence about 1:10,000.
- The etiology is a deficiency of phenylalanine hydroxylase (PH)
- There are varying degrees of deficiency from classical PKU to hyperphenylalaninemia.
- Variant forms exist due to abnormalities of biopterin, which is a cofactor of PH.
- Biopterins are also involved in the metabolism of dopamine and serotonin.
- Dietary treatment: treatment of classical PKU consists of restricting phenylalanine in the diet. Since phenylalanine is an essential amino acid, it should not be completely excluded, otherwise catabolism of endogenous protein would result. The aim of the dietary limitation is to maintain serum phenylalanine level between 3–10 mg/dl (normal 0.5–1 mg/dl). This is usually achieved by limiting dietary phenylalanine intake in the range of 200–400 mg/d. The major source of protein for these patients is in the form of low phenylalanine formula (Lofenalac, Phenylfree, PKU–1). A major practical difficulty is taste. The diet is "topped up" with a measured amount of Similac (which contains 23 mg phenylalanine per fluid ounce) to ensure adequate phenylalanine intake.
- Dietary restrictions:
  Protein: meat, fish, cheese and eggs all have high phenylalanine levels and are not used.
  Vegetables: patients with PKU essentially follow a strict vegetarian diet; however, nuts and legumes should be avoided.
- Maternal PKU: offspring of mothers with PKU have been noted to have mental retardation, microcephaly and other congenital anomalies. These occur even when the baby does not have PKU. Strict dietary limitation, especially before conception, has proved to be helpful in preventing these abnormalities in the newborn.

Renal disease

Because of fluid and electrolyte imbalance, hyperphosphatemia, uremia and hypertension, the patient's dietary intake becomes very important in the management of chronic renal failure. It is complicated by appetite suppression caused by several factors, including taste and smell aberrations associated with chronically elevated BUN, anorexia associated with chronic disease, dialysis induced hyperglycemia. As creatinine clearance decreases, dietary manipulation becomes necessary.

Restrictions to normalize serum levels or control hypertension may be required:
* Phosphate: restrict foods high in phosphorus (e.g. dairy products) and give phosphate binders (e.g. amphogel).
* Sodium: restrict if the child is hypertensive or retains fluid.
* Protein: restrict when BUN is unacceptably high.
* Potassium: to normalize serum K⁺.
* Water: restrict intake in oliguric or anuric children when diuretics are ineffective.

Diabetes mellitus

Good management of the diabetic patient depends more on the amount and timing of meals rather than on dietary restrictions.

The basic aim is to ensure a relatively stable blood sugar throughout the day without episodes of hypo– or hyperglycemia. Dietary input is "smoothed out" by taking three main meals plus three snacks. The final snack should contain protein. This metabolizes slowly to ensure a steady glucose level during the night.

* Calories: daily intake should be 1,000 calories plus 100 calories per year of age.
* Carbohydrate: 45–55% caloric intake. Exclude simple sugars, sweets and fruit juices. Limit fruit intake. Use starches such as vegetables and bread. These are absorbed and metabolized more slowly.
* Protein: 15–20% caloric intake. No restriction.
* Fats: 30–35% caloric intake. Moderate restriction. Limit cream and fat. Use 2% milk or skim milk.

Most patients are taught using the book, *Good Health Eating*, by the Canadian Diabetes Association, which provides practical dietary advice.

Celiac disease

The basic problem is small bowel sensitivity to gliadin (the alcohol soluble portion of gluten), which is present in wheat, rye, barley and oats. The clinical result is mucosal damage, malabsorption and failure to thrive.

The pattern of inheritance is unknown. Incidence is about 1:300 to 1:2,000. Treatment consists of restricting all gluten containing foods and must be continued for life. It is very important to perform a small bowel biopsy before the diet is started or a lengthy delay in diagnosis and repeated biopsies will be necessary.

Common foods that must be avoided are: all bread, rolls, cake, spaghetti and macaroni made from wheat and rye, beer, malted milk and commercial ice–cream. Special gluten–free bread and cake mixes are available, made from rice, corn or a combination of these flours.

Many children will be anemic and lactose intolerant because of the chronic small bowel damage. They often require extra iron and folate supplements plus a lactose–free diet during the initial treatment period. These can be stopped after 3–4 weeks.

Liver disease

Most cases of liver disease are managed without any dietary restrictions but in severe cases some modifications are necessary.

- Mild: no restrictions; a good dietary intake should be encouraged.
- Moderate: when liver cell function falls enough to reduce bile production, malabsorption of long chain fatty acids becomes a problem. Medium chain triglycerides do not need bile acids or pancreatic lipase for absorption so are introduced into the diet, usually in the form of a milk (Portagen, a MCT and protein mixture). Water soluble forms of the fat soluble vitamins (A, D and E) may also be given.
- Severe: eventually some degree of protein restriction may be necessary to avoid hepatic encephalopathy and high serum ammonia levels. A good calorie intake should be maintained. If the patient has ascites, sodium restriction may be necessary.

Food allergy

Food allergy is a contentious subject. A great variety of symptoms have been labelled food allergy often without supporting evidence. It is important to differentiate between a reaction to food associated with disturbed immunological function (food allergy) and the result of other physiological mechanisms (lactose intolerance, celiac disease, etc.).

Food allergies affect 1–3% of the population and reactions vary from life threatening to a minor inconvenience. Children < 3 years of age are more frequently affected than older children and adults.

Parents frequently report "food allergy" as the cause of a variety of symptoms or illnesses for their children. This widespread practice of misdiagnosis or improper labelling is potentially dangerous as it results in unnecessary dietary restriction which can lead to malnutrition. Other consequences are family stress, "misdirected energy" and neglect of the underlying disease.

Any food is capable of causing food allergy but some do so more frequently than others. The most common offenders are milk, egg, wheat, corn, chocolate, citrus fruit, legumes (soybeans, peanuts, peas, beans) and tomatoes.

Causes of suspected food allergy may be subjected to a hypoallergenic (food elimination) diet for a controlled trial period (approximately 2 weeks). Standard procedures must be used to provide objective results.

Diagnosed food allergies are managed by strict dietary avoidance of the offending food(s). Dietary counselling will enable the family to adhere to the necessary restrictions. Careful attention must be given to the nutritional adequacy of the diet, especially when multiple foods are eliminated or if the eliminated food is a major source of nutrients in the diet (e.g. milk, wheat).

Except in cases of anaphylaxis, foods causing allergies may be re–introduced at intervals (q6–12 mo) following a protocol for food challenge to see whether tolerance to the food has developed.

Childhood cancer is a rare disease occurring in 1:8,000 children < 14 years of age. However, it is now curable in the majority of children if diagnosed and treated appropriately. It is therefore imperative that general practitioners and pediatricians understand the principles of diagnosis, treatment, and follow–up of childhood cancer.

- Annual incidence of childhood cancer (ages 0–14 years) is 129 per million (Table I).
- Overall cure rate is approximately 70%.
- Cancer causes more deaths than any other disease in children ages 1–15 years.
- Cancer has a high impact on the cost of health care because of the complexity of its treatment.

Table I: Common childhood malignancies

Malignancy	% Frequency	% Disease free survival with appropriate treatment
Leukemia	30	75
Brain	19	60
Lymphoma	13	75
Wilm's tumor	6	90
Neuroblastoma	8	10–20% (stage 3, 4) 75–90% (stage 1, 2)
Bone cancer	5	65
Soft tissue sarcoma	7	65
Retinoblastoma	3	95
Liver	1	45
Other	8	

PRINCIPLES OF DIAGNOSIS

The diagnosis of childhood cancer is often overlooked or misdiagnosed. Parents do not easily forgive this mistake. Remain alert to the possibility.

Common presenting symptoms

- Tiredness, pallor, lethargy (think about cancer before chronic fatigue syndrome).
- Prolonged bone pain, limp (think about cancer before JRA).
- Weight loss and anorexia (think about cancer before psychological causes of anorexia).
- Recurrent fever and infection.

- Unexplained mass or persistent lymphadenopathy.
- Headache, morning vomiting, visual disturbance, ataxia.
- Recurrent abdominal pain or distension.

Frequent presenting signs

- Pallor, bruises, petechiae.
- Lymphadenopathy, hepatosplenomegaly.
- Abdominal mass, abdominal pain.
- Soft tissue or bony lump (often misdiagnosed as a cyst or infection, often a misleading history of preceding trauma).
- Papilledema (remember to look).
- Other neurological signs.
- Hematuria.
- Always listen to the parents. Investigate persistent symptoms or signs. Parents often suspect cancer but are afraid to voice their concerns.

Diagnostic screening tests

- CBC and differential (for leukemia and other diseases which infiltrate the bone marrow).
- LDH (for lymphoma, leukemia and some solid tumors).
- Liver function test (for hepatic infiltration).
- Alpha$_1$–fetoprotein, β–hCG (for germ cell tumor and liver tumors).
- Chest X–ray (for any solid tumor, leukemia, lymphoma).
- X–ray of extremity (for bone pain or mass).
- Abdominal ultrasound (for suspected abdominal tumor).
- Abdominal CT scan (for suspected abdominal tumor).
- Brain CT or MRI (for suspected brain tumor).

Referral to tertiary care center

If pediatric cancer is suspected or confirmed, the child should be referred to an appropriate tertiary care center for confirmation of the diagnosis, staging investigations and initial management. Whenever possible, a pediatric oncologist should be involved.

Do not arrange for biopsy or surgical resection of a tumor unless:
- It is an emergency.
- You are sure that the appropriate staging workup has been performed.
- The appropriate pathological resources are available to handle the specimen (includes immunohistochemistry, cytogenetics and other genetic analysis, e.g. PCR).
- The appropriate surgeons are available to perform the surgery.

Diagnostic evaluation

1. History
- Detailed history of presenting complaints.

- Associated systemic symptoms, e.g. fever, night sweats, weight loss, anorexia. Recent history of trauma (including cat scratch; cat scratch fever can mimic lymphoma).
- Prenatal history (including maternal illness and exposure to drugs and alcohol).
- Past medical history (including chickenpox, measles and immunizations).
- Developmental history.
- Family history (particularly cancer in close relatives).
- Social history (including support available for family).

2. Physical
- Height, weight, head circumference (plot on growth chart).
- Tanner stage and size of testes.
- Skin: petechiae, bruising, café au lait spots, nodules.
- Lymph nodes: neck, supraclavicular, axillary, epitrochlear, inguinal and femoral.
- Measurement of enlarged organs, lymph nodes or mass.
- Cardiac evaluation: flow murmur, signs of congestive cardiac failure.
- Pulmonary evaluation (including presence of tracheal deviation).

3. Diagnostic tests
- Explain honestly and carefully to the parents and child what each test involves and why it is being performed. Tell them what you suspect, along with appropriate words of encouragement.
- Try to coordinate investigations (including blood tests) to make them as efficient as possible while trying to minimize the stress to the child and family (e.g. if a child is to be sedated for a procedure, try to do all the tests that require sedation at that time).
- Ensure that adequate pathological specimens are obtained.
- Do not "make the diagnosis" or start treatment until you have the final report from the pathologist (unless it is a life threatening emergency).
- Specific investigations will need to be performed depending on the type of cancer. These are listed at the end of the chapter under each disease category.

PRINCIPLES OF TREATMENT

Once the diagnosis and stage of the disease has been established, a treatment plan should be determined and treatment started as soon as possible.

Clinical trials

Childhood cancer is a rare disease. In order to improve the knowledge and therapy, many institutions participate in multicenter clinical trials. These trials compare different treatment regimes and have resulted in improvement in cure rates and reduction in toxicity. Clinical trials are essential to improve quality of care for children with cancer.

Treatment

The pediatric oncologist has several different "weapons" which may be used to treat childhood cancer and a wide range of supportive care treatments.

- Specific treatment: chemotherapy, surgery, radiotherapy, BMT, immunotherapy, maturation agents.
- Supportive care: blood products and hematopoietic growth factors, antimicrobial drugs, nutritional support, venous access, symptom care (pain, nausea, etc.), psychological support, palliation.
- The choice of treatment depends on the type and stage of the cancer and sometimes on the age of the child.

1. Chemotherapy
The use of cytotoxic drugs has resulted in a dramatic improvement in the cure rate for most types of childhood cancer. Unfortunately, cytotoxic drugs also affect normal cells, particularly cells that are dividing and growing rapidly (e.g. hematopoietic cells, endothelium of the gastrointestinal tract and hair follicles).
- Principles of chemotherapy:
  Combination chemotherapy: combinations of drugs are used to minimize drug resistance and enhance cell kill.
  Adjuvant chemotherapy: chemotherapy is most effective when used in patients with a low tumor cell burden.
  High dose intensity: many anticancer drugs have a steep dose response curve. Increasing the dose of the drug results in a significant increase in tumor response.
- Types of chemotherapy drugs:
  Alkylating agents (procarbazine, cyclophosphamide, ifosfamide, carboplatinum, cis platinum).
  Antimetabolites (methotrexate, 6–mercaptopurine, 6–thioguanine, cytosine arabinoside).
  Antibiotics (doxorubicin, daunomycin, bleomycin, dactinomycin).
  Plant alkaloids (vincristine, vinblastine, etoposide).
  Miscellaneous (prednisone, dexamethasone, L. asparaginase).
Chemotherapy is an important component of the treatment for most types of childhood cancer, particularly leukemia, lymphoma, Wilm's tumor, soft tissue sarcomas and bone tumors. Chemotherapy is effective against dividing cells, not cells in the resting phase of the cell cycle.

2. Radiotherapy
- This is the administration of electromagnetic waves or particulate rays to kill tumor cells. It is an effective method of treatment for many childhood cancers. The major disadvantage of radiotherapy in children is its effect on growth of bones and soft tissues.
- Radiotherapy is a particularly important part of the treatment for brain tumors, soft tissue sarcomas, and Ewing's sarcoma.

3. Surgery
Surgical biopsy is frequently necessary in the diagnosis of cancer. Surgical resection alone may be a curative treatment for some cancers (e.g. early stage neuroblastoma and some brain tumors). More often, surgical resection of a tumor results in a significant reduction in the tumor mass, making the residual tumor cells more amenable to cure by chemotherapy or radiotherapy, such as soft tissue sarcomas, Wilm's tumor, neuroblastoma, bone tumors and brain tumors. Second look surgery may be necessary to remove residual tumor following chemotherapy and/or radiotherapy.

4. Bone marrow transplant (BMT)

Bone marrow transplant is used in pediatric oncology to treat the following conditions:

- Definite indications:

  Primary malignant disease of the bone marrow, e.g. ALL after first relapse, AML in first remission, CML in chronic phase.

  Lymphoma (after first relapse).

  Hematological and immunological disorders, e.g. immunodeficiency, aplastic anemia and thalassemia.

- Possible indications:

  Relapsed solid tumor, e.g. Ewing's sarcoma, rhabdomyosarcoma, advanced stage neuroblastoma.

  Bone marrow transplant allows administration of extremely high doses of chemotherapy and/or radiotherapy which would otherwise be lethal because of irreversible damage to the hematopoietic system. Infusion of healthy bone marrow cells after this intensive treatment (either autologous or allogeneic) then "rescues" the bone marrow and allows regrowth of the hematopoietic system.

- Types of bone marrow transplant:

  Syngeneic: that is, from an identical twin.

  Matched related allogeneic: usually from an HLA matched sibling; usual or first choice of donor for leukemia.

  Matched unrelated allogeneic (MUD): donor is usually identified through a donor registry; used if there is no matched related donor available.

  Partially matched related donor: used if there is no matched donor available.

  Autologous purged transplant (i.e. treated ex vivo to remove malignant cells): this type of transplant may be used for leukemia (AML) or neuroblastoma.

  Autologous nonpurged transplant: used for diseases which do not infiltrate the bone marrow to allow ultra high doses of chemotherapy and radiotherapy, e.g. Hodgkin's lymphoma.

  Peripheral blood stem cell transplant (PBSC): this is usually an autologous form of hematopoietic cell rescue for solid tumors.

  Cord blood: the stem cells from cord blood can be used for a matched or partially matched allogeneic bone marrow transplant.

- Common complications of bone marrow transplant:

  Toxicity from the chemotherapy and/or radiotherapy: GI inflammation, liver, renal and lung toxicity.

  Complications of pancytopenia (bleeding, infection and anemia).

  Immunological problems: rejection of the graft, immunodeficiency, graft versus host disease (in this disorder, the bone marrow "graft" recognizes the host as being foreign and "attacks" the host cells, resulting in an autoimmune disease primarily affecting the skin, liver, gastrointestinal tract and joints).

  Long–term toxicity includes: endocrine and growth abnormalities, decreased fertility, learning disabilities and second malignancy.

5. Immunotherapy (biological modifiers)

The use of lymphokines or cytokines in oncology is an area which is being studied extensively. A definite role for these agents in the treatment of childhood cancer has not yet been established, but the role of cell stimulating factors in supportive care is now well established. Lymphokines include: interferons, interleukins, tumor necrosis factor, colony stimulating factors (e.g. GCSF).

6. Maturation agents

The aim of maturation or differentiation therapy is to "mature" the malignant cell to a form that has a lower mitotic potential and which may be more receptive to environmental cues, immune surveillance, or more sensitive to chemotherapy. Maturation agents which may be beneficial in childhood cancer include: cis retinoic acid (in neuroblastoma), all trans–retinoic acid (in acute promyelocytic leukemia).

ADMINISTRATION OF CHEMOTHERAPY

Body surface area (BSA) calculation

Many chemotherapy drugs are calculated according to the child's BSA. This can be calculated as follows:

$$BSA(m^2) = \sqrt{\frac{height\ (cm)\ \times\ weight\ (kg)}{3600}}$$

Slide rule nomograms are often available but are not as accurate. Modification may sometimes be necessary for excessively obese patients. A table for calculating BSA is included in chapter 24 (Appendix).

Intravenous chemotherapy

Most drugs will be mixed in the Pharmacy under a laminar air flow hood and administered according to a specific protocol. Always check the protocol when ordering or administering chemotherapy drugs.

Extravasation of chemotherapeutic drugs

Some drugs, particularly vincristine, vinblastine, doxorubicin, daunomycin, nitrogen mustard and dactinomycin cause severe chemical burns if tissue extravasation occurs.

These drugs are usually given through a central venous catheter, but if administered peripherally:
*   Establish new i.v. with a syringe of normal saline and ensure good backflow of blood.
*   Switch syringes and inject drug (check frequently for blood return).
*   Flush well with normal saline.

If extravasation occurs:
*   Stop drug administration immediately.
*   Aspirate the drug as much as possible via the needle.
*   Inject 1 mL of solucortef (250 mg/0.2 mL) through the needle.
*   For doxorubicin or daunomycin, inject 2.5 mL of $NaHCO_3$ 8.4%.
*   Elevate the limb and apply cold compresses.

Intrathecal administration of chemotherapy

- The following drugs may be given intrathecally:
    Methotrexate (usually diluted in normal saline to a dilution of 1–2 mg/mL).
    Cytosine arabinoside (diluted in sterile water to a total volume of 5–10 mL).
    Hydrocortisone (diluted in normal saline).
    (Ensure that vincristine is not present in the room when administering intrathecal chemotherapy. If vincristine is inadvertently given intrathecally, it will be fatal.)
- Do lumbar puncture in usual way.
- Remove a volume of CSF approximately equal to the volume of drug to be administered. Allow CSF to drip freely into appropriate collection tubes.
- Inject chemotherapy drug slowly through the lumbar puncture needle. (If CSF is heavily blood stained, do not inject chemotherapy drug.) Stop injection if patient complains of excessive back or leg pain.

Specific complications of chemotherapy drugs

1. High dose methotrexate
Toxic effects of high dose methotrexate (8–12 g/m^2) include: mucositis, renal toxicity, CNS toxicity, myelosuppression. Toxic effects can be minimized by:
- Adequate hydration and alkalinization:
    Intravenous fluids D5W + 75 mEq HCO$_3$ /L + 20 mEq KCl/L at 125–150 mL/m^2 per h; give 3 h pre–, during and for 24 h postmethotrexate infusion. Ensure urine pH > 7.0. Increase sodium bicarbonate if necessary.
- Folinic acid "rescue" (leukovorin): toxic effects can be reversed or ameliorated with leukovorin. This is usually started 24 hours after methotrexate and continued until methotrexate levels are within the "safe" range.

2. Cis platinum
Toxic effects of cis platinum include: renal failure and tubular dysfunction, deafness (usually high frequency), severe nausea and vomiting, hypomagnesemia and hypocalcemia, myelosuppression.
- Investigations to be checked prior to cis platinum infusion:
    BUN, creatinine, electrolytes, magnesium, phosphate, calcium, CBC and differential.
    Nuclear medicine GFR or a 24 hour urine creatinine clearance.
    Audiogram.
- Side effects of cis platinum can be minimized by adequate hydration and diuresis as follows:
    i.v. fluids prehydration: D5W/0.5% normal saline + 20 mEq KCl/L + 8 mEq magnesium sulfate/L at 125 mg/m^2 per h × 3 h.
    During cis platinum infusion: add dose of cis platinum to D5W/0.5% normal saline to run at 185 mL/m^2 per h, usually 6–8 h.
    Post–cis platinum: i.v. D5W/0.5% normal saline + 20 mEq KCl/L + 8 mEq magnesium sulfate/L at 125 mL/m^2 per h for 18 h or until tolerating adequate (125 mL/m^2 per h) oral fluids.
- Urine output:
    During cis platinum infusion, the urine output should be > 150 mL/m^2 per h. If it is insufficient, give mannitol 200 mg/kg over 15 min. If no response in one hour, give lasix

0.5 mg/kg.
After cis platinum infusion, urine output should be 125 mL/m² q2h.
Antiemetics: ensure adequate antiemetics are given, usually ondansetron 0.15 mg/kg at hours 0, 4 and 8.

3. Cyclophosphamide and ifosfamide
Toxic effects of cyclophosphamide and ifosfamide include hemorrhage cystitis. This can be prevented by adequate hydration.
- Prehydration: D5W/0.5% normal saline, at 200 mL/m² per h × 2 h.
- During and postinfusion, continue i.v. fluids at 150 mL/m² per h.
- Mesna: this protects the bladder mucosa. Dose is 60–160% of cyclophosphamide or ifosfamide dose. 25% is given concurrently with chemotherapy and the remainder given as 3 bolus doses q3–4h or as a continuous infusion over 8–12 h.

4. Anthracyclines
- These drugs cause cumulative cardiac toxicity.
- Investigations to be done prior to administration: CBC; echocardiogram and assessment of left ventricular function and ECG; calculation of cumulative anthracycline dose.
- Patients should not receive a total life time dose of more than 400 mg/m² except under the guidance of a cardiologist. Cardiotoxicity is enhanced if the heart is irradiated.

SUPPORTIVE CARE

The cure rate of childhood cancer has improved dramatically over the last 20 years because of improvement in therapy of malignancy and improvement in supportive care which allows the patient to cope with increasingly intensive specific therapy.

Blood products and growth factors

- Pancytopenia occurs in children with cancer due to: bone marrow infiltration, bone marrow suppression by chemotherapy or radiotherapy.
- Blood product support is an essential element in the treatment of childhood malignancy but there are significant risks associated. Blood transfusion and blood products should be treated with respect and only used when necessary.

1. Risks of blood transfusion
- Febrile and hemolytic transfusion reactions.
- Alloimmunization and the risk of becoming refractory to transfusion.
- Transmission of infections.
- Graft versus host disease.
- The following measures can be used to reduce the risks of transfusion:
    Avoid transfusions if possible. Do not give "top up" transfusions unless clinically indicated. If several small transfusions are required, split a single unit of red cells into aliquots to reduce donor exposure.
    Irradiate blood products (1,500–3,000 cGy) to prevent graft versus host disease (necessary for severely immunocompromised patients).

Use leukocyte depleted products (leukocyte filters or washed products) whenever possible. These filters are expensive and their use is limited in many institutions to patients who are extremely immunocompromised.

Use CMV negative blood products for severely immunocompromised and CMV seronegative patients.

2. Indications for red cell transfusion
- Acute blood loss: > 15% of blood volume or inadequate tissue oxygenation.
- Chronic blood loss with hemoglobin < 80 g/L.
- Hemoglobin < 80 g/L in a patient prior to the nadir of bone marrow suppression from chemotherapy.
- Hemoglobin < 100 g/L in a patient undergoing radiotherapy (adequate tissue oxygenation is important in determining the dose of radiotherapy).
- Hemoglobin < 80 g/L prior to surgery associated with blood loss or < 70 g/L prior to general anesthetic.

3. Dose of red blood cells
- 10 mL/kg of packed red blood cells over 3–4 h.
- For profound anemia (when not associated with blood loss), give 3–5 mL/kg in repeated aliquots over 3–4 h each, paying attention to the volume status of the patient. The patient may develop congestive cardiac failure.

4. Indications for platelet transfusion
- Well patient with platelet count < 10 × 10^9 /L.
- Patient on induction chemotherapy with platelets < 20 × 10^9 /L.
- Platelets < 20 × 10^9 /L prior to lumbar puncture.
- Patients with brain tumors with platelets < 20 × 10^9 /L.
- Platelets < 50 × 10^9 /L prior to surgery.
- DIC and platelets < 50 × 10^9 /L.
- Bleeding with platelets < 50 × 10^9 /L.
- Septic patient with platelets < 20 × 10^9 /L.

Spontaneous bleeding rarely occurs with a platelet count > 10 × 10^9 /L but is more likely to occur in a sick or septic patient.

5. Platelet dose
- Random donor platelets:

Age	Dose
< 2 yr	2 units
2–6 yr	3 units
6+ yr	5 units

- Single donor platelets (collected by apheresis): used for patients who are refractory to random donors. The platelets collected from a single apheresis are usually approximately equivalent to six random donor units of platelets.

6. Granulocyte transfusions
Granulocyte transfusions are associated with a high risk of alloimmunization, pulmonary leukostasis and transmission of infection. They are rarely, if ever, indicated.

7. Hematopoietic growth factor support
*   Growth factors are cytokines that regulate the growth of hematopoietic progenitor cells. In clinical practice, they are used to:
        Enhance hematopoietic recovery following chemotherapy and bone marrow transplant.
        Mobilize peripheral blood progenitor cells (for future transplant).
*   There are many growth factors available for research and investigative purposes but at present their use is limited to:
        GCSF (granulocyte colony simulating factor):
        GCSF supports mature progenitors committed to the granulocyte lineage.
        Dose: 5–10 µg/kg per d (until the ANC is > 10 × 10^9/L).
        Route: subcutaneous (preferred) or intravenous.
        Toxicity: flushing, hypotension, myalgia, bone pain, chills and fever.
        GMCSF (granulocyte macrophage colony stimulating factor):
        GMCSF supports earlier progenitor cells which give rise to granulocytes, monocytes and eosinophils and have a potential role in regulation of megakaryocytes and red cells.
        Dose: 200–300 µg/m^2 per d.
        Route: subcutaneous (preferred) or intravenous.
        Complications: similar to GCSF but may be more pronounced.
        EPO (erythropoietin):
        EPO supports red blood cell progenitors. It is used for the anemia of chronic disease and occasionally post–bone marrow transplant.

Antimicrobial therapy

Children being treated for cancer are at high risk for infection because of both quantitative and qualitative impairment of their immune systems as follows:
*   Bone marrow suppression due to tumor infiltrate, chemotherapy, and radiation therapy. Neutropenia is the most significant factor. Absolute neutrophil count (ANC) < 1.0 × 10^9/L is associated with increased risk of infection. ANC < 0.5 × 10^9/L is associated with a significantly increased risk of serious infection.
*   Impaired function of neutrophils, lymphocytes and mononuclear cells.
*   Disruption of the normal mechanical barriers to infection by surgery, tumor invasion, radiation therapy (causes breakdown of skin and mucosa), indwelling catheters and chemotherapy (causes breakdown of mucosal barriers).

1. Common infecting organisms in pediatric oncology patients
*   Bacteria:
        Gram positive: staphylococci (coagulase negative and coagulase positive), streptococci (alpha hemolytic), *Streptococcus pneumoniae, Enterococcus.*
        Gram negative: enterobacteriaceae (*E. coli, Klebsiella, Enterobacter* and *Acinetobacter*), *Pseudomonas*, anaerobes.
*   Fungi: *Candida, Aspergillus.*

- Viruses: herpes simplex, varicella zoster, cytomegalovirus.
- Others: *Pneumocystis carinii*.

2. Prevention of infection
- Avoid epithelial penetration:
    No rectal exams, rectal thermometers.
    Keep stools soft.
    Avoid bladder catheterization.
    Strict aseptic technique for all procedures.
    Strict care of central venous catheters.
- Prevent nosocomial infection:
    Strict handwashing and infection control procedures.
    Isolate known infectious patients.
- Prevent specific infection:
    Influenza: give annual vaccine.
    Pneumocystis: give prophylactic trimethoprim/sulfamethoxazole (5 mg TMP/25 µg SMX per kg per 24 h for 3 consecutive days per week).
    Varicella zoster: give zoster immunoglobulin after contact; 1 vial per 10 kg body weight.
    Measles: give i.v. gamma globulin after contact.
    Candida infection: give prophylactic oral nystatin while neutropenic.

3. Management of fever and neutropenia
Fever associated with neutropenia ($< 1.0 \times 10^9$ /L) is an emergency. These patients can rapidly develop septic shock associated with a high mortality rate.
- Assessment must include a careful history and physical. Remember to check:
    Skin: CBC site and recent venepuncture, finger prick, bone marrow and lumbar puncture sites.
    Mouth for ulcers and *Candida* infection.
    Perirectal area for fissures and ulcers.
    Pain may be the only localizing symptom of infection.
- Investigations:
    Blood cultures, both aerobic and anaerobic. If patient has CVC, draw cultures from all lumens. If patient does not have CVC, draw from peripheral vein.
    Urinalysis and urine culture (do not catheterize or "bag" a patient unless there is a strong suspicion of urinary tract infection as this can introduce infection).
    Chest X–ray, if clinically indicated.
    Throat culture and skin cultures, if clinically indicated.
    Stool cultures, if clinically indicated.
    Lumbar puncture, if clinically indicated.

4. Treatment of fever and neutropenia
Empiric broad spectrum antibiotic coverage should be initiated as soon as possible. The choice of antibiotics should be based on the known predominant pathogens and their local sensitivities. A suggested approach is given below for empiric treatment of febrile, neutropenic children:
- Low risk patient: ampicillin (200 mg/kg per d div. q.i.d.) plus cloxacillin (200 mg/kg per d div. q.i.d.) plus tobramycin (7 mg/kg per d div. t.i.d.).

- High risk patient (e.g. post–bone marrow transplant, currently on a relapse protocol): piperacillin (300 mg/kg per d div. q.i.d.) plus cloxacillin (200 mg/kg per d div. q.i.d.) plus tobramycin (7 mg/kg per d div. t.i.d.); add amphotericin (1 mg/kg per d) plus metronidazole (30 mg/kg per d div. t.i.d.) if suspected typhlitis.
- Subsequent management depends on culture results:
  Culture positive:
  Gram positive: if stable, wait for sensitivities; if deteriorating, change cloxacillin to vancomycin.
  Gram negative: change ampicillin to piperacillin or tobramycin.
  Culture negative:
  Febrile: add amphotericin after 4 days negative cultures; earlier if patient is deteriorating.
  Afebrile: continue antibiotics until ANC > 250 or 7 days, whichever is sooner.

Table III: Predisposition to fungal infections

Fungal infection	Predisposing causes
Candida	Neutropenia, hyperglycemia, central venous catheter, disruption of mucocutaneous barriers
Aspergillus	Neutropenia and exposure to dust from old buildings during renovation

- Treatment of fungal infections:
  Amphotericin is the standard treatment, but renal toxicity and hypersensitivity to amphotericin are common.
  Fluconazole may be an effective prophylaxis for *Candida albicans* only.
- Viral infections:
  Varicella zoster:
  Varicella zoster infection can cause fulminant disease in immunocompromised patients with significant morbidity including encephalitis, pneumonitis and hepatitis. In untreated patients, the mortality rate is 7%.
  Prevention: avoid exposure if possible; give varicella zoster immunoglobulin (VZIg), 1 vial per 10 kg of body weight i.m. within 96 h of exposure.
  Treatment: admit patient to hospital in strict isolation; acyclovir 1,500 mg/m^2 per 24 h i.v. div. t.i.d.
  Herpes simplex:
  May cause severe localized infections of oral mucosa, esophagitis, skin and eye, or disseminated infection involving lung, liver or CNS.
  Treatment: acyclovir 750 mg/m^2 per 24 h i.v. div. t.i.d.
  Pneumocystis carinii:
  This is a protozoan infection which can cause fatal pneumonitis in immunocompromised patients.
  Prevention: trimethoprim–sulfamethoxazole (TMP–SMX) 5 mg/kg per d of TMP given 3 consecutive days per week.
  Symptoms: fever, tachypnea.
  Diagnosis: bronchoscopy with bronchial washings or lung biopsy; diagnosis is difficult so

empiric treatment is often started, based on the level of suspicion.
Treatment: TMP–SMX 20 mg TMP/kg per 24 h i.v. or p.o.; pentamidine 4 mg/kg per 24 h i.v. or i.m. daily (second line treatment).

Prevention of tumor lysis syndrome

Any new oncology patient, any patient with bulky disease, or any patient in relapse starting chemotherapy or radiotherapy is at risk for hyperuricemia. Patients at highest risk are those with non-Hodgkin's lymphoma, particularly Burkitt's lymphoma.

To prevent this:
- Allopurinol: if possible, start 2–3 days before chemotherapy as it takes this long to take effect. Dose: 10 mg/kg per d p.o. (i.v. allopurinol is an investigational drug but may be obtained for patients who are unable to take oral medications; dose 10 mg/kg per d i.v.).
- Ensure high urine output: intravenous fluids are usually necessary; for high risk patients, 3,000–4,000 mL/m^2 per d or 2–4 times maintenance fluids.
  Use D5W + 50–70 mEq $NaHCO_3$ /L. Do not add KCl unless patient is hypokalemic. Strict fluid balance records must be kept to ensure patient does not become fluid overloaded.
- Alkalinize urine: add sodium bicarbonate 50–70 mEq/L of D5W. Aim to keep the urine pH > 7. Discontinue alkalinization if patient becomes hypocalcemic. Check uric acid, electrolytes, BUN, creatinine, calcium and phosphate daily or more frequently for several days after starting chemotherapy.
- If there is a high risk of tumor lysis syndrome, contact nephrologist for possible dialysis.

Nutritional support

Malnutrition is common in children undergoing treatment for cancer. Reasons include:
- Nausea and vomiting secondary to chemotherapy and/or radiotherapy.
- Anorexia and altered taste perception, secondary to chemotherapy.
- Mucositis, secondary to chemotherapy, radiotherapy and/or infection (*Candida* and HSV).
- Abdominal surgery and/or radiotherapy.
- Gastrointestinal infection (typhlitis, *Clostridium difficile*).
- Psychological causes, causing anorexia (depression, manipulation).

Nutritional support is essential. Methods include:
- Oral feeding with calorie supplements, e.g. high calorie drinks.
- Nasogastric tube feeding:
    Advantages: simple to start and may be given at home.
    Disadvantages: not suitable for patients with mucositis or severe nausea; tube may require frequent reinsertion.
- Gastrostomy tube feeding:
    Advantages: useful for long–term feeding at home; may be used for patients with mucositis and moderate nausea.
    Disadvantages: requires surgical insertion; may be associated with increased risk of infection.

- Total parenteral nutrition:
   Advantages: may be used for patients with impaired gastrointestinal function.
   Disadvantages: requires central venous catheter access; usually has to be given as an inpatient; less physiologically acceptable as the gastrointestinal tract is not used. Monitor weight daily; try to maintain some enteral feeding to maintain integrity of GI mucosa.

Venous access

Venous access is crucial for administration of chemotherapy and supportive care. Peripheral i.v.'s may be used, but many of the chemotherapy drugs and antibiotics cause sclerosis of the veins and, ultimately, lack of venous access.

1. Central venous catheters (CVC)
These are recommended for the following groups of patients:
- Patients receiving intensive chemotherapy.
- Patients likely to need TPN.
- Patients receiving radiotherapy to the head and neck or abdomen.
- Young patients with difficult venous access.
- Children with "needle phobia".

2. Types of central venous catheters (CVC)
- Right atrial catheters leading to tubing that exits through the skin, usually on the chest or back:
   May have one, two or three lumens; often referred to as Hickmann or Broviac catheter or CVC.
   Advantages: easy access; no needle pokes.
   Disadvantages: requires daily or alternate day heparin flushes, dressing changes 3 times per week; requires parental teaching and cooperation; restricts lifestyle, i.e. no swimming and difficult bathing; requires scrupulous aseptic technique.
- Right atrial catheters that end in a reservoir or port under the skin:
   Often referred to as portacath or VAD (venous access device).
   Advantages: requires minimal care when not accessed; do not restrict lifestyle.
   Disadvantages: access is via a needle and therefore is not suitable for patients with needle phobia; double ports may be difficult to insert in small children.

3. Complications of central lines
- Infection:
   The catheter may become infected (bacteria or fungi) and then act as a reservoir for infection. Clearance can usually be achieved with appropriate antibiotics or antifungal treatment but removal of the catheter may be necessary for persistent infection or very virulent organisms, e.g. *Pseudomonas*.
- Thrombosis:
   Thrombosis is often present around the sheath of the catheter but may occasionally occlude the lumen.
   To clear thrombosis:
   Urokinase (5,000 unit/mL): instill 1.5–3 mL in each lumen for 1 h, then attempt aspiration.
   Urokinase infusion: 200 unit/kg per h into the catheter. If thrombosis cannot be cleared,

the line should be removed.

4. Removal of central lines
- Central lines should be removed for the following reasons:
    CVC is completely occluded and cannot be cleared with urokinase.
    Blood cultures are persistently positive, after 48–72 hours of appropriate antibiotics or antifungal treatment, and there is no other cause of sepsis.
    Severe local "tunnel" infection or cellulitis.
    CVC no longer needed.
- Central lines may be removed for persistent fever, with no other cause, in a neutropenic patient despite use of broad spectrum antibiotics.

Pain control

Adequate pain management is essential. Children may have pain due to:
- Cancer: due to pressure or infiltration, e.g. brain tumor, bone tumor, sarcoma, neuroblastoma, bone marrow infiltration.
- Toxicity of treatment, e.g. mucositis, typhlitis, radiation burns.
- Infection, e.g. abscess, cellulitis.
- Painful procedures, e.g. bone marrow aspirate, lumbar puncture, venepuncture.

1. Methods of pain control
- Psychological: relaxation techniques, reassuring environment, supportive parents and staff.
- Pharmacological:
    Mild pain:
    Acetaminophen 10–15 mg/kg per dose q4–6h p.o. (avoid rectal administration if possible). Acetaminophen may mask fever.
    Nonsteroidal anti–inflammatories (NSAID's), e.g. ibuprofen, naprosyn, are useful for bone pain but should be avoided if possible in patients with thrombocytopenia.
    Moderate pain:
    Codeine 0.5–1 mg/kg per dose q4–6h p.o. (give stool softeners to prevent constipation).
    Severe pain:
    Morphine: usually given initially as an i.v. bolus followed by an i.v. infusion to provide constant analgesia. Bolus dose: 0.05–0.1 mg/kg. Infusion dose: 10–40 µg/kg per h.
    To set up infusion: 1 mg × weight (kg) = morphine (mg) per 100 mL.
    Then each 1 mL/h = 10 µg/kg per h. Titrate infusion rate to control pain.
    To convert i.v. morphine to p.o. for stable patient: add total daily morphine requirement; multiply this dose by 3 to obtain the daily p.o. dose; choose appropriate dosing interval and divide dose accordingly. To convert to long–acting morphine: use same total daily dose as short acting but divide into 2 or 3 doses.

2. Procedure related pain and sedation
- Local anesthesia:
    EMLA cream (lidocaine + prilocane): must be applied 1 hour prior to procedure under occlusive dressing; used for venepuncture, i.m. injections, bone marrow aspiration and lumbar punctures.

Local infiltration of lidocaine or xylocaine: used for bone marrow aspirate and occasionally lumbar punctures.

- Sedation:
  Sedation and/or anesthesia is often required for procedures such as bone marrow aspirates and lumbar punctures which may be extremely frightening to a child. There are many different methods of sedation.

  Midazolam:
  This is a potent imidabenzo diazepine which has hypnotic, anxiolytic, muscle relaxant, anticonvulsant, and amnestic properties.
  Method of administration: intravenously, first dose at minute 0, 0.15 mg/kg; second dose at minute 2, 0.15 mg/kg (if patient well sedated, do not give further doses); third dose at minute 4, 0.15 mg/kg (monitor oxygen saturation with oximeter and blood pressure and heart rate every 2–3 min).
  Complications: respiratory depression, hypotension.
  Oral: 0.5 mg/kg; give 30 min prior to procedure.
  Fentanyl: 1–2 μg/kg dose i.v. over 3–5 min. Antidote is narcan 0.1 mg/kg.
  Ativan: 0.5–1 mg/kg sublingual 20–30 min prior to procedure.
  Morphine: 0.05 mg/kg; may be given with midazolam or ativan.
  Ketamine: 1 mg/kg p.o. 20–30 min prior to procedure.
  General anesthesia may be necessary for children who are extremely anxious or difficult to sedate.

Nausea and vomiting

This is a common problem for patients on chemotherapy. The following drugs cause severe nausea and vomiting: cis platinum, nitrogen mustard, cytosine arabinoside, cyclophosphamide, dactinomycin, high dose methotrexate. Nausea and vomiting should be prevented whenever possible.

Antiemetics:
- Ondansetron (5–HT3 antagonist): this is the most potent antiemetic available and the only licensed drug in this class. It can be combined with dexamethasone and dimenhydrinate for increased efficacy. Dose: 0.15 mg/kg i.v. q8–12h p.r.n., 0.2 mg/kg p.o. q8–12h p.r.n. Disadvantage: very expensive.
- Dimenhydrinate (gravol): 1 mg/kg per dose i.v. q4h p.r.n. Useful for mild nausea and vomiting or in combination with ondansetron.
- Metoclopramide (maxeran): 1 mg/kg per dose i.v. q4h p.r.n. plus diphenhydramine (benadryl), 1 mg/kg per dose i.v. q4h. Benadryl should be given at the same time as metoclopramide to prevent extrapyramidal side effects.
- Dexamethasone: 2–4 mg/m^2 per dose i.v./p.o. q6h. Often used in conjunction with ondansetron.
- Droperidol: 0.1 mg/kg (first dose), then 0.05–0.1 mg/kg to a total of 4 mg/dose q4–8h. Give with benadryl to prevent extrapyramidal side effects.
- Nabilone: if < 18 kg, 0.5 mg p.o. q8–12h; if > 18 kg, 1 mg p.o. q8–12h; if adult, 1–2 mg p.o. b.i.d.

Mucositis

This is mouth ulceration due to delayed cellular turnover of the mucosal lining. It is usually secondary to chemotherapy and/or radiotherapy.

Management:
- Mouth care: chlorhexidene mouthwash, sodium bicarbonate mouthwash; soft toothbrush or sponge to clean gums and teeth; keep lips moist with vaseline.
- Fungal prophylaxis: nystatin suspension 2–5 mL p.o. q6h.
- Pain control: morphine infusion; local anesthetic mouthwash usually causes increased stinging initially and is not acceptable to young children.

Constipation

This is a common problem for patients who are receiving vincristine or narcotics and who are on prolonged bedrest.

Constipation can be prevented or treated by:
- Colace (docusate): 5 mg/kg per 24 h.
- Lactulose: infants, 2–5–10 mL/d; children, 40–90 mL/d.

Suppositories or enemas should be avoided whenever possible, especially in the neutropenic child because of the risk of rectal trauma and bacteremia. However, for the severely constipated child, gentle administration of a suppository or enema may cause less rectal trauma than passage of a hard stool.

Psychological support

Ongoing psychological support is essential for the child and family and will be provided by all members of the team.

From the pediatric resident, the children and parents will expect:
- A caring, encouraging and professional attitude.
- Reasonable knowledge of pediatrics and pediatric oncology and good knowledge of supportive care.
- Honesty: try to answer all questions but do not be afraid to admit that you do not know and need to ask other members of your team. Parents of children with cancer are extremely knowledgeable about their child's disease and will not respect inaccurate or vague information.
- Respect: remember that the child's parents will always know their child better than any of the staff so listen carefully to their observations.

ONCOLOGICAL EMERGENCIES

Emergencies occur frequently in pediatric oncology because of the effects of the underlying disease and the side effects of treatment.

Hematological emergencies in oncology

1. Hemorrhage
- Oncology patients are at risk because of:
    Thrombocytopenia: due to disease causing bone marrow infiltration and treatment causing bone marrow suppression.
    Coagulopathy: due to medications, particularly L. asparaginase, liver disease and leukemia.
- Prevention:
    Thrombocytopenia: transfuse to maintain a platelet count over 10×10^9 /L.
    Coagulopathy: replace as necessary with fresh frozen plasma (10 mL/kg) and specific coagulation factors.
- Treatment of hemorrhage (depends on the site and the cause):
    Platelet transfusion and replacement of fresh frozen plasma and specific coagulation proteins.
    Red cell transfusion or normal saline or other volume expanders, as necessary.
    Specific site management:
    GI tract: for peptic ulcer, treat conservatively with ranitidine and antacids, if possible; surgery may be necessary for severe bleeding.
    Lower GI bleeding: if secondary to infection, treat with antibiotics; surgery only if bleeding uncontrolled.
    CNS bleeding: may require surgery.
    Nose bleeding: nasal pressure for 10–20 min; may need nasal pack and local cocaine.

2. Disseminated intravascular coagulation
This is due to uncontrolled activation of intravascular coagulation and fibrinolysis. This may occur in severe illness (e.g. trauma, burns, sepsis), leukemia (particularly acute promyelocytic leukemia).
- Signs and symptoms: bruising, bleeding and shock.
- Investigations: CBC, platelet count, PT, PTT, fibrin split products or D–dimers, fibrinogen.
- Treatment:
    Treat the underlying disease as a priority.
    Replace platelets, fresh frozen plasma and cryoprecipitate.
    Red cell transfusion.
    Low dose heparin infusion may be needed for acute promyelocytic leukemia (APL).

3. Transfusion emergencies
- Volume: patients with chronic anemia may develop congestive cardiac failure if transfused too quickly. Transfusion should be split into small aliquots and transfused slowly. Give lasix 0.5 mg/kg between aliquots.
- Transfusion reactions:
    Allergic reaction:
    Usually due to "allergenic substances" within the transfused blood.
    Symptoms: urticaria, wheezing and hives; may be treated with antihistamines.
    Febrile transfusion reaction:
    Usually due to white blood cells within the transfusion. An extremely rare cause of febrile

transfusion reaction is infected blood. This usually results in septic shock with a very high mortality rate.

Symptoms: chills and fever.

Treatment: discontinue the transfusion; may need antihistamines. Send a sample of the transfused blood back to the laboratory for investigation.

Prevention: use washed blood cells or leukocyte depletion filters.

Hemolytic transfusion reaction:

Due to intravascular destruction of incompatible red blood cells.

Symptoms: fever, chills, headache, back pain progressing to shock and renal failure.

Treatment: discontinue the transfusion immediately and start forced diuresis.

Allergic or anaphylactic reactions

- In pediatric oncology these reactions may be due to:
    Chemotherapy drugs, particularly L. asparaginase, bleomycin, etoposide.
    Blood transfusion.
    Other drugs, e.g. antibiotics or vitamin K.
- Signs of allergy: urticaria, nasal congestion, wheezing, coughing, stridor, respiratory distress.
- Management:
    Stop infusion of drug.
    Benadryl 2 mg/kg.
    Oxygen as necessary.
    Hydrocortisone 2 mg/kg i.v.
    Adrenalin 1:1,000 0.01 mL/kg subcutaneously.
    If necessary, transfer to ICU for ventilation.

Septic shock

Fever associated with severe neutropenia is an emergency and should be treated as soon as possible. Septic shock occurs very quickly in neutropenic patients, particularly with Gram negative sepsis.

- Symptoms and signs: fever or occasionally low body temperature, hypotension, hypoperfusion, peripheral edema, respiratory distress.
- Management:
    Oxygen.
    Blood pressure support with normal saline, albumen, blood.
    Broad spectrum i.v. antibiotics.
    Low dose dopamine infusion.

Cardiac emergencies

- High output cardiac failure occurs in severe anemia.
- Low output cardiac failure occurs in pericardial restriction due to effusion, fibrosis, infection, arrhythmias, toxic drugs (particularly anthracyclines), metabolic problems and subacute bacterial endocarditis.

- Fluid overload may be seen in patients who are receiving high dose i.v. fluids with borderline renal function.
- Signs of cardiac failure:
  Increased heart rate, increased respiratory rate, hypotension, poor perfusion, gallop rhythm, hepatomegaly.
  Treatment depends on the cause of the cardiac failure.

Superior vena cava syndrome

- Superior vena cava syndrome, i.e. obstruction of the superior vena cava.
- Superior mediastinal syndrome, i.e. obstruction of the superior vena cava and the trachea.
- These syndromes may be caused by malignant tumors within the mediastinum such as non–Hodgkin's lymphoma, Hodgkin's disease, neuroblastoma or germ cell tumor.
- Signs and symptoms of SVC syndrome or SMS syndrome:
  Cough, hoarseness, dyspnea, orthopnea.
  Chest pain.
  Anxiety, confusion, lethargy.
  Headache.
  Visual change.
  Syncope.
  Swelling and plethora of face, suffusion and edema of conjunctivae.
  Wheezing and stridor.
  Increased veins on the chest wall.
- Management:
  Try to keep the patient as quiet and calm as possible.
  Tissue diagnosis may be hazardous and treatment may have to be started empirically with radiotherapy, steroids, or chemotherapy. If empiric treatment is started, a diagnostic biopsy should be performed as soon as it is safe.

Renal emergencies

- Mechanical obstruction: bulky pelvic tumors or tumors around the spinal cord may cause obstruction of the bladder or ureters. Initial treatment is catheterization or nephrostomy.
- Tumor lysis syndrome: this occurs in patients with bulky B–cell lymphoma or T–cell leukemia or lymphoma. It is due to the rapid lysis of blasts, resulting in release of intracellular contents, particularly potassium, phosphorus, and nucleic acid. This results in deposits of uric acid, phosphate, and calcium in the collecting ducts, ureters, and microvasculature of the kidney.
- Signs and symptoms: abdominal pain, back pain, decreased urine output, hypocalcemia.
- Management:
  Hydration: i.v. fluids 2–4 × maintenance, D5W with 50–100 mEq of sodium bicarbonate/L.
  Allopurinol: 10 mg/kg per 24 h p.o. div. q8h. This prevents uric acid synthesis.
  Leukapheresis or exchange transfusion can be used if the white count is over 100×10^9 /L and the patient has signs of uric acid nephropathy.
  Dialysis to be used for progressive renal failure.

Inappropriate antidiuretic hormone (SIADH)

- This may occur in pediatric lymphomas and may be precipitated by cyclophosphamide and vincristine.
- Signs: fatigue, weight increase, lethargy, confusion, seizures and coma.
- Laboratory abnormalities: hyponatremia and hypo–osmolality.
- Treatment: fluid restriction. For severe cases, lasix plus hypertonic saline.

Gastrointestinal complications

- Typhlitis: necrotizing colitis due to infection within the bowel wall. It is associated with severe neutropenia and results in bacterial invasion of the mucosa, causing inflammation and eventually infarction and perforation of the bowel.
- Usual organisms: *Clostridium septicum* and *Pseudomonas aeruginosa*.
- Management: conservative management, if possible, with i.v. antibiotics, nasogastric suctioning and bowel rest. Surgical resection may be necessary for bleeding or bowel infarction.

Central nervous system emergencies

1. Seizures
- May be due to metabolic causes, infection, bleeding, drugs (vincristine, methotrexate, cyclosporine) or raised intracranial pressure (due to tumor or hydrocephalus).
- Management of seizures:
    Airway.
    i.v. glucose.
    i.v. anticonvulsant: diazepam 0.1–0.3 mg/kg, phenytoin 10–15 mg/kg, phenobarbitol 15 mg/kg.

2. Raised intracranial pressure
- May be due to tumor, hemorrhage, edema or infection.
- Increased cerebral spinal fluid may be due to increased production, obstruction of flow or decreased absorption.
- Signs and symptoms of raised intracranial pressure:
    Headache, change in behavior, nausea and vomiting, lethargy.
    Change in pupil reaction, impaired upward gaze.
    False localizing signs, e.g. sixth nerve palsy.
    Seizures.
    Decreased coordination, ataxia.
    Papilledema.
- Management: dexamethasone 2 mg/kg i.v., mannitol 0.25–0.5 g/kg i.v., intubation and ventilation, surgery, radiotherapy.

3. Spinal cord compression
May be due to intradural CNS tumors or extradural tumors causing compression of the spinal cord.
- Signs and symptoms: pain in thighs and back, proximal weakness, sensory changes, bowel

and bladder signs.
- Diagnosis: by CT and myelogram or MRI scan.
- Management: immobilize, analgesia, sedation, dexamethasone, surgery, radiotherapy, chemotherapy if necessary.

MANAGEMENT OF SPECIFIC MALIGNANT DISEASES

Leukemia

Acute leukemia is the most common malignancy in children. It is due to a clonal proliferation of hematopoietic cells.

1. Types of childhood leukemia
- Acute lymphoblastic leukemia (ALL): 75%
- Acute myeloid leukemia (AML): 20%
- Mixed lineage leukemia: 2%
- Chronic leukemia: 3%

2. Common signs and symptoms
- Fever and recurrent infection: due to low white count.
- Easy bruising and bleeding: due to low platelets.
- Lethargy and pallor: due to low hemoglobin.
- Bone pain: due to marrow infiltration.
- Lymphadenopathy and hepatosplenomegaly.

3. Diagnostic evaluation
- Full history: include past medical history, previous infections, any suspected risk factors and family history.
- Full physical examination: include the CNS and testicular examinations; look for chloromas (leukemic mass) in gums and skin.
- CBC and differential: look for blast cells, anemia, thrombocytopenia.
- Chemistry panel: BUN, creatinine, uric acid, electrolytes, calcium, phosphate, liver function tests, LDH. These may all be abnormal, especially with a high cell turnover.
- Coagulation profile: PT, PTT, fibrinogen. There may be coagulopathy, particularly in AML.
- Blood type and cross-match: if there is anemia or thrombocytopenia.
- Chest X-ray: mediastinal mass is often found in T-cell ALL.
- Bone marrow: aspirate and biopsy (essential for diagnosis); cytogenetic evaluation and immunophenotyping (essential for classification).
- Lumbar puncture: send CSF for cell count and cytospin plus chemistry.
- Once the diagnosis is established:
    Infection screen: serology for VZV, hepatitis A, B, and C, CMV, HSV and HIV.
    Cardiac evaluation (often needed pretreatment): ECG and echocardiogram.

4. Acute care and supportive care
- Prevention of tumor lysis syndrome:
    Intravenous fluids 2–3 × maintenance D5W + sodium bicarbonate (50–100 mEq/L).

Allopurinol: dose (10 mg/kg per d).
- Transfusion: platelets or packed red cells if necessary; if possible, wait until diagnosis is established.
- Intravenous antibiotics: if the patient has signs of sepsis.
- Psychological support for the child and parents:
    Explain carefully and honestly the reason for and method of each test.
    If leukemia is suspected but not proven, explain this to the parents along with some appropriate words of encouragement.

5. Specific therapy for ALL
- Classification of ALL: before determining treatment, the type of ALL is subclassified according to morphology, immunophenotype, or risk factors.
    Morphological classification (FAB):
    L1: small cells, regular nuclei, scant cytoplasm.
    L2: large heterogenous cells, one or more nucleoli.
    L3: large homogenous cells, regular nuclei, prominent cytoplasmic vacuoles.
    Immunological classification:
    B-cell: progenitor B-cell, early pre-B ALL, transitional pre-B ALL, B-cell ALL (Burkitt's lymphoma), T-cell ALL.
    Classification according to risk factors: see Table IV.
- Treatment of ALL: treatment is usually stratified according to the known risk factors and/or the immunological and morphological classification.
    Chemotherapy:
    Chemotherapy is the mainstay of treatment. There are many different protocols but they often follow a similar pattern.
    Induction lasts 4–6 weeks. The aim is to achieve bone marrow remission. Commonly used drugs are vincristine, prednisone, L. asparaginase, and/or anthracyclines; 95% achieve remission after induction.
    Consolidation: lasts 4–8 weeks. The aim is to eradicate cells which survived induction. Commonly used drugs are cyclophosphamide, cytosine arabinoside, 6-mercaptopurine, dexamethasone, intrathecal methotrexate.
    Delayed reintensification: lasts 4–8 weeks (for high risk patients). The aim is to eradicate cells which survived initial induction and consolidation. The drugs used are similar to induction and consolidation.
    Maintenance: lasts 2–3 years. The aim is to prevent recurrence of disease. Commonly used drugs are prednisone, vincristine, 6-mercaptopurine, methotrexate, intrathecal methotrexate. This phase is less intensive. Children are usually able to attend school and live relatively normal lives.
    Radiotherapy:
    This is used for prevention and treatment of CNS disease and treatment of testicular relapse. Approximately 20–30% of patients receive cranial radiation in first remission.
    Dose: 1,800–2,400 cGy.
    "Somnolence syndrome", i.e. extreme tiredness and lethargy lasting approximately 1 week may occur 4–8 wk after cranial radiation.
    Bone marrow transplant:
    Only used for patients who have relapsed or ultra high risk patients in first remission.

Table IV: Classification of ALL by risk factors

Risk factor	Good risk	High risk
Age at diagnosis	> 1 yr, < 10 yr	< 1 yr > 10 yr
White cell count at diagnosis	< 50 × 10^9 /L	> 50 × 10^9 /L
Central nervous system disease	Absent	Present
Lymphoma syndrome	Absent	Present
DNA index	> 1.16	< 1.16
Cytogenetics	Hyperdiploidy	Hypodiploidy; specific translocations: t(9:22) t(1:19)

- Prognosis: depends on the presence or absence of multiple risk factors at diagnosis.

High risk patient   Low risk patient
<--->
65%   90%
Disease free   Disease free
survival   survival

6. Specific therapy for acute myeloid leukemia
- FAB morphological classification (this classification is the most commonly used):
    M1: myeloblastic without maturation.
    M2: myeloblastic with differentiation.
    M3: acute promyelocytic (APL); usually has translocation t (15:17).
    M4: myelocytic and monocytic with differentiation.
    M5: monocytic with poorly differentiated ± well differentiated monocytoid cells.
    M6: erythroleukemia.
    M7: megakaryoblastic leukemia (more common in Down's syndrome).
- Treatment of AML:
    Chemotherapy:
    All children with AML (with the possible exception of APL) require intensive chemotherapy and significant bone marrow hypoplasia to achieve remission.
    Induction: intensive. Lasts 4–8 weeks. Useful drugs are daunomycin, ARA–C, VP–16; 80–85% remission.
    Consolidation: often omitted if patient goes on to bone marrow transplant. Lasts 4–6 months. Useful drugs are high dose ARA–C or L. asparaginase, VP–16, daunomycin.
    Maintenance: none; does not improve disease free survival.
    Bone marrow transplant: allogeneic BMT (recommended in first remission if HLA matched sibling available; autologous BMT (advantage over chemotherapy not established).
    Radiotherapy: cranial radiotherapy rarely indicated.
- Prognosis:
    With chemotherapy alone, 5 year disease free survival is approximately 40%.
    With allogeneic bone marrow transplant, 5 year disease free survival is approximately

40–50%.
Down's syndrome patients with M7 AML have a better prognosis than non–Down's syndrome patients.

7. Specific therapy for acute promyelocytic leukemia
• All trans–retinoic acid (ATRA) can induce remission in many patients with APL. It is not yet known whether it is more effective long–term than chemotherapy induced remission.
• DIC is a complication of APL and its treatment. Thromboplastin released from the APL cells stimulates intravascular coagulation. Therefore, monitor coagulation profile frequently. Occasionally low dose heparin therapy is necessary for treatment.

Non-Hodgkins lymphoma (NHL)

This is due to a malignant proliferation of cells of the lymphocytic or histiocytic lineage (Table V):

Table V: Classification of NHL

Subtype	Cell type	Usual site
Lymphoblastic lymphoma	Immature T–cell (occasionally pre–B)	• Anterior mediastinum most common • Cervical and axillary lymph nodes • Occasional abdomen ± bone marrow
Small noncleaved	B-cell (Burkitt's lymphoma)	• Abdomen: 90% ± bone marrow
Large cell (histiocytic)	Immunoblastic B, T, large cell–B, anaplastic large cell (Ki–1 positive) usually T	• Abdomen ± mediastinum skin, CNS, lymph node, testes, GI tract

1. Common signs and symptoms
• Lymphadenopathy.
• Mediastinal mass which may produce superior vena cava syndrome.
• Pleural effusion.
• Abdominal pain, obstruction, intussusception.

2. Diagnostic evaluation
• Full history and physical examination.
• CBC and differential, liver function tests (including LDH), renal function (BUN, creatinine, uric acid, electrolytes).
• Bone marrow aspirate and biopsy. Cytogenetics and immunophenotyping essential. If bone marrow contains > 25% lymphoma cells, it is classified as leukemia.
• Surgical biopsy of lymph node. Cytochemical, immunological, cytogenetic and molecular studies are essential.
• CSF: cell count and cytospin, molecular studies.
• Chest X–ray.
• CT scan of abdomen ± chest.
• Gallium scan (optional).
• Bone scan.

3. Treatment
- Acute and supportive care:
    Tumor lysis syndrome: prevent or treat with fluids and allopurinol.
    Superior vena cava syndrome or superior mediastinal syndrome: attempt to biopsy under local anesthetic if possible. If biopsy is not possible, treat patient with steroids ± radiotherapy and biopsy as soon as possible.
    Bowel obstruction or bleeding: surgical resection if necessary.
- Specific treatment:
    Chemotherapy:
    Chemotherapy is the mainstay of treatment. There are many treatment regimes and the type used depends on the type of NHL and whether or not the disease is localized (most are systemic or advanced at diagnosis).
    Most commonly used chemotherapy agents for NHL are: cyclophosphamide, vincristine, methotrexate, prednisone, adriamycin.
    Intrathecal chemotherapy: patients with nonlocalized disease are at risk for CNS involvement and, therefore, intrathecal chemotherapy is used prophylactically.
    Radiotherapy or radiation therapy: used for emergency treatment in life threatening situations, e.g. SVC syndrome or obstruction of other vital organs. May be used for cranial prophylaxis in high risk patients. Radiation therapy alone is not sufficient to cure NHL.

4. Surgery
Surgical biopsy is usually essential for diagnosis. Localized bowel disease may be completely resected but the patient will still require chemotherapy.

5. Prognosis
This depends on the type and stage but overall, approximately 70% event free survival.

Hodgkin's disease

    Characterized by progressive, often painless, enlargement of lymph nodes.

1. Common signs and symptoms
- Painless lymphadenopathy (cervical lymphadenopathy is most common), splenomegaly.
- Systemic or "B" symptoms: unexplained fever, night sweats, weight loss of 10% or more or failure to gain weight in young children.

2. Diagnostic evaluation
- Full history and physical examination (include "B" symptoms; check for signs of superior vena cava obstruction).
- CBC, ESR, coagulation profile.
- Liver function tests, LDH, renal function.
- Serum copper and ferritin (often elevated).
- Bone marrow aspirate and biopsy.
- Diagnostic surgical lymph node biopsy.
- Chest X–ray.
- Abdominal ultrasound.

- CT scan of chest, abdomen, neck.
- Gallium scan.
- Lymphangiogram (if suspicious of abdominal involvement).

3. Staging
- Stage I: 1 lymph node region positive.
- Stage II: 2 or more lymph node regions on the same side of the diaphragm.
- Stage III: lymph node regions on both sides of the diaphragm.
- Stage IV: involvement of extra lymphatic organs.
- Patients are also classified into "A" (no systemic symptoms) and "B" (systemic symptoms).

4. Treatment
- Acute management: airway obstruction or superior vena cava syndrome.
    May need intubation or tracheostomy.
    May need emergency radiotherapy.
- Specific therapy: treatment depends on staging.
    Radiotherapy:
    May be used alone in stages IA and IIA. Radiotherapy should be avoided in very young children because of its affect on growth; chemotherapy should be used instead.
    Chemotherapy:
    May be used for all stages of disease; always used in advanced stage IIB, III, and IV.
    Most commonly used chemotherapy combinations are: MOPP (nitrogen mustard, vincristine, prednisone, procarbazine), ABVD (adriamycin, bleomycin, vinblastine, DTIC), COPP (cyclophosphamide, vincristine, prednisone, procarbazine) and MOPP/ABV ("Vancouver hybrid").

5. Prognosis
Factors associated with a good prognosis: young age, female sex, absence of systemic symptoms, stage I or II disease; lymphocytic predominant subtype. Overall survival is approximately 75%.

Brain tumors

Brain tumors are the most common "solid tumors" in children.

1. Classification
- Supratentorial: astrocytoma, glioblastoma multiforme, ependymoma, primitive neuroectodermal tumor (PNET).
- Midline (sella or chiasm): optic glioma, craniopharyngioma, pituitary adenoma, germ cell tumor.
- Infratentorial:
    Posterior fossa: medulloblastoma/PNET, astrocytoma, ependymoma.
    Brain stem: astrocytoma, glioma, ependymoma.

2. Signs and symptoms
- Headache and irritability.
- Vomiting.
- Impaired vision (sixth nerve palsy, papilledema).

- Cranial enlargement (in infants).
- Seizures.
- Mental disturbances (somnolence, irritability, personality change).
- Disturbance of balance and gait.
- Endocrine abnormalities.
- Diencephalic syndrome.

3. Diagnostic evaluation
- Full history and physical examination, including detailed neurological and developmental examination.
- CT or MR scan.

4. Treatment
- Surgery: important for diagnosis, resection of tumor and CSF shunts.
- Radiotherapy: most patients with malignant brain tumors require radiotherapy.
  Radiotherapy can cause intellectual and physical impairment which is most severe in younger children. Therefore, whenever possible, radiotherapy is avoided or delayed in children < 3 years of age.
- Chemotherapy: now being used in an adjuvant setting for many brain tumors. The use of chemotherapy has improved survival for medulloblastoma.
  Most commonly used drugs: CCNU, vincristine, prednisone, cis platinum.

5. Prognosis
Depends on type and location of tumor, extent of surgical resection, and age of patient. Overall disease free survival is approximately 50%.

Wilm's tumor

This is a congenital embryonal renal cell tumor.

1. Common signs and symptoms
- Visible abdominal mass (pain is unusual).
- Hematuria.
- Hypertension.

2. Diagnostic evaluation
- Full history and physical examination:
    Look for associated abnormalities (aniridia, hemihypertrophy, genitourinary abnormality, musculoskeletal abnormalities); check blood pressure.
- CBC, BUN, creatinine, electrolytes, liver function tests.
- Coagulation screen (may have acquired von Willebrand's disease).
- Abdominal and chest CT scan.
- Echocardiogram (before adriamycin treatment and for tumors extending into the IVC).

3. Staging
- Stage 1: limited to the kidney and completely excised.

- Stage II: extending beyond the kidney but excised.
- Stage III: residual tumor in abdomen.
- Stage IV: hematogenous metastases; most commonly to lungs and liver.
- Stage V: bilateral renal involvement at diagnosis.

4. Treatment
- Surgery: nephrectomy and removal of tumor usually performed at presentation.
- Radiotherapy: for stages III and IV disease.
- Chemotherapy: all patients require chemotherapy. This has significantly improved the survival from Wilm's tumor.
  Most commonly used drugs: vincristine, actinomycin–D, adriamycin.

5. Prognosis
Overall, approximately 90% disease free survival.

Neuroblastoma

Neuroblastoma is a tumor of the sympathetic nervous system.

1. Common signs and symptoms
- Systemic symptoms: lethargy, anorexia, pallor, weight loss, irritability.
- Bone pain: due to bony metastases.
- Abdominal mass and pain: orbital metastases "racoon eyes".
- Horner's syndrome: spinal cord compression.
- Signs of excess catecholamine secretion: hypertension, flushing and diarrhea.
- Subcutaneous nodules.

2. Staging
Several systems are used, but in general, they may be divided into:
- Localized disease: stage I, stage II.
- Generalized disease: stage III, stage IV.

3. Diagnostic evaluation
- History and physical.
- CBC, differential, BUN, creatinine, liver function tests.
- Ferritin (may be important for prognosis).
- Bone marrow aspirate and biopsy.
- Biopsy of lymph node or mass (measurement of n–myc antigen important).
- CT scan of abdomen.
- Chest X–ray.
- MIBG scan or bone scan.
- 24 hour urine collection for VMA and HVA.
- Echocardiogram pretreatment.

4. Treatment and prognosis
- Stages I and II: surgery alone is often sufficient. Stage II patients may need chemotherapy.

Survival is 70–90%.

- Stages III and IV: surgical resection, chemotherapy, and radiation therapy used in combination. Autologous bone marrow transplant may be used for stage IV disease. Commonly used drugs are cis platinum, VP–16, adriamycin and cyclophosphamide. Survival: stage III, 30%; stage IV, 10%.

Bone tumors

1. Osteosarcoma

This is a malignant osteoid producing tumor which most often occurs during the adolescent growth spurt. It arises most commonly in the metaphysis of a long bone.

- Signs and symptoms:
    Pain, swelling, pathological fracture.
    There is often a history of preceding mild trauma, which is usually blamed for symptoms initially.
- Diagnostic evaluation:
    History and physical examination.
    CBC, BUN, creatinine, liver function tests (include alkaline phosphatase).
    X–ray of involved site.
    MR scan of site.
    Chest X–ray, chest CT scan, bone scan.
    Needle or open biopsy of site after MR scan.
    Prechemotherapy GFR, audiogram, echocardiogram.
    Usual site of metastases: lung and bones.
- Treatment:
    Resection of tumor is essential. This may be achieved by amputation or limb salvage surgery.
    Chemotherapy should be used: neoadjuvant drugs to shrink primary tumor and treat micrometastases; then adjuvant drugs postoperatively to treat micrometastases and residual disease. Use of chemotherapy has significantly improved survival. Commonly used drugs are high dose methotrexate, cis platinum and doxorubicin.
    Radiotherapy: osteogenic sarcoma is not radiosensitive, so radiotherapy is not used.
- Prognosis: for nonmetastatic disease, event free survival is 55–80%.

2. Ewing's sarcoma

This is a small, round cell sarcoma of bone. It may arise in any bone; most commonly arises in the diaphysis.

- Signs and symptoms: pain, swelling, fever.
- Diagnostic evaluation:
    History and physical examination.
    CBC, differential, BUN, creatinine, liver function tests (include alkaline phosphatase and LDH).
    Bone marrow aspirate and biopsy.
    X–ray of involved site.
    MR scan of involved site.
    CT chest.

Bone scan.
Prechemotherapy echocardiogram.
Sites of metastases: lung, bone, and bone marrow.
- Treatment:
  Surgical resection may be used for the primary lesion if resection can be achieved without major functional deficit, or in young children when radiotherapy would result in major growth impairment.
  Radiotherapy: Ewing's sarcoma is radiosensitive, so irradiation of the primary tumor (dose up to 5,500 cGy) is often used to achieve local control.
  Chemotherapy: the use of adjuvant chemotherapy has resulted in a major improvement in survival. Commonly used drugs are vincristine, cyclophosphamide, doxorubicin, VP–16, actinomycin–D and ifosfamide.
- Prognosis: for localized tumors, 60–75% event free survival.

3. Rhabdomyosarcoma and other soft tissue sarcomas

Rhabdomyosarcoma is the most common soft tissue sarcoma of childhood and comprises approximately 50% of all soft tissue sarcomas (Table VI).

Table VI: Cellular origin of soft tissue sarcomas

Soft tissue sarcoma	Cell of origin
Rhabdomyosarcoma	Embryonic mesenchyme that gives rise to skeletal muscle
Fibrosarcoma	Fibroblasts
Neurofibrosarcoma	Schwann cell
Synovial sarcoma	Mesenchyme
Malignant fibrous histiocytoma	Fibroblast

- Most commonly involved sites:
  Head and neck: 40%
  Genitourinary tract: 20%
  Extremities: 20%
  Other sites: 20%.
- Signs and symptoms:
  Visible mass.
  Facial pain, nasopharyngeal obstruction, cranial nerve palsies.
  Genitourinary tract, vaginal bleeding, urinary obstruction, constipation.
- Diagnostic evaluation:
  History and physical examination.
  CBC, electrolytes, BUN, creatinine, liver function tests.
  CT or MR of primary lesion.
  Bone scan.
  Bone marrow aspirate and biopsy.
  Biopsy of mass after MR scan.

Sites of metastases: lymph nodes, lungs, and bone marrow.
- Treatment:
  Surgery: surgical biopsy is usually essential. The tumor should be surgically resected if possible.
  Radiotherapy: rhabdomyosarcoma is radiosensitive and radiotherapy is important for primary tumor control if surgical resection is not possible.
  Chemotherapy: all patients require adjuvant chemotherapy; this has resulted in a significant improvement in survival. Commonly used drugs are cyclophosphamide, actinomycin–D, vincristine, adriamycin, ifosfamide, VP–16.
- Prognosis:
  Localized disease, 70–85% event free survival.
  Nonlocalized disease, 50–70% event free survival.

LATE EFFECTS OF CHILDHOOD CANCER AND ITS TREATMENT

The study of late effects of childhood cancer is still in its infancy as the majority of survivors are under 20 years of age and almost all are under 40. So there is still a lot to learn.

Late effects are caused by:
- The cancer which causes destruction and damage to adjacent tissues.
- The treatment:
  Chemotherapy:
  Cells with a high turnover may have serious acute side effects but these are often reversible. Cells with a low turnover are quite resistant to chemotherapy but once damaged have poor repair mechanisms and may suffer long–term effects, e.g. brain.
  Radiotherapy:
  Most of the effects of radiotherapy are chronic and delayed.
  Surgery:
  May be mutilating or result in loss or damage to organs.
  Immune modulation:
  Can cause graft versus host disease or lymphoproliferative states.
  Maturation agents:
  Late effects not yet known.
- Psychosocial factors: survivors of cancer may be treated differently by society and their expectations of themselves may be less, resulting in difficulty obtaining employment, poor self–esteem, etc.

A full discussion of the late effects of childhood malignancy is beyond the scope of this chapter but the following is a list of the most commonly encountered side effects:
- Impairment of growth.
- Musculoskeletal problems.
- Impairment of neuropsychological and neurological function.
- Impairment of gonadal function.
- Endocrine abnormalities.
- Cardiac abnormalities from anthracycline therapy.
- Second malignancy.

- Respiratory damage.

Ongoing surveillance of survivors of childhood malignancy is essential for:
- Recognition of delayed problems.
- Practical help for the patients.
- So that we may recognize the problems and improve upon our therapy in the future.

INTERFACILITY TRANSPORT

Advances in technology and the delivery of medical care for critically ill neonates and children have resulted in reduced morbidity and mortality and necessitated the development of regionalized neonatal and pediatric intensive care units. Regionalization and rationalization of specialized services have resulted in the need for transfer of the growing number of patients from the institutions where they first received care to these specialised units. Increasingly, this interfacility transfer of patients is managed by transport teams because of the recognition that critically ill and injured children can be extremely vulnerable during interhospital transfers. Transport programs vary considerably, depending on local geography, logistics, and population. However, the priorities for transport teams in different locations are often similar and standard of care has been established to enable the majority of these infants and children to be transported without harm from the inherent risks of the transport process itself.

The safe transport of a child is complicated and requires good communication between the referring and receiving physicians. Stabilization at the referring hospital is important so that the condition of the patient remains as stable as possible during the transfer and no preventable deterioration occurs. Each transport should be coordinated by a transport team director who is experienced in all aspects of transport and responsible for all major decisions regarding interfacility transport.

For continuity of care and safe transfer between one hospital and another, a clear cut sequence of events must occur. Any resident who is contacted regarding a transfer should take the name and telephone number of the referring physician and a brief outline of the patient's problem and then contact the transport coordinator on–call either in the Intensive Care Unit (ICU) for pediatric transports or in the Special Care Nursery (SCN) for neonates.

CRITERIA FOR SAFE TRANSPORT

The criteria for safe transport are:
- Resuscitation.
- Communication.
- Stabilization.
- Appropriate team and escort selection.
- Uneventful transfer.

Resuscitation

For any seriously ill or injured patient, immediate resuscitation and ongoing stabilization are priorities. Individual requirements clearly depend on the nature of the emergency and the systems involved (see appropriate sections).

Communication

The purpose of communication is:
- To provide advice for the initial resuscitation and the beginning of a stabilization process.
- To confirm the necessity for transfer and establish the urgency.
- To enable the receiving physician to select the appropriate personnel, equipment, medication, and priority for the transport.
- To allow notification of the appropriate dispatch team, choice of appropriate vehicles, aircraft, and transport team personnel, and arrangement of journey logistics.
- To ensure that all relevant documentation is ready to accompany the child, along with radiographs, relevant samples, and signed consent forms.

Transport coordinators should be responsible for supervising all interhospital transfers for acutely ill children and neonates. They should also remain available to advise regarding ongoing resuscitation needs and treatment prior to the actual transfer and enroute management of the patient by the transport team. This coordination provides an important measure of safety and continuity and is intended to minimize the inherent risks facing any child needing emergency transport. Continuity of care is important, with most transports taking 4–6 hours to complete and some taking up to 12 hours. Significant clinical changes can occur, requiring reformulation of the care plan.

In making a decision during such a call, the referring and receiving physicians have to decide whether or not the child can receive adequate care at the outlying hospital or whether (s)he should be transported elsewhere. If transport is required, it is important that the transfer is to the closest appropriate hospital. A significant percentage of these calls result in a joint decision to continue managing the child in the outlying hospital.

Stabilization

The key point for safe transport is optimal stabilization of the child prior to leaving the referring hospital. There was a tendency for referring physicians to feel that the sooner a problem was off their territory, the better it was for all concerned. However, this often resulted in hasty transfer of unstable patients who deteriorated enroute or were moribund on arrival. There is no place for truncated handover of an unstable patient in the back of an ambulance on an airport runway. Do not allow an air of anxiety in the referring hospital on arrival of the team to intimidate you into a "scoop and run" situation with the patient. It is important to perform an appropriate history and physical examination, followed by every attempt to stabilize the child prior to departure. Outreach education programs have improved the awareness in outlying hospitals of the importance of stabilization and now transport teams are generally well received. It is common for at least an hour to go by between the arrival of the team and departure from the referring hospital.

This stabilization process should include a thorough review of the history, clinical state of the patient and all laboratory data. There should also be an assessment of which treatment entities suggested by the transport coordinator have been completed successfully and which are outstanding.

Stabilization should concentrate on ensuring that the ABC's can be attended to reliably throughout transport, identifying any potential cause of deterioration or system failure that can be anticipated and acting to minimize or prevent it. Great attention should be paid to oxygen delivery, i.v. access, security of all tubes (ET, i.v., nasogastric, chest, catheters) and treatment to correct all abnormal physiological parameters.

A discussion with the transport coordinator prior to departure will often be beneficial to reassess the diagnosis, the needs of the patient and the clinical and logistic plan for transfer. It is essential for safe transfer that everything is done correctly prior to leaving the relative security of the referring hospital for the unfriendly environment of an aircraft or ambulance.

Appropriate escort team

An uneventful transfer is primarily achieved by a combination of comprehensive stabilization and the use of trained transport personnel who are familiar with the transport environment, particularly the limited space, suboptimal lighting, high background noise, and adverse environmental aspects of many of the transport vehicles. Where aircraft are involved, it is important that the effects of altitude on oxygenation and the volume of trapped gases is understood. In a recent study, the morbidity of transported patients who were seriously ill or injured was shown to decrease five–fold when trained transport personnel were used. The appropriate team is selected by the transport coordinator and usually consists of a mix of specially trained ambulance paramedics or nurses, plus a pediatric fellow or senior resident for more complex calls. Acute neonatal transfers tend to require a higher proportion of physician escorts than pediatric transports. Where assisted ventilation is required, a respiratory therapist can be included to assist with clinical management and the technical aspects of ventilation.

The team should work under the direct supervision of the transport coordinator. Physicians in the referring hospitals, who are unfamiliar with pediatric transports, may be uncertain as to the team's level of training and clinical skills. However, most programs establish a sound reputation through outreach education.

Monitoring equipment is now considered obligatory for transport because of the noise levels in aircraft and the difficulty of clinical examination. It is difficult to auscultate the chest reliably, detect an air leak around an endotracheal tube or listen to heart sounds accurately. The level of lighting is also such that cyanosis or pallor may have to be extreme before it can be recognized by eye. This limitation of physical examination is compensated for by current monitoring equipment which is sophisticated and includes capabilities for following heart rate, ECG, respiratory rate, core and skin temperature, invasive and noninvasive blood pressure, oxygen saturation, and trans-cutaneous PO_2 and transcutaneous CO_2. Familiarity with the operation of this equipment is important for escort team members.

The transport environment depends on the vehicles used. For shorter distances, ground ambulances are used; for longer transports, helicopters or fixed wing aircraft are used. Each vehicle or aircraft has its own characteristics in terms of speed, space, access restrictions, and potential for stress from noise, vibration and gravitational forces. The majority are equipped with mains power (110 volts), oxygen and suction. The aircraft used, like all other equipment supplied for the team, should be kept as consistent as possible.

The transport coordinator and central dispatch organization are responsible for coordinating the air, water, and land links of each transport and will jointly decide the priority of the call, personnel and equipment needed.

Priority assignment is made according to agreed guidelines. A typical system is:
- Priority 1 red: condition is such that any delay would be a serious threat to life or limb.

- Priority 1 green: patient's condition is serious but stable, but the priority 2 (12 hour response) is too long.
- Priority 2: condition is such that the patient should be transferred within 12 hours.
- Priority 3: the patient's condition is stable and does not require specialized treatment or a higher level of care urgently. This priority is usually used for return transports.

Not infrequently, more than one transport will be in progress at any given time. For this reason, the transport coordinator must assign a priority to each call based on his or her discussions with the referring physician. The type of vehicle chosen and the team sent is based on this medical information and the priorities set. Cost effectiveness must also be a consideration, particularly for less urgent transports. Whatever the vehicle, journey time is often variable. Factors such as weather, temperature, darkness, distance and team availability are additional variables.

Communication post–transport should include a phone call to the referring hospital to notify them of safe arrival and to confirm the location of the patient at the hospital. The family should be provided with a telephone number for inquiries about their child if this has not been provided already. Communication is a two way process and the referring physician should be encouraged to keep in contact with his or her patient's progress. Any medical or logistic problems encountered during transport should be reported to the appropriate transport coordinator. Infrequent users are particularly glad to have feedback which may improve their use of the transport service on future occasions. Data should be reviewed from each transport for quality assurance purposes.

TRANSPORT PHYSIOLOGY

During transport, a sick child is exposed to many significant physiological stresses, particularly when air travel is involved. With a progressive rise in altitude, there is a corresponding decrease in atmospheric pressure and partial pressure, and hence, reduced availability of oxygen. If these changes are not anticipated, severe effects on oxygenation and other vital functions result. The child's condition is also likely to deteriorate because of the adverse effects of noise, vibration and temperature. It is important for these effects to be considered when planning the child's needs enroute prior to transport. To do this effectively, an understanding of altitude, physiology and the physical effects of transport is necessary.

Aviation physiology

Altitude causes a number of physical effects which must be understood for transport to be achieved safely.

- Temperature decreases by 1 °C for each 1,000 feet increase in altitude.
- Water vapor decreases.
- Atmospheric turbulence decreases.
- Atmospheric pressure decreases.

Three laws of physics are relevant.

1. Dalton's law
As the atmospheric pressure decreases with altitude, there is a reduction in the available oxygen

partial pressure. The fraction of oxygen (FiO_2) remains constant with altitude but the partial pressure of oxygen falls as atmospheric pressure falls. Consequently, if oxygen is not administered, hypoxia will result as altitude increases. Supplemental oxygen is obviously necessary in any patient without normal oxygen exchange or carrying capacity. Generally speaking, the oxygen requirements of any patient transported will increase, and if oxygenation cannot be improved by an increase in FiO_2, intubation and assisted ventilation should be considered prior to transport.

2. Boyle's law
As atmospheric pressure decreases with altitude, the volume of any gas contained in a closed space will expand. This effect is called dysbarism and the increased volume can be detrimental to respiration (pneumothorax), CNS function (intracranial air) or bowel perfusion (ileus); all cause considerable pain. Clearly, a pneumothorax must be drained prior to flight for this reason, and a nasogastric tube will prevent gastric dilatation.

3. Newton's law
The law relates to the movement and/or stresses caused by acceleration and deceleration. A body at rest tends to remain at rest while a body in movement tends to remain in movement, hence, the need to position patients appropriately and secure all equipment.

Altitude restrictions

Altitude restrictions may be required by your patient's medical condition, and you may be asked to recommend cabin altitude limits. This decision should be based on the patient's condition, primarily the ability to oxygenate and the presence of trapped air. If in doubt, discuss the problem with the transport coordinator. The most extreme needs for low altitude result from gas entrapment in areas which cannot be drained, such as the brain and eye, and decompression sickness. Generally speaking, if the patient can be adequately oxygenated at the referring hospital, (s)he is safe to fly at cabin pressures equal to the altitude of the referring hospital. Remember that many referring hospitals are considerably above sea level. Pressurization to excessively low altitude is often unnecessary, costly in terms of fuel, and may also restrict the operating capabilities of the aircraft.

Pressurization

The main purpose of pressurization is to enable aircraft to fly at higher altitudes while maintaining an environment that is compatible with crew comfort. There is less turbulence at altitude and the aircraft is more fuel efficient. The pressurization process decreases the humidity within the aircraft. In the event of acute decompression, there is an immediate need for supplemental oxygen.

Temperature

The temperature in aircraft and vehicles is often suboptimal. Ambulances are usually insulated and have heaters and, where possible, should be warm prior to loading a patient. Neonates are particularly susceptible to cold stress. With aircraft, request the pilot to run the engine on the opposite side of the aircraft to the door and to begin warming the aircraft prior to loading. Use simple measures like carrying additional blankets and appropriate equipment such as incubators for infants. Request additional environmental temperature from the driver or pilot if necessary. As aircraft altitude increases, the ambient temperature will fall.

Noise and vibration

Different vehicles and aircraft have different noise and vibration characteristics. Noise is stressful and can induce drowsiness, increase anxiety and make auscultation difficult. The use of ear plugs is recommended for long journeys and if noise coupled with turbulence and vibration cause motion sickness, either disqualify yourself from flying if this is a repeated problem or consider antiemetics. All equipment must be safely secured because of the risk of sudden turbulence. Seat belts should be worn.

PATIENT PREPARATION FOR ALTITUDE

Because of the aircraft environment, the clinical effects of altitude may be difficult to see and hear. This means monitoring equipment is essential to detect changes in respiratory pattern, oxygen saturation, heart rate and blood pressure. Because hypoxia and hypocarbia are the commonest causes of cardiac arrest in childhood, a major preoccupation during stabilization is an assessment of the child's oxygen requirements and the provision of measures to secure the airway and provide adequate respiration. In a child with a major respiratory problem, illness or multiple trauma, it is generally safer to intubate and initiate assisted ventilation prior to transfer rather than risk abrupt deterioration and respiratory arrest secondary to transport stress enroute.

All access lines for intravenous fluid resuscitation must be in place prior to the journey and adequate preload and circulatory support be provided prior to leaving. Insertion of nasogastric tubes and urinary catheters is also much simpler in the referring hospital environment. Specific care of cuffed endotracheal tubes and catheters, e.g. Foley catheters which have balloons, includes the filling of these reservoirs with saline rather than air. Unlike air, the saline will not expand. This reduces the risk of rupturing the catheter balloon or pressure necrosis from an ET tube cuff. Other specific equipment needs include the use of collapsible plastic (viaflex) i.v. packs rather than glass bottles and the avoidance of limb splints that inflate or free traction weights. The latter are unstable and the former can cause ischemia at altitude. A Thomas splint is preferable. Heimlich valves should be used on chest tube drains. These one way valves are as effective as an underwater seal and safer during flight. They should be carefully taped to the chest wall.

Endotrachel tube suctioning will likely be required on most transfers. Moisten the suction catheter with saline. Humidification of gases in transit is rarely optimal and dry suction catheters can stick to the wall of the tube and cause accidental extubation. Nasogastric tubes are obligatory for sick patients in transit. They reduce the risk of vomiting and gastric distension. In basal skull fractures, they should be passed through the mouth rather than the nose. Acute gastric dilatation is a common cause of respiratory difficulty in the pediatric age group. A rubber glove attached to a nasogastric tube with a strong rubber band can collect gastric contents enroute. These tubes should not be clamped.

Gravity feed for intravenous fluids is unreliable in the confined space of most transport vehicles, particularly at altitude. Infusion pumps are desirable. If not available, frequent monitoring of intravenous rate is essential. It should be checked particularly carefully after takeoff and landing. All monitoring equipment should be positioned so as to be visible and spare batteries should be carried.

Space limitation

Loading patients in and out of vehicles and aircraft is a period of risk. It is easy for lines, tubes and monitoring equipment to be dislodged. An unstable patient may be subjected to anxiety, pain or stress at these times. Help the personnel with the most expertise to load and secure the patient and equipment. Position the patient in the aircraft where noise is minimal, and lighting and access are optimal. Position yourself where you have best access to the patient. The placement of the patient in the aircraft significantly affects fluid shifts in the body. These effects become most pronounced during takeoff and landing and can also be affected by turbulence. Choose a head to the front of aircraft position for patients requiring positive G–forces, e.g. for head injury, cardiac failure, fluid overload. Use a head to the rear position (negative G–forces) for hypovolemia, spinal shock, and cardiac ischemia. Anticipate some degree of deterioration during the initial acceleration, in early takeoff and during deceleration after landing.

Parents and transport

Parents prefer to travel with their children wherever possible, although most admit this is a difficult and distressing experience. However, the alternatives of setting out to book a scheduled flight or travel long distances by car when the child is enroute by air ambulance and critically ill are even less desirable. Every effort should be made to bring a parent on the transport wherever space constraints in the vehicle and aircraft allow. When it is not possible, the reasons should be explained to parents. On some occasions, more than one patient has to be transported in the transport vehicle; on others, the number of individuals in the transport team may leave no room for the parents to travel as well.

On every transport, the team should make time to speak with the parents before leaving the referring hospital and allow them to see their child. This is a crucial part in the transfer of care responsibilities from one hospital team to another. They should explain what has been done so far, what the transport journey entails and what the tentative care plan for the child involves at the receiving hospital. Parents should be encouraged to telephone for a progress report. When parents arrive, they should be assisted to find temporary accommodation. Usually this can be arranged through the Social Services Department. It may be helpful for the department's telephone number to be given to them at the referring hospital prior to departure. When a child is a patient on one of the regular wards, parents can often stay at the bedside with their child.

Responsibility of physician escort

When a physician is sent with a transport team, this individual has the overall responsibility for patient care decisions. It is important to recognize, however, that the paramedics have considerable experience in the transport environment and are likely to have valuable advice to give regarding many of the logistic decisions. Similarly, the pediatrician of the referring hospital knows the patient better than the transport physician at the time of transfer and effective dialogue is essential to obtain all key elements of the history and care plan and to initiate any additional treatment which is thought necessary. The team physician must also keep in contact with the transport coordinator to provide information about the patient status and to obtain help and support when decisions are difficult or a difference of opinion occurs with the referring physician. Careful records should be kept throughout transport. A comprehensive handover of the patient should occur on arrival at the receiving hospital, and a full note must be written in the hospital chart.

Working in the transport environment does not suit every physician. However, the experience provides valuable opportunities for the physician in training to manage seriously ill infants and children in a way that is closer to the real world of pediatric practice.

Fitness to travel is an important consideration. Upper respiratory tract infection may lead to severe ear or sinus pain. Sedative drugs and alcohol can impair your performance in the transport environment. These should be avoided when on–call for transport.

Clothing should be warm and functional. White coats are not required and their lengths make them unsuitable for rapid access to vehicles. Sixty percent of transports occur out of regular working hours and subzero temperatures occur so it is necessary to dress accordingly. Escorts of either sex should avoid wearing jewelry on clothing which may catch in vehicle equipment.

Equipment

All the basic equipment required for transport should be carried by the team. This must include a full complement of items for airway breathing and circulation support plus miscellaneous equipment, instruments and relevant monitors. Drugs taken are the responsibility of the medical escort and, if special needs are considered, likely these drugs should be drawn from the nurse in charge of the unit coordinating the transport prior to departure. Such drugs might include anticonvulsants, pancuronium, intubation agents, prostaglandin or inotropes.

Aircraft safety

It is important to obey the pilot at all times. If in doubt about any action, check with the pilot. Use your seat belt and secure the patient and all medical equipment carefully. Where indicated, wear your life jacket. Approach all aircraft with care and preferably within view of the pilot. Avoid the engines as exhaust temperatures may be in excess of 600 °F. With helicopters, never go near the tail rotors which are invisible when in motion and anticipate dipping of the main rotor while this is running, particularly when there is a significant wind or when the engine is slowing. It is best to crouch when approaching or leaving a helicopter. Keep clear of flight controls. Keep nonessential conversation to a minimum and, during night operation, avoid exposing the pilot to excess light.

Aircraft emergencies

In the event of sudden decompression, tend to your own oxygen supply first. You have only 15–30 seconds of useful consciousness at 35,000 feet within which to establish your own supplemental oxygen supply. Anticipate a sudden drop in temperature and an increase in condensation within the aircraft. Clamp i.v.'s to avoid rapid infusion rates caused by changing pressures. In the event of impending crash landing, secure yourself tightly; secure the patient optimally and immobilize all equipment. Remove items, such as splints, drug boxes and monitors that may hinder evacuation. Tape scissors onto the stretcher straps for ready access to help extract the patient. If a bulk head is available, lean against it; if not, lean forward and lock your arms under your legs. Once on the ground, exit promptly with the patient to a safe location. If safe to do so, return to the aircraft to remove survival equipment. Then remain in the vicinity of the aircraft for optimal chances of rescue. Remember the advantage of learning basic outdoor survival skills in advance.

Prior to undertaking transport duty, all team members should receive orientation to the vehicles and aircraft used, especially regarding their safety features and evacuation routes.

PEDIATRIC PHARMACOLOGY

The fate of a drug within the body is governed by the pharmacokinetic parameters of absorption, distribution, metabolism and excretion.

Each of these variables changes with age, making rational drug therapy a continual challenge. It is vital to consider drug toxicity, side effects, pharmacokinetics, indications and interactions, and many other variables before giving any medicine to a child. There is no shortage of examples of serious side effects (chloramphenicol, sulfonamide, oxygen toxicity) to illustrate the results of thoughtless "routine" prescribing.

Absorption

Gastric emptying time, intestinal motility, intestinal blood flow and gastric acidity are all poorly developed in infancy. Consequently, enteral absorption is unpredictable and generally slower than it is in adults. Phenytoin and phenobarbital are both absorbed very poorly in children but acid labile drugs may be absorbed better in children than adults.

Topical absorption is much greater in children, especially neonates. Systemic poisoning has been reported after topical application of lindane, hexachlorophene, boric acid and steroid creams.

Distribution

Total body water, especially extracellular water, decreases with age so the loading dose of a water soluble drug like an aminoglycoside will result in a lower peak level in small infants.

Body fat increases with age which affects the fate and toxicity of markedly lipophilic drugs like diazepam and thiopental. Protein binding is decreased in infants due to relative hypoalbuminemia and the lower binding capacity of fetal albumin. Toxicity is possible from increased unbound drug levels. Drug displacement also occurs more easily. Bilirubin displacement by sulfonamides is a classical example.

Metabolism

Neonatal hepatic function is immature. Drugs which are oxidized, like lidocaine, phenobarbital, phenytoin and diazepam, or those undergoing glucuronidation such as chloramphenicol, show prolonged half–lives with increased potential for toxicity. Drugs that are demethylated or sulfated are metabolized normally.

By 1–3 years of age, hepatic function, particularly the oxidase system, is so active that children require higher doses per m^2 of anticonvulsants and theophylline than adults.

Excretion

Renal function is not completely developed in the newborn. Glomerular filtration rate (GFR), renal plasma flow and tubular function reach adult values at about 9–12 months of age. Water soluble drugs like digoxin, penicillin and cephalosporins all show prolonged half–lives in infancy. The maturation of renal and hepatic function occurs so rapidly that dosage increases may be necessary in many drugs, even by the second week of life. Maturation of some pharmacokinetic variables with age are listed in Table I.

Table I: Variation of pharmacokinetic variables with age

Variable	Premature	Newborn	1 year	Adults
Gastric acid (mEq/kg per h)	–	0.015	–	0.2
Gastric emptying (min)	–	87	–	65
Total body water	87	79	67	60
ECF	62	45	27	20
Body fat (% body weight)	3	12	23	12–25
Total serum protein	5.9	6.0	6.4	7.2
Serum albumin (g %)	3.7	4.5	4.9	4.9
GFR (mL/min per m^2)	5	15	50	70

PEDIATRIC DOSING

Most common drugs have a recommended pediatric dosage, usually in mg/kg. Occasionally, however, a child may need a drug for which only an adult dose is available. The simplest conversion is to use the child's weight.

$$\text{Pediatric dose} = \frac{\text{child's weight (kg)}}{70 \text{ kg}} \times \text{adult dose}$$

The child's surface area (SA) is a much better standard since it correlates with several physiological variables like cardiac output, liver and renal blood flow, GFR and body water.

$$\text{Pediatric dose} = \frac{\text{SA of child (m}^2)}{1.7} \times \text{adult dose}$$

Boyd's nomogram (see chapter 24, Appendix) allows surface area to be calculated knowing height and weight. In the absence of a chart, use the following formula:

$$\text{Surface area (m}^2) = \frac{4 \times \text{weight (kg)} + 7}{90 + \text{weight (kg)}}$$

Percentage methods are not valid below 3 months of age. When using new drugs in this age group, with only an adult dose as guidance, great personal bravery is required. When using doses in mg/kg in older chidren, care is necessary not to exceed the stated adult dose. Obese children are also in danger of being overdosed. A reasonable rule of thumb is to give 75% of the calculated dose.

SERUM DRUG LEVELS

Serum levels of many drugs may be measured reliably on < 0.5 mL of blood. However, unless the basic principles of half–life, drug distribution and steady state are appreciated, the results may be seriously misleading.

Pharmacokinetics

Many water soluble drugs like aminoglycosides follow a single compartment model. They distribute rapidly and are excreted predictably. Serum half–life is easily calculated from the log concentration versus time graph. Other drugs like digoxin and salicylates follow a two compartment model with an initial distribution phase followed by elimination.

The dosing interval is usually about one half–life. It takes five half–lives to reach steady state where input equals output. Serum levels oscillate between peak and trough levels within each interval unless a constant infusion is given. In practice, three half–lives are used before serum levels are meaningful. This represents 88% of the steady state value.

Indications for therapeutic drug monitoring

• Close monitoring of potentially toxic drugs like gentamicin and chloramphenicol.
• Drug toxicity or poisoning.
• Drug interactions (particularly among anticonvulsants).
• Drug use in renal or hepatic disease.
• Absent therapeutic response.

Sampling time

Drugs with a long half–life have small fluctuations in serum level so a predose trough sample is sufficient. This also avoids the complication of absorption and distribution phases. All anti–convulsants fall in this category.

Peak and trough levels are taken in toxic drugs having a short half–life. Antibiotics distribute rapidly so levels are taken 30–60 minutes after infusion. Digoxin (8 hours) and ASA (4 hours) have long distribution times. Serum levels taken during this period are falsely elevated since the drug has not equilibrated with tissues.

Pitfalls

Time the blood samples to avoid distribution phases, especially with digoxin and ASA. Do not take samples through the infusion line. Take half–life into account when measuring levels after a dose change. It takes 10 days for phenobarbital to reach steady state. Levels before this are falsely low. Therapeutic range applies to most people but exceptions occur, especially sensitivity to low serum levels. Serum levels do not necessarily reflect tissue levels. Serum to tissue ratios of digoxin vary from 1:5 to 1:50. Treat the patient and not just the drug level.

THERAPEUTIC SERUM CONCENTRATIONS AND SAMPLING GUIDELINES

Drug	Usual sample time	Therapeutic serum concentration	Physician's routine inpatient orders	Comments
Amikacin	Predose: 0–30 min prior to next dose	2.5–10 mg/L	*Initial*: predose and postdose with third regular dose	• Half-life (t½) will be prolonged in patients with renal dysfunction
	Postdose: 30 min after end of infusion	20–35 mg/L	*Maintenance*: predose and postdose once weekly	
Carbamazepine (Tegretol)	Predose: 0–60 min prior to next dose	25–50 µmol/L	*Initial*: predose 3–7 d after final dosing alteration *Maintenance*: predose only if patient still has seizures; if toxicity is suspected, take sample at time of symptoms or 3 hours after the dose	• Enzyme autoinduction occurs so that t½ during chronic dosing may be much shorter than after first dose • Dose should be increased at 5–7 d intervals over a 4–6 wk period and the first serum level measured at 5 wk
Chloramphenicol	Postdose: 30 min after end of i.v. flush or 1 h and 2 h after p.o. administration	15–25 mg/L	*Initial*: postdose on day 2 of therapy *Maintenance*: postdose once weekly	• Pharmacokinetics in pediatric patients are highly variable and unpredictable • Clinical microbiologists will determine if therapeutic drug monitoring is necessary
Cyclosporine	Predose: 0–60 min prior to next dose Renal graft rejection: GVHD prophylaxis in bone marrow transplant Early phase: Maintenance phase:	25–100 µg/L 300–400 µg/L 200–300 µg/L	*Initial*: predose on day 2 of therapy *Maintenance*: predose 3 × weekly during early phase (first 3 weeks); twice weekly thereafter	• Monitoring is necessary to avoid extremely high or low levels which may precipitate nephrotoxicity or therapeutic failure, respectively

THERAPEUTIC SERUM CONCENTRATIONS AND SAMPLING GUIDELINES (cont.)

Drug	Usual sample time	Therapeutic serum concentration	Physician's routine inpatient orders	Comments
Digoxin	Predose: 0–60 min prior to next dose; must be at least 8 h postdose	1.3–2.7 nmol/L	Prelevels should be drawn only if risk factors are present; risk factors include: • suspicion of toxicity • renal or hepatic impairment • poor response • drug interactions • noncompliance • prematurity • hypokalemia	• The correlation between serum levels and therapeutic effect is not clearly defined • Digoxin serum levels are useful when toxicity is suspected • Digoxin therapy should be monitored by clinical effect rather than serum levels • Digoxin serum levels are meaningless after Digibind • Levels may be elevated in neonates due to endogenous digoxin–like substances (EDLS)
Ethosuximide (Zarontin)	Predose: 0–60 min prior to next dose	280–700 µmol/L	*Maintenance*: predose only if patient still has seizures; if toxicity is suspected, take sample at time of symptoms	• Some patients may tolerate and benefit from serum levels that are significantly higher than the recommended maximum level
Flucytosine (5–FC)	Postdose: 2 h postdose	30–70 mg/L	*Initial*: post on day 2 of therapy	
Gentamicin	Predose: 0–30 min prior to next dose	0.6–2 mg/L	*Initial*: predose and postdose with third dose *Maintenance*: predose once weekly in stable patients; predose and postdose as required in patients with unstable renal function	• No monitoring required for (patients with normal renal function): uncomplicated UTI's, surgery prophylaxis < 72 h, empiric therapy < 72 h • t½ will be prolonged in patients with renal impairment
	Postdose: 30 min after end of infusion	5-10 mg/L		

Drug	Usual sample time	Therapeutic serum concentration	Physician's routine inpatient orders	Comments
Methotrexate (MTX)	Dependent upon protocol; usually measured 24 h after the start of the infusion and every 24 h thereafter until levels fall below 10^{-7} mol/L	Not applicable	Dependent upon protocol	• With 4–6 h high dose MTX infusions, plasma levels > 50^{-5} mol/L at 24 h and > 10^{-6} mol/L at 48 h after start of the infusion are often predictive of delayed MTX clearance • Leucovorin therapy normally continues until MTX levels are less than 10^{-7} mol/L
Phenobarbital	Predose: 0–60 min prior to next dose	65–170 µmol/L	*Initial:* predose after 10–14 d, unless toxicity is suspected or patient still has seizures	• Some patients may tolerate and benefit with levels that are significantly higher than the recommended maximum limit
Phenytoin (Dilantin)	Predose: 0–60 min prior to next dose	40–80 µmol/L "free" phenytoin: 4–8 µmol/L	*Initial:* 1 h post–i.v. load; wait 7 d after each oral dosing change to measure prelevel; in acute management of seizures, where patient continues to seizure, measure serum levels (predose) 1 or 2 times daily *Maintenance:* predose only if patient still has seizures; if toxicity is suspected, take level at time of symptoms	• Phenytoin exhibits dose dependent pharmacokinetics: plasma drug concentration may change disproportionately with dosage changes • Phenytoin is highly protein bound • Free phenytoin levels may be useful in monitoring patients with chronic renal failure (hypoalbuminemia) or who are receiving drugs that displace phenytoin from protein (e.g. valproic acid) or in disease states that may displace phenytoin from plasma protein (e.g. hyperbilirubinemia)
Primidone (Mysoline)	Predose: 0–60 min prior to next dose	37–55 µmol/L	*Initial:* predose after 10–14 d, unless patient still has seizures; if toxicity is suspected, take level at time of symptoms	• Phenobarb is an active metabolite and is measured concurrently

THERAPEUTIC SERUM CONCENTRATIONS AND SAMPLING GUIDELINES (cont.)

Drug	Usual sample time	Therapeutic serum concentration	Physician's routine inpatient orders	Comments
Salicylate (ASA)	Predose: 0–60 min prior to next dose JRA: Kawasaki's disease, pericarditis:	1.1–2.2 mmol/L < 2.2 mmol/L	*Initial:* predose on day 3 *Maintenance:* predose once weekly	
Theophylline	Timing depends on route of administration and dosage form	55–110 µmol/L		
Tobramycin	Predose: 0–30 min prior to next dose	0.6–2 mg/L	*Initial:* predose and postdose with third dose *Maintenance:* predose once weekly in stable patients; predose and postdose as required in patients with unstable renal function	• No monitoring required for (patients with normal renal function): uncomplicated UTI's, surgery prophylaxis < 72 h, empiric therapy <72 h • Half-life will be prolonged in patients with renal impairment
	Postdose: 30 min after end of infusion Cystic fibrosis:	5–10 mg/L 10–20 mg/L		
Valproic acid (Depakene)	Predose: 0–60 min prior to next dose	350–700 µmol/L	*Maintenance:* predose only if patient still has seizures; if toxicity is suspected, take sample at time of symptoms	• t½ may be longer in patients with hepatic disease and may be shorter in patients receiving other anticonvulsant drugs • Some patients may tolerate higher levels (≥ 1,000)
Vancomycin	Predose: 0–30 min prior to next dose	5–10 mg/L	*Initial:* predose and postdose with third or fourth dose *Maintenance:* predose and postdose weekly or with each dosage change	• t½ will be longer in patients with renal impairment • Some patients may require an individualized approach • In complete renal failure, patient may only need 1 dose/wk
	Postdose: 60 min after end of infusion	25–40 mg/L		

DRUGS IN RENAL FAILURE

Drug excretion in renal failure is affected in a reasonably predictable fashion.

The patient's volume of distribution is unchanged so the usual loading dose is given, but the maintenance dose must be reduced. Two methods are used: the usual dose can be given less frequently or a smaller dose can be used with a normal interval. The interval extension method is simple, while the dosage reduction method results in smaller swings in drug levels.

Percentage of drug excreted by the kidney

1. Major modification in renal failure
- Aminoglycoside   95
- Penicillin   90
- Gancyclovir   90
- Methotrexate   94
- Penicillin   90
- Thiazides   90
- Ticarcillin   86
- Vancomycin   95

2. Minor modification in renal failure
- Acyclovir   70–80
- Amoxicillin   52
- Cephalosporins   60–80
- Clonidine   62
- Cloxacillin   60
- Digoxin   72
- Doxycycline   40
- Ethambutol   79
- Fluconazole   70
- Flucytosine   84
- Furosemide   74
- Imipenem   60–75
- Methyldopa   63
- Primidone   42
- Ranitidine   70
- Sulphonamides   30–50
- Tetracyclines   48
- Trimethoprim   53

3. No modification in renal failure
- Acetaminophen   3
- ASA   1
- Amphotericin   3
- Benzodiazepines   1

- Carbamazepine   1
- Chloramphenicol   5
- Chlorpromazine   1
- Clindamycin   14
- Erythromycin   15
- Ethosuximide   19
- Heparin   10
- Hydralazine   14
- Indomethacin   15
- Isoniazide   29
- Metronidazole   8
- Minocycline   11
- Narcotics   15–10
- Nifedipine   0
- Nitroglycerine   1
- Phenobarbital   2
- Phenytoin   2
- Prazosin   1
- Prednisolone   7–15
- Propranolol   1
- Rifampin   16
- Theophylline   8
- Valproic acid   1
- Warfarin   1
- Nalidixic acid   10
- Nitrofurantoin   35

DRUGS IN LIVER FAILURE

The hepatic clearance of a drug is the product of hepatic blood flow and the extraction ratio. The extraction ratio is not a constant and depends on hepatic blood flow, protein binding and hepatic drug removal capacity.

Liver disease alters all these factors variably and unpredictably so no general rules are possible for drug dosing. There is also no single test which reliably indicates liver function. However, liver blood flow and cellular function must decrease to a considerable extent before drug levels are affected, therefore, it is not usually a problem except in advanced liver failure.

Commonly used drugs that are metabolized or excreted principally by the liver are:
- Analgesics: ASA, acetaminophen, all opiates.
- Cardiac drugs: β–blockers, digoxin, prazosin, spironolactone, nitroglycerine, verapamil, lidocaine.
- CNS drugs: chlorpromazine, phenytoin, benzodiazepines, barbiturates.
- Antibiotics: chloramphenicol, erythromycin, clindamycin, nafcillin, rifampin.
- Others: theophylline, warfarin, most antimitotics.

DRUGS AND BREAST FEEDING

In most instances, the dose ingested and amount absorbed are small enough to be ignored. It still seems safe, however, for the lactating mother to avoid all drugs unless absolutely necessary. Taking the drug immediately after a feed may result in lower amounts of drug in breast milk by the time of the next feed, but this will depend on how often the baby is breast fed and the pharmacokinetic properties of the drug.

Common drugs that may cause serious effects in the infant are:
• Antibiotics: sulfonamides, fluoroquinolones.
• Cardiac drugs: β–blockers, atropine.
• Endocrine: antithyroid drugs, estrogens, dihydrotachysterol, vitamin D, calciferol.
• CNS drugs: diazepam, lithium, MOA inhibitors.
• Abused drugs: alcohol, narcotics, cannabis, cocaine, LSD, phencyclidine.
• Others: all radioactive drugs such as gallium and iodine, anthraquinones (laxatives), ergot, antineoplastics, iodide.

DRUG INTERACTIONS

This subject is too large to be covered in a handbook. Interactions are common and often unpredictable. For instance, the antabuse effect of flagyl may not be considered in a 6 year old until the child is prescribed a cough medicine containing alcohol.

Unless absolutely certain that drugs are compatible always check them in a specialist handbook.

DRUGS AND G6PD DEFICIENCY

Oxidant substances entering the red cell convert hemoglobin to methemoglobin, then further denature it until the protein precipitates out in visible clumps called Heinz bodies. Finally, the cell is destroyed, producing a hemolytic anemia.

The cell is protected by reducing substances produced in the pentose phosphate pathway (notably reduced glutathione). The first enzyme in this pathway is G6PD. It is transmitted on the X chromosome and about 1,000 variants exist, producing varying degrees of disease.

Ethnic groups commonly affected are Mediterranean races, Sephardic Jews, southern Chinese, Africans, and Filipinos. All these races, and consequently G6PD deficiency, are common in Canada.

Care is necessary with the following drugs in severe forms of G6PD deficiency:
• Antimalarials: primaquine.
• Antibiotics: sulfonamides, dapsone, nalidixic acid, nitrofurantoin.
• Analgesics: ASA, phenazopyridine.
• Others: methylene blue.

TERATOGENIC DRUGS

Transfer across the placenta depends on a drug's lipid solubility, degree of ionization and its molecular weight. Unfortunately, most drugs taken by the mother will cross to the fetus so it is very unwise to prescribe drugs in pregnancy, especially during the first trimester.

There are reports of fetal malformation and loss in conceptuses whose fathers had been exposed to antineoplastics, caffeine, and anesthetic gases. It is always important to ask about drugs taken during pregnancy when examining a child, especially if the child has congenital malformations.

- Drugs known to be dangerous in pregnancy:
    Ace inhibitors (e.g. captopril): oligohydramnios, renal, growth.
    Alcohol: MR heart, face, limbs, CNS.
    Alkylating agents: CNS, skeletal.
    Androgens: masculinization.
    Antithyroid: goiter.
    Diethylstilbestrol: genitourinary anomalies, vaginal adenosis, adenocarcinoma.
    Folate antagonists: CNS, craniofacial, limbs.
    Lithium: heart, neural tube.
    Penicillamine: connective tissue.
    Phenytoin: craniofacial, heart, CNS.
    Tetracycline: teeth and bone staining.
    Thalidomide: limbs, ears, eyes, heart.
    Valproic acid: craniofacial, heart, CNS.
    Vitamin A: CNS, heart.
    Warfarin: small nose, CNS.
- Drugs possibly associated with malformations:
    Caffeine, anesthetic gases, chloroquine, lithium, spermicides, diazepam, zinc deficiency, folate deficiency.
- Drugs that are probably safe:
    Antihistamines, birth control pills, cocaine, LSD, tricyclics, cortisone, phenothiazines.

DRUG DOSAGE GUIDELINES FOR INFANTS AND OLDER CHILDREN

Explanation of table

- Drug: listed by the most common generic name, with common brand names or alternative names in brackets.
- Supplied: dosage forms available.
- Dose: unless otherwise specified, dosages are for children. When dosing on a mg/kg basis, it is usually not advisable to exceed the usual adult dose.
- Comments: these do not necessarily include side effects, just a few important points about each drug.

Sample of a drug dosage table:

Drug	Supplied	Dose	Comments
Amoxicillin (Amoxil)	*Capsule:* 250 mg, 500 mg *Chewable tablet:* 125 mg, 250 mg *Suspension:* 50 mg/mL	40 mg/kg per 24 h p.o. div. q8h	• Achieves serum levels about twice those of oral ampicillin • Absorption not affected by food

Every effort has been made to ensure that the drug dosage schedules are accurate and in accord with standards accepted at the time of printing. The reader is cautioned, however, to check the product information sheet and to verify locations, contraindications, and recommended dosages before using any drug which may be unfamiliar.

Some of the drugs listed are not officially approved for use in children, yet have been shown to be useful in certain circumstances. Dosages for these drugs are based on limited clinical trials and their use should be undertaken very cautiously.

For most drugs listed, a dosage range is provided, that at times is very wide. This reflects the variability of dose responses in the pediatric population. It is prudent to begin with the lowest recommended dose.

Drug	Supplied	Dose	Comments
Acetaminophen (Paracetamol, Tylenol, Tempra, Panadol)	*Chewable tablet:* 325 mg, 80 mg *Elixir:* 32 mg/mL *Drop:* 80 mg/mL *Suppository:* 120 mg, 325 mg, 650 mg	<u>Mild to moderate pain/antipyretic:</u> 10–15 mg/kg per dose p.o. or p.r. q4–6h <u>Postsurgical analgesia:</u> (in normal healthy children, i.e. no hepatic or renal compromise) 20 mg/kg per dose p.o. q6h × 24 h, then reassess *Maximum:* 90 mg/kg per 24 h	• Hepatotoxic in overdose, both chronic and acute • Regular dosing (not p.r.n.) in the postoperative period provides more consistent analgesia • Rectal administration results in unpredictable serum levels and a much slower onset of action compared to oral • If surgical procedure is short (< 30 min), first dose may be given preoperatively
Acetazolamide (Diamox)	*Tablet:* 250 mg, 500 mg Sustained release capsule: 500 mg "sequels" *Injection:* 500 mg/vial	<u>Diuretic:</u> 5 mg/kg per dose p.o. or i.v. daily or every other day <u>Glaucoma:</u> 8–30 mg/kg per 24 h div. q6–8h i.v. or p.o. <u>Hydrocephalus in infancy:</u> *Initial:* 25 mg/kg per 24 h p.o. or i.v. div. t.i.d. *Increment:* 25 mg/kg per 24 h daily *Maximum:* 100 mg/kg per 24 h <u>Seizures:</u> 8–30 mg/kg per 24 h p.o. up to 750 mg/24 h div. q6–12h <u>Urine alkalinization:</u> 5 mg/kg per dose repeated 2–3 times over 24 h	• Diuresis more effective given every other day or 2 out of 3 days only • i.m. injections may be painful • Side effects: renal colic, GI irritation, drowsiness, acidosis, hypokalemia, parethesias, polyuria • Sustained release capsules are dosed q12h
n-Acetylcysteine (Mucomyst, Airbron)	*Oral solution:* 200 mg/mL (20%) 10 mL *Injection:* 200 mg/mL (20%) 10 mL	<u>Acetaminophen overdose:</u> see Poison Manual <u>Mucolytic:</u> 6–10 mL of 10% or 3–5 mL of 20% solution inhaled t.i.d.–q.i.d. <u>Meconium ileus equivalent (distal intestinal obstruction syndrome):</u> 10–15 mL of 20% solution p.o. q.i.d., 100 mL of 10% solution as enema once daily–q.i.d. <u>Irrigation of urinary catheter:</u> 10 mL of a 10% solution (dilute 20% solution with normal saline) into catheter	• Side effects: local irritation, bronchospasm, stomatitis, rhinorrhea, nausea • For oral use, may dilute with water, saline, cola, orange, or grapefruit juice • For inhalation, 20% solution may be diluted with SWI or sterile normal saline

Drug	Supplied	Dose	Comments
ACTH (Corticotropin, Acthar)	*Aqueous injection:* 40 IU/mL *Repository gel:* 40 IU/mL	*Infantile spasms:* *Gel:* 20–80 IU i.m. daily initially; after 1–2 wk, change to alternate day therapy and then reduce over several weeks *Verification of adrenal responsiveness:* (cosyntropin is preferred for verification of adrenal responsiveness) 25–40 IU i.m. (aqueous), 10–25 IU i.v. in 500 mL D5W over 8 h	• Steroid side effects; 1 IU = 1 mg • Aqueous: rapid onset; 2 h duration; i.v. for diagnostic purposes only • Gel: slower onset; up to 3 d duration; do not give i.v.
Acyclovir (Zovirax)	*Tablet:* 200 mg *Suspension:* 200 mg/5 mL *Injection:* 500 mg/vial, 1 g/vial	*HSV (mucocutaneous):* 15 mg/kg per 24 h i.v. div. q8h, 200 mg/dose p.o. 5 × daily *HSV (encephalitis):* 30 mg/kg per 24 h i.v. div. q8h *HSV in immunocompromised patients:* 30 mg/kg per 24 h i.v. div. q8h *Varicella zoster:* 30 mg/kg per 24 h i.v. div. q8h, 80 mg/kg per 24 h p.o. div. q6h × 5 d *Varicella zoster in immunocompromised patients:* 45 mg/kg per 24 h i.v. div. q8h *Treatment of chickenpox:* 80 mg/kg per 24 h p.o. div. q6h × 5 d	• Oral absorption is 15–20% • Keep well hydrated to prevent nephrotoxicity • Minimum dilution for i.v. use is 10 mg/mL • Decrease dose in renal impairment • May cause nausea, vomiting, diarrhea, headache, dizziness, arthralgia, fatigue, rash, insomnia, fever
Adenosine (Adenocard)	*Injection:* 6 mg/2 mL vial	0.05 mg/kg i.v. over 1–2 s; follow with a rapid flush of 2 mL normal saline; dose can be increased by 0.05 mg/kg at 2 min intervals until response achieved *Maximum:* 0.25 mg/kg or 12 mg	• Half-life is 10–15 s • May precipitate bronchodilation
Alcohol, Ethyl 99% (Absolute alcohol)	*Injection:* 10 mL	*Methanol, ethylene glycol intoxication:* *Loading dose:* 0.76 mL/kg i.v. over 30 min *Maintenance:* 0.14 mL/kg per h	• Ethanol must be diluted to a 10% solution before use • Maintain blood ethanol levels > 22 mmol/L

Drug	Supplied	Dose	Comments
Alfacalcidiol (1-α)	*Capsule:* 0.25 µg *Oral liquid:* 0.2 µg/mL	Must be individualized *Children:* 0.01–0.05 µg/kg per 24 h p.o. once daily; increase by 0.005–0.01 µg/kg per 24 h q4–8 wk based on clinical response, up to the usual adult dose of 1–2 µg/24 h; the usual maintenance dose in children is 0.25–1 µg/24 h	• Used for the management of hypocalcemia and osteodystrophy in patients with chronic renal failure and patients with hypophosphatemic D-resistant rickets • Does not require renal activation • Monitor calcium, phosphate, magnesium, and alkaline phosphatase frequently until dose is stabilized
Allopurinol (Zyloprim)	*Tablet:* 100 mg, 200 mg, 300 mg	10 mg/kg per 24 h p.o. or i.v. once daily or div. b.i.d. (i.v. allopurinol is an investigational drug) *Maximum:* 600 mg/24 h	• Maintain alkaline urine flow • Follow serum uric acid levels • Decrease dose in renal impairment • Allopurinol is metabolized to an active metabolite with a long half-life • Daily doses > 300 mg should be div. b.i.d.
Amikacin (Amikin)	*Injection:* 250 mg/mL	*Children:* 15–22.5 mg/kg per 24 h i.v. or i.m. div. q8–12 h *Adults:* 15 mg/kg per 24 h i.v. or i.m. div. q8–12 h	• Ototoxic, nephrotoxic • Adjust dose in renal impairment • Monitor serum levels • Therapeutic peak, 20–30 mg/L; trough, 5–10 mg/L
Aminocaproic acid (Amicar, EACA)	*Tablet:* 500 mg *Oral solution:* 250 mg/mL *Injection:* 250 mg/mL	*Loading dose:* 100–200 mg/kg i.v. or p.o. *Maintenance:* 100 mg/kg per dose q4–6h *Maximum:* 30 g/24 h	• Contraindications: hematuria, DIC

Drug	Supplied	Dose	Comments
Aminophylline (Theophylline ethylene diamine)	*Tablet:* 100 mg, 200 mg *Injection:* 25 mg/mL *PFS:* 25 mg/mL 10 mL	<u>Bronchodilator:</u> *Loading dose:* 6 mg/kg i.v. over 20 min; reduce dose by 50% if patient has had theophylline in previous 24 h *i.v. infusions:* *Infants (1–12 mo):* 0.2–0.9 mg/kg per h *Children (1–9 yr):* 1 mg/kg per h *Children (9–16 yr):* 0.8 mg/kg per h *Children (> 16 yr, healthy nonsmokers):* 0.5 mg/kg per h *p.o. daily maintenance dose:* *Children (1–9 yr):* 20 mg/kg *Children (9–16 yr):* 16 mg/kg *Children (> 16 yr):* 12 mg/kg	• Aminophylline contains 80% theophylline • Daily dose is titrated to maintain serum theophylline level in range of 55–110 µmol/L for bronchodilation • Side effects: restlessness, GI upset, dysrhythmias, seizures • To convert to oral theophylline: multiply aminophylline dose in mg/24 h by 0.8 = theophylline daily dose
5–Aminosalicylic acid tablets (Asacol)	*Enteric coated tablet:* 400 mg (Asacol)	*Adults:* 3–12 tablets daily in div. doses	• Do not crush tablets; swallow whole • Some systemic absorption may occur; use with care in children • No established dosage for children
Amitriptyline (Elavil)	*Tablet:* 10 mg, 25 mg, 50 mg	<u>Depressive disorders:</u> *Children (6–12 yr):* 1–5 mg/kg per 24 h p.o. div. b.i.d. *Adolescents:* 10 mg p.o. t.i.d. and 20 mg at bedtime initially; titrate up as needed to a maximum of 100 mg/24 h *Adults:* *Initial:* 50–150 mg/24 h div. t.i.d.–q.i.d. *Maintenance:* 150–300 mg/24 h div. t.i.d.–q.i.d. <u>Adjunct to analgesia:</u> *Children:* 0.5–1.5 mg/kg per dose p.o. at bedtime	• Side effects: sedation, confusion, weakness, fatigue, tremor, sweating, headache, anticholinergic effects, cardiovascular effects, decreased seizure threshold • Monitor therapy with serum levels and ECG's • Serum level not to exceed 1,000 nmol/L in adults and children

Drug	Supplied	Dose	Comments
Amoxicillin (Amoxil)	*Capsule:* 250 mg, 500 mg *Chewable tablet:* 125 mg, 250 mg *Suspension:* 50 mg/mL	*Children:* 40 mg/kg per 24 h p.o. div. q8h *Adults:* Usual dose 250 mg p.o. q8h	• Achieves serum levels about twice those of oral ampicillin • Absorption not affected by food
Amoxicillin/Clavulanate (Clavulin)	*Suspension:* 125 mg/mL, 250 mg/mL *Tablet:* 250 mg, 500 mg (amoxicillin content)	Based on amoxicillin content: 40 mg/kg per 24 h p.o. div. q8h	• Clavulanate is an inhibitor of β–lactamase • Higher incidence of diarrhea than with amoxicillin alone
Amphotericin B (Fungizone)	*Injection:* 50 mg/vial	0.25 mg/kg per 24 h i.v., increase by increments of 0.125–0.25 mg/kg every 24 h or 48 h, as tolerated, to a maximum of 1 mg/kg per dose Bladder instillation: 15–50 mg/24 h diluted to 0.05 mg/mL in SWI as a continuous irrigation over 24 h	• Fever, chills, nausea, and vomiting are common • Premedication with acetaminophen or diphenhydramine may help • Meperidine may be useful for chills • Hydrocortisone 1 mg/mg amphotericin (maximum: 25 mg) added to infusion bag may help prevent immediate adverse reactions
Ampicillin	*Capsule:* 250 mg, 500 mg *Oral suspension:* 50 mg/mL *Injection:* 125 mg, 250 mg, 500 mg, 1 g, 2 g	Meningitis: 200–400 mg/kg per 24 h i.v. div. q6h Other infections: 100–200 mg/kg per 24 h i.v. div. q6h or 50 mg/kg per 24 h p.o. div. q6h *Adult:* 1–2 g i.v. q6h	• Amoxicillin is preferred for oral therapy except when treating diarrhea caused by *Salmonella* or *Shigella* • Side effects: rash, pruritis, urticaria, nausea, vomiting and diarrhea

Drug	Supplied	Dose	Comments
Antithymocyte globulin (Atgam, ATG, Lymphocyte immunoglobulin)	*Injection:* 250 mg/5 mL amp	*Test dose:* 5 μg intradermally Renal allograft recipients: *Acute rejection:* 10–15 mg/kg per 24 h × 14 d *Delaying onset of rejection:* 15 mg/kg per 24 h × 14 d, then every other day × 14 d, starting within 24 h of transplant Aplastic anemia: 10–20 mg/kg per 24 h for 8–21 doses	• Intradermal sensitivity testing is recommended prior to the administration of the initial dose of ATG • Patients may require pretreatment with acetaminophen, antihistamine, and/or corticosteroid
Aquasol A and D (Water miscible vitamins A and D)	*Drops:* contain vitamin A 40,000 IU/mL, vitamin D 8,000 IU/mL	*Children:* 0.05 mL p.o. daily	• May be mixed in milk, formulas, juices, or cereals • Higher doses are required in children > 4 mo of age with cholestasis but the possibility of overdosage must be considered
ASA (Acetylsalicylic acid, Aspirin)	*Chewable tablet:* 80 mg *Tablet:* 325 mg *Enteric coated tablet:* 325 mg, 650 mg *Suppository:* 150 mg, 650 mg	Antipyretic: 10–15 mg/kg per dose p.o. q4h to a total of 60–80 mg/kg per 24 h Antirheumatic: 60–100 mg/kg per 24 h p.o. div. q6h Kawasaki's disease: *Acute febrile period:* 80–100 mg/kg per 24 h p.o. div. q.i.d. *After fever resolves:* 3–5 mg/kg per 24 h p.o. once daily	• Use cautiously in platelet and bleeding disorders • Follow serum levels when used as an antirheumatic and for treatment of Kawasaki's disease • Therapeutic serum level: 1.5–2 mmol/L • ASA may increase the risk of Reye's syndrome following acute febrile illnesses, especially influenza or chickenpox

Drug	Supplied	Dose	Comments
Atropine	*Injection:* 0.1 mg/mL, 0.4 mg/mL, 0.6 mg/mL	*Preoperative:* *Children:* 0.01 mg/kg per dose s.c., i.v., i.m. or p.o. q4–6h p.r.n. *Maximum:* 0.4 mg/dose *Adults:* 0.5 mg dose i.m., i.v. or s.c. q4–6h p.r.n. *CPR (bradycardia):* 0.02–0.05 mg/kg per dose i.v. q2–5 min × 2–3 p.r.n. minimum dose 0.1 mg *Maximum:* 1 mg for children, 2 mg for adults *Organophosphate poisoning:* *Children:* 0.02–0.05 mg/kg per dose i.v. q10–20 min until atropine effect seen (dry flushed skin, tachycardia, mydriasis, fever), then q1–4h to maintain atropine effect for 24 h *Children (> 12 yr) and adults:* 1–2 mg/dose i.v. q10–20 min until atropine effect seen, then 1–3 mg/dose q1–4h to maintain atropine effect for 24 h	• May give via endotracheal tube • Well absorbed orally; peak plasma concentrations are achieved within 1 h • Injectable form may be given orally • Anticholinergic side effects: Red as a beet (skin flushing), Dry as a bone (dry mouth, urinary retention), Blind as a bat (blurred vision, photophobia), Mad as a hatter (agitation), Hot as a stove (anhidrosis)
Aurothiomalate sodium (Myochrisine, Gold sodium thiomalate)	*Injection:* 25 mg/mL, 50 mg/mL	*Initial:* 0.25 mg/kg per dose i.m. × 1 *Increment:* 0.25 mg/kg per dose i.m., increase with each weekly dose *Maintenance:* 1 mg/kg per dose (maximum: 50 mg/dose) weekly to a total of 20 doses, then q2–4 wk	• Addition of 0.1 mL of 1% lidocaine to each i.m. injection may reduce discomfort • Monitor CBC, platelets, eosinophils, urinalysis with each dose or q2 doses
Azathioprine (Imuran)	*Tablet:* 50 mg *Injection:* 100 mg/vial	*Immunosuppression:* *Initial:* 3–5 mg/kg per 24 h i.v. or p.o. daily *Maintenance:* 1–3 mg/kg per 24 h i.v. or p.o. daily *Rheumatic disease:* 1–3 mg/kg per 24 h p.o. daily	• Bone marrow suppressive • Monitor hematological status • May also cause rash, stomatitis, GI disturbances • Reduce dose in renal impairment or concomitant allopurinol therapy

Drug	Supplied	Dose	Comments
Bacitracin (Baciguent)	*Topical ointment:* 500 unit/g *Eye ointment:* 500 unit/g	Topical: Apply 1–5 × daily Ophthalmic: 0.5–1 cm ribbon q.i.d. to conjuctival sac	
Baclofen (Lioresal)	*Tablet:* 10 mg	*Initial:* 10–15 mg/24 h p.o. div. t.i.d. *Increment:* 5–15 mg/24 h at 3 d intervals *Maximum:* *2–7 yr:* 30–40 mg/24 h p.o. div. t.i.d. *> 8 yr:* 60 mg/24 h p.o. div. t.i.d.	• May cause drowsiness, sedation, weakness, confusion, headache, insomnia, nausea, constipation, frequent urination, hypotension • There is some evidence that baclofen may exacerbate seizures
Beclomethasone (Beclovent, Beclofort, Beconase, Vancenase)	*Inhaler:* 50 µg/puff, 250 µg/puff *Nasal spray:* 50 µg/puff *Rotocaps:* 100 µg, 200 µg	Inhaler: (50 µg/puff) *3–5 yr:* 1 puff q8–12h *6–12 yr:* 1–2 puffs q6–8h *> 12 yr:* 2 puffs q6–8h Rotocaps: *6–14 yr:* 100 µg b.i.d.–t.i.d. *> 14 yr:* 200 µg t.i.d.–q.i.d. Nasal spray: *> 6 yr:* 1 spray into each nostril t.i.d.–q.i.d.	• Metered dose inhalers should be used with a spacer device, especially in young children • Rinse mouth after inhalation • Becloforte (250 µg/puff) may be used if large doses are required to control symptoms • Doses > 400 µg/24 h may be associated with systemic effects • Full effects may not be seen for 4–6 wk
Benzocaine (Hurricaine)	*Spray:* 20%	*> 2 yr:* apply topically as needed	• Not recommended for use in children < 2 yr because absorption of significant quantities (with excessive use) may result in methemoglobinemia
Benzoyl peroxide (Acetoxyl, Dermoxyl, Panoxyl, H₂Oxyl)	*Gel:* 2.5%, 5%, 10%	Apply to acne after skin cleansing daily × 1 wk, then b.i.d.	• Avoid contact with abraded skin, mouth, and eyes • Transient erythema and scaling are common at start of therapy
Benztropine (Cogentin)	*Tablet:* 1 mg, 2 mg *Injection:* 2 mg/2mL	Drug induced extrapyramidal disorders: 0.02–0.05 mg/kg per dose p.o. or i.m. 1–2 × daily	• May cause CNS depression or stimulation, nervousness, dry mouth, blurred vision

Drug	Supplied	Dose	Comments
Benzydamine (Tantum)	*Mouth rinse:* 0.15%	5–15 mL/dose; swish for at least 30 s, then spit; repeat q6–8h p.r.n.	• May be diluted 1:1 with lukewarm water • May initially sting inflammed mucosa due to alcohol content • Do not swallow
Betamethasone, systemic (Betnesol, Celestone)	*Tablet:* 0.5 mg *Injection:* 6 mg/mL	<u>Adrenocortical insufficiency:</u> 0.0175 mg/kg per 24 h p.o. div. q8h or 0.0175 mg/kg per dose i.m. q3 d <u>Anti-inflammatory:</u> 0.02–0.25 mg/kg per 24 h p.o. div. t.i.d.–q.i.d. <u>Asthma:</u> 0.1 mg/kg per dose p.o. b.i.d. <u>Intra-articular:</u> 0.25–2 mL depending on the size of the joint	• Usual steroid effects • 0.5 mg betamethasone = 4 mg prednisone • i.m. injection has a rapid onset of action (1–3 h) and effects may persist for 7 d • For intra-articular use, triamcinolone is preferred
Betamethasone, topical (Betnovate, Betnesol, Celestoderm, Celestone)	*Cream:* 0.05%, 0.1% (valerate) *Ointment:* 0.05%, 0.1% (valerate) *Lotion:* 0.05%, 0.1% (valerate) *Enema:* 5 mg/100 mL (disodium phosphate)	<u>Topical:</u> Apply thinly 2–3 × daily <u>Enema:</u> One enema at bedtime × 2–4 wk	• Topical use may cause burning, itching, irritation, acneiform eruptions, hypopigmentation, thinning of skin • Enema form is occasionally used in left-sided colitis
Bethanechol (Urecholine)	*Injection:* 5 mg/mL	0.15–0.2 mg/kg per 24 h s.c. div. q6–8h	• Do not give i.v. or i.m. • Contraindicated in asthma, mechanical gastrointestinal or genitourinary obstruction, peptic ulcer • May cause hypotension, nausea, bronchospasm, salivation, flushing

Drug	Supplied	Dose	Comments
Bisacodyl (Dulcolax)	*Tablet:* 5 mg *Suppository:* 5 mg, 10 mg *Microenema:* 10 mg/5 mL	p.o.: 0.3 mg/kg per 24 h or 5–10 mg given 6 h before desired effect p.r.: (single daily dose) < 6 yr: 5 mg suppository, 2.5 mL enema > 6 yr: 10 mg suppository, 5 mL enema	• Do not chew tablets • Do not give within 1 h of antacids or milk as tablets are enteric coated • May cause abdominal cramping • Not for use < 1 yr of age • Onset of action: p.o. 6–10 h, p.r. 15–60 min
Bretylium (Bretylate)	*Injection:* 50 mg/mL, 10 mL amp	Acute ventricular fibrillation: 5 mg/kg per dose by rapid undiluted i.v. injection followed by additional doses of 10 mg/kg per dose at 15–30 min intervals until a maximum of 30 mg/kg has been given Other ventricular arrhythmias and maintenance therapy: 5–10 mg/kg per dose by slow diluted i.v. injection or i.m. undiluted q6–8h	• Indicated for life threatening arrhythmias refractory to conventional therapy • Safety and efficacy in children has not been established • Watch for hypotension; patient should be recumbent • Maintenance doses may be diluted in 50 mL D5W and infused over 10–15 min • Requires continuous hemodynamic monitoring
Budesonide (Pulmicort)	*"Turbuhaler" inhaler.* 100 µg/inhalation, 200 µg/inhalation, 400 µg/inhalation *Respiratory solution:* 0.25 mg/mL–2 mL nebule, 0.5 mg/mL–2 mL nebule	Respiratory solution: 0.25–0.5 mg/dose, repeated q12h (may be given q6h in severe cases) Maximum: 3 mg/24 h Turbuhaler: Low dose: < 400 µg/24 h Medium dose: 400–800 µg/24 h High dose: 800–2,000 µg/24 h Average dose: 200 µg b.i.d.	• Dose depends upon severity and response • Systemic side effects are uncommon at low dose but increase with increasing dose • Rinse mouth after each inhalation to prevent candidiasis • Full effects may not be seen for 4–6 wk
Burow's solution (Burosol)	2.2 g tablets or packets for solution	Dissolve 1 or 2 packets or tablets in 500 mL of water (= 1:40 or 1:20 dilution); apply to lesion on a loose wet bandage; apply additional solution as required to keep bandage moist q15–30 min	• May be used as a wet dressing, compress, soak, sitz bath, douche, or earwick • Contains aluminum acetate and benzethonium chloride
Calcitonin (Calcimar)	*Injection:* 200 IU/mL (2 mL vial)	Dose in children is not well established; 20 IU s.c. alternate days for a 50 kg child has been used	

Drug	Supplied	Dose	Comments
Calcitriol (Rocaltrol, 1, 25–Dihydroxychole-calciferol)	*Capsule:* 0.25 µg, 0.5 µg *Injection:* 1 µg/mL	*p.o.:* 0.01–0.05 µg/kg per 24 h p.o. once daily; titrate by 0.005–0.01 µg/kg per 24 h q4–8 wk based on clinical response, up to the usual adult dose of 1–2 µg/24 h (the usual maintenance dose for children is 0.25–1 µg/24 h) *i.v.: Initial:* 0.01 µg/kg per dose i.v. 3 × weekly; titrate by 0.25–0.5 µg q2–4 wk as necessary *Maintenance:* 0.01–0.05 µg/kg per dose i.v. 3 × weekly	• Monitor calcium, phosphate, magnesium, and alkaline phosphatase frequently until dose is stabilized • Does not require renal or hepatic activation • Avoid use with mineral oil
Calcium acetate (Phosex)	*Tablet:* 667 mg	*Children:* 1 g elemental calcium/m² per 24 h div. t.i.d.; titrate dose based on serum phosphorus levels *Adults:* 2 tablets with each meal; may be increased to 4 tablets with each meal, based on serum phosphorus levels	• Calcium acetate binds with twice as much phosphate as calcium carbonate • Each tablet provides 169 mg elemental calcium
Calcium chloride	*Injection:* 100 mg/mL, 10%, vial 10 mL *PFS:* 100 mg/mL, 10%, 10 mL (also with intracardiac needle), 10% solution contains 0.68 mmol Ca²⁺/mL or 27 mg elemental Ca²⁺/mL	*Cardiopulmonary resuscitation:* For hypocalcemia, hyperkalemia, or calcium channel blocker toxicity; 10–30 mg/kg (0.1–0.3 mL/kg) per dose i.v. or intraosseous; inject slowly over 1 min and repeat in 10 min if necessary (dosage in terms of calcium chloride)	• Incompatible with sodium bicarbonate • Avoid extravasation
Calcium disodium edta (Calcium disodium versenate)	*Injection:* 200 mg/mL	*Lead poisoning:* *Children and adults:* 50–75 mg/kg per 24 h i.m. or i.v. div. q4–8h for up to 5 d; may repeat course after a 2 d interval	• May cause renal tubular necrosis • Do not use if anuric • Monitor ECG for arrhythmia when giving i.v. • To decrease pain of i.m. injections, administer with 0.5 mL of 1% procaine

Drug	Supplied	Dose	Comments
Calcium gluconate	*Tablet:* 650 mg (1.5 mmol Ca^{2+}/ tablet) *Injection:* 10% (100 mg/mL) 10 mL vial 10% solution contains 0.23 mmol Ca^{2+}/mL, 9 mg elemental Ca^{2+}/mL	Hypocalcemia: 200–500 mg/kg per 24 h div. q6h i.v. or p.o. Cardiopulmonary resuscitation: For hypocalcemia, hyperkalemia, or calcium channel blocker overdose; 100 mg/kg per dose (1 mL/kg per dose) i.v. q10 min (dosage in terms of calcium gluconate)	• Incompatible with sodium bicarbonate • Monitor for bradycardia or dysrhythmia • Avoid extravasation • Hypercalcemia will precipitate digoxin toxicity
Calcium polystyrene sulfonate (Resonium calcium)	*Powder suspension:* with 25% sorbitol	Acute hyperkalemia: *Children:* 1 g/kg per 24 h p.o. or p.r. div. t.i.d.–q.i.d. (not to exceed usual adult dose) *Maintenance:* 0.5 g/kg per 24 h p.o. or p.r. div. t.i.d.–q.i.d. (not to exceed usual adult dose) Adults: 20 g/dose p.o. or p.r. t.i.d.–q.i.d.	• Exchanges about 1.6 mmol K$^+$/g resin • Do not administer with fruit juices containing K$^+$ • Onset of action of p.o. resin may be delayed 1–2 d, when resin reaches colon; exchange will continue until all resin is voided • p.r. route is less effective than p.o. as retention time is shorter
Calcium supplements (oral) (Oscal, Tums, Calcium Sandoz, Calcium Stanley)	*Chewable tablet:* 200 mg elemental calcium (Tums) *Tablet:* 250 mg, 500 mg elemental calcium (Oscal) *Syrup:* 100 mg elemental calcium or 5 mL (Calcium Stanley) *Effervescent tablet:* 500 mg elemental calcium (Calcium Sandoz)	Maintenance/hypocalcemia: *Infants:* 20–60 mg elemental calcium/kg per 24 h p.o. div. q6h *Children:* 10–30 mg elemental calcium/kg per 24 h p.o. div. q6h	• 1 mEq Ca^{2+} = 20 mg elemental calcium • Calcium carbonate preparations are also used as phosphate binders; the dose depends on the patient's size and degree of phosphatemia • Tums and Oscal are calcium carbonate • Calcium Stanley syrup is sugar free

Drug	Supplied	Dose	Comments
Captopril (Capoten)	*Tablet:* 6.25 mg, 12 mg, 25 mg, 50 mg, 100 mg	*Infants and children:* *Initial:* 0.15 mg/kg per dose p.o. q6–8h; increase as required by 0.15 mg/kg per dose to a maximum of 6 mg/kg per 24 h *Maximum single dose:* 100 mg *Adolescents:* 6.25–12.5 mg/dose p.o. q8–12h *Maximum:* 50–75 mg/dose	• Reduce dose with impaired renal function • Give a test dose (0.1 mg/kg) to determine hypotensive response
Carbamazepine (Tegretol)	*Tablet:* 200 mg *Chewable tablet:* 100 mg, 200 mg *Controlled release (CR) tablet:* 200 mg, 400 mg	*1–12 yr old: < 20 kg:* *Initial:* 50 mg p.o. daily *Increment:* increase by 50 mg/24 h every 5–7 d to a maintenance dose of 20 mg/kg per 24 h div. t.i.d. *> 20 kg: Initial:* 100 mg p.o. daily *Increment:* increase by 100 mg/24 h every 5–7 d to a maintenance dose of 20 mg/kg per 24 h or 600 mg/24 h, whichever is less; divide dose b.i.d. if CR tablets used, otherwise divide dose t.i.d. (doses should be increased above 20 mg/kg per 24 h only if patient still has seizures)	• Dosage should be gradually increased over 1 mo to minimize side effects and to allow development of tolerance to side effects • Because carbamazepine induces its own metabolism, do not measure serum level until final maintenance dose is achieved • Interacts with several drugs • Therapeutic range: 25–50 μmol/L
Cefaclor (Ceclor)	*Liquid:* 50 mg/mL *Capsule:* 250 mg	*Children:* 40 mg/kg per 24 h p.o. div. q8–12h *Adults:* 0.75–1.5 g/24 h	• May cause serum sickness, erythema multiforme, and Stevens–Johnson reactions; may be given with food
Cefazolin (Kefzol, Ancef)	*Injection:* 500 mg, 1 g	*Infants and children:* 50–100 mg/kg per 24 h i.v. or i.m. div. q8h *Adults:* usual dose 1–2 g i.v. or i.m. q8h	• Does not enter CSF
Cefotaxime (Claforan)	*Injection:* 500 mg, 1 g, 2 g	*Infants and children:* 100–150 mg/kg per 24 h i.v. or i.m. div. q8h (meningitis 200 mg/kg per 24 h i.v. div. q6h) *Adults:* usual dose 1–2 g i.m. or i.v. q8–12h	

Drug	Supplied	Dose	Comments
Cefoxitin (Mefoxin)	*Injection:* 1 g, 2 g	*Children:* 80–160 mg/kg per 24 h i.v. or i.m. div. q4–6h *Adults:* Usual dose 1–2 g i.v. or i.m. q6h	
Ceftazidime (Fortaz)	*Injection:* 500 mg, 1 g, 2 g	*Children:* 100–150 mg/kg per 24 h i.v. or i.m. div. q8h Cystic fibrosis: 200–300 mg/kg per 24 h i.v. div. q8h *Adults:* Usual dose 1–2 g i.v. or i.m. q8h	
Ceftriaxone (Rocephin)	*Injection:* 0.25 g, 1 g, 2 g	50–100 mg/kg per 24 h i.v. or i.m. once daily or div. q12h Meningitis: 100 mg/kg per 24 h i.v. or i.m. div. q12h	• i.m. doses can be reconstituted with 1% lidocaine • Good CSF penetration
Cefuroxime (Zinacef)	*Injection:* 750 mg, 1.5 g	100–150 mg/kg per 24 h i.v. or i.m. div. q8h *Adults:* Usual dose 750–1,500 mg i.v. or i.m. q8h	
Cephalexin (Keflex)	*Capsule:* 250 mg, 500 mg *Suspension:* 50 mg/mL	Mild to moderate infections: 25–50 mg/kg per 24 h p.o. div. q6h Severe infections: (stepdown from i.v. therapy for osteomyelitis) 100–150 mg/kg per 24 h p.o. div. q6h *Adults:* 1–4 g/24 h	• More palatable and less GI upset than p.o. cloxacillin • May be given with food

Drug	Supplied	Dose	Comments
Chloral hydrate (Noctec)	*Capsule:* 500 mg *Liquid:* 100 mg/mL	Sedation: 5–15 mg/kg per dose p.o. or p.r. q8h Preprocedural sedation: 20–75 mg/kg per dose p.o. or p.r. 60 min prior to procedure *Maximum dose:* 100 mg/kg per 24 h or 2 g/24 h Hypnotic: 50–75 mg/kg per dose p.o. or p.r. *Maximum:* 1 g/dose, 2 g/24 h	• Oral absorption may vary considerably, particularly in infants in whom absorption may be delayed (≥ 60 min) • Chloral hydrate is generally considered a safe drug but deaths due to respiratory depression have occurred in patients who received a second dose of chloral hydrate or a dose of narcotic when it was felt that adequate sedation had not been achieved • May cause gastric irritation, excitement, delirium • Oral liquid can be given by rectal route
Chloramphenicol (Chloromycetin)	*Injection:* 1 g *Eye drops:* 0.5% *Eye ointment:* 1%	50–75 mg/kg per 24 h i.v. div. q6h Meningitis: 75–100 mg/kg per 24 h i.v. div. q6h Eye drops: 1 drop into the infected eye q3–6h Eye ointment: Small amount placed in the lower conjunctival sac q3–6h; after first 48 h, dose frequency may be decreased; treatment should be continued for at least 48 h after the eye appears normal	• Therapeutic levels: 15–25 mg/L; levels > 50 mg/L are associated with a greater incidence of toxic effects
Chloroquine phosphate (Aralen)	*Tablet:* 250 mg	Malaria prophylaxis: 5 mg base/kg p.o. once weekly Amebiasis, hepatic abscess: 10 mg base/kg (maximum 300 mg)/24 h p.o. 2–3 wk	• Each 250 mg tablet of chloroquine phosphate contains 150 mg of chloroquine base • See hydroxychloroquine
Chlorpheniramine (Chlor–Tripolon)	*Tablet:* 4 mg *Oral liquid:* 0.5 mg/mL *Injection:* 10 mg/mL	0.35 mg/kg per 24 h i.v., s.c., i.m. or p.o. div. q4–6h	• Parenteral administration can cause diaphoresis, pallor, weak pulse, hypotension

Drug	Supplied	Dose	Comments
Chlorpromazine	*Tablet:* 10 mg, 25 mg, 50 mg *Liquid:* 5 mg/mL, 20 mg/mL *Injection:* 25 mg/mL *Suppository:* 100 mg	*Children > 6 mo:* 2.5–6 mg/kg per 24 h i.v. or i.m. div. q6–8 h, 2.5–6 mg/kg per 24 h p.o. div. q4–6h, 1 mg/kg per dose p.r. q6–8h Maximum i.m. dose: *< 5 yr:* 40 mg/24 h *5–12 yr:* 75 mg/24 h	• i.v. route can cause hypotension • Can cause drowsiness, arrhythmias, extrapyramidal symptoms (reversible with diphenhydramine or benztropine), lowered seizure threshold
Chlorthalidone	*Tablet:* 50 mg, 100 mg	2 mg/kg per dose p.o. 3 × wk or 1–2 mg/kg p.o. daily	• Duration of action: 24–72 h
Cholestyramine (Questran)	*Powder:* each 9 g powder contains 4 g anhydrous resin	240 mg resin/kg per 24 h div. t.i.d.; can be increased to 10–12 g resin/24 h in div. doses in infants 6–9 mo and 20–24 g resin in older children for choleresis or pruritis due to cholestasis	• Give as a slurry in water, juice, or milk before meals • Give with plenty of fluids • Use with caution in young children • Due to its anion exchange properties, it may cause hyperchloremic acidosis; follow electrolytes, especially bicarbonate • May also cause constipation, diarrhea, decreased absorption of fat soluble vitamins, and altered absorption of other drugs (take other drugs 1 h before or 6–8 h after cholestyramine)
Cicatrin	*Powder*	Apply to affected area twice daily	• Contains bacitracin 250 unit/g, neomycin 3.3 mg/g, amino acids, cornstarch
Cimetidine (Tagamet)	*Tablet:* 200 mg, 300 mg *Oral liquid:* 60 mg/mL *Injection:* 150 mg/mL	p.o.: 20–40 mg/kg per 24 h div. into 4 doses, before meals and at bedtime i.v.: 20–40 mg/kg per 24 h div. q6h	• May cause diarrhea, rash, myalgia, neutropenia, gynecomastia, dizziness • May increase serum levels of theophylline, phenytoin, and other drugs • Also see ranitidine indications in children
Cisapride (Prepulsid)	*Tablet:* 10 mg *Oral liquid:* 1 mg/mL	0.3 mg/kg per dose p.o. t.i.d.–q.i.d. 15–30 min before meals	• Give prior to meals • Avoid use with ketoconazole, which can inhibit the metabolism of cisapride, resulting in an increased incidence of adverse effects

Drug	Supplied	Dose	Comments
Citrate solution (Bicitra, modified Shohl's solution)	*Oral solution:* contains 1 mEq Na⁺/mL and provides 1 mEq bicarbonate/mL	*Urinary alkalinizer:* 2–3 mEq/kg per 24 h p.o. div. t.i.d.–q.i.d.	• More palatable than plain sodium bicarbonate • Chilling improves palatability; dilute with water before administration • Adjust dose to maintain desired urine pH
Clindamycin (Dalacin–C)	*Capsule:* 150 mg *Injection:* 150 mg/mL *Oral liquid:* 15 mg/mL	*Children:* 25–40 mg/kg per 24 h i.m. or i.v. div q6–8H, 20–30 mg/kg per 24 h p.o. div. q6h *Adults:* 150–450 mg p.o. q6h, 150–900 mg i.v. or i.m. q8h	
Clobazam (Frisium)	*Tablet:* 10 mg	*<20 kg: Initial:* 5 mg/24 h p.o. *Increment:* 5 mg/24 h at 5 d intervals *Maintenance:* 0.5 mg/kg per 24 h; if patient does not respond, dose may be increased to 1 mg/kg per 24 h *>20 kg: Initial:* 10 mg/24 h p.o. *Increment:* 5 mg/24 h at 5 d intervals *Maintenance:* 1 mg/kg per 24 h, to a maximum of 50 mg/24 h	• Do not discontinue therapy abruptly • If daily dose is divided, the higher portion (up to 30 mg) should be taken at night
Clomipramine (Anafranil)	*Tablet:* 10 mg, 25 mg, 50 mg	*Children up to 12 yr old:* dose not established *Adolescents:* 20–30 mg p.o. per d; dose may be increased by 10 mg/d as needed and tolerated *Adults: Initial:* 25 mg t.i.d.; may increase to 150 mg daily or more as required and tolerated *Maintenance:* dose should be kept at lowest effective level	• Dosage must be individualized • Begin treatment at lowest recommended dose and increase gradually • Therapeutic response may not be seen for several days to a few weeks

Drug	Supplied	Dose	Comments
Clonazepam (Rivotril)	*Tablet:* 0.5 mg, 2 mg	*< 30 kg or < 10 yr:* *Initial:* 0.01–0.05 mg/kg per 24 h p.o. div. t.i.d. *Increment:* 0.25 mg/24 h p.o. at intervals of 5 d *Maintenance:* 0.1–0.2 mg/kg per 24 h p.o. div. t.i.d. *> 30 kg: Initial:* 0.5 mg/24 h p.o. div. t.i.d. *Increment:* 0.5 mg/24 h p.o. q5 d *Maximum dose:* 20 mg/24 h p.o.	• Dose should be increased gradually until seizures are controlled • Do not discontinue abruptly
Clonidine (Catapres)	*Tablet:* 0.025 mg, 0.1 mg, 0.2 mg	Hypertension: 5–25 μg/kg per 24 h p.o. div. q6h; allow 5–7 d between dose adjustments Attention deficit hyperactivity disorder: 3–8 μg/kg per 24 h div. q.i.d.	• If drug is discontinued, decrease dose over 2–4 d to avoid withdrawal syndrome which includes rebound hypertension; also used presurgically to potentiate opiate analgesic
Clotrimazole (Canesten)	*Topical cream:* 1% *Topical solution:* 1% *Vaginal tablet:* 100 mg *Vaginal cream:* 1%	Topical: Apply to skin b.i.d. Vaginal candidiasis: 1 tablet or l applicatorful per vagina daily × 6 d	
Cloxacillin (Tegopen, Orbenin)	*Capsule:* 250 mg, 500 mg *Oral liquid:* 25 mg/mL *Injection:* 500 mg, 1 g, 2 g/vial	Mild to moderate infections: 50–100 mg/kg per 24 h p.o., i.v. or i.m. div. q6h Severe infections: 150–200 mg/kg per 24 h i.v. or i.m. div. q6h *Adults:* 1–2 g/dose i.v. q6h	• Give p.o. on an empty stomach • Cephalexin is a better tasting alternative to p.o. cloxacillin
Codeine	*Tablet:* 15 mg, 30 mg *Oral liquid:* 5 mg/mL *Injection:* 30 mg/mL	Analgesia: 0.5–1 mg/kg per dose q4–6h i.m., s.c. or p.o. Maximum: 60 mg/dose Antitussive: *Children: 2–6 yr:* 2.5–5 mg/dose p.o. q4–6h p.r.n. Maximum: 30 mg/24 h *Children: 6–12 yr:* 5–10 mg/dose p.o. q4–6h p.r.n. Maximum: 60 mg/24 h	• Do not give i.v. • If maximum doses are used, risk of toxicity, particularly constipation, is increased

Drug	Supplied	Dose	Comments
Colistimethate (Coly-Mycin, Colistin)	*Injection:* 150 mg/vial	Via inhalation (for *Pseudomonas* infections in cystic fibrosis patients): 50–100 mg/dose b.i.d.–t.i.d. following physiotherapy	• Nephrotoxic when given systemically • Spectrum of activity is similar to polymixin • Injectable form is used for inhalation • Dilute with normal saline
Colonic lavage solution (Golytely, Oral colonic lavage solution)	*Solution:* 1,350 mL bottle	*Children:* 25–40 mL/kg per h p.o., nasogastric tube, or gastrostomy until fluid from rectum is clear (usually 4–10 h) *Adults:* 240 mL p.o. or nasogastric tube q10 min until 4–6 L is consumed	• Chilling makes it more palatable • Use with care and guidance in children with active small or large bowel disease or strictures
Cortisone acetate	*Tablet:* 5 mg, 25 mg *Injection:* 50 mg/mL	Physiological replacement: 15 mg/m² per 24 h p.o. div. q8h Minor stress: 2–4 × physiological replacement Anti-inflammatory: 2.5–10 mg/kg per 24 h p.o. div. q6–8h, 1–5 mg/kg per 24 h i.m. div. q12–24h	• i.m. absorbed slowly over several days • Not suitable for acute stress; use hydrocortisone parenterally
Cortisporin (Hydrocortisone–Neomycin–Polymyxin B compound)	Eye ointment Eye drops Ear drops	Eye ointment: Apply 0.5–1 cm 2–4 × daily Eye drops: 1 drop in conjunctival sac q3–4h Ear drops: 3–4 drops in ear t.i.d.–q.id.	
Cosyntropin (Cortrosyn)	*Injection:* 0.25 mg/mL	Verification of adrenal responsiveness: *Children < 2 yr:* 0.125 mg i.v. or i.m. *Children > 2 yr:* 0.25 mg i.v. or i.m.	• 0.25 mg cosyntropin = 25 unit ACTH

Drug	Supplied	Dose	Comments
Cotrimoxazole (Bactrim, Septra, TMP–SMX, Novo–Trimel)	*Tablet:* TMP 80mg/SMX 400 mg *Oral suspension:* TMP 8 mg/SMX 40 mg per mL *Injection:* TMP 16 mg/SMX 80 mg per mL	Mild to moderate infections: 8 mg TMP/40 mg SMX per kg per 24 h p.o. div. q12h (i.e. 1 mL/kg per 24 h p.o. div. q12h) Severe infections (*Pneumocystis carinii*): 20 mg TMP/100 mg SMX per kg per 24 h i.v. or p.o. div. q6h	• Use i.v. form only when p.o. form cannot be administered • 10 mL oral liquid = 1 tablet
Cromoglycate (Intal, Rynacrom)	*Spincap:* 20 mg (Intal) *Aerosol:* 1 mg/puff (Intal) *Respiratory solution:* 1% (20 mg/2 mL amp) (Intal) *Cartridges:* 10 mg (Rynacrom)	1 spincap or 1 ampoule or 10 puffs via inhalation q.i.d.; interval may be reduced to q8h or q12h when an adequate response has been obtained *Cartridges:* *Children > 5 yr to adults:* 1 cartridge via insufflator into each nostril q.i.d.	• Not for acute asthmatic attacks • Treatment should not be withdrawn abruptly unless substituted by inhaled steroid • Usually takes 4–6 wk before full effect is seen • Aerosol inhaler is an inefficient method of administration, requiring 10 puffs for an adequate dose
Cyclosporine (Sandimmune)	*Capsule:* 25 mg, 50 mg, 100 mg *Injection:* 50 mg/mL *Oral solution:* 100 mg/mL	Bone marrow transplant: 3–6 mg/kg per 24 h i.v. div. q8–12h, 10–15 mg/kg per 24 h p.o. div. q8–12h Renal transplant: 5–15 mg/kg per 24 h p.o. div. q8–12h	• The optimal dose and interval of cyclosporine has not been firmly established in pediatrics; these doses are guidelines only • Due to the erratic absorption of cyclosporine and the increased clearance rate of cyclosporine in infants and young children, cyclosporine levels should be monitored regularly to ensure that a therapeutic range is maintained

Drug	Supplied	Dose	Comments
Dantrolene	*Capsule:* 25 mg, 100 mg *Injection:* 20 mg/vial	Chronic spasticity: *Children > 5 yr:* *Initial:* 0.5 mg/kg per dose p.o. b.i.d. *Increment:* increase frequency to t.i.d.–q.i.d., then increase dose by 0.5 mg/kg *Maximum:* 3 mg/kg per dose p.o. b.i.d.–q.i.d. up to 400 mg/24 h Malignant hyperthermia: *Treatment:* 1 mg/kg i.v.; repeat p.r.n. up to a maximum cumulative dose of 10 mg/kg; then continue at 4–8 mg/kg per 24 h div. q.i.d. for 3 d	• Monitor transaminases to detect hepatotoxicity
Dapsone (Avlosulfon)	*Tablet:* 100 mg	Leprosy: *Children:* 1–2 mg/kg p.o. daily to a maximum of 100 mg daily *Adults:* 100 mg daily Prophylaxis of *Pneumocystis carinii:* *Children:* 1 mg/kg per 24 h p.o. once daily	• Perform frequent CBC with differential and platelet counts
Deferoxamine (Desferal)	*Injection:* 500 mg/vial, 2 g/vial	Chronic iron overload: 20–80 mg/kg per 24 h s.c. or i.v.; dose should be titrated based on iron stores and urinary iron excretion Acute iron overdose: Refer to Poison Manual	• Begin at lower end of dosage range for younger children • s.c. is the preferred route for most patients • i.v. administration may be preferred in patients with massive iron stores and significant organ damage or for patients who do not comply with s.c. infusions

Drug	Supplied	Dose	Comments
Desmopressin acetate (DDAVP)	*Injection:* 4 µg/mL *Nasal liquid:* 0.1 mg/mL *Nasal spray:* 10 µg/spray	Diabetes insipidus: > 3 mo to 12 yr: 5–30 µg/24 h intranasally div. daily or b.i.d. > 12 yr: 10–40 µg/24 h intranasally div. daily or t.i.d. Hemophilia A and von Willebrand's disease type I: *Children:* 0.2–0.4 µg/kg per dose by i.v. infusion, 2–4 µg/kg per dose intranasally Nocturnal enuresis: *Children: Initial:* 20 µg/dose intranasally 1 h before sleep; range 10–40 µg/dose	• Dose must be individualized • Parenteral dose is approximately 1/10 of the intranasal dose • Duration of effect is 8–12 h • For doses < 0.0125 mL, use the injectable form intranasally
Dexamethasone (Hexadrol, Decadron)	*Injection:* 4 mg/mL *Tablet:* 0.5 mg, 0.75 mg, 4 mg *Eye ointment:* 0.1% *Eye drops:* 0.1%	Cerebral edema: *Initial:* 0.5–1.5 mg/kg i.v. or i.m. *Maintenance:* 0.2–0.5 mg/kg per 24 h i.v. or i.m. div. q6h × 5 d, then taper Airway edema: 0.25–0.5 mg/kg per dose i.v. or i.m. q6h p.r.n. for croup or beginning 24 h before elective extubation, then × 4–6 doses Antiemetic: 2–4 mg/m² per dose i.v. or p.o. q6–12h Anti-inflammatory: 0.03–0.15 mg/kg per 24 h i.v., i.m. or p.o. div. q6–12h Meningitis: 0.15 mg/kg per dose i.v. q6h × 4 d Eye drops: 1–2 drops into conjunctival sac q3–6h depending on seriousness of the condition Eye ointment: 0.5–1 cm in the conjunctival sac t.i.d.–q.i.d. initially, then once to twice daily thereafter	• Well absorbed orally • Usual steroid effects

Drug	Supplied	Dose	Comments
Dextromethorphan (Delsym, DM)	*Syrup:* 15 mg/5 mL	*Children:* 1–2 mg/kg per 24 h div. t.i.d.–q.i.d. *Adults:* 60–120 mg/24 h div. t.i.d.–q.i.d.	• May cause nausea, drowsiness • Cough suppression may impair normal mechanism of pulmonary defense
Diavite (Vitamins B and C)	*Tablet*	< 10 yr: ½ tablet daily > 10 yr: 1 tablet daily	• Diavite contains proportions of vitamins suitable for renal patients to minimize potential problems of accumulation
Diazepam (Valium, Diazemuls)	*Tablet:* 2 mg, 5 mg, 10 mg *Injection:* 10 mg/2 mL amp *Injection (emulsion):* 10 mg/2 mL amp *Oral liquid:* 1 mg/mL	Sedative/muscle relaxant: 0.1–0.8 mg/kg per 24 h p.o. div. q6–8h Status epilepticus: 0.3 mg/kg per dose i.v. or 0.5 mg/kg per dose i.v. or p.r., dose may be repeated in 10 min if required *Maximum p.r. or i.v. dose:* 10 mg	• Give undiluted injection over 2 min • Do not mix with i.v. fluids • In status epilepticus, use also a longer acting anticonvulsant such as phenytoin
Diazoxide (Hyperstat, Proglycem)	*Capsule:* 50 mg *Liquid:* 50 mg/mL *Injection:* 15 mg/mL	Hypertensive crisis: *Infants and children:* 2–5 mg/kg per dose i.v. push, injected within 30 s; may repeat in 30 min and q2–4h p.r.n. *Maximum single dose:* 150 mg Hypoglycemia: *Infants:* 8–15 mg/kg per 24 h p.o. or i.v. div. q8–12h *Children:* 3–8 mg/kg per 24 h p.o. or i.v. div. q8–12h	• i.v. extravasation causes severe burning, pain, and inflammation • May cause flushing, hypotension, hyperglycemia • Monitor blood pressure every 1–5 min until stabilized and hourly thereafter
Diclofenac (Voltaren)	*Tablet:* 25 mg, 50 mg	*Adolescents:* dose not well established; 2–3 mg/kg per 24 h p.o. div. b.i.d.–q.i.d. has been used Rheumatoid arthritis: *Adults:* *Initial:* 75–150 mg/24 h in div. doses *Maintenance:* 75–100 mg/24 h in div. doses	• Take with food • Tablets are enteric coated and should be swallowed whole

Drug	Supplied	Dose	Comments
Diethylcarbamazine (Hetrazan)	*Tablet:* 50 mg	*Day 1:* 1 mg/kg p.o. × 1 dose *Day 2:* 1 mg/kg per dose p.o. t.i.d. *Day 3:* 1–2 mg/kg per dose p.o. t.i.d. *Day 4–21:* 6–9 mg/kg per 24 h div. t.i.d.	• If no microfilariae in blood, full doses can be given from day 1 • Headache, lassitude, weakness, or general malaise are common
Digoxin (Lanoxin)	*Tablet:* 0.0625 mg, 0.125 mg, 0.25 mg *Elixir:* 0.05 mg/mL *Injection:* 0.05 mg/mL (1 mL), 0.25 mg/mL (2 mL)	*Digitalizing dose:* Give q8h × 3 doses *Term infants–2 yr:* 17 µg/kg per dose p.o., 12 µg/kg per dose i.v. *> 2 yr:* 13 µg/kg per dose p.o., 10 µg/kg per dose i.v. *Maintenance dose:* Start 12 h after last digitalizing dose *Term infants–2 yr:* 10 µg/kg per 24 h p.o. once daily or div. q12h *> 2 yr:* 8 µg/kg per 24 h p.o. once daily or div. q12h	• May cause GI upset, poor feeding, failure to thrive, blurred vision, cardiac dysrhythmias • Toxicity is enhanced by hypokalemia, hypomagnesemia, hypercalcemia; monitor serum K^+, Mg^{2+}, Ca^{2+}, baseline ECG • Use i.m. only when i.v. or p.o. is not feasible (i.m. digoxin may cause local irritation, pain, and tissue damage) • Doses are based on normal renal function; reduce dose in patients with decreased renal function • i.v. dose is 0.75 × oral dose
Dimenhydrinate (Gravol, Dramamine)	*Tablet:* 50 mg *Syrup:* 3 mg/mL *Suppository:* 50 mg, 100 mg *Injection:* 10 mg/mL (i.v.), 50 mg/mL (i.m.)	*Children < 12 yr:* 5 mg/kg per 24 h p.o., i.m., i.v. or p.r. div. q4–6h p.r.n. *Adults:* 50–100 mg/dose q4–6h p.r.n. p.o., i.m. or i.v. *Maximum p.o. dose:* 2–6 yr: 75 mg/24 h 6–12 yr: 150 mg/24 h *Adults:* 400 mg/24 h *Maximum i.m. or i.v. dose:* 300 mg/24 h	• Drowsiness, dizziness, dry mouth • Irritation at injection site; rotate sites • Paradoxical excitement may occur
Dimercaprol (Bal in oil)	*Injection:* 200 mg/mL	Arsenic, copper, lead, or mercury poisoning: *Children and adults:* 3–5 mg/kg i.m. q4h for the first 2 d, then 3 mg/kg i.m. q6h for 2 d, then 3 mg/kg i.m. q12h for 10 d or until recovery is complete	• Urine must be alkaline • May cause hypertension, GI upset, tachycardia, headache, fever (symptoms can be relieved by antihistamine) • Administer by deep i.m. injection

Drug	Supplied	Dose	Comments
Dimetapp	*Tablet* *Tablet sustained action (extentabs)* *Liquid*	<u>Elixir and tablets:</u> *1–6 mo:* 1.25 mL p.o. t.i.d.–q.i.d. *7–24 mo:* 2.5 mL p.o. t.i.d.–q.i.d. *2–4 yr:* 3.75 mL (½ tablet) p.o. t.i.d.–q.i.d. *4–12 yr:* 5 mL (1 tablet) p.o. t.i.d.–q.i.d. *> 12 yr:* 5–10 mL (1–2 tablets) p.o. t.i.d.–q.i.d. <u>Extentabs:</u> *> 12 yr:* 1 extentab p.o. b.i.d.	• Contains brompheniramine, phenylephrine, and phenylpropanolamine • Give with caution in patients with cardiac disease, hypertension, or concurrent MAOI use; may cause increase in blood pressure
Diphenhydramine (Benadryl)	*Capsules:* 25 mg, 50 mg *Liquid:* 2.5 mg/mL *Injection:* 50 mg/mL (1 mL), 50 mg/mL (PLS)	*Children:* 5 mg/kg per 24 h p.o., i.v. or i.m. div. q6–8h *Maximum:* 300 mg/24 h *Adults:* 10–50 mg/dose p.o., i.v. or i.m. q6–8h *Maximum:* 400 mg/24 h <u>For anaphylaxis or phenothiazine overdose:</u> 1–2 mg/kg i.v. slowly	• Potentiates side effects of anticholinergics and other CNS depressants • Avoid subcutaneous or perivascular injections due to irritating effects
Diphenoxylate (Lomotil)	*Tablet:* 2.5 mg	*Children 2–12 yr:* 0.3–0.4 mg/kg per 24 h div. b.i.d.–q.i.d. *Adults:* 15–20 mg/24 h div. t.i.d.–q.i.d.	• Hepatic metabolism; use with caution in liver disease • Decreased intestinal motility may be detrimental in diarrhea caused by any bacterium or inflammatory bowel disease • Use of antidiarrheal agents in children may cause toxic megacolon and may conceal fluid losses into the gut lumen in diarrhea of any etiology; there are few indications for antidiarrheal drugs in children; use only under expert guidance. • Also see loperamide

Drug	Supplied	Dose	Comments
Dipyridamole (Persantine)	*Tablet:* 25 mg, 50 mg, 75 mg	*Children:* 3–6 mg/kg per 24 h p.o. div. t.i.d. *Adults:* 150–400 mg/24 h p.o. div. t.i.d.–q.i.d.	• May be administered along with ASA 10 mg/kg per 24 h as adjuvant for antiplatelet therapy • May cause excessive vasodilation; use with caution in patients with hypotension
Disopyramide (Norpace, Rythmodan)	*Capsule:* 100 mg, 150 mg	*p.o.:* *< 1 yr:* 10–30 mg/kg per 24 h p.o. div. q6h *1–4 yr:* 10–20 mg/kg per 24 h p.o. div. q6h *4–12 yr:* 10–15 mg/kg per 24 h p.o. div. q6h *12–18 yr:* 6–15 mg/kg per 24 h p.o. div. q6h *Adults:* 200–300 mg/dose p.o. × 1, then 400–800 mg/24 h p.o. div. q6h	• Some anticholinergic side effects may occur (dry mouth, urinary hesitancy)
Divalproex (Epival)	*Enteric coated tablet:* 125 mg, 250 mg, 500 mg	*Children:* *Initial:* 10 mg/kg per 24 h p.o. div. daily–t.i.d. *Increase by:* 5–10 mg/kg per 24 h at weekly intervals *Maintenance:* 20 mg/kg per 24 h div. daily–t.i.d. (monotherapy); higher doses (30–60 mg/kg per 24h) are often required in patients on polytherapy *Adults:* 1–3 g/24 h p.o. div. daily–t.i.d.	• Divalproex dissociates into valproic acid in the GI tract • Valproic acid affects phenobarbital, phenytoin, and carbamazepine serum concentrations which may be monitored when valproic acid is added • Therapeutic levels: 350–700 µmol/L
Dobutamine (Dobutrex)	*Injection:* 12.5 mg/mL 20 mL vial	*Infants, children, and adults:* 2–20 µg/kg per min continuous i.v. infusion	• Tachycardia, dysrhythmias, and hypertension may occur with larger doses • Correct hypovolemia before use

Drug	Supplied	Dose	Comments
Docusate (Colace)	Capsules: 100 mg Liquid: 4 mg/mL Drops: 10 mg/mL	Children: 5 mg/kg per 24 h p.o. div. once daily to q.i.d.	• p.o.: requires 1–3 d to effectively soften stools • p.r.: can be given rectally as enema to older children (add 50–100 mg of oral solution to enema fluid) • Do not administer concurrently with mineral oil as increased absorption of mineral oil may occur (docusate is a surfactant) • Diluting in milk or juice may help disguise bad taste
Domperidone (Motilium)	Tablet: 10 mg	Children: 0.6 mg/kg per dose p.o. t.i.d.–q.i.d. Adults: 10 mg p.o. t.i.d.–q.i.d. Maximum: 80 mg/24 h	• Give dose 15–30 min before meals and at bedtime • Cisapride is a more effective motility modifier
Donnatal	Elixir	Children up to 5 kg: 0.5 mL q4–6h 5–10 kg: 1 mL q4–6h 10–15 kg: 1.5 mL q4–6h 15–20 kg: 2.5 mL q4–6h 20–35 kg: 3.75 mL q4–6h 35–45 kg: 5 mL q4–6h > 45 kg: 5–10 mL q6–8h	• Each 5 mL of elixir = 1 tablet, which contains hyoscyamine sulfate 0.1037 mg, atropine sulfate 0.0194 mg, scopolamine hydrobromide 0.0065 mg, and phenobarbital 16.2 mg
Dopamine (Intropin)	Injection: 40 mg/mL, 5 mL PFS	Infants, children, and adults: 2–20 µg/kg per min continuous i.v. infusion Low dose: < 5 µg/kg per min (renal vasodilator) Medium dose: 5–10 µg/kg per min (increased heart rate and contractility) High dose: > 15 µg/kg per min (increased peripheral vasoconstriction, decreased renal blood flow)	• Correct hypovolemia before use • Avoid extravasation; this can cause tissue necrosis (antidote: phentolamine s.c. around site) • May cause tachydysrhythmias, ectopic beats, hypertension, vasoconstriction

Drug	Supplied	Dose	Comments
Dornase alfa (Pulmozyme)	*Ampoule for inhalation*: 2.5 mg/2.5 mL	*Cystic fibrosis patients ≥ 5 yr*: 2.5 mg by inhalation once daily	• Store in refrigerator • Safety and efficacy has not been established in patients < 5 yr, in patients with FVC < 40%, and when duration of treatment exceeds 1 yr
Droperidol (Inapsine)	*Injection*: 2.5 mg/mL (2 mL)	<u>Premedication</u>: *2–12 yr*: 0.1–0.15 mg/kg per dose i.m. or i.v. *> 12 yr*: 2.5–10 mg/dose i.m. or i.v. <u>Chemotherapy induced emesis</u>: *< 12 yr. Load*: 0.1–0.15 mg/kg i.m. or i.v. × 1 *Maintenance*: 0.05–0.1 mg/kg per dose i.m. or i.v. q4h *> 12 yr. Load*: 10 mg i.m. or i.v. × 1 *Maintenance*: 0.5–2.5 mg/dose i.m. or i.v. q4h	• Diphenhydramine 0.5–1 mg/kg per dose should be given with each dose of droperidol to prevent dystonic reactions when used to treat nausea and vomiting
Edrophonium (Tensilon)	*Injection*: 10 mg/mL	<u>Diagnosis of myasthenia gravis</u>: *Children*: Give 0.04 mg/kg initially as test dose; if no reaction within 1 min, give 1 mg increments to maximum of 10 mg *Adults*: 2 mg as test dose, then 8 mg after 45 s if no reaction	• May cause cholinergic crisis • Keep resuscitation equipment ready • Atropine may reverse bradycardia • Not recommended for treatment of myasthenia gravis due to short duration of action
Ephedrine	*Injection*: 50 mg/mL	<u>Hypotension</u>: *Children*: 3 mg/kg per 24 h i.v., i.m. or s.c. div. q4–6h *Adults*: 5–25 mg/dose i.v.; may repeat once after 5–10 min p.r.n., then q3–4h i.m. or s.c.: 25–50 mg q3–4h	

Drug	Supplied	Dose	Comments
Epinephrine (Adrenalin)	*Injection:* 1:1,000 amp (1 mg/mL), 1:10,000 PFS (0.1 mg/mL); also available with intracardiac needle; 1:1,000 multidose vial, 30 mL (1 mg/mL)	<u>Anaphylaxis:</u> Use 1:1,000 strength for s.c. 0.01 mL/kg per dose up to 0.3 mL s.c. and repeat q10 min for 3–4 doses <u>Cardiopulmonary resuscitation:</u> Use 1:10,000 strength i.v. 0.1 mL/kg i.v. q3–5 min <u>Inotropic agent or hypotension:</u> 0.05–1 µg/kg per min i.v. infusion	• For CPR, may be given by direct instillation into endotracheal tube or intraosseously • May cause necrosis upon injection • May cause tachycardia, dysrhythmias, hypertension, headaches, nervousness • Continuous i.v. infusion in critical care areas only
Epinephrine, racemic (Vaponephrin)	*Respiratory solution:* 2.25%	<u>Croup:</u> 0.5 mL diluted with 2 mL normal saline via nebulizer up to q1'h	• Tachyphylaxis can occur with repeated doses • To be administered by respiratory technologists
Erythromycin (E–Mycin, Erythrocin, Ilotycin, Eryc)	*Tablet:* 250 mg, "sprinkle caps" 250 mg (Eryc) *Suspension (estolate):* 50 mg/mL *Injection:* 500 mg/vial, 1 g/vial *Eye ointment:* 0.5%	<u>p.o.:</u> *Children:* 30–40 mg/kg per 24 h div. q8–12h *Adults:* 1–2 g/24 h <u>i.v.:</u> *Children:* 20–50 mg/kg per 24 h div. q6h *Adults:* 1–4 g/24 h <u>Topical:</u> *Eye infections:* 0.5–1 cm ribbon to affected eye(s) b.i.d.–q.i.d. <u>Prophylaxis of neonatal gonococcal infections:</u> 0.5–1 cm ribbon to each eye × 1	• p.o. estolate form is well absorbed, low GI irritation, and can be given after meals • Rapid i.v. administration causes severe vein irritation (infuse over 20–60 min) • Avoid i.m. route or extravasation • Perform liver function tests with prolonged high doses

Drug	Supplied	Dose	Comments
Erythropoietin (rHu-EPO, Eprex)	*Injection*	Renal failure: Initial: 50–100 unit/kg i.v. or s.c. 3 × weekly Titration: decrease by 25 unit/kg per dose when hematocrit reaches target range or increases by 6% in a 4 wk period; increase by 25 unit/kg per dose if hematocrit is below target range and has not increased by 5–6% after 8–12 wk of therapy HIV positive patients on zidovudine therapy: Initial: 100 unit/kg i.v. or s.c. 3 × weekly × 8 wk Titration: increase by 50–100 unit/kg per dose until hematocrit reaches target range	• Do not shake
Estrogens, conjugated (Premarin)	*Tablet:* 0.3 mg, 0.625 mg, 1.25 mg *Injection:* 25 mg/vial	Female hypogonadism: Doses are gradually increased throughout puberty; dose must be titrated to individual needs	• Consult endocrinologist before initiating therapy
Ethacrynic acid (Edecrin)	*Tablet:* 50 mg *Injection:* 50 mg/vial	Children: p.o.: 25 mg/dose daily; may increase in increments of 25 mg q2–3 d p.r.n. Maximum: 2–3 mg/kg q24 h i.v.: 1 mg/kg per dose; may repeat once in 1 h	• Maximum rate of injection is 10 mg over 1 min; too rapid injection may cause temporary or permanent deafness
Ethambutol (Myambutol)	*Tablet:* 400 mg	Children > 12 yr: 15–25 mg/kg per dose daily or 50 mg/kg per dose twice weekly Maximum: 2.5 g/dose	• Avoid use in children in whom visual acuity and color perception cannot be assessed • Commonly given concurrently with rifampin or other TB drugs

Drug	Supplied	Dose	Comments
Ethinyl estradiol (Estinyl)	*Capsule:* 1.25 µg, 2.5 µg, 5 µg, 7.5 µg, 10 µg *Tablet:* 50 µg	*Female hypogonadism:* Doses are gradually increased throughout puberty; dose must be titrated to individual needs	• Consult endocrinologist before initiating therapy
Ethosuximide (Zarontin)	*Capsule:* 250 mg *Syrup:* 50 mg/mL	*Children 3–6 yr.* *Initial:* 125 mg p.o. daily; increase by 125 mg/24 h at 4–7 d intervals *Maintenance:* 20 mg/kg per 24 h p.o. daily *Maximum:* 1,500 mg/24 h *Children > 6 yr.* *Initial:* 250 mg p.o. daily; increase by 250 mg/24 h at 4–7 d intervals *Maintenance:* 20 mg/kg per 24 h p.o. daily *Maximum:* 1,500 mg/24 h	• Therapeutic levels: 280–700 µmol/L • Mainly hepatic metabolism, t½ approximately 30 h in children and 60 h in adults
Fentanyl (Sublimaze)	*Injection:* 0.05 mg/mL 2 mL, 5 mL amp	*Infants > 3 mo and children:* 1–2 µg/kg per dose i.m. or i.v. q30–60 min p.r.n. *For use as continuous infusion:* 1–4 µg/kg per h (titrate to effect)	• Rapid i.v. injection may cause respiratory depression • Give dose over 3–5 min • The antidote for respiratory depression is naloxone 0.1 mg/kg per dose; repeat p.r.n. • 0.1 mg fentanyl i.v. = 10 mg morphine i.v.
Fluconazole (Diflucan)	*Tablet:* 100 mg *Injection:* 2 mg/mL	*Children > 3 yr.* 3–6 mg/kg per 24 h p.o. or i.v. once daily *Adults:* 100–200 mg p.o. or i.v. once daily	• Dose must be adjusted in renal impairment • Adverse effects include nausea, headache, skin rash, abdominal pain, vomiting and diarrhea • Much higher doses may be required for certain fungi (other than *Candida*)
Flucytosine (Ancotil, 5–FC)	*Capsule:* 500 mg, 100 mg/mL	*Children and adults:* 50–150 mg/kg per 24 h p.o. div. q6h	• Therapeutic levels: 25–100 mg/L • Use caution in patients with any impairment in renal function • Do not use as a single antifungal agent

Drug	Supplied	Dose	Comments
Fludrocortisone (Florinef)	*Tablet:* 0.1 mg	*Infants:* 0.05–0.1 mg/24 h p.o. daily *Children and adults:* 0.05–0.2 mg/24 h p.o. daily	• Titrate dose to suppress plasma renin activity to normal levels • Has primarily mineralocorticoid activity • Monitor BP; decrease dose if BP rises
Flumazenil (Anexate)	*Injection:* 0.1 mg/mL, 5 mL and 10 mL amp	*Pediatrics:* 10–25 µg/kg per dose i.v.; may repeat × 2 p.r.n. *Adults:* Initial: 0.2 mg i.v. over 15 s; may repeat 0.1 mg doses at 60 s intervals to a total dose of 1 mg	• Indicated for treatment of benzodiazepine overdose; not to be used routinely for reversal of benzodiazepine induced conscious sedation • Flumazenil has a short duration of action; repeat doses are often necessary • Patients must be closely monitored until all central benzodiazepine effects have subsided • Seizures may be induced in patients maintained on benzodiazepine therapy
Flunarazine (Sibelium)	*Capsule:* 5 mg	For prophylaxis of migraine headaches: *Children < 40 kg:* 5 mg p.o. at bedtime *Adults:* 5–10 mg p.o. at bedtime	• For prophylactic use only, not for acute attacks • Reduction in migraines may not be evident until 1–3 mo after therapy
Fluoride (Pedi-Dent)	*Drops:* 6.9 mg/mL	< 3 yr: not recommended 3–5 yr: 0.25 mg* p.o. daily ≥ 6 yr: 1 mg p.o. daily (* children who do not use fluoridated toothpaste regularly may be given 0.5 mg daily)	• Most children derive adequate fluoride from fluoridated toothpaste, foods, and drinks • Supplemental fluoride may result in fluorosis which manifests as white flecks on the teeth • Fluoride supplementation should only be given to children at high risk for dental caries • Approximately 1 mg fluoride ion per 8 drops
Fluorometholone (FML)	*Eye drops:* 0.1%	1 drop in eye(s) q3–6h, depending on severity of condition	• Shake well before using

Drug	Supplied	Dose	Comments
Fluoxetine (Prozac)	*Capsule:* 10 mg, 20 mg *Oral liquid:* 20 mg/5 mL	*Adolescents or adults:* *Initial:* 5–20 mg p.o. GAM *Increment:* Gradual dose increase after a trial period of several weeks if expected clinical improvement does not occur *Maximum:* 80 mg/24 h	• A selective serotonin re–uptake inhibitor (SSRI) used for depression, obsessive compulsive disorder, bulemia • It may take 4–5 wk to reach steady state plasma levels • "Wash out" period is approximately 6 wk due to long half–life and active metabolite
Fluphenazine (Moditen)	*Tablet:* 1 mg, 2 mg, 5 mg	Psychotic disorders: *Children:* 0.25–0.75 mg/dose p.o. 1–4 × daily *Adolescents and adults:* *Initial:* 2.5–10 mg/24 h p.o. div. q6–8h; dose may be gradually increased as needed and tolerated *Maintenance:* 1–5 mg/24 h p.o. as a single dose or in divided doses	• May cause dystonias, anticholinergic effects • Dose should be individually titrated to a favorable psychiatric response (within several days to several months) and that dosage continued for about 2 wk, then gradually decreased to the lowest effective maintenance dose
Fluvoxamine (Luvox)	*Tablet:* 50 mg, 100 mg	*Adolescents or adults:* *Initial:* 50 mg p.o. at bedtime *Increment:* 50 mg *Maximum:* 300 mg/24 h (doses > 150 mg should be divided)	• Selective serotonin re–uptake inhibitor (SSRI) • Do not give with MAO inhibitors • Allow a 2 wk "washout" of MAO inhibitor before starting fluvoxamine • Allow a 2 wk "washout" of fluvoxamine before starting MAO inhibitors
Folic acid (Folvite)	*Tablet:* 1 mg, 5 mg *Injection:* 5 mg/mL (10 mL)	*Folic acid deficiency:* *Children:* 0.5–1 mg/24 h p.o. daily *Adults:* 1–3 mg/24 h p.o. div. daily–t.i.d. *Maintenance:* < 1 yr: 30–45 µg/24 h 1–3 yr: 100 µg/24 h 4–6 yr: 200 µg/24 h 7–10 yr: 300 µg/24 h > 10 yr: 400 µg/24 h	• Will not prevent neurological abnormalities due to vitamin B_{12} deficiency, although the hematological effects may be masked • i.v. form can be given orally

Drug	Supplied	Dose	Comments
Furosemide (Lasix)	*Injection:* 10 mg/mL, 2 mL, 25 mL amp *PFS:* 40 mg/4 mL *Tablet:* 20 mg, 40 mg *Oral solution:* 10 mg/mL	*p.o. dose:* 1–2 mg/kg per dose q6–8h p.r.n. *Parenteral:* 0.5–1 mg/kg per dose q6–12h p.r.n. i.m. or i.v. *Maximum single dose:* 6 mg/kg per dose p.o., i.m. or i.v.; may be used by i.v. infusion in critical care areas; 0.1–1 mg/kg per h	• May cause hypokalemia, alkalosis, dehydration, hyperuremia, and increased calcium excretion • Ototoxicity may be associated with large i.v. doses and rapid injection, especially in patients with pre-existing renal impairment or who are taking other ototoxic drugs • Parenteral doses should be infused slowly over 1–3 min or given at a rate not to exceed 0.5 mg/kg per min
Fusidic acid (Fucidin, Sodium fusidate)	*Tablet:* 240 mg *Liquid:* 246 mg/5 mL *Injection:* 500 mg/vial *Cream:* 2% *Ointment:* 2%	<u>p.o.:</u> *Infants–1 yr:* 1 mL oral liquid/kg per 24 h p.o. div. t.i.d. *Children: 1–5 yr.* 5 mL oral liquid/dose p.o. t.i.d. *6–12 yr.* 10 mL oral liquid/dose p.o. t.i.d. *Adults:* 2 tablet/dose p.o. t.i.d. <u>i.v.:</u> *Children:* 20 mg/kg per 24 h i.v. div. q8h *Adults:* 500 mg i.v. q8h <u>Topical:</u> Apply to lesion 3–4 × daily until favorable results seen; may be used less frequently (1–2 × daily) if lesions are covered with gauze dressing	• GI intolerance may occur; administering doses with food may help • Tablets contain 250 mg sodium fusidate = 240 mg fusidic acid • Do not use as a single agent for serious staphylococcal infections as resistance may develop
Gabapentin (Neurontin)	*Capsule:* 10 mg, 300 mg, 400 mg	*Children:* not well established *Adults: Initial:* 300–400 mg daily *Increment:* 300 mg daily *Maintenance:* 900–1,800 mg/24 h div. t.i.d.	• Taper dose prior to discontinuation to prevent withdrawal seizures

Drug	Supplied	Dose	Comments
Ganciclovir (Cytovene)	*Injection:* 500 mg/vial	*Initial:* 10 mg/kg per 24 h i.v. div. q12h × 2–3 wk *Maintenance:* 5 mg/kg per 24 h i.v. once daily × 7 d/wk or 6 mg/kg per 24 h i.v. once daily × 5 d/wk	• Dose reduction required in renal impairment • Considered to be a potential teratogen and carcinogen in humans • Use chemotherapy precautions when handling or disposing
Gaviscon (Alginic acid compound)	*Chewable tablet* *Liquid*	*Children:* 0.5 mL/kg per dose p.o. up to q2h *Adults:* 10–20 mL of liquid or chew 2–4 tablets daily–q.i.d.	• Each 5 mL suspension contains: sodium alginate 250 mg plus aluminum hydroxide 100 mg (30 mg sodium/5 mL) • Each tablet contains: alginic acid 200 mg plus aluminum hydroxide 80 mg plus magnesium trisilicate 20 mg (22 mg sodium/tablet)
Gentamicin (Garamycin)	*Injection:* 10 mg/mL, 40 mg/mL *Eye ointment:* 0.3% *Eye/ear drops:* 0.3% *Topical ointment:* 0.1% *Topical cream:* 0.1%	i.v.: 7.5 mg/kg per 24 h i.m. or i.v. div. q8h *Maximum:* 300 mg/24 h Eye ointment: 0.5–1 cm ribbon to eye(s) b.i.d.–t.i.d. Eye drops: 1 drop to eye(s) q4h Topical: Apply a small amount of cream or ointment to lesion t.i.d.–q.i.d.	• Therapeutic serum levels: predose < 2 mg/L, postdose 6–10 mg/L
Glucagon	*Injection:* 1 mg/vial	Hypoglycemia: *Children:* 0.03–0.1 mg/kg per dose i.m., s.c. or i.v. q5–20 min *Maximum:* 1 mg/dose *Adults:* 0.5–1 mg/dose; repeat in 20 min p.r.n. *Maximum:* 1 mg/dose	• Do not delay initiation of glucose infusion while awaiting the effects of glucagon • 1 unit = 1 mg • Bolus glucagon therapy in idiopathic hyperinsulinism produces rebound hypoglycemia

Drug	Supplied	Dose	Comments
Glyburide (Diabeta, Euglucon)	*Tablet:* 5 mg	Must be individualized *Adults:* *Initial:* 5 mg p.o. daily; increase or decrease by 2.5 mg daily, depending on response *Maximum:* 20 mg/24 h	• Give dose with breakfast • If more than 10 mg/24 h is required, take excess with evening meal
Granulocyte colony stimulating factor (G–CSF, Filgrastim, Neupogen)	*Injection:* 300 µg/mL, 1 mL vials	*Adults and children:* 5 µg/kg per 24 h i.v. or s.c. for up to 14 d, or until ANC of 10,000/mm³; if inadequate response is seen, dose may be doubled in subsequent courses	• Endpoints of G–CSF therapy vary between different chemotherapy protocols • May cause bone pain, fever, and rash
Griseofulvin (Grisovin–FP)	*Tablet:* 250 mg fine particle	*Children:* 15 mg/kg per 24 h p.o. once daily	• Take with food; fat enhances absorption • Usual treatment is 3–6 wk; may extend to several months
Growth hormone (Somatropin = Humatrope, Somatrem = Protropin)	*Somatrem:* 5 mg/vial *Somatropin:* 5 mg/vial	0.18–0.3 mg/kg per wk s.c. or i.m. in 3–7 div. doses	• Somatropin is produced by a recombinant DNA process and has the same amino acid sequence as pituitary derived somatropin • Somatrem is also produced by a recombinant DNA process but differs from recombinant somatropin by the addition of an extra amino acid • Somatropin and somatrem are not interchangeable
Guaifenesin (Robitussin)	*Syrup:* 20 mg/mL	*Children: 2–6 yr:* 50–100 mg (2.5–5 mL) q4h *6–12 yr:* 100–200 mg (5–10 mL) q4h *> 12 yr:* 200–400 mg (10–20 mL) q4h	• Each 5 mL of raspberry flavored syrup contains guaifenesin 100 mg, alcohol 3.5%, sodium 1.96 mg, and sugar

Drug	Supplied	Dose	Comments
Haloperidol (Haldol)	*Tablet:* 0.5 mg, 1 mg, 2 mg, 5 mg *Solution:* 2 mg/mL *Injection:* 5 mg/mL–1 mL	*Children 3–12 yr.* Agitation: 0.01–0.03 mg/kg per 24 h p.o. daily Psychosis: 0.05–0.15 mg/kg per 24 h p.o. b.i.d.–t.i.d. Tourette's syndrome: 0.05–0.075 mg/kg per 24 h p.o. div. b.i.d.–t.i.d. *Children > 12 yr.* Acute agitation: 2–5 mg i.m. or 1–15 mg p.o.; repeat in 1 h p.r.n. Psychosis: 2–5 mg/dose i.m. q4–8h or 1–15 mg/24 h p.o. div. b.i.d.–t.i.d. *Maximum:* 100 mg/24 h Tourette's syndrome: 6–15 mg/24 h p.o. div. b.i.d.–t.i.d.	• Safety and efficacy have not been established in children < 3 yr • Extrapyramidal symptoms can occur
Heparin	*Injection:* 100, 1,000, and 10,000 unit/mL 1 and 2 mL amp, 1, 5, 10 mL vials	Anticoagulant: *Loading dose:* 75 unit/kg i.v. bolus *Initial maintenance:* ≤ 1 yr: 25 unit/kg per h > 1 yr: 20 unit/kg per h	• Adjust dose to maintain APTT in range of 1.5–2.5 times control • Major toxicities are bleeding, allergy, thrombocytopenia • Antidote is protamine sulphate 1 mg/100 unit heparin received in previous 4 h
Hydralazine (Apresoline)	*Tablet:* 10 mg, 25 mg, 50 mg *Injection:* 20 mg/mL–1 mL	Chronic hypertension: *Children:* 0.25–1 mg/kg per dose p.o. div. q6–8h *Maximum:* 7 mg/kg per 24 h (not to exceed adult dose) *Adults:* 10–75 mg p.o. q.i.d. Hypertensive crisis: *Children:* 0.1–0.5 mg/kg per dose i.m. or i.v. q6–8h *Adults:* 10–50 mg/dose i.m. or i.v. q3–6h p.r.n.	• Maximum effects with p.o. doses not achieved until after 3–4 d • i.v. hydralazine should be given slowly over 3–5 min

Drug	Supplied	Dose	Comments
Hydrochlorothiazide (HydroDiuril, HCTZ)	*Tablet:* 25 mg, 50 mg	*Infants < 6 mo:* 2–3 mg/kg per 24 h p.o. div. b.i.d. *Children:* 1–2 mg/kg per 24 h p.o. div. b.i.d. (not to exceed adult dose) *Adults:* 25–100 mg/dose p.o. daily	• Monitor serum electrolytes; may deplete potassium
Hydrocortisone (Cortef, Cortenema, Unicort, Hydrocortone, Solu–Cortef)	*Tablet:* 10 mg, 20 mg *Injection (as sodium succinate):* 100 mg/vial, 250 mg/vial, 500 mg/vial *Cream:* 0.5%, 1% *Ointment:* 0.5%, 1% *Eye ointment:* 2.5% *Retention enema:* 100 mg/60 mL *Suppository:* 10 mg, 25 mg	Anti-inflammatory: 0.8–4 mg/kg per 24 h i.v. or p.o. div. q6h Status asthmaticus: *Loading dose:* 4–8 mg/k per dose i.v. *Maintenance:* 2–4 mg/kg per dose i.v. q6h Acute adrenal insufficiency: *Loading dose:* 70 mg/m² per dose i.v., followed by 70 mg/m² per 24 h i.v. div. q4–6h, then wean to required maintenance Physiological replacement: 14–20 mg/m² per 24 h p.o. div. q8h *Topical:* Apply 2–3 times daily *Eye ointment:* Apply 0.5–1 cm into conjunctival sac t.i.d.–q.i.d.; may reduce frequency to daily or b.i.d. when favorable response is seen Enema: *Adults:* One 60 mL enema daily × 2–3 wk	• A corticosteroid with less mineralocorticoid activity is recommended for prolonged use • Usual steroid side effects • 4 mg hydrocortisone = 1 mg prednisone

Drug	Supplied	Dose	Comments
Hydroxychloroquine sulfate (Plaquenil)	*Tablet:* 200 mg (= 155 mg hydroxychloroquine base)	(Doses in terms of mg hydroxychloroquine base) *Children:* <u>Juvenile rheumatoid arthritis or SLE:</u> 3–5 mg/kg per 24 h p.o. daily–b.i.d. *Maximum:* 6 mg/kg per 24 h or 400 mg/24 h <u>Acute malaria attack:</u> 10 mg/kg p.o. initially, followed by 5 mg/kg p.o. 6 h after first dose, then 5 mg/kg p.o. 18 h after second dose, then 5 mg/kg p.o. 24 h after third dose <u>Malaria prophylaxis:</u> 5 mg/kg weekly	• Prophylactic dose should begin 1 wk before exposure and continue for 4 wk after leaving endemic area • Chronic use requires color vision and visual field monitoring every 6 mo
Hydroxyzine (Atarax)	*Capsules:* 10 mg, 25 mg *Syrup:* 2 mg/mL *Injection:* 50 mg/mL, 1 mL amp	<u>p.o.:</u> *Children:* 2 mg/kg per 24 h p.o. div. q6h *Adults:* 25–100 mg/dose t.i.d.–q.i.d. <u>Parenteral:</u> *Children:* 0.5–1 mg/kg per dose i.m. q4–6h p.r.n. *Adults:* 25–100 mg/dose i.m. q4–6h p.r.n.	• i.m. injections may produce local discomfort, erythema, sterile abscesses, and tissue necrosis • Not to be given by i.v. or s.c. routes
Hyoscine butylbromide (Buscopan)	*Tablet:* 10 mg *Injection:* 20 mg/mL	*Children:* 0.3 mg/kg per dose s.c., i.m., i.v. or p.o. q8h p.r.n. *Adults:* 10–20 mg/dose to a maximum of 100 mg/24 h	• A semi-synthetic derivative of scopalamine but doses are not equivalent (for hyoscine hydrobromide, see scopalamine) • Infants and children are more susceptible than adults to the adverse effects of anticholinergics
Ibuprofen (Motrin, Advil)	*Tablet:* 200 mg, 300 mg, 400 mg, 600 mg	<u>Antipyretic:</u> *Children:* 20 mg/kg per 24 h p.o. div. q8h <u>Juvenile rheumatoid arthritis:</u> 20–35 mg/kg per 24 h p.o. div. q8h <u>Anti-inflammatory:</u> *Adults:* 400–800 mg/dose p.o. q6–8h <u>Pain, fever, or dysmenorrhea:</u> 200–400 mg/dose q4–6h	• Use caution in patients with aspirin hypersensitivity • Take with food or milk to lessen GI upset

Drug	Supplied	Dose	Comments
Idoxuridine (Herplex, Stoxil)	*Eye ointment:* 0.5% *Eye drops:* 0.1%	Ointment: Apply 0.5–1 cm ribbon to eye(s) q4h (5 × daily); continue for 3–5 d after healing is complete Solution: One drop in eye(s) q1h during day and q2h at night until improvement is seen, then reduce daytime dose to 1 drop q2h and q4h at night	• May cause light sensitivity • Do not co-administer with boric acid containing solutions
Imipenem–Cilastatin (Primaxin)	*Injection:* 500 mg imipenem and 500 mg cilastatin per vial	*Children:* 40–60 mg/kg per 24 h i.m. or i.v. div. q6h *Maximum:* 500 mg q6h *Adults:* 1–4 g/24 h	• Cilastin blocks the metabolism of imipenem in the kidney • Dose must be reduced in renal failure
Imipramine (Tofranil)	*Tablet:* 10 mg, 25 mg, 50 mg	Antidepressant: *Children (> 6 yr): Initial:* 1.5 mg/kg per 24 h p.o. div. t.i.d.; increase by 1–1.5 mg/kg per 24 h q3–4 d *Maximum:* 5 mg/kg per 24 h Enuresis: *Children (> 6 yr): Initial:* 10–25 mg at bedtime (1 h prior to bedtime); increase by 10–25 mg/dose q1–2 wk until effect or maximum dose is achieved; continue optimal dose for 2–3 mo, then slowly taper	• Maximum dose for enuresis: age 6–12 yr: 50 mg/24 h age 12–14 yr: 75 mg/24 h • Serum levels and ECG's should be used to monitor patients
Indomethacin (Indocid)	*Capsule:* 25 mg, 50 mg *Sustained release capsule:* 75 mg *Suppositories:* 50 mg, 100 mg *Injection:* 1 mg/vial	Anti-inflammatory: *Children > 14 yr:* 1–3 mg/kg per 24 h p.o. div. t.i.d.–q.i.d. *Maximum:* 200 mg/24 h	• Take with food or milk to lessen GI upset • Up to 90% absorbed by rectal route • Use caution in patients with ASA allergy or impaired renal function • Sustained release capsule can be dosed once daily–b.i.d. after dosage is established with regular capsules

Drug	Supplied	Dose	Comments
Ipecac	*Syrup:* 15 mL	*Children 6–12 mo:* 10 mL p.o. *Children 1–12 yr:* 15 mL p.o. *Children > 12 yr:* 30 mL p.o. Repeat dose once in 20–25 min if no emesis occurs	• Follow each dose with 10–20 mL/kg of water; do not give milk or carbonated beverages • If emesis does not occur within 30 min after the second dose, gastric lavage should be performed
Ipratropium (Atrovent)	*Respiratory solution:* 0.025% (250 µg/mL): 20 mL bottle, 1 mL amp *Inhaler:* 20 µg/puff	*Inhaler:* *Children:* 4 puffs t.i.d.–q.i.d. *Respiratory solution:* *Children 5–12 yr:* 1 mL of solution diluted in 3 mL of normal saline and administer via nebulizer q4–6h p.r.n.	• Inhaler is used for maintenance therapy only, not for acute asthmatic attacks • Respiratory solution may be mixed with salbutamol in mask prior to treatment for acute asthma
Iron preparations [Ferrous gluconate (Fergon, Fertinic), Ferrous sulfate (Fer-In-Sol)]	Ferrous gluconate: *Tablet:* 300 mg (35 mg elemental Fe) *Syrup:* 60 mg/mL (7 mg elemental Fe); Ferrous sulfate: *Tablet:* 300 mg (60 mg elemental Fe) *Syrup:* 30 mg/mL (6 mg elemental Fe) *Drops:* 125 mg/mL (25 mg elemental Fe)	Iron deficiency anemia: 3–6 mg elemental Fe/kg per 24 h p.o. div. t.i.d. Prophylaxis: *Term infants and children:* 1–2 mg elemental Fe/kg per 24 h p.o. div. q8–24h *Maximum:* 15 mg/24 h elemental Fe *Adults:* 100 mg elemental Fe/24 h p.o. div. q12–24h	• Avoid tetracycline and antacids; may decrease iron absorption • Liquid iron may stain teeth; give with dropper or drink through a straw • Give with or after meals to decrease GI irritation
Iron sorbitol (Jectofer)	*Injection:* 50 mg Fe/mL, 2 mL amp	1.5 mg elemental Fe/kg per 24 h i.m., up to 2 mL (100 mg); this can be given daily or every other day until hemoglobin value reaches the normal range	• For i.m. use only • Inject using the Z-track injection technique

Drug	Supplied	Dose	Comments
Isoniazid (INH)	*Tablet*: 100 mg, 300 mg *Liquid*: 10 mg/mL	<u>Prophylaxis</u>: *Children*: 10 mg/kg per 24 h p.o. daily *Maximum*: 300 mg/24 h <u>Treatment</u>: (should not be used alone for treatment; combine with other antitubercular agents) *Children*: 10–20 mg/kg per 24 h p.o. daily. *Maximum*: 300 mg/24 h or 20–40 mg/kg per dose twice weekly (not more than 900 mg/dose)	
Isoproterenol (Isuprel)	*Injection*: 0.2 mg/mL–1 mL amp *Injection*: 1 mg/5 mL PFS	For use by continuous infusion in critical care areas <u>Chronotrope or inotrope</u>: 0.025–0.1 µg/kg per min <u>Bronchodilation</u>: 0.1–1 µg/kg per min	• May cause tachycardia, dysrhythmias, and hypertension, especially when combined with other inotropic agents
Itraconazole (Sporanox)	*Capsule*: 100 mg	*Children*: 3–5 mg/kg per 24 h p.o. once daily *Maximum*: 100 mg/24 h *Adults*: 100–400 mg p.o. daily	• Administer immediately after a full meal for maximal absorption • Less potential to interfere with cytochrome p450 enzyme system (compared to ketoconazole)
Ketamine (Ketalar)	*Injection*: 10 mg/mL, 50 mg/mL–10 mL vials	<u>Dissociative analgesic</u>: <u>i.v.</u>: 0.5–2 mg/kg per dose as undiluted injection over 1 min; may be given by continuous i.v. infusion in critical care areas; 20–40 µg/kg per min <u>Conscious sedation</u>: 10 mg/kg per dose p.o.	• Hypertension, tachycardia, respiratory depression, laryngospasm • May be combined with a benzodiazepine to prevent emergent reactions • Watch airway closely • Onset of sedation after an oral dose is 30–40 min

Drug	Supplied	Dose	Comments
Ketoconazole (Nizoral)	*Tablet:* 200 mg *Suspension:* 20 mg/mL	*Children > 2 yr:* 5–10 mg/kg per 24 h p.o. daily or div. b.i.d. *Adults:* 200–400 mg/24 h p.o. daily	• A potent inhibitor of the cytochrome p450 enzyme system; concomitant use with drugs metabolized by this system (especially astemizole, terfenidine, cisapride) will result in increased plasma concentrations of these drugs and possibly increased incidence of adverse effects • Administration with food will decrease GI upset but may also decrease drug absorption • Do not administer with antacids
Ketoralac (Toradol)	*Injection:* 30 mg/mL	*Children/adolescents:* *Loading dose:* 1 mg/kg i.v. *Maintenance:* 0.5 mg/kg per dose i.v. q6h p.r.n. or 0.3–0.5 mg/kg per dose i.m. q6h p.r.n. *Maximum:* 30 mg/dose	• Ketoralac is a nonsteroidal anti-inflammatory agent (NSAID) and therefore has the potential to cause nausea, GI toxicity, and inhibition of platelet function
Labetolol (Trandate)	*Injection:* 5 mg/mL, 20 mL amp	0.2–1 mg/kg per dose i.v. over 2 min; may be repeated at 10 min intervals until desired BP has been achieved or a total of 4 mg/kg has been given; 0.25–1.5 mg/kg per h by continuous i.v. infusion Maximum infusion rate: 4 mg/kg per h	• Can cause postural hypotension • Contraindicated in asthma or bronchospasm, > 1° heart block, cardiogenic shock, severe bradycardia, uncontrolled CHF • To be given in critical care areas only
Lactulose (Cephulac)	*Syrup:* 667 mg/mL	Laxative or portal systemic encephalopathy (PSE): *Infants:* 2.5–10 mL/24 h p.o. div. t.i.d.–q.i.d. *Children:* 40–90 mL/24 h p.o. div. t.i.d.–q.i.d. *Adults:* 30–40 mL/dose p.o. t.i.d.–q.i.d. For hepatic coma, adjust dose daily to produce watery diarrhea	• Laxative onset within 12–24 h • Use with caution in diabetics due to the lactose and galactose released from drug • May cause flatulence, abdominal distension, and discomfort

Drug	Supplied	Dose	Comments
Leucovorin (Folinic acid, Citrovorum factor)	*Tablet:* 5 mg *Injection:* 3 mg/mL (1 mL), 50 mg/vial	Adjunctive with antimicrobials (e.g. trimethoprim): 2–15 mg/24 h p.o. daily × 3 d or until blood counts are normal; minimum of 6 mg/24 h required for patients with platelet counts < 100,000/mm^3 Rescue dose after methotrexate: 10 mg/m^2 per dose p.o. or i.v. q6h × 72 h; start within 24 h of methotrexate administration; if serum creatinine is increased by > 50% above the pretreatment level 24 h after methotrexate administration, increase leucovorin dose to 100 mg/m^2 per dose q3h until serum methotrexate is < 5 × 10^{-8} molar	• Hematological effects of vitamin B$_{12}$ deficiency may be masked with the administration of leucovorin, but neurological abnormalities will not be prevented
Levothyroxine sodium (Eltroxin, Synthroid, Thyroxine, T$_4$)	*Tablet:* 0.025 mg, 0.05 mg, 0.10 mg, 0.15 mg, 0.20 mg *Injection:* 500 µg/vial	p.o.: *Infants and children:* 100 µg/m^2 per dose once daily i.v.: *Infants and children:* give 75% of oral doses recommended above	• Doses should be titrated to obtain normal serum T$_4$ and TSH levels as well as a clinically euthyroid state • Very unstable in solution; if oral liquid must be given, administer dose immediately after mixing
Lidocaine, systemic (Xylocaine)	*Injection:* 1% (20 mg/2 mL) 20 mL vial, 2% (100 mg/5 mL) PLS, 5 mL amp, 20 mL vial, 20% (1 g/5 mL) PLS, 1 g/250 mL D5W bag	Anti-arrhythmic: *Loading dose:* 1 mg/kg per dose by slow i.v. or endotracheal injection; may repeat q5–10 min up to 5 mg/kg *Continuous infusion:* 20–50 µg/kg per min Head injury protocol: 1 mg/kg per dose by rapid (over 1–2 s) i.v. injection; wait 2 min before suctioning endotracheal tube Endoscopy: 1–1.5 mg/kg per dose i.v. to prevent coughing and laryngospasm during passage of endoscope	• Monitor to maintain drug levels in therapeutic range of 4.5–21 µmol/L • Decrease dose in presence of hepatic or renal failure or CHF • Toxicity includes seizures, anxiety, euphoria, drowsiness, agitation, hypotension, heart block, cardiovascular collapse

Drug	Supplied	Dose	Comments
Lidocaine, topical (Xylocaine, Xylocaine viscous)	*Jelly:* 2% *Jelly:* 2% urological syringe *Ointment:* 5% *Viscous:* 2% *Topical solution:* 4% *Endotracheal spray:* 10%	*Lidocaine 2% jelly:* Used for surface anesthesia and lubrication (e.g. for urethral catheter insertion) *Lidocaine 5% ointment:* Used for temporary relief of pain associated with minor burns and abrasions of the skin *Lidocaine 2% viscous:* Used to provide relief of pain and discomfort of the mouth and pharynx *Children > 3 yr:* 5 mL gargled and may be swallowed q3h *Children < 3 yr:* 1.25 mL applied with a cotton swab q3h	• Topical anesthesia in the mouth may impair swallowing and thus enhance the danger of aspiration; food should not be ingested for 60 min following the use of lidocaine in the mouth or throat • Significant systemic absorption does not occur with normal topical use but amount absorbed increases as the surface area and frequency of application increases
Lindane (Kwellada, gBH, Gamma benzene hexachloride)	*Lotion:* 1% *Shampoo:* 1%	*Lotion:* Apply liberally to affected areas; leave on 6–12 h; wash thoroughly; repeat in 4 d if necessary *Shampoo:* Massage thoroughly into the hair; leave in place for 4–10 min before rinsing and drying; repeat in 7 d if necessary; remaining nits should be removed with a fine comb	• Avoid use in children < 2 yr due to risk of toxic effects from systemic absorption • Avoid contact with eyes, nose, mouth and other mucous membranes • Itchiness due to scabies may persist for 2 wk even when treatment has been successful • Permethrin is the drug of choice for the treatment of scabies in infants and young children
Lithium carbonate (Lithane, Carbolith)	*Capsule:* 150 mg, 300 mg	*Children:* *Initial:* 15–60 mg/kg per 24 h p.o. div. t.i.d.–q.i.d. *Maintenance:* adjust p.r.n. to achieve therapeutic levels *Adults:* *Initial:* 300 mg p.o. t.i.d. *Maintenance:* adjust p.r.n. to achieve therapeutic levels	• Therapeutic levels: 0.6–1.2 mEq/L • Increased sodium intake will decrease lithium levels • Obtain levels twice weekly until patient is clinically stable; then obtain levels every 1–2 mo

Drug	Supplied	Dose	Comments
Loperamide (Imodium)	*Capsule:* 2 mg *Liquid:* 0.2 mg/mL	<u>Acute diarrhea:</u> *Children:* 0.4–0.8 mg/kg per 24 h p.o. div. q6–12h until diarrhea resolves *Maximum:* 7 d <u>Chronic diarrhea:</u> *Children:* 0.08–0.24 mg/kg per 24 h div. b.i.d.–t.i.d. *Maximum:* 2 mg/dose	• Use of antidiarrheal agents in children may cause toxic megacolon and may conceal fluid losses into the GI tract in diarrhea of any etiology • There are few indications for antidiarrheal drugs in children; use only under expert guidance • Also see diphenoxylate
Lorazepam (Ativan)	*Sublingual tablet:* 0.5 mg, 1 mg, 2 mg *Injection:* 4 mg/mL (1 mL)	<u>Anxiolytic:</u> 0.05 mg/kg per dose q4–8h p.o. or sublingually <u>Premedication:</u> 0.05 mg/kg per dose sublingually or i.m. 2 h before procedure *Maximum:* 4 mg/dose <u>Status epilepticus:</u> *Infants and children:* 0.05 mg/kg per dose p.r. or i.v. *Maximum:* 4 mg/dose; may repeat once in 15–20 min	• Injectable products may be given rectally, but p.r. absorption is erratic and may be incomplete • Sublingual tablets dissolve in about 20 s; patients should not swallow for at least 2 min to allow time for absorption • Sublingual tablets can be given orally
Loxapine (Loxapac)	*Oral solution:* 25 mg/mL *Tablet:* 5 mg, 10 mg, 25 mg *Injection:* 50 mg/mL	*Adolescents/adults:* *Initial:* 5–10 mg p.o. b.i.d. *Increment:* Increase over 7–10 d to effective control of psychotic symptoms *Maximum:* 100–200 mg/24 h in 2–4 div. doses *Usual i.m. dose:* 12.5–50 mg/dose q4–6h	• High potency antipsychotic • Causes a high incidence of extrapyramidal symptoms, moderate sedation, moderate effect on the cardiovascular system and a low incidence of anticholinergic side effects • 10 mg p.o. loxapine approximately = 100 mg chlorpromazine or 2 mg haloperidol

Drug	Supplied	Dose	Comments
Magnesium/Aluminum hydroxide (Gelusil, Diovol, Maalox)	*Tablet* *Liquid* *Liquid plus* (contains simethicone)	*Children:* Tablet: chew ½–1 tablet 20 min to 1 h after meals and at bedtime Suspension: 0.5 mL/kg per dose, up to 5–10 mL 20 min to 1 h after meals and at bedtime *Adults:* Tablet: chew 1–2 tablets 20 min to 1 h after meals and at bedtime Suspension: 10–20 mL 20 min to 1 h after meals and at bedtime	• Suspensions may be mixed with water or milk • Can interfere with the absorption of iron preparations and tetracyclines
Magnesium citrate (CitroMag)	*Solution:* 15 g/300 mL	*Children:* 4 mL/kg per dose p.o.; repeat q4–6h until liquid stool results *Maximum dose:* 200 mL *Adults:* 240 mL p.o. daily p.r.n.	• Up to 20% absorbed • Onset of action 0.5–3 h • Serve chilled • Give with plenty of water
Magnesium sulfate	*Injection:* 50% (500 mg/mL)–10 mL	*Hypomagnesemia or hypocalcemia:* *i.m. or i.v.:* 25–50 mg/kg per dose q4–6h × 3–4 doses, repeat p.r.n. *Maintenance:* i.v.: 30–60 mg/kg per 24 h i.v.	• Each mL contains 500 mg magnesium sulfate = 4 mEq Mg (2 mmol) • Use with caution in renal failure • Rapid i.v. administration may cause arrhythmias, hypotension, respiratory, and CNS depression • Maximum infusion rate: 1 mEq/kg per h
Magnesium supplements (oral) (Magnesium Rougier, Magnesium glucoheptonate, Magnesium gluconate)	*Oral solution:* 10% (Rougier) *Tablet:* 500 mg (gluconate)	*Children:* 3–6 mg elemental Mg/kg per 24 h p.o. div. t.i.d.–q.i.d. *Maximum:* 400 mg/24 h *Adults:* 200–400 mg elemental Mg/24 h p.o. div. t.i.d.–q.i.d.	• Each mL of solution contains 100 mg magnesium glucoheptonate = 5 mg elemental Mg = 0.21 mmol Mg = 0.4 mEq Mg • Each tablet contains: 29 mg elemental Mg = 1.2 mmol Mg = 2.4 mEq Mg • Large doses may cause diarrhea • Use with caution in renal failure

Drug	Supplied	Dose	Comments
Magnolax (Magnesium hydroxide plus mineral oil)	*Suspension*	*Infants and children:* 1.25–10 mL p.o. once daily *Adults:* 7.5–15 mL p.o. once daily	• May interfere with the absorption of iron preparations or tetracycline antibiotics • Each mL contains 60 mg of magnesium hydroxide
Mannitol	*Injection:* 25%–50 mL	*Anuria/oliguria:* (test dose) 0.2 g/kg per dose i.v. over 3–5 min; discontinue if no diuresis within 2 h *Cerebral edema:* 0.25 g/kg i.v. push; repeat q5 min p.r.n.; may increase gradually to 1 g/kg per dose if necessary	• 25% mannitol contains 25 g in 100 mL = 250 mg/mL • May give furosemide concurrently or 5 min before mannitol for cerebral edema • May cause circulatory overload, electrolyte disturbances, hypovolemia
Mebendazole (Vermox)	*Chewable tablet:* 100 mg	*Children >2 years and adults:* 100–200 mg p.o. b.i.d. × 3–20 d	• Dose and duration of treatment depend upon parasite being treated
Medroxypro–Gesterone acetate (Provera, Depo–Provera)	*Tablet:* 5 mg, 10 mg *Injection:* 100 mg/mL	Modulation of the menstrual cycle: 5–10 mg/24 h p.o. × 7–14 d of each menstrual cycle	• Depo–Provera is for i.m. injection only
Meperidine (Demerol, Pethidine)	*Tablet:* 50 mg *Injection:* 50 mg/mL, 75 mg/mL	p.o., i.m., i.v or s.c.: *Children:* 1–1.5 mg/kg per dose q3–4h p.r.n.; maximum 100 mg/dose *Adults:* 50–150 mg/dose q3–4h p.r.n.	• 75 mg i.v. meperidine = 10 mg i.v. morphine; use with caution in renal failure: metabolite of meperidine has CNS effects (tremors, seizures)
Methotrimeprazine (Nozinan)	*Tablet:* 5 mg *Oral liquid:* 5 mg/mL *Injection:* 25 mg/mL	*Children: Initial:* 250 µg/kg per 24 h p.o. div. b.i.d.–t.i.d.; increase gradually as needed to a maximum of 40 mg/24 h; 62.5–125 µg/kg per 24 h i.m. in single or div. doses *Adults:* 6–25 mg/24 h p.o. div. t.i.d.; increase gradually as needed; in severe cases, begin with 50–75 mg/24 h p.o. div. b.i.d.–t.i.d. Psychosis or severe pain: 75–100 mg/dose i.m. q6–8h p.r.n. Premedication prior to surgery or postoperative analgesia: 10–25 mg i.m. q8h	• Dosage should be adjusted according to condition being treated and patient's individual requirements • Excessive daytime sedation may be resolved by lowering daytime dose and increasing bedtime dose

Drug	Supplied	Dose	Comments
Methyldopa (Aldomet)	*Tablet:* 125 mg, 250 mg *Injection:* 50 mg/mL	*Children:* i.v.: 5–10 mg/kg per dose q6–8h Maximum: 65 mg/kg per 24 h p.o.: Initial: 10 mg/kg per 24 h div. q6–12h; increase by 5–10 mg/kg per 24 h p.r.n. q2 d Maximum: 65 mg/kg per 24 h *Adults:* i.v.: 250–1,000 mg q6–8h p.o.: 250–750 mg q6–12h	• i.v. use for hypertensive crises only (other agents are preferred) • May require 7 d to achieve maximum effects with p.o. use
Methylphenidate (Ritalin)	*Tablet:* 10 mg *Sustained release tablet:* 20 mg	Attention deficit hyperactivity disorder: *Children > 6 yr: Initial:* 0.3 mg/kg per dose p.o. b.i.d. *Increment:* if tolerated, increase by 0.1 mg/kg per dose at weekly intervals until maintenance dose is reached *Maintenance:* 1–2 mg/kg per 24 h *Maximum dose:* 60 mg/24 h or 2 mg/kg per 24 h	• Discontinue use if no improvement is seen within 1 mo • Give as a single dose in the morning or as divided doses with breakfast and lunch
Methylprednisolone (Medrol, Depo–Medrol, Solu–Medrol)	*Tablet:* 4 mg *i.m. Depo injection:* 40 mg/mL (acetate) *i.m. or i.v. injection:* 40 mg/vial, 125 mg/vial, 500 mg/vial, 1 g/vial (sodium succinate)	Anti-inflammatory or immunosuppressive: 0.16–0.8 mg/kg per 24 h p.o. or i.v. div. q6–12h Status asthmaticus: *Children:* Load: 1–2 mg/kg per dose i.v. × 1 *Maintenance:* 0.5–1 mg/kg per dose i.v. q6h *Adults:* 10–250 mg/dose q4–6h i.v. or i.m. "Pulse therapy:" Up to 30 mg/kg per 24 h i.v. × 1–3 d may be given for various conditions (e.g. polyarticular and systemic juvenile arthritis, SLE, severe glomerular nephritis, and dermatomyositis)	• Acetate form may be used for intra-articular or intralesional injection • 4 mg methylprednisolone = 5 mg prednisone

Drug	Supplied	Dose	Comments
Metoclopramide (Maxeran, Reglan)	*Tablet:* 5 mg, 10 mg *Injection:* 5 mg/mL (2 mL, 10 mL) *Liquid:* 1 mg/mL	GI hypomotility and GE reflux: *Children (i.v., p.o. or i.m.):* 0.2–0.4 mg/kg per 24 h div. q.i.d. *Maximum:* 0.5 mg/kg per 24 h *Adults:* 10 mg/dose q.i.d. Chemotherapy induced nausea and vomiting: (when given in high doses, administer diphenhydramine, 1 mg/kg per dose, concurrently to prevent dystonic reactions) 1–2 mg/kg per dose q2–6h i.v. *Maximum:* 10 mg/kg per 24 h	• Cisapride is a more efficacious agent for hypomotility and GE reflux; cisapride does not act on the CNS and has fewer side effects • Chronic tardive dyskinesia has been described with use of metoclopramide for longer than 3–6 mo • Parenteral metoclopramide may be used to facilitate passage of GI tubes or pre- or postanesthesia for nausea and vomiting
Metolazone (Zaroxolyn)	*Tablet:* 2.5 mg, 5 mg	*Children:* 0.2–0.4 mg/kg per 24 h p.o. div. daily–b.i.d. *Adults:* Edema: 5–20 mg/24 h Hypertension: 2.5–5 mg/24 h	• Concurrent administration of metolazone and furosemide may cause excessive electrolyte depletion; use caution when both are used together
Metoprolol (Betaloc, Lopresor)	*Tablet:* 50 mg, 100 mg	*Children:* 1–5 mg/kg per 24 h p.o. div. b.i.d. *Adults: Initial:* 50 mg p.o. b.i.d.; increase at weekly intervals to 100–450 mg/24 h div. b.i.d.–t.i.d.	• Allow at least 3 d between dose adjustments
Metronidazole (Flagyl)	*Tablet:* 250 mg *Injection:* 5 mg/mL (100 mL) *Vaginal insert:* 500 mg *Vaginal cream:* 10%	p.o.: 15–35 mg/kg per 24 h p.o. div. q8h i.v.: 30 mg/kg per 24 h i.v. div. q6–8h *Clostridium difficile:* 20 mg/kg per 24 h i.v. or p.o. div. q6h *Vaginal therapy:* One insert or 1 applicator PV nightly × 10–20 d	• Avoid alcohol containing preparations for 24 h after dose to prevent disulfuram–like reactions • May be used i.v. or p.o. for *Clostridium difficile* infections • Well absorbed orally
Miconazole (Micatin, Monistat)	*Topical cream:* 2% *Vaginal cream:* 2%	*Topical:* apply to affected area b.i.d. for 2–4 wk *Vaginal:* insert contents of one applicator of vaginal cream at bedtime × 7 d	

Drug	Supplied	Dose	Comments
Midazolam (Versed)	*Injection:* 5 mg/mL 1 mL vial, 10 mL vial	*Preoperative sedation:* 0.08 mg/kg i.m. 30–60 min prior to surgery, 0.5–1 mg/kg per dose p.o. 20–60 min prior to surgery *Maximum:* 20 mg/dose *Intranasal:* 0.2 mg/kg per dose; onset of action: 10 min *Conscious sedation:* 0.1 mg/kg i.v. over 2–3 min; may repeat dose × 3 at 2 min intervals *Maximum total dose:* 8 mg Sedation in ICU by continuous *infusion:* 1–6 µg/kg per min; lower dose by 25% when used with narcotics	• Rapid, direct i.v. administration is associated with respiratory depression, apnea and hypotension • Avoid the use of midazolam in patients with unstable hemodynamics, especially after cardiac surgery; close cardiorespiratory monitoring is required • Be prepared to resuscitate • Injection may be used orally, may be mixed with apple juice or Kool–Aid • Patients receiving midazolam for conscious sedation should have pulse oximetry in place for at least 1 h after administration • Risk of respiratory depression increases when used in combination with narcotics
Minoxidil (Loniten)	*Tablet:* 2.5 mg, 10 mg	*Children:* 0.2–1 mg/kg per 24 h p.o. div. daily–b.i.d.; start with small doses and increase slowly at intervals of not < 3 d *Adults:* start with 5 mg/24 h daily, doubling the dose until blood pressure is controlled *Maximum:* 100 mg/24 h	• Full effects are not usually seen within 3–7 d • Effects on blood pressure may persist for up to 75 h • Must be given with a β-blocker and a diuretic to minimize reflex tachycardia and fluid retention
Moclobemide (Manerix)	*Tablet:* 100 mg, 150 mg	*Adolescents or adults:* *Initial:* 100 mg p.o. t.i.d. *Increment:* increase gradually to clinical effect; usual dose is 450 mg/24 h *Maximum:* 600 mg/24 h	• A reversible inhibitor of monamine oxidase • Less tyramine potentiation compared to older MAO inhibitors, but should be taken after meals to minimize risk of hypertensive response to dietary tyramine • Cimetidine significantly increases serum concentrations of moclobemide
Mometasone (Elocom)	*Scalp lotion:* 0.1%, 30 mL	Apply a few drops to affected skin and/or scalp sites once daily	• Massage lotion gently into skin or scalp until lotion disappears

Drug	Supplied	Dose	Comments
Morphine (M-Eslon, MOS)	*Oral solution:* 1 mg/mL, 5 mg/mL *Injection:* 2 mg/mL, 10 mg/mL, 15 mg/mL, 100 mg/4 mL, 500 mg/5 mL amp *Injection (no preservative):* 5 mg/5 mL amp *Capsule sustained release:* 10 mg, 30 mg, 60 mg, 100 mg	*Infants 1–12 mo:* *Intermittent:* 0.04–0.1 mg/kg per dose q4h i.m. or s.c. *Continuous infusion:* *Infants > 3 mo:* 0.01–0.05 mg/kg per h *Children > 1 yr:* *Intermittent:* i.v., s.c. or i.m. 0.05–0.2 mg/kg per dose q3–4h *Infusion:* 0.02–0.06 mg/kg per h average dose; higher doses may be required especially in palliative care situations *p.o.:* 0.15–0.6 mg/kg per dose p.o. q3–4h	• Respiratory depression is a risk in nonventilated patients; monitor ventilation and be prepared to assist • Antidote for narcotic overdose is naloxone 0.1 mg/kg per dose i.v. or i.m. p.r.n. • For patients being converted from parenteral to oral, p.o. dose is 3 × i.v. dose • Contents of slow release capsules may be mixed with soft foods
Mupirocin (Bactroban)	*Ointment:* 2%	Apply a small amount to affected area t.i.d.	• Due to cost, mupirocin should not be used when polysporin would suffice
Muromonab–CD3 (Orthoclone OKT3)	*Injection:* 5 mg/5 mL	< 30 kg: 2.5 mg i.v. daily × 10–14 d > 30 kg: 5 mg i.v. daily × 10–14 d	• The optimal dose and duration of OKT3 has not been established in pediatrics • These doses are guidelines only
Nabilone (Cesamet)	*Capsule:* 1 mg	*Children:* < 18 kg: 0.5 mg p.o. q8–12h ≥ 18 kg: 1 mg p.o. q8–12h *Adults:* 1–2 mg p.o. b.i.d. *Maximum:* 2 mg p.o. t.i.d.	• Give the first dose the night before chemotherapy and continue for up to 48 h after chemotherapy
Naloxone (Narcan)	*Injection:* 0.4 mg/mL, 1 mg/mL	Reversal of narcotic induced respiratory depression: *Children < 20 kg:* 0.01–0.1 mg/kg per dose i.m., i.v. or s.c.; repeat p.r.n. q3–5 min *Children ≥ 20 kg:* 2 mg/dose; repeat p.r.n. q3–5 min Continuous infusion to prevent itching or urinary retention during epidural morphine administration: 0.001 mg/kg per h (= 1 µg/kg per h)	• Short duration of action (1–4 h), may require multiple doses

Drug	Supplied	Dose	Comments
Naproxen (Naprosyn, Anaprox)	*Tablet:* 125 mg, 250 mg (Naprosyn) *Tablet:* 275 mg (Anaprox) *Suspension:* 25 mg/mL *Suppository:* 500 mg	*Children:* Analgesic: 10 mg/kg per dose p.o. or p.r. b.i.d. Juvenile rheumatoid arthritis: 15 mg/kg per 24 h p.o. or p.r. div. b.i.d. Maximum: 1 g/24 h *Adults:* Analgesic: 500–1,250 mg/24 h p.o. b.i.d. Dysmenorrhea: 500 mg/dose × 1, then 250 mg/dose p.o. q12h	• Take with food to avoid GI upset • Avoid in patients who have had asthma reactions (bronchoconstriction) from ASA; may cross-react with aspirin • Suppositories should be dosed to the nearest 250 mg • May cause photosensitive vesicular rash (pseudoporphyria)
Neo-Cortef	*Topical ointment:* 0.5%, 1% (containing neomycin 0.5% and hydrocortisone 0.5% or 1%)	*Topical ointment:* A small amount rubbed gently into affected area q8–24h	• Topical neomycin may induce contact dermatitis
Neomycin (Mycifradin, Myciguent)	*Tablet:* 500 mg *Oral solution:* 25 mg/mL *Ointment:* 0.5%	Enteropathogenic *E. coli* diarrhea: *Infants, children and adults:* 100 mg/kg per 24 h p.o. div. q6h Hepatic encephalopathy: *Children:* Acute: 2.5–7 g/m² per 24 h p.o. div. q6h × 5–7 d Chronic: 2.5 g/m² per 24 h p.o. div. q6h Bowel preparation: *Children:* 90 mg/kg per 24 h p.o. div. q4h × 3 d	• Avoid use in ulcerative bowel disease or intestinal obstruction • About 3% of oral dose is absorbed but impaired GI motility may increase absorption and subsequently toxicity

Drug	Supplied	Dose	Comments
Neosporin	*Eye/ear drops:* (polymixin, neomycin, gramicidin) *Topical cream:* (polymixin, neomycin, gramicidin) *Topical ointment:* (polymixin, neomycin, bacitracin) *Spray:* (polymixin, neomycin, bacitracin)	Ear drops: 1–2 drops in affected ear b.i.d.–q.i.d. Topical cream/ointment: Apply a small quantity 2–5 × daily Spray: 1 s spray from a distance of about 20 cm, b.i.d.–q.i.d.	• Topical neomycin may induce contact dermatitis • Not recommended for use in eye
Neostigmine (Prostigmin)	*Injection:* 0.5 mg/mL, 1 mL, 10 mL	Myasthenia gravis: *Diagnosis* *Children:* 0.04 mg/kg i.m. × 1 *Adults:* 0.02 mg/kg i.m. × 1 *Treatment* *Children:* 0.01–0.04 mg/kg per dose i.m., i.v. or s.c. q2–3h p.r.n. *Adults:* 0.5–2.5 mg/dose i.m., i.v. or s.c. q3–4h p.r.n. to maximum 10 mg/24 h Reversal of nondepolarizing neuromuscular blocking agents: *Infants:* 0.025–0.1 mg/kg per dose i.v. with atropine or glycopyrrolate *Children:* 0.025–0.08 mg/kg per dose i.v. with atropine or glycopyrrolate *Adults:* 0.5–2 mg/dose i.v. with atropine or glycopyrrolate	• Dose must be titrated to avoid excessive cholinergic effects
Niclosamide	*Tablet:* 500 mg	*Children: 11–34 kg:* 1 g/dose p.o. × 1 *> 34 kg:* 1.5 g/dose p.o. × 1 *Adults:* 2 g/dose p.o. × 1	• Tablets should be chewed thoroughly

Drug	Supplied	Dose	Comments
Nifedipine (Adalat, Adalat PA)	Capsule: 5 mg, 10 mg Prolonged action tablet: 10 mg, 20 mg	Hypertension: Infants: 0.1–0.3 mg/kg per dose p.o. q6h or sublingual q8h Children: 0.2–0.5 mg/kg per dose p.o. q6h or sublingual q8h (prolonged action tablets should be given b.i.d.)	• To prepare sublingual doses or doses < 5 mg: 5 mg capsules contain 0.1 mL (concentration in capsule = 50 mg/mL); use a 22 or 23 gauge needle attached to a 1 mL tuberculin syringe; pierce capsule with needle and withdraw desired dose volume • For sublingual use: instill drug in buccal pouch • Nifedipine is very light sensitive; prepare dose just prior to administration; discard any unused drug • Absorption is faster if capsules are bitten and swallowed than if given sublingually • Nifedipine PA tablets may be split but not crushed or chewed
Nitrazepam (Mogadon)	Tablet: 5 mg	Anticonvulsant: Children up to 30 kg: 0.3–1 mg/kg per 24 h p.o. div. t.i.d.	• Begin therapy at low dose, gradually increase to effect/tolerance • Higher doses may cause excessive drowsiness
Nitrofurantoin (Macrodantin)	Capsule: 25 mg, 50 mg Liquid: 5 mg/mL	Children: Treatment: 5–7 mg/kg per 24 h p.o. div. q.i.d. Prophylaxis: 1–2 mg/kg per 24 h in one dose Adults: Treatment: 200–400 mg/24 h p.o. div. q.i.d. Prophylaxis: 50–100 mg/24 h p.o. once daily	• Contraindicated in infants < 1 mo of age • Administration with food or milk may lessen GI upset

Drug	Supplied	Dose	Comments
Nitroglycerine (Nitrostat, Nitropaste)	*Injection:* 5 mg/mL amp *Ointment:* 2%	Continuous i.v. infusion: 0.5–10 µg/kg per min Topical: Dose not well established in children but can be approximated by calculating total daily i.v. dose and converting this amount to cm of ointment and dividing into two daily doses	• Administer continuous infusions via a syringe pump with non-PVC tubing • When converting from i.v. to topical: 1 cm of 2% ointment contains approximately 7.5 mg of nitroglyercin
Nitroprusside (Nipride)	*Injection:* 50 mg/vial	Continuous i.v. infusion: 0.5–6 µg/kg per min	• To be administered by infusion control devices only in intensive care areas where facilities are available for invasive hemodynamic monitoring • Monitor thiocyanate levels if used in high doses (> 3 µg/kg per min) for longer than 2 or in patients with renal impairment; keep thiocyanate levels < 0.8 mmol/L • Overdose will cause hypotension, metabolic acidosis and CNS symptoms
Nystatin (Mycostatin, Nilstat)	*Suspension:* 100,000 univ/mL *Topical ointment and cream:* 100,000 unit/g *Vaginal cream:* 25,000 unit/g *Vaginal tablet:* 100,000 unit *Topical powder:* 100,000 unit/g	Suspension: *Infants:* 200,000 unit/dose p.o. q.i.d. *Children and adults:* 400,000–600,000 unit/dose p.o. q.i.d. Topical ointment and cream: Apply liberally to affected area q6–24h Vaginal cream and tablet: One applicator of cream or 1 tablet vaginally once or twice daily × 14 d Topical powder: Apply to lesion b.i.d.–t.i.d.	• Oral suspension should be swished around mouth for 30–60 s and then swallowed • Nystatin is not appreciably absorbed when given orally • Topical cream is preferred to ointment in diaper areas
Octreotide (Sandostatin, somatostatin analogue)	*Injection:* 50 µg/mL, 100 µg/mL, 500 µg/mL	*Children:* 1–10 µg/kg per 24 h s.c. div. b.i.d.–t.i.d.	• Monitor blood glucose at onset of therapy and periodically • Local reaction at the injection site may be reduced by allowing solution to reach room temperature and administering slowly

Drug	Supplied	Dose	Comments
Ondansetron (Zofran)	*Tablet:* 4 mg, 8 mg *Injection*	*Children:* 0.15 mg/kg per dose i.v. or 0.2 mg/kg per dose p.o.; doses may be repeated q8–12h; give oral doses 60–90 min prior to chemotherapy; give i.v. doses 15 min prior to chemotherapy *Adults:* 8 mg p.o. q8h	• Indicated for the treatment of chemotherapy and radiation induced nausea and vomiting only • A very expensive product: use a minimum effective dose (start with q12h dosing); use tablets whenever possible • Dexamethasone may enhance antiemetic activity with highly emetogenic chemotherapy
Opium and Belladonna (B & O suppositories)	*Suppository:* containing 65 mg powdered opium and 15 mg dry extract of belladonna	*Children:* doses not well established < 5 yr: ⅓–½ suppository p.r. q6h p.r.n. > 5 yr: 1 suppository p.r. q6h p.r.n. Adults: 1 suppository p.r. q6h p.r.n.	
Orciprenaline (Alupent, Metaproterenol)	*Syrup:* 2 mg/mL *Respiratory solution:* 50 mg/mL *Inhaler:* 750 μg/puff	p.o.: *Children:* 0.3–0.5 mg/kg per dose p.o. q6–8h *Adults:* 20 mg/dose p.o. q6–8h Inhaler: 1–3 puffs q3–4h to a maximum of 12 puff/24 h Respiratory solution: Dilute 0.1–0.3 mL in 2.5 mL normal saline via nebulizer q4–6h or up to q1h for severe bronchospasm	• May cause tachycardia, palpitations
Ovral	*Tablet*	"Morning After" dose: 2 tablets p.o. within 72 h of intercourse followed by 2 tablets p.o. 12 h later	• Each tablet contains 250 μg d-norgestrel and 50 μg ethinyl estradiol
Oxazepam (Serax)	*Tablet:* 10 mg, 15 mg, 30 mg	*Children 6–12 yr:* dose not well established; 1 mg/kg per 24 h p.o. in divided doses has been used *Adults: Mild to moderate anxiety:* 10–15 mg t.i.d. or q.i.d.	• Peak serum levels 3–4 h after p.o. dose • Half-life is about 11 h • Do not discontinue abruptly after prolonged (several months) therapy

Drug	Supplied	Dose	Comments
Oxybutynin (Ditropan)	*Tablet:* 5 mg *Liquid:* 1 mg/mL	*Children <5 yr:* 0.4–0.8 mg/kg per 24 h p.o. div. b.i.d.–q.i.d. *Children >5 yr:* 10–15 mg/24 h p.o. div. b.i.d.-t.i.d. Adults: 10–20 mg/24 h p.o. b.i.d.–q.i.d.	• Atropine–like side effects (dry mouth, blurred vision, dizziness and drowsiness are most common)
Oxymetholone (Anapolon)	*Tablet:* 50 mg	*Children, adolescents and adults:* 1–2 mg/kg per 24 h p.o.; treatment of refractory anemias may take 3–6 mo	• Use with caution in children and adolescents because of possible premature epiphyseal closure, precocious sexual development in males and virilisation in females
Pancreatic enzymes (Pancrease, Pancrease MT, Cotazyme ECS)	*Pancrease Pancrease MT4, MT10 and MT16 Cotazyme plain (not enteric coated) ECS 8, ECS 20*	Must be titrated to minimize steatorrhea and maintain good nutritional status; these are guidelines, expressed in units of lipase; dosages should be adjusted according to the response of the patient. *Usual dosage range:* 500–1,500 unit/kg per meal	• For infants and small children, contents of capsules may be mixed with soft food; sweep child's mouth with finger after administration to ensure no beads remain as these are irritating to the mucosa • Give at the beginning of meal or snack • Colonic strictures have been reported in patients receiving massive doses (> 8,000 unit/kg per meal)
Pancuronium (Pavulon)	*Injection:* 2 mg/mL	*Children > 1 mo to adults:* *Initial:* 0.04–0.1 mg/kg per dose i.v. *Maintenance:* 0.02–0.1 mg/kg per dose i.v. q30–60 min as needed	• Ventilation must be supported during neuromuscular blockade • Antidote: neostigmine and atropine

Drug	Supplied	Dose	Comments
Paraldehyde	*Injection:* 1 g/mL–10 mL amp	*Seizures:* p.r.: 0.3 mL/kg per dose q2–4h p.r.n. seizures; dilute dose in normal saline, mineral oil or olive oil to make a 50% solution *i.v.:* *Loading dose:* 0.15 mL/kg (diluted to a 5% solution") over 15–20 min *i.v. continuous infusion:* 0.4 mL/kg per h of 5% solution (" to make a 5% solution, add 2.5 mL paraldehyde to 47.5 mL D5W, normal saline or ⅔ and ⅓)	• Will dissolve plastic equipment and rubber stoppers • Do not admix with other drugs • Protect infusion from light • Change i.v. infusion set q8h • Discard solution if it has a brown color or sharp odor of acetic acid • For p.r. use, give immediately after dilution
Paroxetine (Paxil)	*Tablet:* 20 mg, 30 mg	*Adolescents or adults:* *Initial:* 20 mg p.o. q a.m. *Increment:* 10 mg at 1–2 wk intervals *Maximum:* 50 mg daily	• Selective serotonin re-uptake inhibitor (SSRI) • Therapeutic response may not be obtained until third or fourth week of treatment • Do not use with MAO inhibitors • Allow a 2 wk "washout" of MAO inhibitor before starting paroxetine • Allow a 2 wk "washout" of paroxetine before starting MAO inhibitor
Pediazole (Erythromycin/ Sulfisoxazole)	*Liquid:* 200 mg erythromycin plus 600 mg sulfisoxazole per 5 mL	*Children (based on erythromycin component):* 40 mg/kg per 24 h p.o. div. q6–8h (i.e. 1 mL/kg per 24 h p.o. div. q6–8h)	• Contains erythromycin ethylsuccinate • Not recommended for infants < 2 mo old due to sulfisoxazole component
Pemoline (Cylert)	*Tablet:* 18.75 mg, 37.5 mg, 75 mg	*> 6 yr. Initial:* 37.5 mg p.o. once daily *Increment:* 18.75 mg at 1 wk intervals to desired clinical effect *Maintenance:* 0.5–3 mg/kg per 24 h; usual effective dose is 56.25–75 mg *Maximum:* 112.5 mg daily	• Dose should be given in the morning • Significant benefit from therapy may not be evident until the third or fourth wk

Drug	Supplied	Dose	Comments
Penicillamine (Cuprimine)	*Capsule:* 125 mg, 250 mg	Wilson's disease: *Infants < 6 mo:* 250 mg/dose p.o. once daily *Children < 12 yr:* 250 mg/dose p.o. b.i.d.–t.i.d. *Adults:* 250 mg/dose p.o. q.i.d. Cystinuria: *Infants/young children:* 30 mg/kg per 24 h p.o. div. q6h *Older children/adults:* 1–4 g/24 h p.o. div. q6h Rheumatoid arthritis: Start with a low dose (125–250 mg/24 h) and increase to 10 mg/kg per 24 h over a 3 mo period *Maximum:* 750 mg/24 h Arsenic or lead poisoning: *Children:* 100 mg/kg per 24 h p.o. div. q6h × 5 d *Maximum:* 1 g/24 h; allow 3–5 d before rasuming therapy if symptoms recur; second course of therapy should be 40 mg/kg per 24 h p.o. div. q6h	• Give doses 1 h before or 2 h after meals • Patients treated for Wilson's disease or cystinuria should be supplemented with pyridoxine • Check CBC and urinalysis q1–2 wk during first 6 mo of therapy
Penicillin G benzathine (Megacillin, Bicillin)	1,200,000 IU/2 mL PLS	Streptococcal pharyngitis: *< 27 kg:* 600,000 units i.m. × 1 dose *> 27 kg:* 1,200,000 units i.m. × 1 dose Rheumatic fever prophylaxis: *< 27 kg:* 600,000 units i.m. once a mo *> 27 kg:* 1,200,000 unit i.m. once a mo	• Provides sustained serum levels for 2–4 wk • Do not give i.v. • Warning to room temperature will lessen pain on injection

Drug	Supplied	Dose	Comments
Penicillin G sodium	*Injection:* 1 mu/vial, 5 mu/vial, 10 mu/vial	100,000–250,000 unit/kg per 24 h i.m. or i.v. div. q4–6h Meningitis: 250,000 unit/kg per 24 h i.v. div. q4h	• For oral therapy use penicillin V (1 mg = 1,600 units)
Penicillin procaine (Wycillin)	*Injection:* 500,000 unit/mL– 10 mL vial	25,000-50,000 unit/kg per 24 h i.m. in 1–2 doses	• Contains 120 mg procaine/300,000 unit • Do not give i.v. • Provides sustained serum levels for 2–4 d
Penicillin V (Phenoxymethyl penicillin, V–Cillin K, Ledercillin–VK)	*Tablet:* 300 mg (500,000 units) *Solution:* 60 mg (100,000 unit/mL)	*Children:* 25–50 mg/kg per 24 h p.o. div. q6–8h Prophylaxis for asplenia: < 5 yr: 125 mg p.o. b.i.d. > 5 yr: 250 mg p.o. b.i.d.	• GI absorption is better than penicillin G • 1,600 units = 1 mg • Take on an empty stomach (1 h before or 2 h after meals)
Pentamidine (Pentacarinat)	*Injection:* 300 mg/vial	Systemic (treatment): 4 mg/kg per 24 h i.m. or i.v. daily × 12–14 d Inhalation/*Pneumocystis* prophylaxis: ≥ 5 yr: 60 mg via nebulizer q2 wk or 300 mg q4 wk	• i.v. route preferred over i.m. • Adverse effects include hypoglycemia, nephrotoxicity, hypotension, increased liver function tests, leukopenia, neutropenia, thrombocytopenia • Cough and bronchospasm may occur with inhalation therapy; pretreatment with bronchodilator may be beneficial
Pentobarbital (Nembutal)	*Capsule:* 100 mg *Injection:* 50 mg/mL	Hypnotic: *Children:* 2–6 mg/kg per dose i.m. or p.o. to a maximum of 100 mg/dose *Adults:* 150–200 mg/dose i.m. Barbiturate coma: *Initial:* 10–15 mg/kg per dose i.v. over 1–2 h *Maintenance:* 1 mg/kg per h by i.v. infusion, may increase to 2–3 mg/kg per h (monitor blood levels and maintain at 25–35 mg/L)	• May be used as an adjunct to decrease intracranial pressure • Barbiturate coma may also be used for intractable seizures • Short–acting; very rapid onset of action • Injection may be used orally, add dose to juice just prior to administration

Drug	Supplied	Dose	Comments
Permethrin (Nix)	*Creme rinse:* 1% *Cream:* 5%, 30 g tube	*Children and adults:* apply after hair has been washed with shampoo, rinsed and towel dried; apply sufficient permethrin to saturate hair and scalp; leave on hair for 10 min, then rinse with water. Topical cream: 2–23 mo: ⅛–¼ tube 2–5 yr: ¼ tube 5–12 yr: ½ tube > 12 yr: 1 tube Thoroughly massage cream into the skin from the head to soles of feet; remove by washing after 12–14 h	• A single treatment is sufficient to eliminate head lice or scabies; however, if live lice or mites are observed 7 d or more following initial treatment, a second application can be given • Combing of nits is not required for therapeutic efficacy • Creme rinse is indicated for head lice • Topical cream is indicated for scabies
Phenazopyridine (Pyridium)	*Tablet:* 100 mg	*Children 6–12 yr:* 12 mg/kg per 24 h p.o. div. t.i.d. *Adults:* 200 mg p.o. t.i.d.; administer until symptoms are controlled	• Colors urine orange; stains clothing and is difficult to remove • Administer with food
Phenobarbital (Luminal, Phenobarbitone)	*Tablet:* 15 mg, 30 mg, 60 mg, 100 mg *Injection:* 30 mg/mL, 120 mg/mL *Elixir:* 5 mg/mL	Status epilepticus: *Children:* 15–18 mg/kg per dose i.v. × 1 then 5 mg/kg per dose q15–30 min p.r.n. *Maximum total dose:* 30 mg/kg Chronic anticonvulsant: < 1 yr: 5–6 mg/kg per 24 h div. q12–24h 1–5 yr: 6–8 mg/kg per 24 h div. q12–24h 6–12 yr: 4–6 mg/kg per 24 h div. q12–24h > 12 yr: 1–3 mg/kg per 24 h div. q12–24h	• May cause paradoxical hyperactivity in children • Rapid i.v. injection may cause respiratory depression or hypotension, therefore, i.v. rate must not exceed 1 mg/kg per min • Elixir is very unpalatable; use tablets if possible • Therapeutic range is 65–170 µmol/L

Drug	Supplied	Dose	Comments
Phenoxybenzamine (Dibenyline)	*Injection:* 10 mg/0.2 mL	*Children:* Loading dose: 1 mg/kg i.v. in 4 div. doses over a 1–4 h period, depending on BP response Maintenance: 1 mg/kg per 24 h i.v. div. q6h	• Investigational drug to be used in ICU only
Phentolamine (Rogitine)	*Injection:* 5 mg/vial	*Children:* 0.05–0.1 mg/kg per dose i.m. or i.v., repeat q5 min until hypertension is controlled, then q2–4h p.r.n. *Adults:* 2.5–5 mg/dose i.m. or i.v., repeat q5 min until hypertension is controlled, then q2–4h p.r.n. <u>Treatment of α–adrenergic drug extravasation:</u> 0.1–0.2 mg/kg up to 10 mg, infiltrated into area of extravasation within 12 h	• Monitor blood pressure and heart rate continuously
Phenytoin (Dilantin)	*Injection:* 50 mg/mL *Tablet:* 50 mg (chewable) *Capsule:* 100 mg *Suspension:* 6 mg/mL, 25 mg/mL	<u>Status epilepticus:</u> 18 mg/kg per dose i.v. <u>Maintenance for seizure disorder:</u> *Infants and children:* 5–10 mg/kg per 24 h i.v. or p.o. div. q12–24h *Adults:* 300–400 mg/24 h i.v. or p.o. div. q12–24h <u>Anti-arrhythmic:</u> *Children:* 2–4 mg/kg per dose i.v. over 5 min or 2–5 mg/kg per 24 h p.o. div. q12–24h *Adults:* 100 mg i.v. q5 min; repeat in 2 h p.r.n. *Maximum total dose:* 500 mg	• For oral dosing, chewable tablets are preferred over liquid dosage forms • Oral dosage changes should be in 25 mg increments to accommodate tablet size • Increases in maintenance dosage should not exceed 25 mg/24 h unless serum concentration is < 30 mmol/L; at higher serum concentration small dosage increases can result in disproportionally high serum levels • Therapeutic serum concentration: 40–80 mmol/L

Drug	Supplied	Dose	Comments
Phosphate (Potassium phosphate, Phosphate sandoz, Sodium phosphate)	Tablet: 500 mg elemental phosphorus (Sandoz), 16 mmol phosphorus Injection: 3 mmol phosphorus/mL, 4.4 mEq potassium/mL (potassium PO_4), 4 mEq sodium/mL (sodium PO_4)	Hypophosphatemia: Children: 0.15–0.33 mmol/kg per dose (5–10 mg/kg per dose) i.v. over 6 h Maintenance: Children: 0.5–1.5 mmol/kg per 24 hr i.v., 2–3 mmol/kg per 24 h p.o. Adults: 40–70 mmol/24 h i.v., 100–150 mmol/24 h p.o.	• Injectable phosphate should be ordered by mmol of phosphate • Oral absorption is about 60% • Each tablet contains 3.1 mmol K^+ and 20.4 mmol Na^+ • Tablets must be dissolved in water prior to administration (125–250 mL)
Phosphate enema (Fleet)	Enema: 65 mL (pediatric), 130 mL (adult)	Children: ≤ 14 kg: 30 mL 14–27 kg: 60 mL 27–40 kg: 90 mL Adults: 120 mL	• Not recommended for infants < 1 yr • Contains sodium phosphate 16 g/100 mL and dibasic sodium phosphate 6 g/100 mL • Overdose may cause hypocalcemia and tetany
Physostigmine (Antilirium)	Injection: 1 mg/mL	For life threatening situations only Anticholinergic toxicity: Children < 5 yr: 0.02 mg/kg i.v. q5 min until therapeutic effect or until total dose of 2 mg has been given Children > 5 yr: 1–2 mg/dose i.v.; repeat in 10 min if ineffective Maximum: 4 mg in 30 min	• Atropine must be available to reverse excess cholinergic side effects; give 0.5 mg atropine for each 1 mg of physostigmine just given
Pimozide (Orap)	Tablet: 2 mg, 4 mg	Children > 12 yr and adults: Initial dose: 2–4 mg p.o. q a.m. Increment: 2–4 mg/wk until therapeutic effect Average maintenance: 6 mg daily (range 2–12 mg) Tourette's disorder: Initial: 1 mg/24 h p.o. Maximum: 0.2 mg/kg per dose	• May cause extrapyramidal side effects, anticholinergic side effects

Drug	Supplied	Dose	Comments
Piperacillin (Pipracil)	*Injection:* 2 g/vial, 3 g/vial, 4 g/vial	*Severe infections:* *Children:* 200–300 mg/kg per 24 h i.m. or i.v. div. q4–6h *Adults:* 3–4 g/dose i.v. q4–6h *Cystic fibrosis patients:* 600 mg/kg per 24 h i.v. div. q6h	• Contains 1.85 mEq Na$^+$/g
Pivampicillin (Pondocillin)	*Tablet:* 500 mg *Suspension:* 35 mg/mL	*Mild to moderate infections:* *Children:* 20–50 mg/kg per 24 h p.o. div. q12h *Otitis media:* 40–50 mg/kg per 24 h p.o. div. q12h *Severe infections:* 40–100 mg/kg per 24 h p.o. div. q8h	• Pivampicillin is a pro-drug of ampicillin • 1.3 mg pivampicillin provides 1 mg ampicillin
Polymyxin B (Aerosporin)	*Sterile powder.* 50 mg/vial	*Inhalation:* 1–20 mg/dose via inhalation q4–6h	• Dose for inhalation should be dissolved in 1–2 mL of sterile normal saline or D5W • Injectable form is used for inhalation
Polysporin	*Cream:* (polymyxin B plus gramicidin) *Ointment:* (polymyxin B plus bacitracin) *Eye ointment:* (polymyxin B plus bacitracin) *Eye/ear drops:* (polymyxin B plus gramicidin)	*Topical cream or ointment:* apply a small amount 2–5 × daily *Eye/ear drops:* 1 drop into each affected eye or ear, q3–6h *Eye ointment:* apply q3–4h, depending on severity of condition	• More specific therapy should be prescribed for use in eye

Drug	Supplied	Dose	Comments
Potassium chloride (Slow K, Micro–K, K–Dur, Extencaps, KaoChlor, K–Lyte)	*Tablet:* slow release 600 mg [8 mEq] (Slow–K), slow release 20 mEq (K–Dur), effervescent 25 mEq (K–Lyte) *Capsule:* slow release 600 mg [8 mEq] (Micro–K Extencap) *Elixir:* 1.3 mEq/mL *Injection:* 2 mEq/mL	*Children:* 1–4 mEq/kg per 24 h continuous i.v. infusion or div. b.i.d.–t.i.d. p.o., as required to maintain normal serum potassium *Adults:* 10–15 mEq/dose t.i.d.–q.i.d.	• Gastric irritation may be relieved by administering after meals • Do not crush, break or chew Slow–K tablets • Contents of Micro–K extencaps may be sprinkled on soft foods • K–Dur tablets may be broken to facilitate swallowing or an aqueous suspension can be prepared as follows: place tablet in about 100 mL of water; allow 2–3 min to disintegrate, then stir for 30 s and drink immediately
Pralidoxime (Protopam, 2–PAM)	*Injection:* 1 g/vial	Organophosphate poisoning: *Children:* 25–50 mg/kg per dose i.v.; repeat in 30 min and at 8–12 h intervals if cholinergic signs recur *Adults:* 1–2 g/dose i.v.; repeat in 30 min p.r.n.; if no improvement after second dose, pralidoxime may be infused at 0.5 g/h	• For organophosphate insecticide poisoning only; for best results administer within 3 h of exposure • For severe cases, patient should be premedicated with atropine 2–4 mg (adults) and 0.05 mg/kg (children), repeated q30–60 min p.r.n. • This drug should be reserved for use in facilities where intubation and ventilation is available • Reduce dose in renal impairment
Praziquantel (Biltricide)	*Tablet:* 600 mg	75 mg/kg per 24 h p.o. div. q8h × 1–2 d	• Do not chew tablets due to bitter taste • Take with meals

Drug	Supplied	Dose	Comments
Prazosin (Minipress)	*Capsule:* 1 mg, 2 mg, 5 mg	*Children:* *Initial dose (to assess hypotensive effect):* 1 mg p.o. *Maintenance:* 0.01–0.05 mg/kg per dose p.o. q6–8h *Maximum:* 0.1 mg/kg per dose *Adults:* *Initial:* 0.5–1 mg p.o. b.i.d.–t.i.d. *Maintenance:* 3–20 mg/24 h p.o. div. b.i.d.–q.i.d.	• Orthostatic hypotension may occur after initial dose
Prednisolone	*Tablet:* 5 mg	Same as prednisone	• Prednisone is more commonly used (except in hepatic disease) as more dosage forms are available
Prednisolone eye drops (Pred–Forte, Pred–Mild)	*Eye drops:* 0.12% (Pred–Mild), 1% (Pred–Forte)	*Initial therapy in severe cases:* (Pred–Forte) 1 drop into the conjunctival sac q3–6h depending on severity of condition Mild–moderate inflammation or when favorable response is attained in severe cases: (Pred–Mild) 1 drop q3–6h; the lowest effective concentration should be used	

Drug	Supplied	Dose	Comments
Prednisone (Deltasone)	*Tablet:* 1 mg, 5 mg, 50 mg, 2 mg/mL, 5 mg/mL	<u>Physiological replacement:</u> 4–5 mg/m^2 per 24 h p.o. div. b.i.d. <u>Asthma:</u> *Acute exacerbation:* 0.5–2 mg/kg per 24 h p.o. (maximum: 20–40 mg/24 h) div. b.i.d. × 3–5 d *Chronic refractory asthma:* 5–10 mg/dose p.o. daily or 10–30 mg p.o. every other day (attempt to taper and/or wean to aerosol corticosteroid) <u>Anti-inflammatory or immunosuppressive:</u> 0.5–2 mg/kg per 24 h or 25–60 mg/m^2 per 24 h p.o. div. q6–12h <u>Immune thrombocytopenia purpura:</u> 4 mg/kg per 24 h p.o. div. q8–12h × 6 d, then taper <u>Nephrotic syndrome:</u> *Initial:* 1–2 mg/kg per 24 h or 60 mg/m^2 per 24 h p.o. div. t.i.d.–q.i.d. (maximum 90 mg/24 h) until urine is protein–free × 5 d (to a maximum of 28 d) *Maintenance:* 1–2 mg/kg per dose or 60 mg/m^2 per dose p.o. every other day × 28 d, then taper as appropriate	• Methylprednisolone (i.v.) or prednisolone (p.o.) are preferred in hepatic disease as prednisone is hepatically metabolized to prednisolone • For severe refractory asthma, alternate day therapy (given in morning) is preferred • 4 mg of hydrocortisone = 1 mg of prednisone
Primaquine	*Tablet:* 15 mg	To prevent relapse of malaria after treatment of acute attack: 0.3 mg/kg per 24 h p.o. × 14 d *Maximum dose:* 15 mg/24 h	• May cause hemolysis in patients with G6PD deficiency

Drug	Supplied	Dose	Comments
Primidone (Mysoline)	*Tablet:* 125 mg, 250 mg	*< 8 yr:* *Initial:* 125 mg/24 h p.o. once daily *Increment:* 125 mg/24 h p.o. weekly *Maintenance:* 10–25 mg/kg per 24 h p.o. div. t.i.d.–q.i.d. *> 8 yr–adult:* *Initial:* 250 mg/24 h p.o. once daily *Increment:* 250 mg/24 h p.o. weekly *Maintenance:* 0.75–1.5 g/24 h p.o. div. t.i.d.–q.i.d.	• Metabolized to phenobarbital • Monitor both primidone and phenobarbital levels • Therapeutic range: Primidone: 37–55 μmol/L Phenobarbital: 65–170 μmol/L
Procainamide (Pronestyl)	*Capsule:* 250 mg, 375 mg *Injection:* 100 mg/mL for i.v. use	*Children:* p.o.: 15–50 mg/kg per 24 h div. q3–6h i.v. *(initial dose):* 3–6 mg/kg per dose over 5 min (maximum: 100 mg/dose); may repeat q5 min to a maximum of 15 mg/kg per load i.v. *maintenance:* 20–80 μg/kg per min by i.v. infusion *Adults:* *Loading:* 100–200 mg/dose; repeat q5 min p.r.n. to maximum of 1,000 mg *Maintenance:* 1–6 mg/min by continuous infusion p.o.: 250–500 mg/dose q3–6h	• Monitor i.v. administration for BP, ECG, QRS; widening of QRS > 0.02 s suggests toxicity • May cause lupus-like syndrome, hypotension, heart block, arrhythmias, GI complaints, thrombocytopenia
Prochlorperazine (Stemetil)	*Tablet:* 5 mg, 10 mg *Liquid:* 1 mg/mL *Injection:* 5 mg/mL *Suppository:* 10 mg	*Children (> 10 kg or > 2 yr):* 0.4 mg/kg per 24 h p.o. or p.r. div. t.i.d–q.i.d.; 0.1–0.15 mg/kg per dose i.m. or i.v. t.i.d.–q.i.d. *Adults:* 5–10 mg/dose p.o. or i.m. q4–6h; 25 mg/dose p.r. b.i.d.	• Extrapyramidal reactions are common in children • Use i.v. route with caution

Drug	Supplied	Dose	Comments
Procyclidine (Kemadrin)	*Tablet:* 5 mg	For drug induced extrapyramidal symptoms: *Adolescents and adults:* *Initial:* 2.5 mg p.o. t.i.d. *Increment:* 2.5 mg p.o. daily *Usual maintenance:* 10–20 mg p.o. daily	• Anticholinergic side effects (red as a beet, dry as a bone, etc.)
Promethazine (Phenergan)	*Tablet:* 10 mg, 25 mg *Liquid:* 2 mg/mL *Injection:* 25 mg/mL	Antihistamine: *Children:* 0.1 mg/kg per dose p.o. q6h during the day and 0.5 mg/kg per dose p.o. at bedtime *Adults:* 12.5 mg p.o. t.i.d. and 25 mg p.o. at bedtime Antiemetic: *Children:* 0.25–0.5 mg/kg per dose p.o., i.v. or i.m. q4–6 h p.r.n. *Adults:* 12.5–25 mg/dose i.m. q4–6h p.r.n.	• Use with caution in children < 2 yr due to possible respiratory depression • May cause sedation, hypotension, anticholinergic effects, extrapyramidal effects
Propranolol (Inderal)	*Tablet:* 10 mg, 40 mg *Injection:* 1 mg/mL	Arrhythmias: *Children:* 0.01–0.1 mg/kg per dose i.v. up to 1 mg/dose q6–8h p.r.n. *Adults:* 1 mg/dose q5 min i.v. to total of 5 mg Hypertension: *Children: p.o.:* 0.5–1 mg/kg per 24 h div. q6–12h *Adults:* 10–20 mg/dose p.o. b.i.d.–t.i.d. up to 400 mg p.o. daily Migraine prophylaxis: *Children:* < 35 kg: 10–20 mg p.o. t.i.d. > 35 kg: 20–40 mg p.o. t.i.d. Tetralogy spells: 0.15–0.25 mg/kg per dose i.v.; repeat once in 15 min p.r.n. *Maximum:* i.v. 10 mg/dose *Maintenance:* 1–2 mg/kg per dose p.o. q6h p.r.n.	• Administer with continuous ECG monitoring when given i.v. • Give by slow i.v. push at a rate not > 1 mg/min

Drug	Supplied	Dose	Comments
Propylthiouracil (Propyl–Thyracil)	*Tablet:* 50 mg, 100 mg	*Children: Initial:* 5–7 mg/kg per 24 h p.o. div. q8h *Maintenance:* ⅓–⅔ of the initial dose, q8h *Adults: Initial:* 300–400 mg/24 h p.o. div. q8h *Maintenance:* 100–150 mg/24 h p.o. div. q8h	• Begin maintenance when patient is euthyroid • Adjust dose to achieve T_3, T_4 and TSH serum levels in the normal range
Protamine	*Injection:* 50 mg/5 mL amp refrigeration required	Heparin reversal: 1 mg for each 100 unit of heparin given in the last 3–4 h *Maximum dose:* 50 mg; give by slow i.v. push not faster than 5 mg/min	• May cause severe hypotension and anaphylactoid reactions if given by rapid i.v. injection • Large doses can produce a paradoxical anticoagulation • Monitor effects on anticoagulation by means of a PTT
Pseudoephedrine (Sudafed)	*Tablet:* 60 mg *Liquid:* 30 mg/5 mL	*Children:* 4 mg/kg per 24 h p.o. div. q6h *Adults:* 30–60 mg/dose p.o. q6–8h	• May cause restlessness, nervousness, insomnia • Use with caution in patients with hypertension, hyperglycemia, cardiac disease
Psyllium hydrophylic mucilloid (Metamucil)	*Powder:* unflavored *Instant mix:* flavored	*Children > 6 yr:* 2.5 mL powder or ½ package of instant mix in at least 120 mL of fluid 1–3 × daily *Adults:* 5 mL powder or 1 package of instant mix in at least 240 mL of fluid 1–3 × daily	• Takes 2–3 d to become fully effective • Instant mix contains 11 mmol of sodium per package
Pyrantel pamoate (Combantrin)	*Tablet:* 125 mg *Suspension:* 50 mg/mL	Pinworms or roundworms: *≤ 11 kg:* 1 tablet or 2.5 mL × 1 dose *12–23 kg:* 2 tablets or 5 mL × 1 dose *24–45 kg:* 4 tablets or 10 mL × 1 dose *46–68 kg:* 6 tablets or 15 mL × 1 dose *> 68 kg:* 8 tablets or 20 mL × 1 dose Hookworms: same dosage as above is given once daily for 3 d	• It is recommended that all family members be treated

Drug	Supplied	Dose	Comments
Pyrazinamide	*Tablet:* 500 mg	*Children:* 20–40 mg/kg per 24 h p.o. once daily or 2 g/24 h or 50 mg/kg per dose p.o. twice weekly. *Maximum dose:* 2 g	• Should not be given alone in the treatment of TB
Pyridostigmine (Mestinon, Regonol)	*Tablet:* 60 mg *Tablet:* slow release 180 mg *Injection:* 10 mg/2 amp	Myasthenia gravis: *Children:* p.o.: 7 mg/kg per 24 h div. 5 or 6 doses i.m. or i.v.: 0.05–0.15 mg/kg per dose by slow i.v. injection *Adults:* p.o.: 60–1,200 mg/24 h i.m. or i.v.: 2–5 mg/dose by slow i.v. injection	• Poorly absorbed; oral dose is 30 times parenteral dose • Effects of oral dosage changes may not be seen for several days • Doses should be divided equally throughout the day at 3–4 h intervals (6–8 h for slow release tablets) • Antidote for toxicity (cholinergic crisis): atropine 0.01–0.04 mg/kg per dose i.v.
Pyridoxine (Vitamin B$_6$)	*Tablet:* 25 mg, 100 mg *Injection:* 100 mg/mL	Deficiency: 5–10 mg/24 h *Maintenance:* 20 μg/g of dietary protein Drug induced neuritis: *Treatment:* 10–50 mg/24 h *Prophylaxis:* 1–2 mg/kg per 24 h With oral contraceptives: 25–30 mg/24 h Sideroblastic anemia: 200–600 mg/24 h × 1–2 mo, then 30–50 mg daily Seizures: 50 mg/dose i.v. acutely under EEG; 200 mg/24 h × 2 wk to check for B$_6$ response to seizures Metabolic disorders: 100–500 mg daily	• May be given i.m., i.v. or s.c. if oral administration is not possible • Long–term (> 2 mo) therapy with large doses (≥ 2 g/24 h) can cause sensory neuropathy or neuropathy syndromes
Quinine	*Capsule:* 200 mg, 300 mg	Malaria: 25 mg/kg per 24 h p.o. div. q8h × 3 d *Maximum:* 650 mg/dose	• Toxicities: cinchonism (tinnitus, headache, nausea, abdominal pain, visual disturbances), blood dyscrasias, arrhythmias, hypotension, hemolysis

Drug	Supplied	Dose	Comments
Ranitidine (Zantac)	*Tablet:* 150 mg *Liquid:* 15 mg/mL *Injection:* 50 mg/2 mL	Acid peptic disease in children: p.o.: 3–4 mg/kg per 24 h div. q12h i.v.: 1–2 mg/kg per dose q6–8h *Maximum:* 50 mg i.v. q6h Stress ulcer prophylaxis in ICU patients: *Children:* i.v.: 1–2 mg/kg per dose q6h or 0.1 mg/kg per h in patients following cardiopulmonary bypass *Adults:* p.o.: 150 mg q12h i.v.: 50 mg q6–8h	• The daily dose of ranitidine may be added to TPN and infused continuously over 24 h • Keep intragastric pH $\geq$ 4 when used for stress ulcer prophylaxis • Reduce dose in patients with renal impairment • i.v. ranitidine may be used in the acute phase of GI bleeding until etiology of bleeding/pain is determined by endoscopy and biopsy • Most peptic ulcer disease in children is H. pylori related, therefore definitive treatment is not acid suppression
Ribavirin (Virazole)	*Powder:* for inhalation	Delivered via small particule aerosol generator (SPAG) 1 vial/d; administered over 24 h for 3–5 d	• Costs approximately $3,500 per treatment course
Rifampin (Rifadin, Rimactane, Rofact)	*Capsule:* 150 mg, 300 mg	Maximum single dose: 600 mg Tuberculosis: 10–20 mg/kg per dose p.o. daily or twice weekly Meningitis prophylaxis: *H. influenzae:* < 1 mo (dose not well established): 10 mg/kg per 24 h p.o. × 4 d > 1 mo: 20 mg/kg per 24 h p.o. × 4 d *N. meningitidis:* < 1 mo: 10 mg/kg per 24 h p.o. div. q12h × 2 d > 1 mo: 20 mg/kg per 24 h p.o. div. q12h × 2 d Other infections: 10–20 mg/kg per 24h p.o. once daily or div. q12h Pruritis due to cholestasis: 10–20 mg/kg per 24 h div. q12h	• Will discolor body fluids (urine, saliva, tears) and soft contact lenses red • Taken 1 h before or 2 h after meals • Use in liver disease only under guidance; rifampin may increase cholestasis in some patients and require concomitant use of choleretic drugs

Drug	Supplied	Dose	Comments
Salbutamol (Ventolin, Albuterol)	*Oral solution:* 0.4 mg/mL *Nebulizer solution:* 5 mg/mL *Inhaler:* 100 μg/puff *Rotacap:* 200 μg/cap, 400 μg/cap *Injection:* 0.5 mg/mL– 1 mL amp, 10 mL amp 0.05 mg/mL– 5 mL amp	*Bronchodilator:* p.o.: 0.3–0.6 mg/kg per 24 h div. t.i.d.–q.i.d. *Nebulizer:* dilute 1 mL in 3 mL normal saline and nebulize at 6–8 L/min over 10 min q20 min–6 hr (< 6 mo of age: 0.5 mL/3.5 mL normal saline) *Puffer:* 1–2 puffs q.i.d. *Rotocaps:* 200 μg via Rotahaler q.i.d. (adolescents or adults may require 400 μg q.i.d.) *Infusion:* for use in ICU only; 0.2–10 μg/kg per min	• i.v. infusions and high dose inhalation therapy of salbutamol will cause hypokalemia • Other side effects: tachycardia, tremor, nervousness, GI symptoms and headaches • Possible exacerbation of chronic asthma with continuous long–term use • The use of spacer devices may enhance efficacy of administering metered dose inhaler doses
Scopolamine hydrobromide (Hyoscine)	*Injection:* 0.4 mg/mL, 0.6 mg/mL	*Preoperative:* *Children:* 6 μg/kg per dose s.c., im., i.v. or p.o.	• Avoid use in patients with glaucoma, urinary or GI obstruction • Well absorbed orally; peak concentration achieved in 1 h • Injectable form may be given orally
Seattle mouthwash	*Contains:* Maalox 0.4 mL/mL, diphenhydramine 1 mg/mL, lidocaine viscous (2%) 0.2 mL/mL	2.5–10 mL/dose (depending on size of child) q4–6h p.r.n.; swish and spit	• Should be swished around mouth for 1–2 min and then spit out; not to be swallowed
Selenium (Sodium selenite)	*Liquid:* 200 μg/5 mL	*Children:* *Repletion:* 2 μg/kg per 24 h p.o. or i.v. (in TPN) once daily *Maintenance:* 1 μg/kg per 24 h p.o. or i.v. (in TPN) once daily	• Repletion doses should not be used unless facilities are available to measure serum selenium levels • Toxicities can develop with prolonged high doses • Selenium therapy may vary with the degree of depletion

Drug	Supplied	Dose	Comments
Senna glycosides (Glysennid, Senokot, X-Prep)	*Tablet:* 8.6 mg, 12 mg *Liquid:* 1.7 mg/mL	*Children (1–5 yr):* 3–6 mg/dose p.o. at bedtime *Children (6–12 yr):* 8.6–12 mg p.o. at bedtime *Adults:* 12–24 mg p.o. at bedtime	• Onset of action is 6–24 h • Senna glycosides should be taken with plenty of fluid • Abdominal cramping is common • Do not use in active bowel disease or GI bleeding except under expert guidance
Sertraline (Zoloft)	*Capsule:* 50 mg, 100 mg	*Adolescents/adults:* *Initial:* 50 mg p.o. daily *Increment:* 50 mg at weekly intervals *Maximum:* 200 mg/24 h	• Serotonin re–uptake inhibitor • Full antidepressant effect may not be seen until 4 wk of treatment have been given • Administer with food to increase absorption
Silver sulfadiazine (Flamazine)	*Cream:* 1%, 30 g tubes, 500 g jars	Apply topically in a 3–5 mm thick layer; burns should be treated daily; other wounds at least 3 × weekly	• In burn therapy, jars should be reserved for the exclusive use of one patient
Simethicone (Ovol)	*Tablet:* 40 mg *Drops:* 40 mg/mL	*Infants:* 0.25–0.5 mL/dose with or after each meal *Adults:* 1–2 tablets/dose q.i.d.	• Drops may be added to formula or given directly from dropper
Sodium bicarbonate (NaHCO₃, Sodamint)	*Tablet:* 325 mg (3.9 mmol) *Injection:* 8.4% 10 mmol/10 mL PFS, 8.4% 50 mmol/50 mL PFS, 4.2% 5 mmol/10 mL PFS *Injection:* 7.5% 45 mmol/50 mL vial, 8.4% 50 mmol/50 mL vial	Cardiopulmonary resuscitation: 1–2 mmol/kg per dose; repeat q10–15 min for prolonged arrest or documented metabolic acidosis Oral therapy: 1–10 mmol/kg per 24 h in divided doses Cystic fibrosis: 1–4 tablet/meal with enzymes	• Use 8.4% concentration for children, 4.2% concentration for neonates and infants • Incompatible with catecholamines, calcium salts • Use with adequate alveolar ventilation • May be used as an adjuvant to pancreatic enzymes in cystic fibrosis

Drug	Supplied	Dose	Comments
Sodium polystyrene sulfonate (Kayexalate)	Powder suspension: (with 25% sorbitol) 0.25 g/mL	Children: 1 g/kg per dose p.o. q6h p.r.n. (not to exceed usual adult dose). 1 g/kg per dose p.r. q2–6h p.r.n. (not to exceed usual adult dose) Adults: 20 g p.o. q.i.d., 30–50 g as retention enema	• Rectal administration effective in about 30 min; oral administration may take 12 h • Do not administer with fruit juices containing K^+, or with antacids or laxatives containing Mg^{2+} or Al^{3+}. • Exchanges about 1 mmol K^+/g of resin • Provides 4.1 mmol Na^+/g
Sofracort	Eye/ear drops: containing framycetin, gramicidin and 0.5% dexamethasone	Ear: 2–3 drops in the ear canal t.i.d.–q.i.d.	• To avoid the possibility of reinfection, do not touch ear with dropper • Not recommended for eyes
Sotalol (Sotacor)	Tablet: 160 mg	Arrhythmias: 2–10 mg/kg per 24 h p.o. div. b.i.d.	• Reduce dose in renal impairment
Spironolactone (Aldactone)	Tablet: 25 mg, 100 mg	Children: 1–4 mg/kg per 24 h p.o. div. b.i.d.–q.i.d.	• Watch for hyperkalemia especially when combined with potassium supplementation • Avoid use in renal failure
Streptokinase (Streptase)	Injection: 250,000 unit/vial	Children: Dose not well established. Loading dose: 4,000 IU/kg i.v. over 30 min Maximum: 250,000 IU Maintenance: 2,000 IU/kg per h × 24 h; maximum recommended duration Adolescents and adults: Loading dose: 250,000 IU i.v. over 30 min Maintenance dose: 100,000 IU/h × 24–72 h (length of therapy varies with condition treated)	• Monitor for signs of bleeding • Avoid i.m. injections and arterial sticks • Recent strep. infection or streptokinase treatment may produce increased levels of streptokinase antibodies which neutralize the effects of streptokinase • Do not use if streptokinase has been used previously
Streptomycin	Injection: 500 mg/mL	Severe infections: Children: 20–30 mg/kg per 24 h i.m. div. q12h Adults: 1–2 g/daily	• A toxic drug; monitor auditory status • May also cause myocarditis, serum sickness or toxic epidermal necrolysis • For TB, to be given with other anti–TB drugs

Drug	Supplied	Dose	Comments
Sucralfate (Sulcrate)	*Tablet:* 1 gm *Suspension:* 200 mg/mL	*Children:* 40–80 mg/kg per 24 h p.o. div. q.i.d. *Adolescents and adults:* 1 g p.o. q.i.d.	• Give doses 1 h before meals and at bedtime • Sucralfate contains aluminum, which may accumulate in patients with renal impairment
Sulfacetamide (Sodium sulamyd)	*Eye drops:* 10%, 30% *Eye ointment:* 10%	10% drops (mild–moderate infections): Instill 1 drop into the lower conjunctival sac q3–6h during the day; less frequently at night 30% drops (severe infections): Instill 1 drop into the lower conjunctival sac q3–6h Ointment: Place a 0.5–1 cm ribbon in the conjunctival sac q.i.d. and at bedtime	• Ointment may be applied at night in conjunction with the daytime use of eye drops
Sulfasalazine (Salazopyrin)	*Tablet:* 500 mg *Enteric coated tablet:* 500 mg *Suspension:* 50 mg/mL	*Children > 2 yr:* *Initial:* 40–60 mg/kg per 24 h p.o. into 3–6 div. doses *Maintenance:* 30 mg/kg per 24 h p.o. in 2–4 div. doses *Maximum:* 4 g/24 h	• Patients experiencing GI side effects with the uncoated tablets should use the enteric coated tablets, a lower dose or a different 5–ASA preparation
Sumatriptan (Imitrex)	*Tablet:* 100 mg *Injection:* 6 mg/0.5 mL	*Adults:* 100 mg p.o. or 6 mg s.c. as a single dose *Maximum:* 3 × 100 mg p.o. or 2 × 6 mg s.c./24 h	• Avoid sumatriptan 6 h before or 24 h after ergot administration due to potential additive vasoconstriction • Not for i.v. administration • Contraindicated in patients receivng MAO inhibitors (i.e. moclobemide) or selective serotonin re–uptake inhibitors (i.e. sertaline, paroxetine, fluvoxamine, fluoxetine)

Drug	Supplied	Dose	Comments
Terfenidine (Seldane)	*Tablet:* 60 mg *Suspension:* 6 mg/mL	*3–6 yr:* 15 mg p.o. b.i.d. *7–12 yr:* 30 mg p.o. b.i.d. *> 12 yr–adults:* 60 mg p.o. b.i.d.	• Less sedating than other antihistamines • Avoid use in patients with liver disease or dysfunction, pre-existing cardiac disease, metabolic diseases which may cause electrolyte imbalance, or those patients receiving ketoconazole or erythromycin concurrently, as these situations may predispose to serious cardiac effects from terfenidine
Tetracycline	*Capsule:* 250 mg *Suspension:* 25 mg/mL	*Children > 8 yr:* 25–50 mg/kg per 24 h p.o. div. q6h *Adults:* 1–2 g/24 h p.o.	• Responsible for staining of developing teeth • Do not give with dairy products or with any divalent cations (Fe^{2+}, Ca^{2+}, Mg^{2+})
Theophylline (Quibron–T)	*Oral liquid:* 10 mg/mL	<u>Asthma:</u> *p.o. maintenance dose:* *0–2 mo:* 3–6 mg/kg per 24 h div. q8h *2–6 mo:* 6–15 mg/kg per 24 h div. q6h *6–12 mo:* 15–22 mg/kg per 24 h div. q6h *1–9 yr:* 22 mg/kg per 24 h div. q6h *9–12 yr:* 20 mg/kg per 24 h div. q6h *12–16 yr:* 18 mg/kg per 24 h div. q6h *> 16 yr:* 13 mg/kg per 24 h div. q6h *Maximum:* 900 mg/24 h	• To convert from i.v. therapy, multiply aminophylline dose in mg/kg per 24 h × 0.8 = theophylline dose; divide dose by an appropriate interval • Monitor drug levels to maintain serum theophylline in range of 55–100 μmol/L
Thiabendazole (Mintezol)	*Tablet:* 500 mg	50 mg/kg per 24 h p.o. div. b.i.d.	• Length of therapy depends upon parasite being treated • Adverse GI effects are common; give with meals • Use with caution in renal or hepatic disease

Drug	Supplied	Dose	Comments
Thiamine (Vitamin B₁)	*Tablet:* 10 mg, 25 mg, 50 mg *Elixir:* 0.05 mg/mL *Injection:* 100 mg/mL	Deficiency: 10–25 mg/dose i.m. or i.v. daily (if critically ill) or 10–50 mg/dose p.o. daily × 2 wk, then 5–10 mg/dose p.o. daily × 1 mo Wernicke's encephalopathy: 50 mg i.v. and 50 mg i.m. × 1 dose each, then 50 mg i.m. daily until patient resumes a normal diet *Dietary supplement:* *Infants:* 0.3–0.5 mg p.o. daily *Children:* 0.5–1 mg p.o. daily *Adults:* 1–2 mg p.o. daily	• Absorption is an active process and the total amount absorbed following oral administration of a large dose is 4–8 mg • Very large doses may be used in certain metabolic disorders
Thioridazine (Mellaril)	*Tablet:* 10 mg, 25 mg, 50 mg, 100 mg *Solution:* 30 mg/mL *Suspension:* 2 mg/mL	*Children 2–12 yr:* 1–2.5 mg/kg per 24 h p.o. div. q6–12h; increase gradually. *Adults:* *Initial:* 150–300 mg/24 h p.o. div. q6–12h; increase gradually	• Extrapyramidal side effects are common in children
Ticarcillin (Ticar)	*Injection:* 1 g, 3 g, 6 g	*Children:* 200–300 mg/kg per 24 h i.v. or i.m. div. q4–6h *Adults:* 12–24 g/24 h Cystic fibrosis patients: 600 mg/kg per 24 h i.v. div. q6h	• Contains 5.2 mEq of sodium/g
Tobramycin	*Injection:* 10 mg/mL, 40 mg/mL	Moderate to severe infections: *Children:* 7.5 mg/kg per 24 h i.m. or i.v. div. q8–12h *Adults:* 3–5 mg/kg per 24 h Cystic fibrosis: 12 mg/kg per 24 h i.v. div. q8h; dose may be higher based on serum levels	• Therapeutic serum levels: Predose < 2 mg/L. Postdose 6–10 mg/L (up to 20 mg/L in CF) • Use gentamicin unless *Pseudomonas aeroginosa* is suspected or confirmed

Drug	Supplied	Dose	Comments
Tolmetin (Tolectin)	*Tablet:* 200 mg, 400 mg	*Children:* 30 mg/kg per 24 h p.o. div. t.i.d. *Adults:* *Initial:* 400 mg p.o. t.i.d. *Maintenance:* titrate to desired effect; usually 600–1,800 mg/24 h p.o. div. t.i.d.	• GI upset may be lessened by administration with meals or milk
Tranexamic acid (Cykokapron, AMCA, Trans AMCA)	*Tablet:* 500 mg *Injection:* 500 mg/5 mL	*Pediatric:* i.v.: 10–20 mg/kg per dose i.v. b.i.d.–t.i.d. p.o.: 25 mg/kg per dose t.i.d.–q.i.d. *Adolescents:* i.v.: 10–15 mg/kg per dose 2–3 times/24 h p.o: 1–1.5 g 3–4 times/24 h	• Reduce dose in patients with renal impairment • Absorption from GI tract is about 40%
Triamcinolone (Aristocort, Aristospan, Kenalog, Triaderm)	*Cream:* 0.025%, 0.1% *Ointment:* 0.025%, 0.1% *In orabase:* 0.1% *Injection:* 10 mg/mL (acetonide [Kenalog]). 20 mg/mL (hexacetonide [Aristospan]), 40 mg/mL (acetonide)	*Topically:* Apply a small amount of cream or ointment t.i.d.–q.i.d. Triamcinolone in orabase: Press a small dab (about 6 mm) to oral lesion until a thin film develops, do not rub in; may be applied b.i.d.–t.i.d. depending on the severity of symptoms *Intra–articular:* use hexacetonide (Aristospan) Large joints: 40 mg (2 mL) Small joints: 20 mg (1 mL) Intralesional: use 5 mg/mL or 10 mg/mL dilution of acetonide (Kenalog); amount injected depends on size of lesion	• Injectable forms are not for i.v. use

Drug	Supplied	Dose	Comments
Trifluoperazine (Stelazine)	*Tablet:* 1 mg, 2 mg, 5 mg, 10 mg *Solution:* 10 mg/mL	Psychosis or behavior disorders: *Children (6–12 yr):* usual starting dose is 1 mg p.o. once or twice daily, depending on the size of the child; dose may be gradually increased until symptoms are controlled or side effects become troublesome; it is rarely necessary to exceed 15 mg daily, but some older children may require, and tolerate, higher doses *Adults:* usual dose is 1–2 mg twice daily (may be much higher in hospitalized patients)	• Extrapyramidal symptoms are common in children
Trihexyphenidyl (Artane)	*Tablet:* 2 mg	Drug-induced Parkinsonism: Dose must be determined empirically; start with 1 mg daily; if extrapyramidal symptoms are not controlled within a few hours of dose, subsequent doses may be progressively increased until satisfactory control is achieved. *Usual adult dose:* 5–15 mg/d	• Anticholinergic side effects (red as a beet, dry as a bone, etc.)
Trimeprazine (Panectyl)	*Tablet:* 2.5 mg, 5 mg *Liquid:* 2.5 mg/mL	*Children:* 6 mo–3 yr: 1.25 mg p.o. at bedtime or 1.25 mg p.o. t.i.d. p.r.n. >3 yr: 2.5 mg p.o. at bedtime or 2.5 mg p.o. t.i.d. p.r.n. *Adults:* 2.5 mg p.o. q.i.d. Preoperative sedation: *Children:* 2–4 mg/kg p.o. 90 min preoperative	• Extrapyramidal symptoms are common in children
Urokinase (Abbokinase open–cath)	*Injection:* 5,000 unit/vial 250,000 unit/vial	Systemic thrombolytic therapy: *Loading dose:* 4,000 unit/kg *Maintenance:* 4,000 unit/kg per h via continuous infusion *Maximum recommended duration:* 24 h	• Monitor patients for signs of bleeding • Use urokinase instead of streptokinase in patients < 3 mo old or if streptokinase has been used previously

Drug	Supplied	Dose	Comments
Ursodiol (Actigall, Ursofalk, Ursodeoxycholic acid)	*Capsule:* 250 mg	*Infants and children:* 10 mg/kg per 24 h p.o. div. b.i.d.; can be increased to 20 mg/kg per 24 h with care (20 mg/kg per 24 h is often required in cystic fibrosis patients) *Adults:* 8–10 mg/kg per 24 h p.o. div. b.i.d.	• Doses > 10 mg/kg per 24 h should be used cautiously and with expert guidance (20 mg/kg per 24 h is often required in cystic fibrosis patients) • May cause diarrhea and worsen malabsorption by decreasing bile salt pool • Aluminum–based antacids (Amphogel, Gelusil, Maalox) can bind to ursodiol and decrease its absorption; do not use antacids within 2 h of ursodiol dose
Valproic acid (Depakene)	*Capsule:* 250 mg *Enteric coated capsule:* 500 mg *Syrup:* 50 mg/mL	*Children:* *Initial:* 10 mg/kg per 24 h p.o. div. daily–t.i.d. *Increment:* 5–10 mg/kg at weekly intervals *Maintenance:* 20 mg/kg per 24 h div. daily t.i.d. (monotherapy); higher doses (30–60 mg/kg per 24 h) are often required in patients on polytherapy	• Valproic acid may not achieve its full effect for 1–2 mo • Therapeutic serum levels: 350–700 µmol/L • Valproic acid affects phenobarbital, phenytoin and carbamazepine serum concentrations, which may be monitored when valproic acid is added.
Vancomycin (Vancocin)	*Capsule:* 125 mg, 250 mg *Injection:* 500 mg/vial	Systemic infections: *Children:* 40 mg/kg per 24 h i.v. di.v. q6–8 h *Adults:* 1–2 g/24 h i.v. Severe infection and meningitis: *Children:* 40–60 mg/kg per 24 h i.v. div. q6–8h *Adults:* 2–4 g/daily i.v. Pseudomembranous colitis: 10–50 mg/kg per 24 h p.o. div. q6h up to 500 mg/24 h, or 1,000 mg/24 h in critically ill patients	• Dose adjustments are required for renal impairment • Metronidazole is preferred therapy for antibiotic associated colitis; if vancomycin is indicated, use oral form only as parenteral vancomycin does not achieve adequate concentrations in gut • Desired serum levels: Prelevel: 5–10 mg/L Postlevel: 25–40 mg/L

Drug	Supplied	Dose	Comments
Vasopressin (Pitressin)	*Injection:* tannate 5 unit/mL amp *Aqueous:* 10 unit/0.5 mL amp, 100 unit/5 mL amp	<u>Diabetes insipidus:</u> *Aqueous:* 2.5–10 unit i.m. or s.c. b.i.d.–q.i.d. *Tannate:* 1.25–2.5 unit i.m. q2–3 d *i.v. infusion:* 0.001–0.015 unit/kg per h; begin at low dose and increase at 30–60 min intervals until urine output < 2 mL/kg per h <u>Gastrointestinal hemorrhage:</u> By continuous i.v. infusion 0.002–0.01 unit/kg per min. *Maximum:* 0.9 unit/min	• Tannate must not be given i.v. or s.c. • Side effects occur more frequently at doses > 0.01 unit/kg per min • Side effects include hypertension, electrolyte abnormalities, fluid overload, cardiac dysrhythmias, urticaria, anaphylaxis
Vecuronium (Norcuron)	*Injection:* 10 mg/vial	*Infants > 7 wk–1 yr:* *Initial:* 0.08–0.1 mg/kg per dose i.v. *Maintenance:* 0.05–0.1 mg/kg per h i.v. p.r.n. *Children > 1 yr:* *Initial:* 0.08–0.1 mg/kg per dose i.v. *Maintenance:* 0.05–0.1 mg/kg per h p.r.n.	• Caution in severe liver disease • Elimination not affected by renal impairment • Reverse effects with neostigmine and atropine • Infants are more sensitive to vecuronium and may have a longer recovery time • Children may require higher and more frequent doses than adults
Vidarabine (Vira–A)	*Eye ointment:* 3%	<u>Herpetic keratitis:</u> Apply 1 cm ribbon to lower conjunctival sac q3h, 5 times in 24 h	• Continue for 7 d after lesion has healed
Vigabatrin (Sabril)	*Tablet:* 500 mg	*Children:* Give in 1 or 2 div. doses daily. *Initial:* 40 mg/kg per 24 h *Maximum:* 100 mg/kg per 24 h *Increment:* increase by 250 mg every 7 d to desired clinical response *Adults:* usual dose is 2–3 g/24 h given o.d. or div. b.i.d. *Maximum:* 4 g/24 h	• Useful in refractory partial epilepsy • Used as adjunct therapy with standard anticonvulsants • Vigabatrin dose should be tapered when therapy is stopped • Infantile spasms may require doses up to 150 mg/kg per 24 h

Drug	Supplied	Dose	Comments
Vitamin C (Ascorbic acid)	*Tablet:* 100 mg, 250 mg, 500 mg *Chewable tablet:* 100 mg, 500 mg *Injection:* 250 mg/mL	Deficiency (scurvy): *Infants and children:* 100–200 mg/24 h p.o. for at least 2 wk *Adults:* 500–1,000 mg/24 h p.o. for at least 2 wk *Maintenance:* *Children:* 35–45 mg/24 h *Adults:* 50–100 mg/24 h Deferoxamine adjunct: 150–250 mg/24 h p.o.	
Vitamin D (Ostoforte, D–Vi–Sol, Drisdol, Ergocalciferol)	*Capsule:* 50,000 unit *Solution:* 8,300 unit/mL (Drisdol), 400 unit/0.6 mL (D–Vi–Sol)	Nutritional rickets and osteomalacia: *Children and adults:* 2,000–5,000 unit/24 h × 6–12 wk Children with malabsorption: 10,000–25,000 unit/24 h Familial hypophosphatemia: *Children:* *Initial:* 40,000–80,000 unit/24 h *Increment:* 10,000–20,000 unit at 3–4 mo intervals until adequate response is obtained *Adults:* 10,000–60,000 unit/daily	• Consider dietary intake when calculating vitamin D dosage • 1 μg of ergocalciferol = 40 units
Vitamin E (D–alpha Tocopheral Acetate, Aquasol E)	*Capsule:* 100 IU, 200 IU, 400 IU *Drops:* 50 IU/mL	Recommended dietary allowance (RDA): *Infants up to 1 yr:* 4–6 units *Children 1–10 yr:* 7–10 units *Adult males:* 15 units *Adult females:* 12 units Treatment of deficiency: 4–5 times the RDA Supplementation in cystic fibrosis: 100–400 unit/24 h	• Oil miscible preparations (as in capsules) may be used in cystic fibrosis

Drug	Supplied	Dose	Comments
Vitamin K (Phytonadione, Aqua–Mephyton, Menadiol, Menadione)	*Injection (phytonadione, K_1):* 1 mg/0.5 mL, 10 mg/mL	*Neonatal hemorrhagic disease:* *Prophylaxis and treatment:* 0.5–1 mg/dose i.m., s.c., i.v. × 1 *Liver disease or malabsorption:* 2.5–25 mg/24 h p.o., i.v., i.m., s.c. *Vitamin K deficiency:* *Infants and children:* 1–2 mg/dose i.v. × 1 or 2–5 mg/24 h p.o. *Adults:* 5–25 mg/24 h p.o.	• Injectable form may be given orally • Hyperbilirubinemia and hemolysis have been reported in newborns (especially premature infants) • The risk is much less with phytonadione than other vitamin K preparations unless high doses (10–20 mg) are given • Use i.v. route only when other routes of administration are not feasible (i.v. may cause flushing, dizziness, hypotension, anaphylaxis)
Warfarin (Coumadin)	*Tablet:* 1 mg, 2 mg, 2.5 mg, 5 mg	*Children:* *Initial:* 0.2 mg/kg per dose p.o.; subsequent doses should be adjusted to maintain INR in desired range *Maximum:* 10 mg/dose	• Peak effect on patient occurs after 36–72 h • INR should be measured q24–48h during first week of therapy or until maintenance dose is established • Many drugs interact with warfarin
Xylometazoline (Otrivin)	*Spray:* 0.05%, 0.1%	*Children < 6 yr:* 1 (0.05%) spray into each nostril q8–10h *Children > 6 yr:* 1–2 (0.05%) spray into each nostril q8–10h *Adults:* 1–2 (0.1%) sprays into each nostril q8–10h	• Prolonged or excessive use may lead to rebound congestion when the drug is discontinued
Zidovudine (Retrovir)	*Capsule:* 100 mg *Oral syrup:* 50 mg/5 mL *Injection:* 200 mg/amp	*0–2 wk:* 2 mg/kg per dose p.o. q6h *2–4 wk:* 3 mg/kg per dose p.o. q6h *4 wk–13 yr:* 180 mg/m² per dose p.o. q6h If n.p.o.: 120 mg/m² per dose i.v. q6h *Minimum:* 75 mg/m² per dose q6h	• Anemia, leukopenia, neutropenia occurs in up to 30% of patients and is dose related • Onset is 4–8 wk

Drug	Supplied	Dose	Comments
Zinc	*Tablet (gluconate):* 10 mg Zn²⁺ *Injection:* 5 mg Zn²⁺/mL	Zinc deficiency: *Infants and children:* 0.5–1 mg Zn²⁺/24 h p.o. daily *Adults:* 25–50 mg Zn²⁺/dose p.o. t.i.d.	• 70 mg of zinc gluconate = 10 mg elemental zinc • Approximately 20–30% of p.o. zinc is absorbed

RENAL   **CHAPTER 19**
James Carter

HEMATURIA

Hematuria may be macroscopic (gross) or microscopic. Hematuria is defined as > 5 red blood cells (RBC's) per high power field on two separate analyses.

The reagent stick test is based on the peroxidase activity of hemoglobin. It is very sensitive and can detect 5 RBC/µL. Concentrated urine samples and high levels of vitamin C reduce the test's sensitivity.

Causes of positive dipstick screen

- Hematuria.
- Hemoglobinuria.
- Myoglobinuria.
- False positive: urinary tract infection (bacterial peroxidase), iodides.

There are many causes of red urine apart from hematuria.

Causes of "dipstick negative" red brown urine

- Endogenous: bile pigments, porphyrins, urates.
- Drugs: trinitrophenol, phenolphthalein, laxatives, pyridium, phenothiazines, cascara, rifampicin, desferrioxamine.
- Foods: beetroot, rhubarb, blackberries, red dyes.

A positive reagent stick reaction must be checked by microscopic urinalysis. The presence of red cells confirms hematuria. Also, note the presence of red cell casts which suggests a renal origin for hematuria (the urine must be freshly examined). The absence of red cells suggests hemoglobinuria, myoglobinuria, lysis of red cells in stored dilute urine or a false positive reagent test due to oxidizing agents, e.g. hypochlorite and peroxidases of bacteria. Table I may help in the differential diagnosis.

Table I: Differential diagnosis of positive dipstick test

Pathology	Reagent sticks	Color of spun serum	Urinalysis	Urine color
Microscopic hematuria	Positive	Clear	RBC's	Clear
Hemoglobinuria	Positive	Pink	No RBC's	Red
Myoglobinuria	Positive	Clear	No RBC's	Dark red

Transient hematuria is not uncommon in children, especially in those with a fever, so the initial step is to repeat the test in a few days if the child is asymptomatic. Hemoglobinuria and myoglobinuria are potentially serious problems and must be investigated without delay. The difference between the two is usually obvious on clinical grounds. They can be differentiated spectroscopically by the laboratory.

History

- Symptoms of urgency, swelling abdominal or loin pain and a history of trauma. Obtain information on urine volumes and type of stream.
- Family history of stones, renal disease, hypertension, or visual or hearing deficits, e.g. Alport's syndrome, cystic kidneys.
- Bleeding defects, excessive exercise, previous renal disease or urinary tract infection, sickle cell disease.
- Drug history (particularly analgesics).
- Type of hematuria: bright red urine, clots and varying degrees of hematuria during urination suggest lower tract disease. Constant red but brown urine throughout the stream suggests upper tract disease.

Examination

- A good physical examination to include: height, weight, blood pressure, presence or absence of edema, wasting and anemia.
- Check hearing (Alport's syndrome) and abdomen (renal mass, e.g. cystic kidney or tumor).
- Check for skin rash and arthritis (Henoch–Schönlein purpura, SLE).
- Check the eyes for retinitis, etc. (nephrophthisis, interstitial nephritis).
- Examine the external genitalia.

Causes

Subsequent investigations depend on the most likely diagnosis.

The major causes of hematuria in children are:
- Glomerular disease: glomerulonephritis (postinfectious nephritis, IgA nephropathy).
- Hereditary: polycystic kidneys, Alport's syndrome (nephritis and deafness), benign familial hematuria.
- Systemic disease: vasculitis (SLE, polyarteritis nodosa, Henoch–Schönlein purpura).
- Vascular disease: renal vein or artery thrombosis, malformation, hemolytic uremic syndrome.
- Neoplasm: Wilm's tumor.
- Trauma: including excessive exercise, march hematuria.
- Infection: bacterial, viral (adenovirus), tuberculosis, schistosomiasis.
- Nephrolithiasis or nephrocalcinosis, hypercalcinemia.
- Others: subacute bacterial endocarditis (SBE), sickle cell disease, coagulopathies, foreign body, drugs.

Table II helps to differentiate between upper and lower tract bleeding.

Table II: Determining the source of hematuria

Observation	Upper	Lower
Urine color	Brown	Bright red
Variation	Same throughout stream	Alters (may be terminal only)
Casts, protein	Sometimes	No
Clots	No	Sometimes
Red blood cells	Dysmorphic	Normal
Systemic (edema, rash, hypertension)	Frequent	Rare

Investigations

- Basic labwork should include:
    CBC and platelets plus thin smear.
    ESR, PT, PTT.
    Complete urinalysis (remember to test the parents and siblings as well for hematuria), urine culture, throat culture, ASOT, urea and creatinine.
- More detailed investigations include: additional blood tests such as serum proteins, immunoglobulins, complement levels and serological studies for SLE and hepatitis.
- Ultrasound, IVP or renogram, and a renal biopsy.
- Isolated hematuria of low intensity (RBC's 5–15/HPF) may be followed. Microscopic hematuria with substantial amounts of red cells (> 100/HPF) or associated with episodes of gross hematuria, proteinuria or a positive family history should be further investigated.

Myoglobinuria

Hemoglobin and myoglobin are probably not nephrotoxic but act as markers for a tissue substance which is toxic (possibly thromboplastin).

The major causes are:
- Trauma: especially extensive crush injuries.
- Muscular: polymyositis and muscular dystrophy, phosphorylase deficiency.
- Metabolic: hypokalemia, hypernatremia, hypophosphatemia.
- Others: alcohol poisoning, influenza.

Hemoglobinuria

When hemoglobin binding is exceeded, hemoglobin appears in the urine. Spun serum is pink as opposed to being clear in myoglobinuria. It is mostly a sign of intravascular hemolysis.

Causes include:
- Immune: paroxysmal cold and paroxysmal nocturnal hemoglobinuria.

- Others: malaria, burns, severe exercise, especially running.
- Spurious: lysis of RBC's in a dilute urine.

PROTEINURIA

Several methods are used to measure protein. The commonest is a buffered reagent strip that depends on a color change with pH. The sticks are reasonably specific for albumin but will not detect globulins like hemoglobin, myoglobin or Bence–Jones protein. The sensitivity is about 10 mg protein/100 mL.

- A dipstick screen is usually negative but may read trace on a concentrated sample.
- The average urinary protein loss is:
    0–1 month: 250 mg/m^2 per 24 h.
    1 month–9 years: 140 mg/m^2 per 24 h
    $\geq$ 10 years: 100 mg/m^2 per 24 h
- False positives can be produced by acetazolamide, bicarbonate and skin cleaning fluids that contaminate the sample.
- A positive screen should be checked by a precipitation method in the laboratory. Several drugs, notably penicillins, cause false positives in this test.

History

- Ask about symptoms of nephrosis (puffy eyes, edema, poor growth).
- Take a full family history (congenital renal disease, cystic kidneys).
- Take a medical history, e.g. hepatitis, syphilis, malaria, drugs (especially gold, penicillamine).

Examination

- A full examination to include: height, weight and blood pressure.
- Note the presence of edema, ascites, rash, arthritis, loin tenderness and abdominal masses.

Causes

Subsequent investigations depend on the most likely diagnosis.

The major causes of proteinuria are:
- Prerenal: fever, severe exercise, pregnancy, benign orthostatic proteinuria, venous congestion (especially heart failure, constrictive pericarditis).
- Renal:
    Glomerulonephritis, nephrotic syndrome (1°: minimal change, focal glomerulosclerosis, crescentic; 2°: diabetes, SLE, syphilis, malaria).
    Pyelonephritis, cystinosis, Wilson's disease.
    Drugs: penicillamine, gold salts.
    Congenital nephrosis.
- Postrenal: cystitis, contamination (e.g. vaginal secretion, skin cleaning fluids).

Investigations

- Transient proteinuria is not uncommon so check initial result. Fever and exercise may cause proteinuria. If still positive, rule out orthostatic proteinuria. Midday or evening urine contains protein, while first sample after waking in the morning should be completely clear. This diagnosis carries a benign prognosis. If persistent proteinuria, quantify with a 24 hour urine collection.
- Basic labwork should include:
    24 hour urine for protein and creatinine (the creatinine estimation is used to check the completeness of the sample).
    Serum albumin and globulin.
    Urinalysis and culture, serum lipids, C3 and C4, urea, creatinine.
    Urine electrophoresis to determine selectivity of the proteinuria is sometimes done.
- A poor prognosis in the nephrotic syndrome is indicated by age less than 1 year or more than 10 years, unselective proteinuria, abnormal urine sediment (e.g. casts and hematuria), low complement, hypertension and raised urea or creatinine. Many of these patients will eventually come to renal biopsy.
- If a child is nephrotic (massive edema, hypoalbuminemia—i.e. serum albumin < 2 g %, proteinuria—i.e. urine > 2 g/24 h with hyperlipidemia) and between 1 and 10 years of age, the most likely diagnosis is nephrotic syndrome (in childhood). Biopsy will show minimal changes. First determine if steroid responsive by giving prednisone 2 mg/kg per d until response obtained or for a maximum of 4–6 weeks. If no response in 4–6 weeks, consider renal biopsy. If the child is < 1 year of age or postpubertal, other diseases become more likely, therefore, a renal biopsy must be considered to guide therapy.

HYPERTENSION

Hypertension is quite common in childhood and easily missed. Average rates are 1–2% in preterm infants and children, 5–10% among adolescents and as high as 15% among African adolescents; 10% will have severe hypertension. The majority of hypertension in children will be secondary to renal disease.

Several potential areas of error exist, especially inadequate cuff size and patient anxiety or distress. A single raised reading in an otherwise asymptomatic child must be checked repeatedly and carefully before labelling a patient as hypertensive. Table III gives a guide to the definition of hypertension with different ages.

History

- Family history of hypertension, cerebral or coronary vascular disease, myocardial infarcts.
- Presence of renal disease, e.g. glomerulonephritis, cystic kidneys, Henoch–Schönlein purpura.
- Systemic disease: SLE, PAN, diabetes.
- Past history of renal trauma, radiation, umbilical catheterization, cardiac surgery, coarctation, drugs (steroids, methysergide, amphetamines).
- Symptoms: headache, epistaxis, palpitations.

Classification of hypertension

Table III: Definitions of hypertension with ages

Age	Significant hypertension	Severe hypertension
7 d	Systolic BP ≥ 96	Systolic BP ≥ 106
8–30 d	Systolic BP ≥ 104	Systolic BP ≥ 110
Infant (< 2 yr)	Systolic BP ≥ 112 Diastolic BP ≥ 74	Systolic BP ≥ 118 Diastolic BP ≥ 82
Children (3–5 yr)	Systolic BP ≥ 116 Diastolic BP ≥ 76	Systolic BP ≥ 124 Diastolic BP ≥ 86
Children (6–9 yr)	Systolic BP ≥ 122 Diastolic BP ≥ 78	Systolic BP ≥ 130 Diastolic BP ≥ 86
Children (10–12 yr)	Systolic BP ≥ 126 Diastolic BP ≥ 82	Systolic BP ≥ 134 Diastolic BP ≥ 90
Adolescents (13–15 yr)	Systolic BP ≥ 136 Diastolic BP ≥ 86	Systolic BP ≥ 144 Diastolic BP ≥ 92
Adolescents (16–18 yr)	Systolic BP ≥ 142 Diastolic BP ≥ 92	Systolic BP ≥ 150 Diastolic BP ≥ 98

Examination

A good examination to include:
- Blood pressure (lying and sitting), height, weight, anemia, edema and other evidence of chronic renal disease.
- Look particularly for the clinical pictures of Cushing's syndrome and hyperthyroidism.
- Conscientiously check for abdominal bruit of renal artery stenosis, delayed or absent femoral arteries of coarctation or abdominal mass (cystic kidneys, Wilm's tumor, neuroblastoma).

Causes

- Renal: HUS, HSP, dysplasia, polycystic kidneys, glomerulonephritis, hydronephrosis (obstructive uropathy), chronic pyelonephritis and reflux nephropathy, diabetes, acute or chronic renal failure, Wilm's tumor.
- Vascular: coarctation, hypoplastic aortic arch, renal artery stenosis or occlusion due to previous umbilical catheterization, fibromuscular dysplasia, neurofibromatosis, arteritis, etc.
- Endocrine: Cushing's syndrome (primary or secondary), pheochromocytoma, neuroblastoma, hyperaldosteronism.
- Drugs: steroids, amphetamines, hypotensive drug withdrawal.
- Others: chronic lead poisoning, hypervolemia, raised ICP, pregnancy, hypercalcemia.
- Essential or idiopathic: by far the commonest cause in adolescents and young adults. Related obesity and a positive family history are important clues.

Laboratory

- A good history and physical examination will reveal most of the secondary causes.
- The basic workup should include: urinalysis and urine culture, CBC, electrolytes, BUN, creatinine.
- More detailed investigations will include: renal scans, ultrasound, renal arteriogram, renal vein renin sampling, 24 hour urine for catecholamines and 17–ketosteroids.

Treatment outline

See chapter 18 (Pharmacology and Drug Dosage Guidelines) for doses. Acute hypertension is also covered under chapter 3 (Emergencies). Many treatment regimens exist.

The following approaches are suggested:
- Hypertensive crisis: control with sublingual nifedipine, i.v. labetalol, i.v. diazoxide or i.v. nitroprusside. Long–term management as for significant hypertension.
- Significant hypertension: start with propranolol ± hydralazine or captopril ± diuretic.
- Mild hypertension: begin with diet and exercise. If no control, add a thiazide diuretic and then propranolol, atenolol or nifedipine.

URINARY TRACT INFECTIONS

Urinary tract infections are among the commonest of pediatric infection. About 1–2% of female children of all ages have asymptomatic bacteriuria. This rate is 10 times greater than males except in infancy when the incidence of infection is equal.

Infection usually ascends via the urethra. Hematogenous spread is rare except in neonates or occasional older children with SBE or septicemia.

Pathogens

- Gram negatives: *E. coli*, *Klebsiella*, *Proteus*, *Pseudomonas*.
- Gram positives: *S. epidermidis* (if catheterized); *S. aureus* rarely.
- Anerobes: *Cl. perfringens*, bacteroides, fusobacterium (especially if bladder stasis).
- Others: tuberculosis, viruses (adenovirus), fungi rarely.

History

- Ask about family history of UTI.
- The medical history includes previous infections, neurological disease (especially spina bifida), catheterization or other instrumentation of the urinary tract.
- Presentation is very variable.
- Classical symptoms are urgency, frequency, loin pain, dysuria, incontinence in a previously dry child and dribbling.
- Nonspecific complaints like vomiting, failure to thrive and poor feeding are found in younger children.
- Symptoms in infancy include jaundice, lethargy, hypothermia and even apneic spells.

Examination

A good examination to include:
• Height, weight and blood pressure.
• Neurological screen, e.g. spina bifida, lower limb function and incontinence.
• Abdomen for renal masses and palpable bladder.
• Genitalia for abnormalities.

Causes

• Stasis: stones, congenital abnormalities, urethral valves, neurogenic (e.g. spina bifida).
• Mechanical: catheterization, surgery, instrumentation, foreign body.
• Hematogenous spread: SBE, neonates.
• Sterile pyuria (hematuria and pyuria without bacterial infection): viral, cyclophosphamide, catheterization, high fever and dehydration.

Laboratory

• UTI is defined as more than 10^6 colonies/L of urine. This correlates well with one or more bacteria per oil field in uncentrifuged urine.
• Collecting a clean urine specimen from children is not always easy:
    Midstream: clean external genitalia well. Quite good for children > 5 years of age.
    Collection bag: clean perineum well. Contamination from stool, etc., is common. Remove bag immediately after child produces urine. Negative result rules out UTI but a positive result may be difficult to interpret.
    Catheter: reasonably easy, small chance of contamination; probably above 10^3 colonies/mL significant.
    Suprapubic: safe if done carefully. Any bacterial count is significant.
• Several methods have been tried to differentiate between upper and lower tract disease such as B_2 microglobulin, LDH, antibody coated bacteria and others. They are not reliable enough for clinical work. Currently, the most reliable study is the DMSA renal scan.
• Most people investigate any child, male or female, after one well documented urine infection to look for reflux or anomalies. However, in female children > 5 years, the yield may be low and thorough investigation is carried out only after repeat infections. Transient urinary reflux is common during acute infections so a voiding cystourethrogram is performed at least 3–4 weeks after treatment. A renal ultrasound may be performed earlier than this.

Treatment

• Most infections respond to a 10 day course of oral antibiotics. Refer to chapter 10 (Infectious Diseases) for choice of drug.
• Single dose treatment is rarely used in children < 10–12 years of age.
• For infants with pyelonephritis and unusual organisms like *Pseudomonas*, a course of intravenous antibiotics is most often advised. The newer quinolone derivatives should not be used in prepubertal children.

ACUTE RENAL FAILURE (ARF)

Acute renal failure is defined as an abrupt decline in renal function so that retention of nitrogenous waste results. It is not now tied to urine output because of recognition of nonoliguric renal failure. However, oliguria usually accompanies ARF with urine output below 180 mg/m² per 24 h. Ten to 20% of cases maintain an output above this level despite renal failure.

The inability to excrete waste products leads to a complex array of problems, notably acidosis, hyperkalemia, water retention, hypertension and uremia.

The underlying cause is often determined by a good history and physical examination.

Evaluation

- A good examination takes into account drug history, toxic exposure, sepsis, hypoxia (especially in the neonate), dehydration (burns, diarrhea), surgery (especially cardiac bypass), preceding renal disease, recent bloody diarrhea (hemolytic uremic syndrome).
- The precipitating cause is often very obvious on examination: sepsis, DIC, hypotension, shock, hemorrhage, surgery and burns. Assess hydration, blood pressure, IVP and perfusion.

Causes

- Prerenal: hypovolemia (shock, sepsis, third space losses, nephrotic syndrome with low circulating volume).
- Renal: venous or arterial thrombosis, hypoxia, drugs (sulfas, penicillins), toxins (ethylene glycol, carbon tetrachloride), increased uric acid, toxic lysis syndrome, glomerulonephritis (including HUS).
- Postrenal: stones, clots, pelvi–ureteric obstruction or posterior urethral valves.

Laboratory

- The kidneys can still concentrate urine with prerenal failure. While in intrinsic renal failure, any urine formed is just filtered plasma. Based on these facts, several tests are used to differentiate prerenal and renal failure (Table IV). They are of little value if a dose of lasix has been given.
- If still in doubt, insert a central line to measure the venous pressure. An abdominal ultrasound will help in the differentiation between intrinsic renal failure and urinary tract obstruction.

Management

- Prerenal: rapidly restore volume with colloid, preferably with a CVP monitor. If no urine output, try 1 dose of mannitol (0.5–1.0 g/kg) or 1 dose of furosemide (1.0–2.0 mg/kg).
- Postrenal: temporarily bypass posterior urethral valves with a catheter. Other causes may require surgical intervention.
- Water retention: limit input to 300 mL/m² per 24 h plus urine output.
- Hyperkalemia and hypertension: see chapter 3 (Emergencies).
- Uremia: limit protein intake to 1 g/kg per d.
- Nutrition: high calorie low protein diet, orally or via central line. See chapter 15 (Nutrition).
- If hyperkalemia, fluid overload or symptoms of uremia become unmanageable, acute dialysis

is indicated.

Table IV: Differentiating renal from prerenal failure

Measured variable	Child		Newborn	
	Prerenal	**Renal**	**Prerenal**	**Renal**
Urinary osmolarity	> 500	< 350	> 400	< 400
Urinary osmolarity or plasma osmolarity	> 1.3	< 1.1	> 1.3	≤ 1.0
Urinary urea/plasma urea	> 8	< 8	–	–
Urinary creatinine/plasma creatinine	> 40	< 20	> 30	< 10
Urinary sodium	< 20	> 50	–	–
Fractional excretion (Na)	< 1	> 2	< 2.5	> 2.5
Urine flow rate	Variable	Variable	Variable	Variable

$$\text{Fractional excretion (Na)} = \frac{(\text{urinary sodium/plasma sodium})}{(\text{urinary creatinine/plasma creatinine})} \times 100$$

CHRONIC RENAL FAILURE (CRF)

Chronic renal failure in children is relatively rare: 3–4 cases (require dialysis) per million population per year. However, frequent admissions make CRF a common ward management problem. The difficulties associated with CRF and the long list of medications prescribed to deal with them are not so daunting when considered logically and one at a time.

Causes

- Structural: obstruction (UP junction, urethral valves), dysplastic or polycystic kidney, reflux plus chronic pyelonephritis.
- Immune: glomerulonephritis (crescentic, SLE, PAN, etc.).
- Others: cystinosis, oxalosis, radiation, trauma, drugs, toxins, HUS, hereditary nephritis, nephrectomy for malignancy, renal vein thrombosis, papillary or cortical necrosis, hypoxic or ischemic damage.

Management problems

1. Sodium
- Most patients have a "no added salt" restriction, mainly to control hypertension and fluid retention. Occasionally, some children are salt wasters and require added sodium.
- Measure urine sodium for guidance.

2. Potassium
- Potassium excretion is usually preserved until dialysis is required, as long as reasonable dietary allowances are observed (no fruit juices, cocoa, chocolate).

- Diuretics or poor intake may induce hypokalemia while hyperkalemic crises may complicate acute illnesses.

3. Acidosis
- Decreased acid excretion and decreased bicarbonate reabsorption lead to acidosis.
- About 2 mEq/kg per 24 h of alkali may be needed as a buffer.
- Bicitra solution contains 1 mEq/mL. Adjust dose by urine pH or serum bicarbonate level.

4. Water
A difficult balance exists between dehydration and edema. Usually requires about 400 mL/m^2 plus urinary output.

5. Osteodystrophy
An imprecise term covering osteomalacia, rickets, osteitis fibrosa and impaired bone growth. The combined effects of renal failure on bone metabolism are summarized in Table V.

Table V: The effects of chronic renal failure on bone

Cause	Effect
Low 1:25 vitamin D	Hypocalcemia, osteomalacia, rickets
Hyperphosphatemia	Hypocalcemia from decreased absorption, vitamin D inhibition; metastatic calcification
Acidosis	Decreased bone mineralization
Hypocalcemia	Hyperparathyroidism, bone cysts and pain
Malnutrition	Poor bone growth

- Treatment consists of three approaches:
    Hyperphosphatemia: phosphate binders such as calcium carbonate or acetate (avoid magnesium and aluminum containing antacids). Decrease phosphate intake.
    Low vitamin D: high doses of vitamin D or one of its metabolites. Danger of hypercalcemia and reduced renal function if not followed closely.
    Hypocalcemia: oral calcium tablets. (Dairy products contain a lot of phosphate.)

6. Nutrition and growth
- Good nutrition is essential for growth and to decrease catabolism. Added calories and amino acid solutions are used. See chapter 15 (Nutrition).
- Occasionally, sugar intolerance occurs probably due to insulin resistance. Watch sugar levels if pushing calories.
- Recombinant growth hormone shown to have possible effects on linear growth.

7. Anemia
- Poor production of erythropoietin is probably the major cause.
- Hemoglobin is maintained better by peritoneal dialysis.
- Children on hemodialysis also lose blood in the membrane and often require a regular

transfusion.
- Recombinant erythropoietin is now available.

8. Neurological
Patients with uremia have a complex array of neurological complaints, including peripheral neuropathy, irritability, failure to concentrate and seizures.

DIALYSIS

Temporary renal failure is a common complication following a wide range of serious illnesses, particularly complex cardiac surgery. Consequently, dialysis is a common procedure in any PICU. Fortunately, most cases of acute renal failure in children recover well after a few days of dialysis support.

Indications

- Hyperkalemia: a rapidly rising potassium level that has not been controlled by potassium restriction and ion exchange therapy; dictates the urgent institution of dialysis.
- Hypervolemia: fluid overload and pulmonary edema are common complications of cardiac surgery. Dialysis is sometimes used in grossly fluid overloaded children even though renal function might be normal. Continuous lasix infusions are also used in this situation.
- Poisons and toxins: dialysis can be used to enhance the elimination of some poisons (salicylates, methanol, ethylene glycol and several others). It can also be used to increase the clearance of ammonia in children with an acute exacerbation of an underlying metabolic disease.
- Uremia: there is no absolute value of BUN that dictates dialysis, but if the child is developing neurological symptoms from uremia or if the urea level is rising rapidly, then dialysis is indicated.

Methods of dialysis

There are several types of dialysis, each of which has advantages and disadvantages.

1. Peritoneal dialysis
This technique uses the peritoneal lining as a dialysis membrane. Following insertion of a catheter into the peritoneal space, dialysis fluids are introduced to the peritoneal cavity and allowed to equilibrate. Standard solutions that contain fixed quantities of electrolytes and varying concentrations of dextrose between 1.25% and 4.5% are available. Higher concentrations of dextrose are more efficient at removing fluid from the child but run the risk of inflaming the peritoneal membrane. After a dwell time that can vary from half an hour to about 4 hours, the fluid is run out of the peritoneum into a collecting bag. Strict records of input and output are required to calculate the amount of fluid that is being removed. When instituting this technique in a child with an unstable cardiovascular system, great care must be used to drain the ascitic fluid slowly following catheter insertion or marked hypotension can result. Peritoneal dialysis is considerably simpler than the other available techniques, but it is not as efficient in removing fluids or solutes. Apart from peritoneal infection, the main practical problem is partial or complete obstruction of the

peritoneal catheter by abdominal contents.

2. Hemodialysis

Hemodialyis equipment is expensive and requires well trained technicians. Patients requiring chronic hemodialysis first require the creation of an arteriovenous shunt. When hemodialysis is used for an acute indication such as poisoning, it is more useful to access the vascular system using large double lumen cannulas. These may be venovenous or arteriovenous catheters. Some machines are able to use a single lumen venous catheter by alternately aspirating and infusing blood. Hemodialysis achieves the best fluid and solute clearance, but it is expensive and requires invasive vascular access.

3. Continuous hemofiltration

The acronyms used to describe the various forms of hemofiltration can be very confusing. Earlier techniques consisted of putting a dialysis filter in the circuit between an arterial and venous catheter. Blood was pushed through the circuit by the patient's own blood pressure. This was called continuous arteriovenous hemofiltration (CAVH). A dialysis countercurrent was sometimes used with the filter, further complicating the acronym to CAVHD. The simplicity of the system was attractive but children who require dialysis quite frequently have poor cardiac output. Consequently, the circuits would frequently thrombose even though the children were heparinized. The circuit also required arterial and venous catheters. Subsequently, venovenous circuits were developed that included a small pump. They can be used with or without a dialysis countercurrent (CVVH or CVVHD). Commercial machines are now available and many PICU's use the technique routinely, particularly on fluid overloaded postsurgical patients. The technique requires large two lumen venous access and also requires full heparinization of the child. The total blood flow through the circuit is only a small percentage of the child's cardiac output so clearance of solutes is not as high as can be achieved in hemodialysis. However, close control of the patient's volume status is possible.

The key element of your training should be a progressive increase in the level of independent action in all aspects of patient care while still in a situation where you can receive guidance from more experiencd physician peers. This process inevitably involves elements of supervision and direction and relies, for its successful completion, on your motivation and effective involvement. Ultimately, you are the one who determines how well you are trained. The program can only provide the structure on which you build your clinical experience and knowledge. A sense of responsibility for your education and your role in patient care is a key element. Taking appropriate responsibility enhances self-esteem, and your self–esteem has a considerable bearing on how good or bad you decide each day has been. Whatever you feel about your postgraduate training, you will inevitably have moments of extreme doubts. Be reassured that this time is a finite "rite of passage" and with thoughtful management, it can be both a rich and rewarding experience.

Communication

No human being, including the best physician, can get on well with everyone. Though some communication skills are innate, many others can be learned. Residents and fellows with good communication skills are more likely to thrive during training. Clear communication, both spoken and written, improves relationships with other physicians, nurses, children and parents as well as with family and significant others. Communicating the key details of a child's hospitalization to the family physician and/or referring pediatrician is an essential component of good care, particularly at the time of discharge and following emergency transfer.

Beware of individuals with whom communication is impossible (at least for you at that particular time). Individuals who see themselves as complex, fascinating and informed may in fact be difficult, ignorant and dogmatic. Give each person the benefit of the doubt, but do not allow your confidence to be destroyed by individuals who complain about everything. When your best efforts to communicate fail, you must delegate the responsibility to others. This is important for your own morale, for good patient care and for medicolegal reasons. If communication with a parent is difficult, involve another colleague and tell the physician in charge. If problems occur with a senior physician, seek discrete advice from another resident or staff physician.

Harassment

There must be a clear distinction between what constitutes appropriate behavior and what is rude or threatening. You should expect to be challenged during training to acquire new skills and more knowledge and to provide comprehensive, well rounded care. Whether you interpret such "challenges" as appropriate or inappropriate depends on numerous factors, many of them personal.

Life involves moral and cultural standards; medicine involves risk and urgency. To avoid becoming a society of victims, we must improve our ability to share concerns, give and receive apology and, above all, retain an element of common sense and good will. It is easy to make hasty assumptions and more difficult to unravel formal accusations. The most important step with any perceived harassment is to talk the matter through calmly with a suitable third party.

Some physical contact can be as unwelcome as other aspects of behavior. Be mindful of this but do not abandon touch altogether. Touch remains a key element in intuitive diagnosis, effective communication and compassionate care.

Emotional support

During your training, try to identify a pediatrician to whom you can turn for emotional and intellectual support. This informal mentoring arrangement provides a safety net for the doubts, uncertainties and dilemmas which always arise during training. If you can, cultivate such a relationship before major problems arise. A staff physician with an aura of huge personal success may appeal to you, but in the long run, an interested listener with uncommon good sense will help you most. In turn, try to listen sympathetically to patients, colleagues, senior physicians and nurses. All of these individuals have expectations of you. If these expectations are unclear to you or in conflict with your own goals, the rift between you and them will cause disappointment, conflict and unhappiness (as well as a bleak assessment).

Some rotations are more frustrating than others, but all eventually come to an end. Your written reviews and positive suggestions should follow each rotation. Spontaneous verbal suggestions are not as effective as facts put in writing. Simple, nonjudgmental assessments are more likely to result in change. Your expectations of your senior supervising colleagues are important too and also benefit all concerned if they are written and mutually agreed upon.

Living by the clock

Time management is important. Your tardiness will upset other people and waste time. To avoid wasting your own time, keep meetings brief and end them on schedule. Try to complete tasks without interruption. This is particularly important during ward rounds, clinical examination of patients and order writing. If you complete one task before moving on, you avoid having to come back later. This discipline fosters better organization and ensures that fewer tasks are overlooked.

As you move beyond your teens, your sense of responsibility increases while your brain cells begin their inevitable decline. Make lists and set priorities. Each day, or period on–call, should be divided into issues of greater and lesser importance. Set deadlines, especially when reading or writing. Deadlines are more difficult to follow when they involve patient care, but your available time must be divided reasonably among the priorities you have identified.

Manage your free time even more aggressively. An efficient system for taking over responsibility in the morning and for evening sign out rounds should be put in place. Scheduled appropriately, these measures improve patient care and get off–duty residents out of the hospital on time. Cultivate a full life away from the hospital; this will make you more efficient and committed while at work. Your recreation should be fun, stimulating and completely different from your normal work regimen.

Your physical well being is as important as your mental morale. Exercise relieves stress, enhances efficiency, and improves sleep. It is very tempting to avoid exercise if you are frantically busy, but it makes you feel better and helps you to focus your life. Try to eat sensibly, especially when you are at the hospital cafeteria. Avoid putting on too much weight; some transport programs will not let residents fly if they weigh more than 185 pounds!

Stress

"Burn out" and "critical incident stress" are genuine entities. Multiple patient deaths, demoralizing rotations or a clustering of on–call nights or weekends can precipitate depression. More subtle problems (chronic dissatisfaction or strained personal relationships) can also cause real unhappiness. Awareness of potential problems, as well as deliberate attempts to improve your morale, can ease some of the strain. Mental health breaks are sometimes essential for your well being. Work together with your colleagues to create a flexible, compassionate schedule for all of you.

In spite of your own best effort, the very nature of the pediatric residency and fellowship training will bring you into situations where you are unable to manage the effects of stress on your own. What overwhelms one individual may only appear mildly to another. We each react differently to life's stressful events, and there is good evidence that much of our response originates from our emotional experience prior to a critical incident. Unfortunately, stress is cumulative and major events such as the death of a child or an important professional error will usually result in most of us developing stress related symptoms within about 24 hours. Some of us who believe we feel no consequences from stress are in denial, although a small proportion of individuals do seem largely immune.

The concept of intervention to reduce the effects of critical incident stress was originally developed by Mitchell, based on evidence that there is a window of opportunity for effective intervention following a critical incident of something like 72 hours. The first step is to talk to someone about what has occurred and what you feel. This may be your official mentor, a close professional colleague or a member of your family. Sometimes this is all that is required; on other occasions, more is needed. Hospitals increasingly have trained individuals who form teams to assist with critical incident stress debriefing. The process itself has a number of recognized steps which explain the process, allow the recall of thoughts related to the incident, discuss the reaction experienced and symptoms that have resulted, and help the individual with a series of measures aimed at providing insight and identifying coping strategies. We also recognize that our families are exposed to the effects of critical incidents through us, and the debriefing process can, when necessary, include our significant other.

If your private life is as physically and emotionally demanding as your work, you will soon fall apart. Late parties and hangovers will not prepare you well for the next night on–call. When returning home after a difficult night at work, warn your family that you are ragged and irritable. Avoid unrealistic expectations of yourself; the night after call is not the time to cook dinner for your in–laws.

Families need insight into your hospital experience. Most of us are not articulate when we try to express our feelings. You may be tempted to say, "I am fine; I had a good day," when in fact you had burst into tears three times. Resist the temptation to gloss over your feelings. While constant talk about medicine will alienate your family, you must tell the truth. If you do not make an effort to communicate, your relationships will be shallow or very transient. Ask your family or friends to visit while you are on–call. It might help them to understand the stress of a night at work.

The Agony of exams

Being a good doctor and sailing through exams do not necessarily go together. Academic growth is as important to your training as acquiring clinical skills. Books are better read a little at a time rather than as a gargantuan effort just before exams. Remember that the patients you meet from the beginning to the end of your training provide the experience upon which your skills are based. It is a salutory lesson to realize that the less call you do, the less wisdom you acquire.

Never underestimate the value of teaching others while you are trying to learn. It may seem a chore at the time, but there is no better way to organize your thoughts or discover the gaps in your understanding. Research, too, is often undervalued by residents. In its purest form, research simply asks the question why and then looks for an answer in a logical way. Those who never ask questions will always have to use other people's answers.

Attitude

Nearly everyone survives and completes his or her specialty training, but life should be more than mere survival. Take a firm grasp of all the opportunities you are offered. You will be surprised how many of them prove to have been useful once you are out in practice. Taking responsibility for your training and for your role within the hospital is an integral part of maintaining your self–esteem and preparing you for the complex but rewarding job of being a pediatrician. Compassion and humor will enrich your life both during and beyond your residency. Celebrate the strengths and positive attributes of your colleagues and your lot in life. With these insights and your own creativity, you can make much of your training enjoyable and some of it truly memorable.

Michael Seear

INTRODUCTION

A good working knowledge of respiratory medicine is essential for anyone practicing hospital pediatrics. The top three causes of acute admission to any Children's Hospital in North America are all respiratory diseases (bronchiolitis, asthma and pneumonia), while one of the commonest causes for chronic admission is cystic fibrosis. In addition, many patients admitted under other disciplines, such as Oncology, Intensive Care and Special Care Nursery, will frequently have major respiratory complications.

Respiratory medicine is not an esoteric subject. The lung has very few ways of expressing its displeasure, so most complaints will be a permutation of cough, wheeze or shortness of breath. With judicial use of common sense and a knowledge of basic physiology, most respiratory problems can be diagnosed and managed effectively.

ASSESSMENT OF LUNG FUNCTION

Respirologists are fortunate in having a large number of tests at their disposal for the evaluation of a child with a respiratory disease. These can range from peak flow readings to lung MRI. If common sense is abandoned, it is easy to waste a lot of money. Apart from a detailed history and physical examination, a standard workup should include a chest X–ray plus pulmonary function tests in children old enough to cooperate (usually an intelligent 5 year old in a good mood).

Spirometry

The use of acronyms and technical jargon makes pulmonary function testing seem a good deal more complex than it really is. Spirometry is simply a means of measuring static lung volumes, as displayed in Figure I. The volume between total lung capacity and residual volume is called vital capacity and can be measured reproducibly and accurately. The effects of chronic diseases such as cystic fibrosis or muscular dystrophy upon lung function are manifested by a slow but steady drop in vital capacity. This simple measurement allows the severity of disease to be assessed by a single number. The volume of air expelled at maximal effort in one second is called FEV_1 and is a good first order of approximation of the degree of small airway obstruction. The ratio between FEV_1 and FVC is sometimes used to classify lung diseases into two broad groups: restrictive (> 75%) and obstructive (< 75%).

Flow volume loops

By plotting flow rate against instantaneous lung volume, a closed flow volume loop is obtained. The expiratory limb should be a straight line (Figure II), which is largely independent of patient effort. The shape of the curve is useful diagnostically and changes predictably with several diseases. In asthma, it takes a characteristically scooped pattern since instantaneous flows are less than normal for a given lung volume. Peak flow (PEF) and mid–expiratory flow (FEF_{25-75}) are used as estimates of small airway obstruction in the same way as FEV_1 (which is a volume not a flow).

Figure I: Spirometric lung volumes

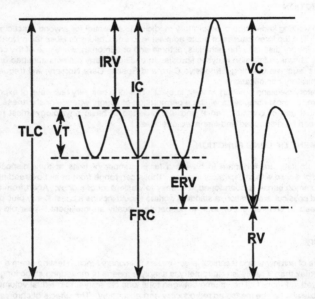

VC: vital capacity
RV: residual volume
FRC: functional residual capacity
V_T: tidal volume
TLC: total lung capacity
IC: inspiratory capacity
ERV: expiratory reserve volume
IRV: inspiratory reserve volume

Figure II: Flow–volume loop

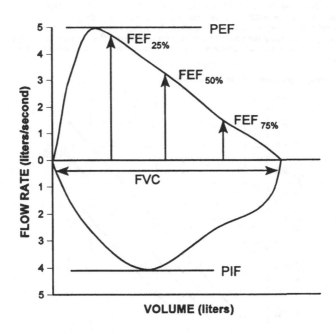

PEF: peak expiratory flow
FVC: forced vital capacity
PIF: peak inspiratory flow
FEF: forced expiratory flow (at 25%, 50% or 75% of expiration)

Diffusion capacity

The diffusion of carbon monoxide across the lung (D_LCO) can be measured in most well equipped pulmonary function laboratories. It is dependent on a number of physiological factors, including lung volume, V/Q mismatch, diffusion thickness, pulmonary capillary blood volume and cardiac output. The final result is a very sensitive indicator of lung disease and should probably be interpreted in the same way as an erythrocyte sedimentation rate, that is, if it is abnormal, then there is certainly something wrong but it gives no indication to the cause of the problem.

Peak flow meter

The simplest test of pulmonary function is a portable peak flow meter; several cheap commercial makes are available. When used in conjunction with a daily diary, they are of some value in assessing the degree of asthmatic control. They also offer some degree of early warning for the occasional patient who deteriorates rapidly. However, the devices are strongly effort dependent and many physicians prefer to rely on symptom diaries. Normal values are shown in Figure III.

Figure III: Normal values for peak expiratory flow

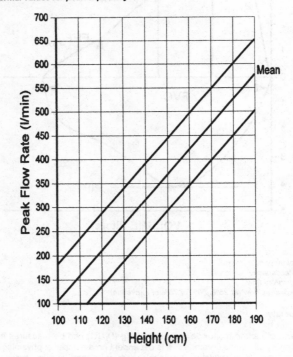

Other tests of pulmonary function

- Airway resistance: (Raw) can be measured directly in a body plethysmograph or, in the form of impedance, using an impulse oscillometer. In practice, these offer no advantage over the more easily measured FEV_1 and FEF_{25-75}. Functional residual capacity and, consequently, residual volume (Figure 1) can be measured by helium dilution or body plethysmography and are of some value in the occasional asthmatic.
- Measures of oxygenation: pulse oximetry is the simplest method to assess the adequacy of oxygen saturation. The normal level is above 95%, although children with cyanotic cardiac lesions can survive and grow with saturations in the 70's. The reading has no value unless there is a good pulse signal. Arterial blood gases are usually only of value in the Intensive Care Unit since the practical problems of arterial puncture preclude their regular use on the ward. Modern machines measure pH, PCO_2 and PO_2 with small volumes of blood using individual electrodes. Saturation is derived from a standard dissociation curve and is not measured. The bicarbonate is calculated by the Henderson–Hasselbalch equation. Capillary blood gases are often used on the ward and provide a reasonable indication of pH and PCO_2. The value of PO_2 is too unreliable to be of any clinical value. Transcutaneous monitors exist to measure both oxygen and carbon dioxide partial pressures. Unfortunately, they have not proved to be reliable outside the neonatal age range.
- Radiology: a chest X–ray is certainly the single most useful diagnostic test for pulmonary disease. A basic approach needs to be developed for viewing the films so that lesions are not missed. This includes assessment of the film technique, evaluation of the chest wall (including bones and soft tissues), diaphragm and pleura, examination of the thoracic and hilar areas and, of course, the lung fields. Upper GI studies are sometimes used to give information regarding mediastinal structures, presence of reflux and other esophageal anomalies. CT scans of the lung are being used more commonly in the assessment of lung disease, especially now that rapid scan times are possible. Ventilation perfusion scans and lung MRI scans are occasionally used.
- Bronchoscopy: the upper and central airways can be viewed either with a rigid or flexible bronchoscope. The rigid scope provides the best visualization but requires a general anesthetic. It is most useful for therapeutic procedures such as extraction of foreign bodies. Much diagnostic information can be provided somewhat less invasively using a flexible bronchoscope in sedated infants or children. Many respiratory departments have a flexible bronchoscopy suite where the procedures can be performed on an outpatient basis. Transbronchial lung biopsy specimens can be taken through the flexible scope but require fluoroscopic guidance for safety. Bronchoalveolar lavage specimens can be obtained using either technique and often provide useful information on the etiology of lung infections.
- Lung biopsy: occasionally, it is necessary to take a biopsy of the lung to diagnose conditions such as interstitial lung disease and obscure pulmonary infections. The severely ill child may require ventilation following the procedure.

DISEASES OF THE UPPER AIRWAY

Diseases of the upper airway produce prolongation of the inspiratory time, inspiratory stridor, frequently a barking cough, and aphonia if the disease process involves the vocal cords. Apart from a foreign body, which is usually diagnosed by history, the differential diagnosis of acute stridor is usually between three infectious diseases: croup, epiglottitis and bacterial tracheitis. The diameter of the airway in a typical child with these conditions is usually no more than half a centimeter. The resistance to flow increases as the fourth power of the radius so that 1 or 2 mm of mucosal swelling can produce a life threatening obstruction.

Viral croup

Viral croup is the commonest cause of acute upper airway obstruction. It is generally caused by parainfluenza type 1, although other respiratory viruses can cause an identical syndrome. Subglottic mucosal edema is the cause of the signs of upper airway obstruction. Roughly 5% of affected children will require hospital admission and a small percentage of this group will require intubation. Management is supportive. Croup tents do not help and generally simply upset the child. Added oxygen should not be necessary in pure upper airway obstruction. If desaturation is present in room air, then it is a sign of another urgent problem (most likely hypercarbia or pneumonia). At that point, oxygen should be administered but further investigations (chest X–ray and blood gas) should be instituted urgently. The average child should be disturbed as little as possible, compatible with careful observations. If necessary, nebulized epinephrine (0.5 mL made up to 3 mL of normal saline) may be given. If the drug is needed more than hourly, then admission to an ICU should be considered. Fashions for the use of steroids change about every 5 years. At present, the trend is to give a single intramuscular dose of dexamethasone (0.6 mg/kg) early in the course of the disease.

Spasmodic croup is a poorly defined condition that produces recurrent croup–like episodes in children of all ages. It is probably in the allergy spectrum and responds well to a short course of prednisone and nebulized adrenalin. It can cause significant obstruction even in older children. The combination of parental anxiety and a tendency to try less conventional therapies makes the management of this chronic, poorly understood disease a bit of a challenge. It is fortunately rare.

Bacterial tracheitis

This condition probably represents a severe form of viral croup, complicated by a bacterial superinfection. It is also known as bacterial croup or pseudomembranous croup. The commonest organism isolated from the trachea is *S. aureus* but *H. influenzae*, group A *Streptococcus* and other organisms are found. There is usually a viral prodrome that shows rapid deterioration with fever and toxicity. Occasionally, it is possible to see irregularity in the tracheal shadow on X–ray, indicating pseudomembrane formation in the airway. The best investigation for a child with fever and stridor is an examination under anesthetic by skilled personnel. Most children require intubation for several days until the thick tracheal secretions subside. Management consists of high dose antibiotics, adequate humidification, frequent suctioning and careful observation.

Epiglottitis

Bacterial infection of the epiglottis and other supraglottic structures is generally caused by *Haemophilus influenzae* type B and is becoming less common following the advent of HIB vaccination. The patient usually presents with sudden onset of fever, inspiratory respiratory obstruction, a sore throat and sometimes a change in voice. The swollen epiglottis can cause acute respiratory obstruction at any time but particularly if the child is irritated, examined or made to lie flat. A lateral neck film will often show the typical enlarged epiglottitis, often compared to a thumb print. However, the clinical picture may not allow the luxury of taking an X–ray. Although occasional centers, continuously staffed by anesthetic trained ICU fellows, will manage children conservatively; most physicians prefer to secure an airway in the Operating Room under direct vision. The child with suspected epiglottitis should be managed gently and left undisturbed as much as possible, preferably on the mother's lap. Continuous observation by a person able to intubate is vital. A team consisting of an anesthetist and surgeon, who are able to pass a pediatric rigid bronchoscope and perform a tracheostomy, should be assembled and accompany the child to the Operating Room. Following an inhalational anesthetic and intubation, the child should be managed in ICU. Most children can be extubated after about 48 hours of antibiotic treatment (usually cefotaxime). Rifampin prophylaxis must be given to family members and household contacts if there is another child under the age of 48 months.

Chronic inspiratory stridor

The first consideration should always be a missed foreign body. Once this has been excluded, the commonest cause of chronic inspiratory stridor is laryngomalacia. This is generally a benign condition caused by poorly developed supraglottic structures. As the cartilaginous support structures strengthen with age, the obstruction settles. Most children are better by 2 years of age. Other problems that should be considered in a child with chronic stridor are: subglottic stenosis secondary to previous intubation or trauma, laryngeal papillomas, tracheomalacia (usually secondary to tracheoesophageal fistula repair) and vascular rings.

DISEASES OF THE LOWER AIRWAY

The classical signs of lower airway intrathoracic disease are wheeze and prolonged expiratory phase. The commonest causes are asthma and bronchiolitis. These two diseases are so common that it is easy to forget that there is a large differential diagnosis of wheeze in a young child, including foreign body, cystic fibrosis, immune defects and airway compression by lymph nodes or vascular abnormalities. This list is incomplete but the important point is to remember that wheezing does not necessarily mean asthma.

Bronchiolitis

Bronchiolitis is the commonest single admission diagnosis in most North American pediatric hospitals. It is an important cause of morbidity in small children around the world. When combined with malnutrition in developing countries, it is a lethal disease. In the developed world, mortality is mainly associated with children who have underlying diseases such as BPD, cardiac abnormalities and cystic fibrosis. A vaccine is currently under investigation.

Following a viral prodrome, the inflammation of small airways produces a predictable syndrome consisting of lung hyperinflation, respiratory distress and wheeze. The commonest cause is respiratory syncytial virus (RSV) but an identical picture can be produced by parainfluenza and adenovirus. Apart from clinical examination, some guidance to hospital admission may be gained by oximetry. It is unwise to send any child home who is even marginally desaturated (92% or less) in room air or who has given a history of apnea. Roughly 5% of those admitted will require intubation and ventilation. The overall mortality is low, even among children with underlying medical problems. Management is largely supportive and includes oxygen by nasal prongs when needed and intravenous fluids. If the respiratory effort is impeding feeding, some of these children will be helped by a nasogastric tube. Some children (particularly the older infants) obtain symptomatic relief with bronchodilators. There is evidence in the literature that nebulized adrenalin is more effective than pure beta agonists such as salbutamol. Oral steroids have clearly been shown to be ineffective in this disease. There is no firm evidence on the value of inhaled steroids but they are frequently used in an attempt to reduce the pulmonary inflammation. Although the specific antiviral drug (ribavirin) has been endorsed by several worthy committees, recent collaborative studies have shown no beneficial effect from the drug. Due to the drug's expense and its unproven efficacy, those who use it usually reserve the drug for children with underlying medical problems.

Asthma

The ancient story of seven philosophers trying to describe an elephant in a dark room is usually used to display the dangers of a narrow mind; each sage claims possession of absolute truth but in reality is simply holding onto the tip of the elephant's tail. The analogy works well with asthma. The literature is vast and frequently contradictory; there is not even an accepted definition of the disease that satisfies everybody. There is no shortage of experts representing a range of therapeutic options from magnetic therapy to inhaled steroids, but there are still a lot of children with asthma. In fact, a state of therapeutic confusion is not at all unusual among the parents of asthmatic children. The recommendations in this chapter are clearly based on the Western medical tradition. Although this is certainly not the last word in asthma management, it should be stressed that careful use of modern inhaled drugs will allow the great majority of asthmatics to lead a completely normal life.

The following criteria offer a reasonably inclusive working definition of asthma:
- Episodic or chronic wheeze, with or without a cough, noted on examination.
- Exacerbation of cough and wheeze by upper respiratory tract infections, exercise or airborne allergens.
- Favorable response to conventional asthma therapy.

1. Pathogenesis
- Asthma is a chronic inflammatory disorder. Macroscopically, the respiratory mucosa is reddened and edematous while histologically there is usually a mixture of epithelial damage and obvious inflammation deep to the basement membrane. This consists of eosinophils, lymphocytes and plasma cells with degranulated mast cells. The inflammation is mediated by a complex chemical soup which includes oxygen radicals, lipid degradation mediators, eosinophilic granules (including eosinophil peroxidase and major basic protein), macrophage cytokines such as tumor necrosis factor, platelet activating factor and interleukins. The end result is airway constriction, epithelial edema and denudation, transepithelial exudation, mucous hypersecretion and airway hyper-responsiveness.
- Once in motion, the system is probably self-perpetuating, e.g. epithelial shedding exposes nerve endings which release inflammatory neuropeptides. In addition, there is a consequent reduction in epithelial derived relaxant factor (EpDRF) and loss of the enzyme NEP (neuroendopeptidase), which normally provides some protection against bronchoconstriction.

Many other examples of amplifying circuits exist, and the total picture is probably fathomlessly complex.

2. Asthmatic triggers
- By far, the commonest trigger is a viral respiratory tract infection. The lay expression that a cold goes to the chest is quite appropriate.
- Irritants such as pollution (particularly cigarette smoke), exercise, emotional stress and some airborne allergens can also trigger attacks. Many children with persistent asthma have positive type 1 skin reactions to a number of allergens, including dust mites and animal dander. These exposures may contribute to the chronic nature of the inflammation, but acute asthmatic attacks generally follow an acute respiratory tract infection.

3. Patterns of asthma
The clinical manifestations of asthma are enormous and each child seems to be different in some small way. However, for ease of description, there are three broadly identifiable clinical patterns of asthma.
- Well over half of all asthmatics will have relatively benign intermittent asthma. The trigger is almost always a viral infection and associated allergic problems such as hay fever, allergies and eczema are not common. With good control early in life, many of these children grow out of the problem with age. In between acute attacks, these children are generally completely normal and usually well managed with intermittent medication.
- Roughly a quarter of the children seen in a referral clinic will have persistent asthma. Even at their best, in between acute attacks, these children still have some degree of limitation in the form of wheeze, cough, exercise limitation or pulmonary function abnormalities. Allergic disease is much commoner in this subgroup. Some of these children will go on to be asthmatic adults but the pessimistic outlook often quoted in textbooks is usually based on older information. The advent of modern inhaled steroids and early efficient treatment of these children may well effect the long–term outlook. The chronic cycle of inflammation can often be broken with a month or two of inhaled steroids so that the children can subsequently be managed simply on an intermittent basis. However, some of these children will require continuous therapy, particularly during the winter months.
- A small percentage (usually $\leq$ 5%) will have severe chronic asthma that requires continuous high dose inhalation therapy and, in some cases, the use of alternate day steroids. It should be stressed that with the use of modern drugs, such cases are unusual and the prognosis for the average asthmatic patient is very good.

4. Investigations
- A careful history and physical examination, combined with standard pulmonary function tests, will enable the diagnosis of asthma to be made in the great majority of cases.
- Methacholine or histamine are irritating substances that cause bronchoconstriction in many normal people. Challenge tests have very poor sensitivity and have little value in clinical work. They are of some value in asthma research.
- The use of exercise tests is occasionally useful in managing some asthmatics. Serum IgE levels are usually raised but there is too much overlap with normal values for the test to be of any value.
- Skin prick tests and RAST tests are performed in some clinics. They are frequently positive.

- If doubt about the diagnosis of asthma exists, it is usually because the child shows no abnormalities at the time of examination. Rather than pursue the diagnosis with provocation tests or nonspecific tests of allergy, it is better to ask the parents to return whenever the child exhibits respiratory problems (usually when they contract a viral URTI).

5. Management of acute asthma
- The management of acute asthmatic attacks is fairly standardized. Initial therapy in most Emergency Rooms consist of high dose beta agonists with early use of oral steroids. After observation, many of these children can be discharged and managed at home with follow–up in the Respiratory Clinic.
- Those children who are admitted to the ward are usually treated with intravenous steroids, intravenous theophylline infusions and, occasionally, the addition of inhaled anticholinergic agents. Fortunately, most children avoid the need for mechanical ventilation. The overall mortality of asthmatic children who manage to reach hospital is very low. Examination of asthma mortality has shown that many deaths occur at home before medical help can be reached. Consequently, hospital staff rarely see a child die from asthma and tend to underestimate the potentially lethal nature of this disease when treated inappropriately.

6. Management of chronic asthma
- This is where most of the arguments begin. The reader, who is confused by competing asthma therapies, is probably best advised to apply a single question to any new therapy, "Has this been tested by a prospective double blind randomized study?" If the answer is "no", then a more traditional route might be advisable.
- The single most important aspect of asthma management is education, and any referral clinic should have a full–time clinical specialist who does nothing except educate parents about asthma and its treatment, so allowing them to take charge of the child's management. This person also acts as a first contact for parents when they have a number of questions about a child's management.
- The first step in asthma management is to remove any known triggers. Unfortunately, a clear history of cause and effect is rarely obtained. Occasionally, exposure to a definite allergen (frequently animal dander) is obtained and avoidance is worthwhile. Skin prick tests are frequently used in an attempt to define asthmatic triggers. The relevance of the results of a type 1 response in the forearm to the diagnosis and management of a complex inflammatory response within the parenchyma of the lung is not universally accepted. The commonest skin sensitivities are to house dust mite and grass pollen. Maneuvers designed to reduce mite exposure are commonly used (mostly consist of trying to achieve a spotlessly clean, dust free bedroom). The clinical value of dust control is about the same as the chance of a child keeping his/her bedroom clean.
- Devices designed to improve the quality of the bedroom air such as air filters, ionizers, humidifiers and dehumidifiers have no clinical value. Cigarette smoke and air pollution both have a significant effect on a child's asthma and should be avoided. Persuading people to stop smoking is a frustrating and frequently futile exercise. At the very least, they should be counselled to smoke outside the house and never to smoke in the car with the child. About 20% of asthmatics are sensitive to the effect of aspirin and, in the absence of a simple test, it is best to avoid the drug altogether. The value of trying to avoid some other food additives such as sodium metabisulfite, monosodium glutamate and tartrazine dyes is less well defined.

Hyposensitization or allergy shots have a long tradition, but the results of numerous clinical trials are less than encouraging.

- Two general groups of drugs are used in the medical management of asthma: bronchodilators and anti–inflammatory agents. Of the bronchodilators, there are three groups of drugs: beta agonists, theophylline compounds and anticholinergic drugs. Theophylline compounds are used very little for chronic asthma because of side effects such as hyperactivity and gastrointestinal upset. Absorption from the intestinal tract is erratic even with the newest sustained release preparations. Atropine–like drugs offer no advantage over beta agonists at the expense of side effects such as tachycardia, drying of respiratory secretions and occasional gastrointestinal side effects. Beta agonists such as ventolin have recently come under scrutiny from studies based on adults who abused the drug. The results of such studies should not be extrapolated uncritically to children. When used carefully at appropriate times, beta agonists are safe drugs to use in children. A small dose of ventolin prior to the use of inhaled steroids probably improves the delivery of the steroid and is not associated with side effects when used on a once or twice a day schedule.
- There are several drugs with anti–inflammatory action used in the treatment of asthma, the most powerful of which are the steroids; others include sodium cromoglycate, nedocromil and ketotifen. Ketotifen was brought out some years ago as a platelet activating factor antagonist, but subsequent experience has shown very limited value from this drug. It is an antihistamine and most of its benefit may be in children with hay fever in addition to their asthma. Sodium cromoglycate and nedocromil are often used as first line drugs in the treatment of mild intermittent asthma. Some children do obtain relief but many in this group will require inhaled steroids during winter. Both drugs are quite safe. The first of the inhaled steroids was beclomethasone but, more recently, budesonide and fluticasone have been added. The newer steroids are claimed to be cleared in a first pass through the liver so minimizing the effect of any absorbed drug. They are powerful drugs and most children respond to them. Although there is always a worry about effects on adrenal suppression, growth retardation and cataracts, these complications usually occur in patients on very high doses, often in combination with oral steroids, for prolonged periods. Extensive research has failed to show any serious side effects in children taking short intermittent courses at the usually stated doses.

Chronic or persistent bronchitis

The classification of children with chronic or recurrent wheezing episodes has always been a contentious issue. In the past, such terms as asthmatoid bronchitis, chronic bronchitis and wheezy bronchitis were used to describe poorly defined conditions with common clinical features of cough and wheeze. The confusion probably contributed to the well reported underdiagnosis and poor treatment of asthma. The terms have fallen out of favor and wheezing children are generally squeezed into a single diagnosis of asthma. However, controversy does exist and can probably be divided into "lumpers", who would include all wheezy children within the umbrella of asthma, and "splitters", who feel there are definable subgroups of wheezing children that deserve separate diagnostic terms.

Anyone working on a large pediatric respiratory ward will soon notice a chronic respiratory pattern of productive cough, usually among socially disadvantaged children, that probably justifies a separate diagnostic term. A typical child is usually a boy from a poor social background who is below the age of 1 year and who has a history of admission to hospital for a serious viral lung infection. Subsequently, each time the child catches another respiratory tract infection, a syndrome of productive cough, wheeze and respiratory distress develops. The children often grow quite normally. Chronic otitis media and purulent nasal discharge are frequent coexisting findings. In North America, Native American Indian children are over represented. The condition exists around the world and has been termed "Glasgow lung" and "London lung" in Britain. The older Scottish term "wee snotterer" might be a more widely accepted term.

The combination of severe respiratory tract infections in early life and poor social conditions probably produce, in some children, chronic pulmonary inflammation that becomes self–sustaining and manifests as a productive cough with frequent exacerbations. A similar picture can be found among children who have had major medical interventions at a young age (e.g. chemotherapy, cardiac surgery, prolonged mechanical ventilation, tracheoesophageal fistual repair). It is important to remember that social class has a profound effect on the respiratory health of young children. Whether this is due to parental smoking, air pollution, poor access to health care, poor nutrition, or a dozen other reasons, is difficult to establish. Whatever the exact cause, it is reasonable to assume that an early respiratory insult will tend to produce more severe disease among a segment of a population living in poor social conditions and is more likely, in some of them, to produce a degree of chronic lung injury that might well last into adulthood.

PARENCHYMAL DISEASES

The last group is loosely described as diseases of the lung parenchyma, although this is stretching the point a bit for cystic fibrosis. The classical sign of parenchymal disease is bronchial breathing due to the acoustic effects of consolidation. Of course, there will also be tachypnea, cough, grunting and, in severe cases, cyanosis.

Pneunomia

Infection of the pulmonary parenchyma is the commonest major infection in children. Its maximum incidence is in the toddler age range when it reaches a cumulative rate of 40:1,000 per year. The mortality is considerably higher than asthma and is roughly 1:10,000 per year. A strict definition is impossible because there is a good deal of clinical overlap with a number of respiratory problems, including acute asthma and aspiration. However, the presence of fever, tachypnea, increased sputum and alar flare, combined with bronchial breathing and chest X–ray findings of consolidation, allow a definite diagnosis to be made in most cases.

It is often difficult to determine the etiology of a child's pneumonia, and treatment is frequently based on guesswork. Pathogens depend on the patient's age, season of the year, social class and the presence of other diseases such as leukemia or AIDS. The simplest classification is based on the child's age.

- Neonates: commonest organisms are group B *Streptococcus* and Gram negative organisms (*E. coli* and *Klebsiella*). *Listeria*, CMV, herpes and *Chlamydia* are other possibilities. There are claims that *Ureaplasma* and occasionally *Pneumocystis* are pathogens, but this is not universally accepted.
- Under five years of age: the commonest organism in the toddler range group is respiratory syncytial virus, both as a cause of pneumonia and bronchiolitis. Other common viral infections are parainfluenza, influenza and adenovirus. Bacterial infection is usually either pneumococcal

or *H. influenzae*. Superinfection of any viral pneumonitis with *Staphylococcus* is possible and should be considered if a child deteriorates rapidly.
- School age: the commonest organisms in this age group are *Mycoplasma* and the pneumococcus, but relatively recent work has shown that a subgroup of *Chlamydia* (*C. pneumoniae*) may be another common pathogen in this age range. Other possibilities in this group are influenza, adenovirus and group A *Streptococcus*.

There is no radiological or clinical finding that can reliably differentiate between bacterial and viral agents. Pertussis and RSV can both produce a definable clinical syndrome but even in these cases, several other organisms can produce an identical picture. Even if a viral agent such as adenovirus has been isolated, it is still possible for bacterial superinfection to occur. Pediatric pneumonia is one of the few areas of medicine where it is fair to invoke two etiologies.

Following history and examination, the most useful investigation is a chest X–ray. Blood cultures are specific but only positive in about 5–10% of cases (using transthoracic needle aspiration as a gold standard). Collections of pleural fluid should always be sampled. Infection is not the only cause of pleural fluid collections and, occasionally, surprises do occur (lymphoma, tuberculosis and hemothorax). If purulent fluid is obtained by needle aspiration, most people would subsequently attempt to drain the chest completely using a large bore chest tube; otherwise organization with multiple pleural abscesses is a possibility.

Sputum cultures only reflect the causative organism in cases of bronchiectasis and cystic fibrosis. Throat cultures are of no value. Subsequent testing will depend on the clinical situation but can include skin testing for tuberculosis and serological testing for Q fever, *Chlamydia*, Legionnaires' disease and a variety of viruses. Rapid diagnostic viral panels now exist. The best known test is for RSV but several other respiratory pathogens are covered.

Apart from supportive care, antibiotic therapy is usually given on an empirical basis. For the neonatal age group, a mixture of ampicillin and gentamicin has stood the test of time and is commonly used. Although the organism in the toddler age range is usually viral, most physicians will use intravenous antibiotics if a child is sick enough for hospital admission. Cefotaxime (often combined with cloxacillin if there is suspicion of staphylococcal infection) is a good starting point. Penicillin or ampicillin is usually the initial drug in school age patients. Oral erythromycin or tetracyline is used if *Mycoplasma* or *Chlamydia* is suspected.

Cystic fibrosis

1. Pathophysiology
- Cystic fibrosis is an autosomal recessive disorder associated with a wide range of problems; the most important of which is suppurative lung disease. Its incidence varies with different ethnic communities but is diagnosed in roughly 1:2,500 live births in Caucasians. It is caused by a mutation within the CF gene situated on chromosome 7, which codes for the cystic fibrosis transmembrane regulator (CFTR). This protein is a transmembrane chloride channel that is activated by ATP. Roughly 75% of the mutations involve position 508 (delta F508). However, there are over 300 mutations found in the remaining 25%.
- The CFTR is involved with correct hydration of exocrine secretions, making them easier to clear. Abnormalities of the CFTR produce viscid secretions that are difficult to clear. Subsequent obstruction within the lung, pancreas and liver is probably the common factor in the final clinical picture of cystic fibrosis. About 10% of patients preserve their pancreatic

function. This group usually has milder respiratory disease.
- Chronic airway obstruction and superinfection lead to a slow downhill course over many years marked by intermittent acute exacerbations. The median survival in many clinics is now 30 years for males. It is usually a few years less for females. However, outcome in cystic fibrosis depends on many factors, particularly committed family support and general social conditions. It does not just depend upon medical care. Gender differences and median survivals vary widely around the world.

2. Traditional therapy
- In young children, the airway is initially colonized with *H. influenzae* or *S. aureus*. Later, many patients begin to acquire *Pseudomonas*. The aim of respiratory treatment is to clear infected secretions from the lungs. The most important part is to encourage the child to lead a physically active life within the limitations imposed by the lung disease. Percussive physiotherapy and antibiotics are also very important. Many children have obstructive disease and bronchodilators are used in these children. Recently, the lessons learned from asthma therapy have been applied to cystic fibrosis. Studies of the use of anti–inflammatory drugs, particularly oral or inhaled steroids, are becoming more common. Unfortunately, oral steroids are associated with numerous side effects including poor control of serum glucose and reduced growth rates. Intermittent admission to hospital for intravenous antibiotics, bronchodilators and intensive physical therapy are necessary in most patients. The choice of antibiotic is usually guided by the result of sputum cultures from previous hospital visits. Outpatient intravenous therapy is becoming more common.
- About 90% of patients with cystic fibrosis have exocrine pancreatic insufficiency, leading to the usual signs of malabsorption such as abdominal distention, greasy stools and failure to thrive. The basis of treatment is supplementation with pancreatic granules. The dose varies widely and must be titrated against stool frequency, stool consistency and weight gain. Some patients still fail to absorb despite adequate supplementation with pancreatic granules. These children may be helped by the addition of an antacid. An unrestricted high energy diet should be encouraged, usually with vitamin supplementation and extra salt (at least 1 g/d) during hot weather.
- Poor caloric intake and weight loss are common problems in children with severe lung disease. There are usually several factors involved such as chronic ill health, an adolescent diet and problems at home. Attempts to improve the nutritional state by dietary supplementation are an obvious therapeutic route but have numerous practical problems. Overnight nasogastric tube feeding usually only produces a short–term benefit. It inhibits the patient's cough and probably makes gastroesophageal reflux worst. A better option is overnight feeding through a button gastrostomy. Apart from occasional surgical problems, these are fairly well tolerated. Whether improved weight gain can improve respiratory disease is not clear.
- Gastroesphogeal reflux has only fairly recently been widely accepted as being a contributory problem in cystic fibrosis. Following pH monitoring and upper GI studies, conventional therapy such as cisapride has been shown to have some benefit. Fundoplication is used in some patients.
- Several other gastrointestinal problems associated with cystic fibrosis are found: intermittent bowel obstruction, also called meconium ileus equivalent, occurs when poor attention is paid to pancreatic supplementation. This is often a problem of adolescents and older children. Acute attacks can usually be managed with laxatives or, in some cases, enemas. Avoidance

of the problem requires careful attention to nutrition and supplementation. Rectal prolapse can occur in some children and is usually associated with poor nutrition and lung health. Complete obstruction of the bowel in infancy with thick meconium is a fairly common presenting feature of cystic fibrosis. The obstruction is cleared in some children with the use of hypotonic contrast solutions such as gastrografin, but other children will require surgery. As the median age of survival of cystic fibrosis increases, more individuals are presenting with cirrhosis and the effects of portal hypertension. Complications such as advanced liver damage and esophageal varices are fortunately rare in children.

3. Newer therapies

Several new therapies have been introduced in the last few years and their clinical value is still under review. Heart lung transplantation is performed for advanced cystic fibrosis in some centers but it is very expensive and the 2 year survival rate is usually below 50%. Once the CF gene was cloned in 1989, the chance for inserting this gene using a viral vector became an obvious avenue of research. Unfortunately, gene therapy is easier said than done and it will probably be years before it becomes a realistic option. Recombinant deoxyribonuclease (DNAase) has been introduced in nebulized form. Purulent secretions are thick and difficult to clear due to the high concentration of DNA derived from neutrophils and bacteria. Cleaving this DNA reduces sputum viscosity and has been shown to produce clinical improvement. The effect may be more significant in the sickest group of patients. $Alpha_1$–antitrypsin has been used in aerosol form in an attempt to inhibit the action of neutrophil elastase upon the lung. Amiloride has also been given in nebulized form in an attempt to block cellular reabsorption of sodium and consequently improve hydration of airway secretions. The drug certainly alters the transepithelial potential in cystic fibrosis but there appears to be no associated clinical improvement.

Interstitial lung disease

This ragbag contains many diseases that are often assumed to have an immunological basis. It includes: fibrosing alveolitis and its subdivisions, the pulmonary vasculitides (primary pulmonary hemosiderosis, Goodpasture's syndrome, Wegener's granulomatosis), pulmonary eosinophilia and its subdivisions, secondary causes of pulmonary hemosiderosis (SLE, PAN, pulmonary veno–occlusive disease), allergic alveolitis and many others. Individually, they are all rare but taken as a group they are certainly not uncommon in a referral center. Children of all ages can be affected. Initial presentation is often breathlessness, fatigue and weight loss. Clinical signs include desaturation in room air, tachypnea and clubbing. Auscultation may reveal an end inspiratory crackle but is often normal.

If old enough, pulmonary function testing reveals a restrictive defect with a marked reduction in lung diffusion and SaO_2. Chest X–ray and CT scan usually leave little doubt of the diagnosis of interstitial lung disease. The differential diagnosis is so large that a biopsy is usually considered. High quality CT scans make this less necessary with some clinical presentations, especially since therapeutic options are limited.

These diseases are all too rare to allow extensive therapeutic trials. Steroids are the usual mainstay of treatment, although hydroxychloroquine is becoming more popular. In desperation, azathioprine and cyclosporine are sometimes used.

MUSCULOSKELETAL PAIN (MSP) AND ARTHRITIS

MSP is a common and usually benign childhood complaint often related to trauma. In a young child, the site of pain may be difficult to localize. It may manifest as a limp or refusal to use a limb. Arthritis is an uncommon cause of MSP and it should be distinguished from other causes of MSP by paying attention to the history and the specific clinical signs.

Historical evaluation should pay special heed to the mode of onset and duration of the pain. Trauma is the most likely cause of acute onset pain. Less obvious "traumatic" stresses include "pulled elbows", foot splinters from wearing no shoes, new shoes and unusual or excessive physical activity. Strains and sprains are relatively uncommon in young children; always consider child abuse especially in multiple soft tissue or bony injuries. With subacute onset, it is vital to exclude infection (septic arthritis or osteomyelitis). Specific diagnoses for hip pain (slipped capital femoral epiphysis, Legg–Calvé–Perthes' disease, sepsis) should always be excluded early if sequelae are to be minimized (Table I). For a more insidious onset of pain with a chronic course, consider malignancy (leukemia, neuroblastoma, bone tumor), inflammation and noninflammatory pain syndromes.

Table I: Differential diagnosis of hip pain

Feature	Septic arthritis	Transient synovitis	Legg–Calvé–Perthes' disease	Slipped capital femoral epiphysis	Juvenile ankylosing spondylitis
Peak age at onset	< 2 (50%)	3–10	4–9	11–16	> 10
M:F ratio	2:1	4:1	4:1	2:1	7:1
Bilateral	4.4%	4%	13%	30%	50%
Pain	Severe thigh	Hip, knee thigh	Hip, knee	Hip	Hip, back chronic
Associated disorders	Usually febrile	Preceding URI: 50%	None	Obesity	Arthritis enthesitis
Acute phase reactants	Usually elevated	Usually normal	Normal	Normal	Often elevated

50% of children with septic arthritis at any joint are < 2 yr old.
4.4% of children with septic arthritis at one site have multiple sites involved.

Most patients presenting with chronic MSP and/or complaints of swelling do not have arthritis. Swelling described as lasting only a few hours is almost never due to arthritis. Arthritis is considered chronic if it persists beyond 6 weeks. It should not be diagnosed in the absence of objective findings.

Objective signs of arthritis:
* Joint swelling or effusion.
  or
* At least two of the following signs at the joint:
  Limitation of range.
  Pain on motion.
  Increased heat.

Differential diagnosis of chronic arthritis in childhood

The principle groups of childhood chronic arthritis are juvenile rheumatoid arthritis (JRA) and the seronegative spondyloarthropathies (SSA's) which include seronegative enthesopathy and arthropathy (SEA) syndrome. Other rheumatic diseases are uncommon or uncommonly present with arthritis and/or MSP without other characteristic features. The noninflammatory pain syndromes are more common than chronic arthritis, may cause even greater dysfunction and have distinctive features. Infection and malignancy should always be considered in the differential diagnosis of chronic MSP and arthritis, but in the absence of any systemic features over a longer period, they may be less likely. A systemic approach to history taking and examination will best distinguish these conditions.

Selected differential diagnosis of arthritis and conditions that may mimic arthritis:
* Infectious: septic arthritis (pyogenic, *Mycoplasma*, gonococcus, tuberculosis); viral arthritis; osteomyelitis.
* Rheumatic: juvenile rheumatoid arthritis (JRA), seronegative spondyloarthropathies (SSA's), reactive arthritis (rheumatic fever, post–immunization), systemic lupus erythematosus (SLE), MCTD; dermatomyositis, vasculitis (Henoch–Schönlein purpura, serum sickness, Kawasaki's disease).
* Noninflammatory pain syndromes: "mechanical" and pain amplification syndromes.
* Traumatic/orthopedic: traumatic arthritis, nonaccidental injury, slipped capital femoral epiphysis (SCFE), Legg–Calvé–Perthes' disease.
* Neoplastic: leukemia, neuroblastoma, bone tumors.
* Hematological: sickle cell disease, hemophilia.
* Metabolic or endocrine: storage diseases, diabetes, thyroid diseases.
* Other: skeletal dysplasias (usually associated with contractures).

APPROACH TO THE CHILD WITH POSSIBLE ARTHRITIS

History

* Night pain and morning stiffness relieved by activity are characteristic of chronic inflammatory arthritis. The symptoms are persistent over several weeks although juvenile ankylosing arthritis may have an episodic onset. Elicit which joints are painful, stiff or swollen and whether there is also pain at other sites. The severity of the pain is best estimated by considering sleep disturbance, school absenteeism and recreational disruption.
* Preceding or current associated symptoms (fever, anorexia, weight loss, rash, bleeding or bruising, oral or genital ulcers, dysuria, painful or red eyes, diarrhea, etc.) or associated events

(immunization, sexual activity, travel, contact with infectious illness) will help in formulating a differential diagnosis or classifying the type of arthritis.

- A family history of arthritis, especially of spondyloarthropathies (ankylosing spondylitis or chronic back pain, inflammatory bowel disease, psoriasis) or bleeding disorders is diagnostically relevant.
- A social history to determine family or school stresses, level of school performance, behavioral changes and unusual personality traits is essential.

Examination

- Look for swelling, deformity, asymmetry and muscle wasting around the sites of complaint.
- Palpate for tenderness over bone, the joint margins, entheses (sites of insertion of tendons, ligaments and fascia to bone) and soft tissue "fibrositis" sites.
- Distinguish arthralgia (joint pain alone) from arthritis where there may be heat, swelling or effusion, reduced range and/or pain with motion of the joint. Determine the extent of the problem by examing all joints, including the temporomandibular joint, spine and sacroiliac joints.
- Look for limb length discrepancy and examine gait and stance.
- General examination should determine whether there are more widespread manifestations with growth disturbance or evidence of multisystem disease.

Investigations

- CBC, differential and ESR may help identify infection, malignancy or systemic inflammation; normal values do not exclude arthritis.
- X–rays or bone scan of involved sites may be necessary to define infection, fracture or mass (depending on the degree of suspicion).
- Synovial fluid analysis to exclude sepsis is almost mandatory for an acute or subacute monoarthritis but less imperative for multiple joint disease.
- Antinuclear antibodies (ANA) are not diagnostic of arthritis but are required for a diagnosis of SLE.
- Rheumatoid factor (RF) has no value as a screening test for arthritis.
- Ophthalmological slit–lamp examination to detect uveitis is imperative in the young child with pauciarticular arthritis.
- Further specific testing should be guided by the above findings with a presumptive or focused differential diagnosis.

JUVENILE RHEUMATOID ARTHRITIS (JRA)

JRA is chronic arthritis (> 6 weeks) developing in a child under 16 years of age, without evidence of other rheumatic disease. It is subclassified according to the type of onset in the first 6 months of the disease as follows: oligoarticular (four or fewer joints), polyarticular (five or more joints), systemic (arthritis associated with fever and other systemic features such as rash, serositis and organomegaly). Characteristic features of these onset types are shown in Table II.

SERONEGATIVE ENTHESOPATHY AND ARTHROPATHY (SEA) SYNDROME

SEA syndrome describes children who are seronegative for ANA and rheumatoid factor, have enthesitis (inflammatory pain and tenderness at sites of insertion of tendons, ligaments and fascia to bone) and arthralgia or arthritis. Patients with this syndrome are more similar to patients with juvenile ankylosing spondylitis (JAS) than those with JRA (Table III). They may not have back symptoms or signs, do not have radiographic sacroiliitis but do have a high probability of developing JAS within 5–10 years, especially if they are HLA–B27 positive. Children who have pauciarticular onset JRA type II are generally the same group of children. These children should be considered to have an early SSA.

Table II: Characteristics of onset types of JRA

Feature	Oligoarticular	Polyarticular	Systemic
Frequency	50%	40%	10%
F:M ratio	5:1	3:1	1:1
Onset age	1–3	1–3, > 10	None
Systemic signs	None	Moderate	Prominent
Chronic iritis	20%	5%	Rare
ANA	80% (if iritis)	45%	10%
RF	Rare	10%	Rare
Outcome	Excellent except if iritis	Variable; poor if RF positive	Poor to moderate

Table III: Comparison of JRA, SEA syndrome, JAS and JPsA

Feature	JRA	SEA	JAS	JPsA
F:M ratio	4:1	1:9	1:7	2.5:1
Mean onset age	5	10	> 10	6
Enthesitis	Rare	100%	Common	Uncommon
Uveitis	Chronic	Acute	Acute	Chronic
ANA positive	60%	0%	0%	50%
RF positive	15%	0%	0%	0%
HLA–B27 positive	15%	72%	90%	15%

Acute uveitis is usually symptomatic.
Chronic uveitis is usually asymptomatic.

SERONEGATIVE SPONDYLOARTHROPATHIES (SSA's) OF CHILDHOOD

The SSA's—juvenile ankylosing spondylitis (JAS), arthritis associated with inflammatory bowel disease (IBD), Reiter's syndrome (RS) and juvenile psoriatic arthritis (JPsA)—are named because of the absence of rheumatoid factor and presence of axial skeleton disease). Children with SEA syndrome also share these features.

Most children with SSA do not have arthritis of the spine. Inflammatory disease of the sacroiliac joints is an infrequent or late finding. Children with SEA syndrome, the most frequently diagnosed SSA, may not develop axial symptoms and signs for 5–10 years after onset. Children with JAS account for less than one-fifth of the SSA's. Reactive arthritis uncommonly progresses to JAS in childhood; most patients have peripheral arthritis with or without enthesitis resolving in the relatively short–term. The arthritis associated with IBD is more commonly peripheral than axial. Axial disease in JPsA is very common.

Characteristics of the juvenile spondyloarthropathies:
- Familial occurrence of spondyloarthropathies.
- High frequency of HLA–B27.
- Male preponderance.
- Late childhood onset.
- Frequent enthesitis.
- Peripheral arthritis asymmetrically involving lower limbs.
- Inflammatory low back pain.
- Acute, asymptomatic uveitis.
- ANA and IgM rheumatoid factor negative.

Juvenile ankylosing spondylitis (JAS)

JAS is relatively uncommon in childhood. Using adult criteria, a definite diagnosis of JAS cannot be made until there is radiological sacroiliitis. In many children, peripheral arthritis may precede axial arthritis for many years and a specific diagnosis of JAS will be delayed. Children with this early spondyloarthropathy are often identified as having SEA syndrome.

- Diagnostic criteria for AS:
    Limitation of lumbar spine motion in three planes.
    Pain, or a history of pain, at dorsolumbar junction of spine.
    Limitation of chest expansion to 2.5 cm or less.
- Definite AS:
    Grade 3–4 bilateral sacroiliitis on X-ray plus one criterion.
    Grade 3–4 unilateral or grade 2 bilateral sacroiliitis plus criterion 1 or criteria 2 and 3.
- Probable AS:
    Grade 3–4 bilateral sacroiliitis and no clinical criteria.

Juvenile psoriatic arthritis (JPsA)

Arthritis may precede development of psoriasis by many years, but there are criteria for diagnosis of JPsA in the absence of rash. Psoriatic arthritis is usually grouped with the SSA's, however, JPsA patients may be ANA positive, HLA–B27 negative, develop chronic uveitis and follow a course more similar to JRA.

Vancouver criteria for the diagnosis of juvenile psoriatic arthritis are:
- Definite JPsA:
    Arthritis with a typical psoriatic rash.
    or
    Arthritis with three of the following minor criteria:
    Dactylitis.
    Nail pitting or onycholysis.
    Psoriasis in 1° or 2° relative.
    Psoriatic–like rash (atypical in location or appearance).
- Probable JPsA:
    Arthritis with two of the four minor criteria.

MANAGEMENT OF CHRONIC ARTHRITIS OF CHILDHOOD

The principles of managment include:
- Treatment of inflammation and the pain of inflammation.
- Maintenance or recovery of range of motion, muscle strength and function.
- Detection of complications of the disease or therapy.
- Educational and psychosocial support for patients and families and career counselling for the older child.
These aims are best met in the multidisciplinary setting.

In each patient, the aims of drug therapy should be defined (analgesia, anti–inflammatory) and the risks and benefits discussed with the patient and family.
- Start with single agent NSAIDS at anti–inflammatory doses (naproxen 15 mg/kg per d div. b.i.d. for JRA; tolmetin sodium 30 mg/kg per d div. t.i.d. for SSA's). Wait 6–8 weeks for an objective response before trying an alternate single agent.
- Use of multiple drugs or second line agents (e.g. systemic or intra–articular corticosteroids, sulfasalazine, hydroxychloroquine, methotrexate, gold) should be guided by a rheumatologist. Early intra–articular triamcinolone hexacetonide therapy may benefit patients with limited large joint involvement.

CHRONIC UVEITIS

Chronic uveitis as a complication of JRA is most frequent in young girls with early age of onset of oligoarticular arthritis and who have antinuclear antibodies. It also occurs in patients with JPsA. The risk persists even if the arthritis becomes inactive; it is highest at the time of onset of arthritis and then becomes small by 5 years of age. Chronic uveitis has an insidious, asymptomatic onset and, if untreated, can lead to blindness. Early detection and treatment improves the prognosis considerably. Frequent (every 3–4 months) ophthalmologic slit–lamp screening of patients with oligoarticular or polyarticular JRA or JPsA should be continued for 5 years and subsequently every 6–12 months.

NONINFLAMMATORY PAIN SYNDROMES

These are diagnosed more commonly than chronic arthritis and may cause even greater dysfunction. Pain amplification syndromes are so named because symptoms are out of proportion to physical findings and their organic basis in unknown; they may be primary or complicate organic conditions.

1. Noninflammatory pain syndromes
- Hypermobility: generalized/local (recurrently dislocating patella, pes planus, genu recurvatum).
- Overuse syndromes: chondromalacia patella, Osgood–Schlatter's disease, stress fractures, shin splints, plica syndromes, tenosynovitis.

2. Pain amplification syndromes
- Growing pains.
- Reflex sympathetic dystrophy (syn. reflex neurovascular dystrophy, algodystrophy, causalgia, Sudeck's atrophy).
- Primary fibromyalgia syndrome.

Noninflammatory, mechanical pain syndromes

Hypermobile individuals develop musculoskeletal pains more frequently than those who are less flexible. Symptomatic "hypermobile" patients are often dramatically improved by use of custom made insoles and selective muscle strengthening exercises.

The earlier age of starting competitive athletic pursuits may be making overuse syndromes more common. These patients may also benefit from physical and occupational therapy and possibly orthopedic advice. Always consider that complaints of MSP may be a manifestation of a desire to quit competition that is being principally driven by parents.

Growing pains (GP)

Growing pains are a common complaint in children of ages 4–12 years. The pain is very distressing but poorly localized or between the joints in the lower limbs. It occurs in the evenings or after falling asleep and never persists to the morning. They may be precipitated by exercise or relieved by massage or simple analgesics. The children, at other times, have no physical disability and normal history, examination, laboratory studies and radiographs. Serious rheumatic disease or malignancy should always be considered, but persistence over several years make these unlikely. Parents should be assured that there are no sequelae. Prophylactic bedtime simple analgesics may be helpful in children with obvious precipitants or frequent nightly occurrences.

Reflex sympathetic dystrophy (RSD)

RSD is a condition found predominantly in females in late childhood and adolescence. They present with constant pain and complete disability of a distal extremity; continued disuse exacerbates the problem which may generalize to other limbs. While there is usually no underlying pathology or significant precipitating trauma, there may be psychological factors. Patients are usually highly motivated and high achievers but are indifferent to their dysfunction.

On examination of the affected part, there is an abnormal, immobile posture, diffuse swelling, exquisite tenderness to even light touch, coolness and mottled blue discolouration. Passive and active movements are painful. Laboratory tests are normal. X-rays may show osteoporosis. Nuclear imaging may be normal or show diffuse increase or decrease in intake, but its usefulness is in excluding underlying precipitating causes such as stress fractures.

Treatment involves a graduated program of tactile desensitization and remobilization, using simple analgesics, transcutaneous nerve stimulation, sympathetic and informative approach. The patient and family must contract to undertake frequent, rigorous, intensive physiotherapy and appropriate psychotherapy. The prognosis is excellent with early treatment by an experienced physiotherapist and if they make an early return to school and normal activity.

Primary fibromyalgia syndrome

Fibromyalgia is a well recognized, poorly understood, noninflammatory condition that also occurs in the pediatric population, usually teenage girls. They present with diffuse musculoskeletal pains and stiffness, constant fatigue and disturbed sleep patterns. They have "jump" tenderness at characteristic symmetric sites, particularly around the neck, scapula and upper posterior pelvis. All investigations are normal. Withdrawal from activity promotes sleeplessness and exacerbates a fatigue, depression, pain and inactivity cycle. Treatment is difficult and involves sympathy, assurances, simple analgesics and topical modalities for pain control; a graduated return to normal activities and sleep patterns with the help of a physical therapist is beneficial.

KAWASAKI'S DISEASE

Kawasaki's disease (KD) is an acute systemic vasculitis of infants and young children with 1–2% acute mortality from myocarditis, myocardial infarction and ruptured coronary artery aneurysm. Diagnosis requires fulfilling diagnostic, clinical criteria. Early treatment with high dose intravenous γ–globulin decreases the incidence of coronary artery abnormalities.

Diagnostic criteria for Kawasaki's disease

Diagnosis requires four of five criteria in a child with unexplained fever (> 38.3 °C) for at least 5 days:
- Bilateral, bulbar, nonexudative conjunctivitis (85%).
- Acute cervical lymph node enlargement > 1.5 cm (70%).
- Polymorphous rash primarily on trunk (80%).
- Any of the following changes to the extremities (70%): erythema of palms and soles, edema of hands and feet, periungual desquamation in convalescent phase.
- Any of the following changes to lips and oral cavity (90%): dry and red fissured lips, diffuse oropharyngeal erythema, "strawberry tongue".

Disease course

It is usually a triphasic illness. The diagnostic features usually manifesting in the acute febrile phase (5–10 days). The child is typically irritable, may have evidence of myocarditis (up to 50%), other multisystem manifestations and elevation of acute phase reactants.

In the subacute phase (11–24 days), there may be desquamation of the rash, characteristic extreme thrombocytosis (up to $1,200 \times 10^9$). Coronary artery dilatation is usually detected during this period; defervescence and the return of the platelet count to normal ends this phase.

In the chronic illness (> 24 days), the child appears well but there is evolution of the coronary artery abnormalities; half may have resolved by 30 days but new aneurysms may develop up to 3 months post–onset. Boys < 12 months of age wih prolonged fever are at greatest risk for coronary artery disease.

Other manifestations

Gall bladder hydrops (rare) or any erythematous, desquamative perineal eruption (67%) are almost unique associations. Other features include arthritis, peripheral artery aneurysms, uveitis, aseptic meningitis, focal neurological signs, otitis, pneumonitis, dysuria, sterile pyuria, proteinuria, hepatitis, gastroenteritis, generalized lymphadenopathy.

Diagnosis

Differential diagnosis may include Stevens–Johnson's and Reiter's syndromes, scarlet fever, scalded skin syndrome, leptospirosis, measles, infectious mononucleosis and toxoplasmosis.

Atypical disease may occur especially in infants under 6 months of age. The diagnostic criteria may be incomplete or be present only briefly and out of phase. In an irritable infant with prolonged unexplained fever, specific testing for sterile pyuria, elevated liver enzymes, uveitis, hydropic gall bladder and early coronary artery dilatation my be helpful in defining a multisystem disease, and even with incomplete criteria for Kawasaki's disease, treatment with γ–globulin should be considered.

Management

- Admit all children with suspected or definite Kawasaki's disease.
- Order CBC, ESR, platelets, blood and throat cultures, urinalysis, liver function tests.
- Clinical monitoring for myocarditis and cardiac failure. Early EKG, chest X-ray and an echocardiogram may be necessary.
- Intravenous γ–globulin (2 g/kg) is given as soon as possible.
- Aspirin therapy: high dose ASA (60–100 mg/kg per d in 4 doses) in the acute phase as an anti–inflammatory, antipyretic agent. Low dose ASA (2–5 mg/kg per d single dose) as an antiplatelet agent when the fever falls or the platelets rise. With coronary artery dilatation, continue low dose ASA indefinitely; otherwise continue until the platelet count and ESR normalize.
- Corticosteroid therapy is associated with an increased risk of coronary artery dilatation and is usually contraindicated.
- Consult rheumatologist and cardiologist.

SYSTEMIC LUPUS ERYTHEMATOSUS

SLE is a diagnosis often considered in patients presenting with persistent systemic symptoms such as fever, malaise, anorexia and weight loss. The differential diagnosis may include infections, malignancy, inflammatory bowel disease and other "rheumatic" diseases such as systemic onset JRA and polyarthritis nodosa. SLE is distinguished by its characteristic multisystem involvement and the presence of specific antinuclear antibodies (ANA). The presence of four of the 10 classification criteria supports the diagnosis of SLE, although organ involvement may be more diverse than these criteria suggest. It is difficult to make a diagnosis of SLE in the absence of autoantibodies, specifically antibodies to native, i.e. double stranded DNA (anti–nDNA, anti–dsDNA); on the other hand, the presence of antibodies alone is insufficient for diagnosis. Treatment of SLE often includes the use of corticosteroids and other immunosuppressive agents. Because significant morbidity may be associated with either disease or treatment, management is best monitored by physicians with specific training and experience with this relatively infrequent disease.

Criteria for classification of SLE:
- Malar rash, butterfly rash; discoid rash.
- Photosensitivity.
- Oral or nasal mucosal ulcers
- Arthritis.
- Renal disease (proteinuria > 0.5 g/d or cellular casts).
- Serositis (pleuritis or pericarditis).
- Neurological manifestations (seizures or psychosis).
- Hematological disorder (leukopenia, lymphopenia, thrombocytopenia, hemolytic anemia).
- Presence of specific autoantibodies (anti–dsDNA, anti–Sm, false positive test for syphilis).
- Positive ANA.

Blood products are potentially the most dangerous "pharmaceutical" that most physicians will ever prescribe. Transfusions can result in serious injury or death very soon after transfusion, within weeks or months of transfusion, or many years after the date of transfusion. In general, physicians have not approached transfusion with this type of philosophy and, in part, the tragedy of transfusion transmitted infection is a consequence of inappropriate transfusion practice. In the current climate, each transfusion episode should be approached very carefully and the benefits and possible complications of a transfusion carefully weighed in an individual clinical situation. The risks must be carefully explained to the patient or family. These stipulations apply to elective and nonurgent transfusions, but even in urgent clinical situations, the use of blood products should always be preceded by careful thought.

BLOOD PRODUCT COLLECTION, PREPARATION AND TESTING

Blood donors should be healthy adults. For first time donors, the age limits are 17 to 60 years; for established donors the upper age limit is 71 years. Donors are required to complete a questionnaire and undergo a face–to–face interview regarding their physical well being and past medical history and behavior. In most centers, donors are also required to complete a confidential exclusion or self–designation form. This form allows those donors who may in the past have engaged in high risk sexual and other activities to exclude themselves from the donor pool and ensures that their blood is used for research purposes only. Using strict asepsis, the donations are collected from an antecubital vein into sealed plastic packs. The donors are required to rest after the collection of the 450–500 mL donation while fluid replacement in the form of oral liquids is given. The donations are handled carefully because of the danger of damage to plastic bags and are usually stored at 4 °C until further processing can be performed.

All blood donations are ABO and Rh grouped, and the donor's serum is screened for the presence of atypical red cell antibodies. Infectious disease marker screening is performed. This consists of serological testing for syphilis, hepatitis B antigen, HIV I/II, hepatitis C and HTLV–I infection. In centers providing large volumes of blood for pediatric and neonatal units, a significant number of the donors are also subjected to serological testing for cytomegalovirus (CMV) antibodies. CMV negative blood is used for premature neonates and other groups such as CMV seronegative transplant recipients. Only those units which have proved negative in the syphilis, hepatitis and retroviral screening can be released from a blood center to a hospital. Since blood is an excellent storage medium, blood and blood products must be handled with great care and with all manipulations performed by trained staff under controlled conditions. If infusion has not started, packs of red cells which have remained at room temperature for 30 minutes must be returned to a properly controlled blood bank refrigerator. Particular care should be taken when leaving red cells at room temperature for long periods of time in a warm ICU or Operating Room. Domestic refrigerators, which are often used on nursing stations and in Operating Rooms for the storage of medications, must not be used for the storage of blood and blood products.

Immunohematological testing

The basic test in immunohematology is the agglutination test. Hemagglutination is the process by which immunoglobulin molecules link adjacent erythrocytes when these cells carry antigens corresponding to the serological specificity of the antibody. The larger immunoglobulin molecules, IgM, are capable of causing agglutination of red cells in a saline medium and are often called saline antibodies. These antibodies always fix complement. IgM antibodies are the first to form following an antigenic challenge, and many of the cold red cell alloantibodies of dubious clinical significance such as anti–P_1, anti–M, anti–N and anti–Lewis antibodies belong to this category. The smaller immunoglobulin molecules, IgG, are usually not capable of causing red cell agglutination in a saline medium because they are not physically capable of spanning the distance between two adjacent red cells. IgG antibodies form as a secondary response to an antigenic challenge and may or may not fix complement. The IgG blood group antibodies usually form in response to some clear antigenic challenge such as an injection or infusion of blood, or a blood product, or pregnancy. Since the antibodies act optimally at 37 °C, this class of antibody may cause severe hemolytic transfusion reaction and may also cause alloimmune hemolytic disease in the newborn. It is critical, therefore, that antibodies of this type are detected in a patient's serum, but because these antibodies cannot react in a saline medium, some type of enhancement is necessary to facilitate antibody detection. The most common enhancement technique is the use of an antiglobulin bridge to link and agglutinate adjacent IgG coated cells. This immunoglobulin "bridge" is usually an antihuman immunoglobulin raised in another species. This procedure, which traditionally has been called the Coombs' test, should be more correctly named the antiglobulin test.

Direct antiglobulin test (DAT, direct Coombs' test)

When an antiglobulin reagent is added directly to red cells which have been well washed in saline, and a positive result occurs, the patient is said to have a positive direct antiglobulin (Coombs') test. Such a positive DAT occurs during hemolytic transfusion reactions, in autoimmune hemolytic anemia, alloimmune hemolytic disease of the newborn or as an immune complication of recently administered medication.

Indirect antiglobulin test (IAT, indirect Coombs' test)

The indirect antiglobulin test is performed by mixing the patient's serum with screening red cells. These screening cells are chosen because they express, in significant dosage, the antigens from the major blood group systems. After incubation, the screening cells are washed to remove unbound immunoglobulin and the antiglobulin reagent is added. If hemagglutination occurs, the patient's serum is said to have a positive IAT test. This positive result implies the presence of atypical antibodies in the patient's serum which have reacted with the screening cells. In this way, the technologist and transfusion medicine physician are alerted to the presence of atypical red cell antibodies and further investigation to identify the nature of the antibodies is required. The IAT is the central test in the type and screen and the red cell cross–match.

Type and screen

In order to avoid the needless cross–match of large volumes of blood for surgical and medical procedures which only rarely require red cell transfusion, most hospital blood banks operate a type and screen policy. When a type and screen is ordered, the patient is ABO and Rhesus grouped and his/her serum is subjected to an indirect antiglobulin test. If no atypical antibodies are found, then no further action is needed. If unexpected complications occur and excessive bleeding results at the time of procedure, then the infusion of group specific unmatched red cells is considered to be a safe and acceptable practice. If, during a type and screen, an atypical red cell antibody is detected, this antibody must be identified and appropriately grouped antigen negative units must be available before the procedure can proceed.

Maximal surgical blood ordering schedule (MSBOS)

Many hospitals, in addition to type and screen, operate an MSBOS system. Such a system designates a maximum order for a specific surgical procedure such as 3 units of blood may be ordered for correction of a tetralogy of Fallot in a 2 year old child. The MSBOS system and the proper use of type and screen obviate needless over ordering by residents, interns and medical students for complicated surgeries, yet at the same time assures the anesthetist and surgeon of sufficient blood for the time of surgery. In order for a MSBOS system to work, it is essential that the schedules are agreeable to the surgeon, anesthetist and the transfusion medicine physician.

BLOOD PRODUCTS

Whole blood

Whole blood is not generally available since almost all blood donations now have the plasma removed for further processing and fractionation. The indications for whole blood infusion are few but include exchange transfusion for hemolytic disease of the newborn. For clinical use, whole blood is usually reconstituted from red cell concentrate and frozen plasma. This is rarely done and doubles the risk for the recipient since it involves two donor exposures.

Red blood cells

1. Red cell concentrate
Red cell concentrate, also called packed red cells, is the main form of red cell product available from a hospital blood bank. A unit contains approximately 200 mL of red cells. Red cell concentrate can be used whenever red cell infusion is required and has the advantage of reduced risk of circulatory overload and reduced transfusion reactions to donor antibodies or plasma components. Red cell concentrate must be filtered through a standard blood infusion filter (with a nominal pore size of 170 µm) or through a filter of higher efficiency. Red cell concentrate should be stored at 4 °C and has a shelf–life of at least 35 days. The shelf–life varies depending on the particular blood preservative system used locally.

2. Leukocyte poor red blood cells
This product is required when patients have had repeated severe febrile reactions directed

against the leukocytes, which are inevitably present in a red cell concentrate. Such reactions typically occur in massively transfused patients such as patients with hemoglobinopathy who require frequent red cell infusion. Various methods can be used to remove the leukocytes, including washing and filtration. The drawback to washing is that inevitably there is a loss of red cells and it is difficult, even with automated instrumentation, to remove more than 85% of the leukocytes. Various filtration techniques can be used and the most efficient of the filters removes 99.99% of leukocytes. Such filters are expensive and should not be used for all patients but should be reserved for specially selected patients in whom the use of leukocyte poor blood is critical. Such patients would include patients with lifelong transfusion requirements and those in whom the infusion of leukocytes will speed up the appearance of alloantibodies against HLA and platelet antigens. Such alloantibodies seriously affect the utilization of and response to random donor platelet products in patients with acute myeloblastic leukemia, aplastic anemia and bone marrow transplant candidates and recipients.

3. Frozen red cells

Red cells can be frozen in a mechanical freezer using glycerol as a cryoprotectant. This process is expensive and should be reserved for the storage of red cell units of unusual phenotype or for autotransfusion to patients with multiple red cell antibodies. Reconstituted frozen blood can also be used as a means of providing deleukocyted blood for patients with high titer HLA antibodies who are having unpleasant febrile reactions. However, the use of high efficiency levodepletion filters is now preferred for these patients. Frozen red cells can be stored for years at −70 °C but require deglycerolization prior to infusion, consequently they are not immediately available for the patient.

Platelet infusion

Platelet infusions are required for the prevention and treatment of thrombocytopenic bleeding, particularly in the amegakaryocytic patient. They are used extensively for the support of patients with oncological and hematological disorders. Platelets should not be used other than in very rare and special circumstances for patients with destructive thrombocytopenia such as immune thrombocytopenia, drug induced immune thrombocytopenia, hemolytic uremic syndrome and thrombotic thrombocytopenic purpura. Platelet infusion may also be occasionally required to treat hemorrhagic complications in patients with disorders of platelet function, even when they are not thrombocytopenic. The decision to infuse platelets should always be taken in conjunction with a hematologist or transfusion medicine physician and is contingent on the platelet count, the diagnosis and the specific clinical situation. The infusion of one unit of platelets will usually cause a platelet increment of $35–50 \times 10^9$ /L per 10 kg of body weight, and this formula should be used in calculating the dosage required. When platelets are infused, it is very important that the platelet count be checked either immediately or 1 hour after the infusion has been completed to determine the increment in platelet count. By following platelet count increments, the hematologist and transfusion medicine service can usually determine when a patient is becoming refractory to random donor platelets.

Platelets are typically available as single pack platelet concentrate, containing $> 60 \times 10^9$ /L (>60,000/μL) platelets in a volume of approximately 50 mL of plasma. Platelets must be infused through a standard infusion filter or a filter of higher efficiency. Special high efficiency deleukocyting filters are available for platelet concentrate. These decrease the rate of sensitization to random donor platelets but are expensive and should be reserved for specific clinical indications similar to those in which high efficiency red cell deleukocyting filters are used.

1. Random donor platelets
Random donor platelets are collected from one random donor unit of whole blood. The unit is centrifuged and a platelet–rich plasma is transferred to a satellite pack. This platelet–rich plasma is centrifuged and the supernatant plasma is transferred to a third pack for further processing, leaving the platelet concentrate behind. Random donor platelet concentrate should be stored at room temperature, ideally at 22 °C, and subjected to constant agitation to prevent damage to the platelets which impairs platelet function. Random donor platelet concentrate has a shelf–life of up to 5 days, depending on the type of donor pack that is used.

2. Single donor platelet concentrate
Single donor platelet concentrate is collected by thrombocytopheresis from a single donor. This product is reserved for those patients who become refractory to random donor platelets and is used almost exclusively for patients with oncological and hematological disease. Such products are only available following a consultation with a hematologist or transfusion medicine physician.

Anti–CMV nonreactive products

Cellular products which have been shown to be nonreactive for anti–CMV should be used only in special clinical circumstances. Since approximately 50% of donor blood is CMV seropositive, these products are in short supply and must be reserved for specific patient groups. Appropriate indications include bone marrow transplant recipients, anti–CMV nonreactive neonates of < 1,500 grams body weight and anti–CMV nonreactive pregnant females in the second trimester of pregnancy. A case can also be made for the infusion of anti–CMV nonreactive cellular products to CMV seronegative patients with various oncological disorders such as AML, high risk ALL and those who have a significant risk of progressing to allogeneic bone marrow or solid organ transplantation.

Plasma

Various types of plasma products were traditionally available: stored, frozen and fresh frozen. Only fresh frozen and frozen plasma are currently available in Canada because of concerns regarding the accumulation of plasticizer derived from the plastic pack used for storing liquid plasma. Frozen plasma can be used for plasma volume expansion when other products are not available or for infusion of multiple clotting factors typically in a patient with disseminated intravascular coagulation (DIC). This, however, is suboptimal therapy. Concentrated coagulation factor preparations are, however, the treatment of choice for coagulation factor deficiencies. Plasma can also be used for replacement during plasmapheresis, but albumin is preferred in most circumstances.

Plasma is stored frozen at –30 °C for up to 3 months and should be thawed at 37 °C immediately before use. Liquid plasma, which has not been used within 24 hours, should be returned to a transfusion center. Plasma, inevitably, contains red cell fragments which can sensitize the recipient to red cell antigens. Rhesus negative girls and females in the childbearing age must, therefore, always receive plasma which has been collected from Rh negative individuals. If plasma from Rh negative donors is not available and a patient within this group requires plasma, plasma from donors of any Rh type may be given, provided that Rh immunoglobulin (anti–D) prophylaxis is given at the same time.

Cryoprecipitate

Cryoprecipitate is prepared from frozen plasma which has been thawed. When frozen, plasma thaws under standardized conditions; fibrinogen and factor VIII remains as a cold insoluble precipitate which can be separated from the rest of the plasma by centrifugation. This cryoprecipitate has a small volume (5–10 mL) and contains significant amounts of factor VIII and fibrinogen from a single donor unit. Cryoprecipitate is stored at –300 °C for up to 3 months and has been used for treating mild cases of hemophilia A or von Willebrand's disease, for replacing fibrinogen and factor VIII in patients with DIC and as a means of replacing fibrinogen in patients with acquired or congenital fibrinogen deficiency. The dose of cryoprecipitate varies with the patient's clinical condition and weight. Dosage should be calculated in conjunction with a hematologist or transfusion medicine physician. The optimal treatment for hemophilia A and von Willebrand's disease is respectivey recombinant factor VIII and specially processed and treated factor concentrates.

Fractionated products

By collecting large volumes of plasma which are then subjected to ethanol fractionation, various concentrated blood protein fractions can be achieved. The disadvantage of fractionated products is that one contaminated donor may infect an entire pool with an infectious agent. Not all fractionated products, however, can transmit infectious agents. Albumin is pasteurized and does not transmit hepatitis or HIV infection. Intravenous gamma globulin has been shown to transmit hepatitis C in some situations but the risk is small. This product is now prepared using a viral inactivation step and some manufacturers test the plasma pools for hepatitis C using PCR technology.

Viral transmission is a particular risk with clotting factor concentrates and large numbers of hemophiliacs have been infected with HIV derived from factor VIII concentrate. Factor concentrates are now subjected to a wet–heat and solvent detergent treatment which inactivates the virus.

1. Albumin

Albumin is available in 5% and 25% preparations. These have a physiological pH and a sodium concentration of approximately 145 mmol/L. Albumin is used for blood volume expansion, particularly in an emergent situation before cross–matched blood is available. The 25% product draws extravascular fluid into the intravascular space and can promote diuresis in patients with hypoproteinemia but should be given with caution because of the risks of rapidly expanding the intravascular volume. Albumin can be stored for long periods of time at room or refrigerator temperature and should be filtered through a standard infusion filter.

2. Intravenous gamma globulin (IVIg)

This is an expensive blood product with specific clinical indications. IVIg may be used for patients with inherited immunodeficiency, during the management of acute immune thrombocytopenic purpura and Kawasaki's disease, and for CMV prophylaxis at the time of bone marrow transplantation. This product is used experimentally in a large variety of conditions, but because of the expense involved, it should only be used following consultation with an immunologist, hematologist or transfusion medicine physician.

3. Rhesus immunoglobulin (anti–D)
This product is collected from rhesus negative females who have been immunized to the Rh (D) antigen. It is used in the prophylaxis of Rh sensitization during and after pregnancy and to prevent sensitization to the Rh antigen during inadvertent or unavoidable infusion of Rh positive cellular products or plasma to Rh negative patients. This type of prophylaxis is particularly important in female children and adult females of childbearing age. The product comes in 120 and 300 µg doses. A 300 µg dose is considered sufficient to prevent sensitization by 30 mL of Rh positive cells.

4. Other immunoglobulin products
Other specific immunoglobulins are available for the prophylaxis of hepatitis B (hepatitis B immunoglobulin–HBIg), for varicella zoster (varicella zoster immunoglobulin–VZIg), and CMV hyperimmunoglobulin. No doubt in the future, other specific immunoglobulin products will also become available.

5. Clotting factor concentrates
Factor VIII and factor IX concentrates are both available. Both are high potency products which in the past have been responsible for transmitting hepatitis and retroviruses to recipients. These products should be reserved for the management of severe bleeding or surgery in patients with hemophilia A or B and must be used in consultation with a hematologist or transfusion medicine physician. These products are lyophilized and can be stored at refrigerator temperature for long periods of time. Complications include viral transmission (which has now been significantly minimized) and immune hemolysis (the fraction also contains high titer anti–A and anti–B isoagglutinins).

NONHUMAN PRODUCTS

Products produced by recombinant DNA technology

Recombinant DNA technology has been used to produce factor VIII concentrate and albumin. Factor VIII concentrate is currently available and is the preferred product for most hemophiliacs. These products have the advantage of considerable purity and zero risk for transmission of viral disease. They are very expensive.

Growth factors

Hematopoiesis is controlled by a variety of growth factors. Several of these growth factors can now be produced by recombinant DNA technology and can be used to manage cytopenias in particular situations. Recombinant human erythropoietin is used to manage the chronic anemia of renal failure and may also have benefits in the management of anemia following chemotherapy and bone marrow transplantation. The usefulness of erythropoietin in the management of neonatal anemia has been established as further studies are needed to clarify the precise clinical indications. If successful, this strategy will minimize the need for neonatal red cell transfusion and multiple donor exposure. GM–CSF produced by recombinant DNA technology is also being used in an experimental basis in the management of severe neutropenic patients following intensive chemotherapy or bone marrow transplantation. In the future, the use of this type of therapy will be more prevalent and minimize the need for patients to be exposed to human blood products.

Nonhuman plasma expanders

Several types of nonhuman plasma expanders have been used clinically and these include starch derivatives (particularly hydroxyethyl starch and penta starch), gelatin derivatives, (particularly modified fluid gelatin) and dextran products of varying molecular weight. The advantages of these products are zero risk for transmission of infectious disease, easy availability, (particularly in times of natural or other disaster) and a relatively low cost of manufacture. These products have been extensively used in Europe with success. The literature describing their use in the pediatric age group is almost nonexistent and research in this regard is required. Complications to these factors include allergic reactions and coagulopathies due to dilution and alteration of hemostatic function.

Blood substitutes

Considerable research is ongoing into the development of satisfactory oxygen carrying blood substitutes. Various types of fluorocarbon molecule have been tried, however, the oxygen carrying capacity of these products to date has not been significantly greater than that of plasma.

AUTOLOGOUS BLOOD TRANSFUSION

Wherever possible, reinfusion of a patient's own blood is much preferred to the infusion of a homologous product from a random donor. There are several different approaches to autologous transfusion: preoperative deposit, preoperative hemodilution and venesection, and intraoperative salvage. In some centers, autologous blood transfusion programs for children exist. Predeposit autologous donation can be used successfully for teenage patients but can also be used for children as young as 4 years and in selected cases for infants as young as 18 months. The principle use of this type of program is for patients undergoing reconstructive elective surgery. No untoward effects occur with this type of approach and the procedure is well accepted by patients and parents. Intraoperative salvage can be used for clean surgeries, typically thoracic surgery. Blood is aspirated by the surgeon and anticoagulated. The salvaged blood can be reinfused, ideally, after it has been washed and filtered. Various types of commercially available salvage and washing instrumentation exist. Preoperative hemodilution and venesection can also be used for patients undergoing major reconstructive surgery. Immediately after induction of anesthesia, the anesthetist infuses a large volume of saline and simultaneously phlebotomizes the patient from another limb. In this way, 2–3 units of blood can be obtained and during surgery, as blood loss occurs, the units are reinfused in reverse order.

Autologous transfusion programs, although beneficial, are limited for the most part to elective procedures and to patients who are relatively fit and capable of undergoing a phlebotomy without long–term transfusion requirements.

COMPLICATIONS OF TRANSFUSION

Many complications of transfusion exist and are best categorized as immune or nonimmune.

Immune mediated transfusion reactions

1. Hemolytic transfusion reaction
- This type of reaction occurs when red cells are infused to a patient whose serum contains an antibody which recognizes a foreign antigen on the infused erythrocytes. Lysis of the infused donor cells results. When the hemolysis occurs immediately, as is seen when ABO incompatible blood is infused, there is intravascular hemolysis which may result in hemoglobinemia and hemoglobinuria. There is also a release of vasoactive products, resulting in shock. Circulating cell debris and immune complexes often trigger the coagulation cascade to produce disseminated intravascular coagulation. The combination of hemoglobinuria, shock and disseminated intravascular coagulation (DIC) often causes acute renal failure. In the anesthetized patient, the first sign of an acute hemolytic transfusion reaction may be DIC, which manifests itself as oozing from sites at which hemostasis had previously been achieved. Acute hemolytic transfusion reactions typically occur from infusion of ABO incompatible blood. This is a rare event and usually results from a clerical error either in the transfusion laboratory or the clinical setting at the time the blood product is infused.
- In patients in whom the infusion of foreign red cells stimulates an anamnestic antibody response, the production of IgG antibodies directed against the donor red cells results in a less aggressive extravascular destruction of donor red cells. This phenomenon, the delayed hemolytic transfusion reaction, classically presents as unexpected anemia and jaundice several days following a transfusion. Very rarely a delayed hemolytic transfusion reaction can be accompanied by renal failure.
- Investigations of a hemolytic transfusion reaction include a direct antiglobulin test on the patient, a review of all clerical, laboratory and nursing data regarding the identity of the cross–match sample, the blood product and the patient, together with an antibody investigation to detect and identify any atypical red cell antibodies.
- Hemolytic transfusion reactions can also occur when the red cell product has been subjected to thermal stress, as occurs with a faulty blood warmer or when the blood has been refrigerated inappropriately or inadvertently frozen. Severe hemolytic reactions associated with shock may also occur when bacterially contaminated blood is infused.

2. Febrile reactions
These are common and usually occur when a patient who has antibodies to leukocyte antigens receives a blood product, usually red cells, containing leukocytes carrying the offending antigen. The clinical reaction is mild but consists of fever without shock, which may be accompanied by rigors. A limited investigation is usually warranted as this type of reaction can be avoided by infusion of leukocyte depleted blood (as described above).

3. Allergic reactions
This is the most common type of immune mediated transfusion reaction and, in its mildest form, consists of urticaria. In its most severe form, urticaria can be associated with bronchospasm and even anaphylactic shock. Allergic reactions occur in patients who are allergic to an allergen

present in the infused product. Occasionally, this type of reaction occurs because an atopic person has given a blood donation and the passively transfused atopic antibody reacts with the corresponding allergen which is present in the patient. The most severe type of allergic (anaphylactic) reactions occur in patients who are IgA deficient. These patients develop antibodies against foreign immunoglobulin A molecules. IgA related allergic reaction can be severe and even life threatening. In patients who are IgA deficient, all blood products should be either plasma free, or when plasma products are required, these should be prepared from donations taken from IgA deficient donors.

Other complications of transfusion

Nonimmune transfusion reactions include the transmission of disease and septic shock due to the infusion of blood which is contaminated with bacteria. Embolism (particle debris, air) or fluid overload may also occur.

Although the risk of transmission of an infectious agent is small, this risk must always be borne in mind when contemplating a transfusion in any patient. This risk is of great importance to parents of sick children who will invariably raise the matter with the attending and treating physicians. The possibility of infusing a blood product infected with bacteria is very remote but remains a potential problem when infusing platelet concentrate, which is stored at 22 °C and is often infused to a severely immunosuppressed oncology patient. Of much greater concern, particularly when giving an infusion of red cell concentrate, is the transmission of a viral agent. The risk of infusing blood that can contain infectious HIV particles but is anti–HIV negative is very small but has been calculated at approximately 1:250,000 units. Of greater concern has been the risk of transmitting viruses which can cause hepatitis, which in turn can cause chronic hepatitis and even cirrhosis. Since the advent of hepatitis C testing, the risk of infusing a unit containing hepatitis C has dropped to 1:6,000, but the total elimination of transfusion associated viral hepatitis remains unlikely until some type of physical or chemical antiviral treatment of blood products is introduced. When considering the risks of disease transmission by blood products, it should always be remembered that the risk increases with the number of donor exposures.

Massive transfusion

Massive transfusion is defined as the infusion of transfusion fluids with a volume equal to or exceeding the patient's blood volume within a 24 hour period. Massive transfusion typically occurs in the seriously ill, traumatized patient and is accompanied by a variety of specific complications. These include coagulopathies, citrate toxicity, microembolization, hypothermia and other metabolic changes. Citrate toxicity occurs because of the infusion of large amounts of citrate. Citrate is an essential ingredient in the anticoagulant mixture used to preserve the donor blood. Hypocalcemia may occur but only results when very rapid infusions of blood occur. Liver disease and hypothermia can exacerbate the effects of citrate toxicity. Citrate toxicity can be prevented by the infusion of 10% calcium gluconate, 10 mL for every litre of blood infused. In practice, infusion of too much calcium may cause more problems than citrate toxicity. Calcium gluconate must never be administered through the same line as a blood product, unless it is preceded and followed by a saline flush. Wherever possible, drugs should never be mixed with blood products but should be infused separately through a different venous line. The recommended solution to mix with red cells is normal saline. Five percent dextrose solution and

Ringer's lactate must not be infused at the same time as red cells.

Various coagulopathies can complicate massive transfusion. These include thrombocytopenia and reduced levels of all coagulation factors, particularly the labile clotting factors due to dilution by large amounts of donor blood which is depleted in platelets and clotting factors. Various "rules of thumb" exist to infuse platelet concentrate and frozen plasma at specific intervals during a massive transfusion episode. If at all possible, these rules should be avoided and if the hematology laboratory is capable of providing rapid turnaround for platelet counts and coagulation tests, then platelets and plasma should be used empirically when indicated by laboratory parameters.

The infusion of large amounts of stored blood invariably results in infusion of large amounts of accumulated particulate debris. This debris may be filtered out in the pulmonary capillary bed and to avoid this, the use of microaggregate filters is advised for the massive transfusion episode, particularly for the patient with impaired pulmonary function.

Since blood is stored at 4 °C, rapid infusion of large volumes of stored blood can result in central cooling, but the use of properly regulated and controlled blood warming devices can prevent this complication. It should be remembered that poorly maintained or faulty blood warming devices may result in excessive warming and hemolysis of donor red cells which may cause the patient even greater problems than hypothermia.

Various other metabolic complications may occur in the massive transfusion situation. These include altered acid–base balance, typically acidosis and impaired oxygen release. Acidosis is usually a consequence of impaired tissue perfusion rather than the infusion of large amounts of acidified, stored blood and usually corrects itself once adequate tissue perfusion has been restored. Depletion of 2,3 DPG in donor erythrocytes in stored blood may interfere with oxygen release by hemoglobin. Levels of 2,3 DPG recover within 24 hours of transfusion. Nonetheless, whenever possible, the infusion of large volumes of older, stored blood should be avoided. In the massive transfusion situation, if at all possible, the bulk of infused red cells should be not more than 7–10 days old.

In the massive transfusion situation, the risk for clerical mix up is significantly increased and particular care must be taken at these times to maintain the clerical records relating to when and which blood products were infused. Particular vigilance must be exerted in relation to compatibility and identity of the infused blood products. This is of even greater importance after major disasters when multiple massive transfusion incidents may be occurring simultaneously within an Emergency Room or Operating Room.

Table I: Dental eruption/shedding

Primary teeth	Eruption		Shedding	
	Maxillary	**Mandibular**	**Maxillary**	**Mandibular**
Central incisors	6–8 mo	5–7 mo	7–8 yr	6–7 yr
Lateral incisors	8–11 mo	7–10 mo	8–9 yr	7–8 yr
Canines	16–20 mo	16–20 mo	11–12 yr	9–11 yr
First molars	10–16 mo	10–16 mo	10–11 yr	10–12 yr
Second molars	20–30 mo	20–30 mo	10–12 yr	11–13 yr

Secondary teeth	Maxillary	Mandibular
Central incisors	7–8 yr	6–7 yr
Lateral incisors	8–9 yr	7–8 yr
Canines	11–12 yr	9–11 yr
First premolars	10–11 yr	10–12 yr
Second premolars	10–12 yr	11–13 yr
First molars	6–7 yr	6–7 yr
Second molars	12–13 yr	12–13 yr
Third molars	17–22 yr	17–22 yr

Table II: Arm span and upper/lower segment ratio

Age	Male		Female	
	Span	U/L	Span	U/L
Birth	48.5	1.60	48.3	1.73
6 mo	64.5	1.61	63.0	1.60
12 mo	71.9	1.54	70.4	1.52
18 mo	78.2	1.51	76.4	1.47
2 yr	83.1	1.44	81.5	1.42
3 yr	91.9	1.33	89.1	1.32
4 yr	98.6	1.27	96.8	1.25
5 yr	105.2	1.21	103.4	1.19
6 yr	111.8	1.14	110.0	1.13
7 yr	117.3	1.10	116.8	1.09
8 yr	123.4	1.06	122.4	1.05
9 yr	129.5	1.03	128.0	1.02
10 yr	135.6	1.02	133.6	1.01
11 yr	141.2	0.99	140.5	1.00
12 yr	147.1	0.98	146.1	0.99

Span represents the 50th percentile measured in centimeters.
U/L = upper to lower segment ratio measured to the symphysis pubis.

Table III: Triceps skin–fold thickness (millimeters)

Age (yr)	Male percentiles			Female percentiles		
	5th	50th	95th	5th	50th	95th
0–0.5	4	8	15	4	8	13
0.5–1.5	5	9	15	6	9	15
1.5–2.5	5	10	14	6	10	15
2.5–3.5	6	9	14	6	10	14
3.5–4.5	5	9	14	5	10	14
4.5–5.5	5	8	16	6	10	16
5.5–6.5	5	8	15	6	10	15
6.5–7.5	4	8	14	6	10	17
7.5–8.5	5	8	17	6	10	19
8.5–9.5	5	9	19	6	11	24
9.5–10.5	5	10	22	6	12	24
10.5–11.5	6	10	25	7	12	29
11.5–12.5	5	11	26	6	13	25
12.5–13.5	5	10	25	7	14	30
13.5–14.5	5	10	22	8	15	28
14.5–15.5	4	9	26	8	16	30
15.5–16.5	4	9	27	8	15	27

Modified from A. Frisancho, Am J Clin Nutr 1974;27:1052.

Table IV: Mid–arm muscle circumference (centimeters)

Age (yr)	Male percentiles			Female percentiles		
	5th	50th	95th	5th	50th	95th
0–0.5	8.1	10.6	13.3	8.6	10.4	12.8
0.5–1.5	10.0	12.3	14.6	9.7	11.7	13.5
1.5–2.5	11.1	12.7	14.6	10.5	12.5	14.3
2.5–3.5	11.4	13.2	15.2	10.8	12.8	14.6
3.5–4.5	11.8	13.5	15.7	11.4	13.2	15.2
4.5–5.5	12.1	14.1	16.6	11.9	13.8	16.0
5.5–6.5	12.7	14.6	16.7	12.1	14.0	16.5
6.5–7.5	13.0	15.1	17.3	12.3	14.6	17.5
7.5–8.5	13.8	15.8	18.5	12.9	15.1	18.6
8.5–9.5	13.8	16.1	20.0	13.6	15.7	19.3
9.5–10.5	14.2	16.8	20.2	13.9	16.3	19.6
10.5–11.5	15.0	17.4	21.1	14.0	17.1	20.9
11.5–12.5	15.3	18.1	22.2	15.0	17.9	21.2
12.5–13 5	15.9	19.5	24.2	15.5	18.5	22.5
13.5–14.5	16.7	21.1	26.5	16.3	19.3	23.4
14.5–15.5	17.3	22.0	27.1	16.6	19.5	23.2
15.5–16.5	18.6	22.9	28.1	17.1	20.0	26.0

The ideal mid–arm muscle circumference (MAMC) is calculated from measurements of mid–arm circumference (MAC) and triceps skin–fold thickness (TSF) by the equation:

$$MAMC = MAC \ (cm) - 0.1314 \cdot TSF \ (mm)$$

Modified from data of A. Frisancho.

Table V: Burn surface area chart (% BSA)

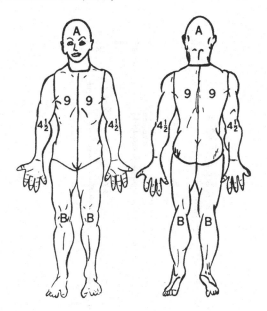

AGE RANGE	A = HEAD AND NECK	B = LOWER LIMB
0 - 2	9 1/2	6 1/2
3 - 5	8 1/2	7
6 - 8	7 1/2	7 1/2
9 - 11	6 1/2	8
12 - 14	5 1/2	8 1/2
15 +	4 1/2	9

The relative proportions of arms and head change with age. Use columns A and B to adjust estimates of burn area for different ages.

Table VI: Body surface area nomogram (m²)

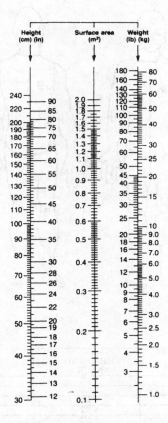

A straight line joining the child's weight and height indicates body surface area at its intersection with the center line.

Modified from data of E. Boyd.

Table VII: Intrauterine growth chart for weight (both sexes)

Grams

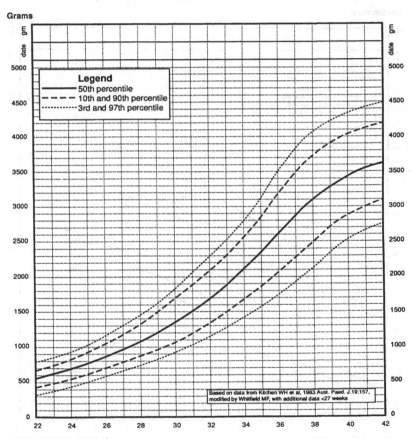

Gestational Age (weeks)

Table VIII: Intrauterine growth chart for length and head circumference (both sexes)

Centimetres

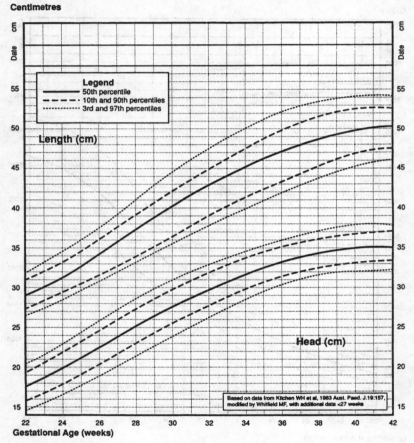

Legend
— 50th percentile
– – 10th and 90th percentiles
······ 3rd and 97th percentiles

Length (cm)

Head (cm)

Based on data from Kitchen WH et al, 1983 Aust. Paed. J.19:157, modified by Whitfield MF, with additional data <27 weeks

Gestational Age (weeks)

Table IX: Position of umbilical artery catheter tip

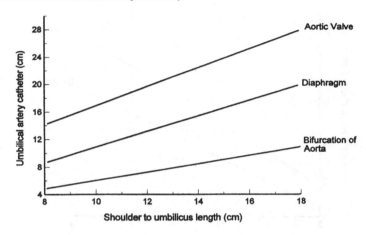

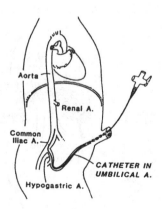

Table X: Position of umbilical venous catheter tip

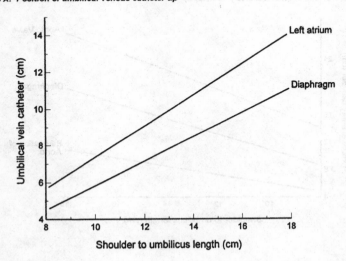

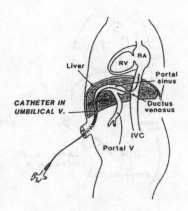

Table XI: Height and weight percentiles – girls, birth–36 months

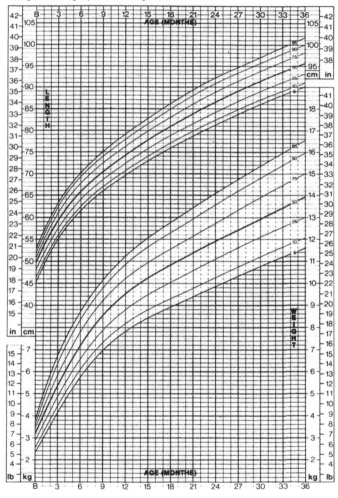

Table XII: Height and weight percentiles – boys, birth–36 months

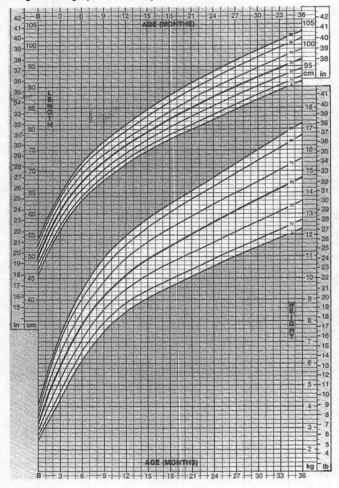

Table XIII: Height and weight percentiles – girls, 2–18 years

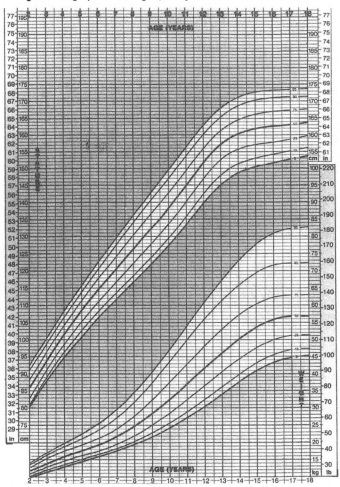

Table XIV: Height and weight percentiles – boys, 2–18 years

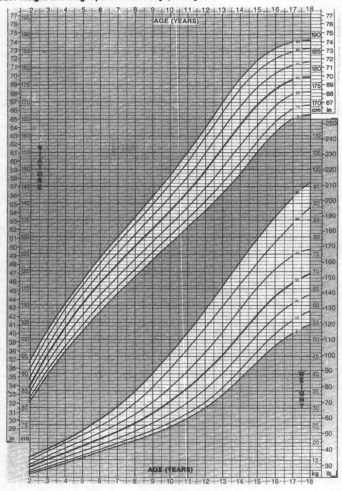

Table XV: Height velocity – girls

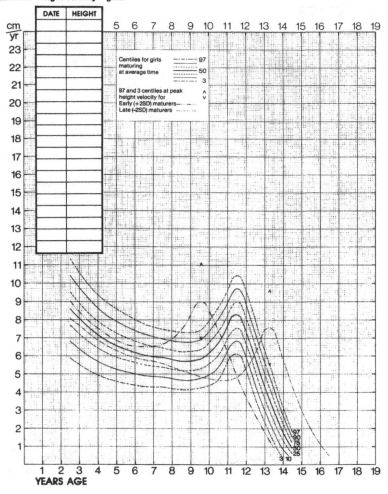

Table XVI: Height velocity – boys

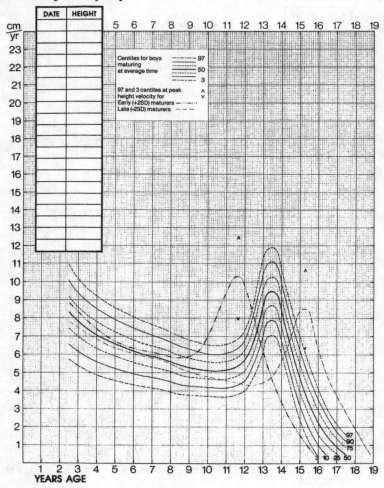

Table XVII: Weight for height – girls

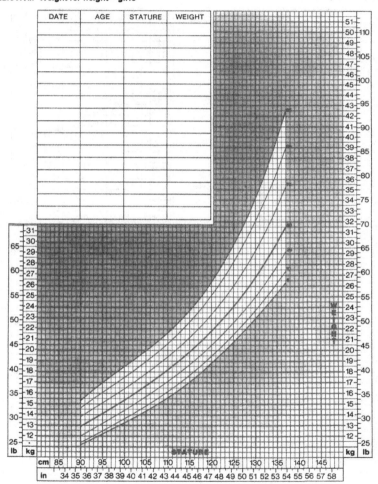

Table XVIII: Weight for height – boys

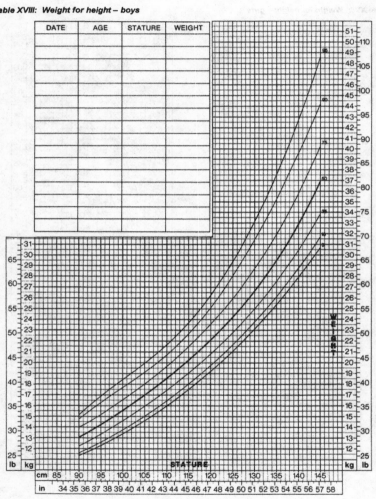

Table XIX: Head circumference – girls

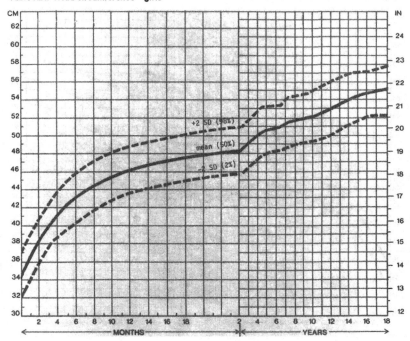

Table XX: Head circumference – boys

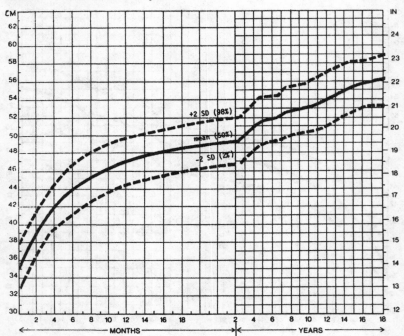

INDEX

Numbers in bold type refer to main discussions

calcitonin 65, **441**
calcitriol 442
calcium (Ca)
  oral supplements 443
  requirements 61, 291
  see also hypercalcemia; hypocalcemia
calcium acetate 442
calcium chloride 201, 244, 442
calcium disodium edta 442
calcium gluconate 65, **443**
  in acute renal failure 35
  i.v. infusion 244
  in massive transfusion 569
  in neonates 291, **329–30**, 348
calcium polystyrene sulfonate 330, 443
calories, see energy
Campylobacter (jejuni) infection 82, 83,
    85, 176
Canadian Medical Association (CMA),
    code of ethics 125
Canadian Pediatric Society (CPS) 129,
    131
cancer, childhood **378–410**
  chemotherapy 381, 383–5
  emergencies 394–8
  late effects 409–10
  principles of diagnosis 378–80
  principles of treatment 380–3
  supportive care 385–94
Candida infections 388, 389
candidiasis, chronic mucocutaneous 156
captopril 330, 444
carbamazepine 423, 444
carbenicillin 171
carbon dioxide
  clearance, mechanical ventilation 218
  tension, arterial (P_aCO_2) 213, 226
  transport 215
carbon monoxide
  diffusion capacity 537
  poisoning 239
cardiac arrest 18–19, **200–2**
cardiac axis 9
cardiac catheterization 12
cardiac failure, *see* heart failure
cardiac massage, external (ECM) 18,
    201
  newborn infants 270

cardiac murmurs 5
cardiac output (CO) 198
  and shock 202, 203
cardiology **1–12**
cardiomyopathies 207
cardiopulmonary arrest 18–19, 200–2
cardiopulmonary resuscitation (CPR)
    18–19, 201–2
  do not resuscitate (DNR) orders 128,
    130–1
  presence of parents 14
cardiovascular system **198–200**
  in infants 199–200
  physiology 198–9
cathartics, in poisoning 39
caustic ingestion 107–8
cefaclor 170, 444
cefazolin 92, 170, **444**
  in neonates 326, 351
cefixime 170
cefotaxime 149, 170, **444**
  in epiglottitis 28
  in meningitis 32
  in neonates 326, 351
cefoxitin 92, 170, **445**
ceftazidime 171, 326, 351, **445**
ceftriaxone 171, 445
cefuroxime 170, 445
celiac disease 376
cell mediated immunity
  defects of 156
  in malnutrition 364
cellulitis 175
central nervous system (CNS) **225–33**
  complications in cancer 398
  crises in sickle cell disease 148
  infections 174–5
  monitoring 227–8
  pathophysiology 226
  physiology 225
central venous catheters (CVC)
  in cancer patients **391–2**
  parenteral nutrition via 364–5
central venous pressure 199
cephalexin 170, 445
cephalosporins 170–1
cerebral blood flow (CBF) 225
  control 225–6

rectal prolapse 549
red blood cells (RBCs)
    decreased survival 144
    disorders **136-54**
    enzyme defects 146-7
    failure of formation 141-2
    frozen 563
    leukocyte poor 562-3
    membrane defects 144-5
    osmotic fragility test 145
    packed 562
    preparations **562-3**
    transfusions 140, 386
red cell concentrates 562
reflex sympathetic dystrophy (RSD)
    556-7
regurgitation 77
rehydration, oral 84-5
renal disease **518-30**
    fluid losses 60, 290
    in sickle cell disease 148
renal failure
    acute (ARF) 34-5, **526-7**
    chronic (CRF) **527-9**
    anemia in 142-3, 528-9
    drugs in **427-8**
    fluid requirements 61, 290
    nutrition in 35, 372, **375-6**, 528
renal function 58, 287-8, 420-1
research **133-5**
    innovative therapy as 135
    using children 134-5
residents
    junior 122
    senior 122
    training **531-4**
residual volume (RV) 536, 539
Resonium calcium (calcium polystyrene
    sulfonate) 330, 443
resources
    competition for scarce 133
    microallocation 132
    unethical use of precious 132
respiration, in neonates 268, 269
respiratory arrest 18-19, 200-2
respiratory distress, surgical causes in
    newborn 98-9
respiratory distress syndrome (RDS)

adult (ARDS), *see* acute lung injury
    neonatal 273-4
respiratory failure **215-21**
    in acute asthma 31
    alternative therapies 219
    intubation techniques 219-21
    management 217-19
respiratory syncytial virus (RSV) 180,
    186, 541, 547
respiratory system **212-25**
    anatomy 212-13
    diseases in neonates **273-9**
    physiology 213-15
respiratory tract infections
    asthma and 543
    lower 180-1
respirology **535-49**
resuscitation
    in adrenal insufficiency 24
    brain 228-9
    in burns 40, 239-40
    cardiopulmonary, *see*
        cardiopulmonary resuscitation
    in coma 230
    interfacility transport and 411
    neonatal 3, **267-73**, 348
    in trauma 20-1, 234-5
reticulocytes
    in anemia 137, 138
    in aplastic anemia 139
    in hemolytic anemia 144
    in newborn 304
retinoblastoma 378
rhabdomyosarcoma 408
Rhesus (anti-D) immunoglobulin 152,
    160, **566**
Rhesus isoimmunization 151-2
rheumatic fever 5-6
rheumatoid arthritis, juvenile (JRA) 551,
    552, 553, 555
rheumatoid factor (RF) 552, 553
rheumatology **550-9**
rhinovirus 186
ribavirin 180, 223, **345**, 504, 542
rifampin 32, 327, **504**
rotavirus infections 83, 176, 186
rubella 184
    congenital 158, **298**

Printed in the United States
By Bookmasters